Therapy with Botulinum Toxin

NEUROLOGICAL DISEASE AND THERAPY

Series Editor

WILLIAM C. KOLLER

Department of Neurology
University of Kansas Medical Center
Kansas City, Kansas

Therapy with Botulinum Toxin

edited by

Joseph Jankovic
Baylor College of Medicine
Houston, Texas

Mark Hallett
National Institute of Neurological Disorders and Stroke
National Institutes of Health
Bethesda, Maryland

Marcel Dekker, Inc.　　　　　New York•Basel•Hong Kong

Library of Congress Cataloging-in-Publication Data

Therapy with botulinum toxin / edited by Joseph Jankovic, Mark
Hallett.
    p. cm. — (Neurological disease and therapy ; 25)
   Includes bibliographical references and index.
   ISBN 0-8247-8824-9 (alk. paper)
   1. Botulinum toxin—Therapeutic use. 2. Spasms—Chemotherapy.
3. Dystonia—Chemotherapy. 4. Voice disorders—Chemotherapy.
I. Jankovic, Joseph. II. Hallett, Mark. III. Series: Neurological
disease and therapy ; v. 25.
   [DNLM: 1. Botulinum Toxins—therapeutic use. 2. Muscular
Diseases—drug therapy.   W1 NE33LD v.25 1994 / QV 132 T3985 1994]
RC935.S64T48 1994
616.7'4061—dc20
DNLM/DLC
for Library of Congress   93-45267
                                                 CIP

The publisher offers discounts on this book when ordered in bulk quantities. For more information, write to Special Sales/Professional Marketing at the address below.

This book is printed on acid-free paper.

Marcel Dekker, Inc.
270 Madison Avenue, New York, New York 10016

Current printing (last digit):
10 9 8 7 6 5 4 3

PRINTED IN THE UNITED STATES OF AMERICA

To our wives and children

Series Introduction

Therapy with Botulinum Toxin by Drs. Jankovic and Hallett discusses many aspects related to the important discovery of the use of this substance in human disease. The basic science of botulinum and its mechanism of action are thoroughly discussed in 11 chapters dedicated to the basic science. Twelve chapters are devoted to the discussion of dystonia; dystonia in general; how to assess patients with dystonia; and the role of botulinum toxin in the treatment of cervical dystonia. The uses of electromyographic guidance are discussed. Several chapters are devoted to focal dystonias of the hand and limb dystonia. Also discussed is clinical experience of botulinum toxin F in the treatment of focal dystonias. Three chapters discuss hemifacial spasm and the use of botulinum toxin for this disorder as well as for oral mandibular spasms and bruxism; three chapters are devoted to the use of botulinum toxin in strabismus. Voice disorders such as spasmodic dysphonia and voice tremor are discussed from a variety of aspects, including assessment and the use of botulinum toxin for treatment. The last section discusses miscellaneous disorders such as botulinum treatment for tremors, tics, cerebral palsy, and spasticity, as well as other clinical disorders.

Rarely in neurological disease is a new treatment introduced that has such a profound effect as that seen with botulinum toxin therapy. Dystonic disorder was basically an untreatable condition, with a minority of patients responding to drug therapy. Botulinum toxin has dramatically changed this. Now dystonia and several other disorders have changed from the ranks of untreatable diseases to disorders that now can be managed adequately. The change in quality of life for dystonic patients, now that botulinum toxin is available, is dramatic. Clearly, this is a major advance in the therapeutics of neurological disease. *Therapy with Botulinum Toxin* discusses these advances in both highly scientific and practical terms.

William C. Koller, M.D.

v

Foreword

Advances in medical therapy seldom develop at an even pace, often occurring stepwise. This book is a timely recounting of the treatment of various clinical motor disorders in the aftermath of such a step, the introduction of direct intramuscular injection of botulinum toxin. Nearly all authors and editors were involved as clinical investigators in the initial application of the drug to their particular topic area and therefore speak with special authority. While a few were recruited by me, most sought out this investigational opportunity to advance their field, their patients, their careers, their departments. This energy and creative effort were present both during the investigational phase and at the National Institutes of Health (NIH) Consensus Development Conference at which most of this material was first presented in summary form, and it is reflected in this volume.

The approach of using botulinum toxin began in 1970-1971. We were seeking ways to influence strabismus by directly altering the extraocular muscles. Surgery for this had been employed since 1840, with development of many variations, but this was still imprecise, with strabismus surgical reoperation rates as high as 45% in some categories. We had been injecting small amounts of local anesthetics to paralyze individual extraocular muscles in alert human volunteers for physiological studies. For this we developed portable electromyographic equipment and electrode injection needles and used the electrical activity of the muscle to localize injection. This delivery system is still current for eye, laryngeal, and many other injections. An important observation just then was that eye muscles were active or even hyperactive under ketamine anesthesia. This allowed drug injection and localization and testing in animals. It further encouraged us by showing an anesthetic technique for eventual clinical use in childhood strabismus. With this approach we found alcohol unreliable; local anesthetics, alpha bungarotoxin, and saxitoxin too transient; and cholinesterase inhibitors systematically toxic.

The idea of using botulinum toxin had been considered for several years but it seemed too wild to consider seriously. Bach-y-Rita, Crone, Jampolsky, and Maumanee probably all had the idea independently, too. Indeed, Crone (Amsterdam) relates that he once ordered some botulinum toxin from England but the package arrived broken and leaking. In 1971 Simpson's book *Neuropoisons* appeared. The chapter by Daniel Drachman showed that he could induce local changes in animal muscles with botulinum toxin, just what we wanted! Schantz supplied Drachman and nearly the whole experimental world with crystalline toxin, using at the University of Wisconsin's Food Research Institute the crystallization techniques developed at Fort Detrick by Lamanna and others. Schantz generously supplied us with botulinum toxin to do the experiments in animals on extraocular muscle, which were published in 1973. These showed paralysis could be localized to the target muscle, its duration and depth controlled by dose, and all without systemic side effects. While the focus of this paper was on strabismus treatment and the persistence of eye alignment change after the paralysis wore off, we explicitly identified the potential utility of the drug in blepharospasm, and in other neurological conditions where ablation of unwanted tonus or movement was the goal. Schantz continued to send us crystalline toxin upon request with which we established pharmaceutical methods: buffering with human albumin, freeze drying, stability studies, determination of safe vial dosage, and so on. Our application to the Food and Drug Administration (FDA) to issue an IND for clinical trials languished for years. I finally asked David Cogan, who had moved from Harvard to the NIH, to put a word in to the FDA. His distinguished reputation did the trick. We injected the first strabismus patient in 1977, 12 in 1978, and by 1982 we had injected the eye muscles for strabismus and nystagmus, the lid muscles for blepharospasm, hemifacial spasm, and lid retraction, the gastrocnemius and thigh adductors for spasm due to central nervous system disease, and the neck for torticollis, all as predicted in 1973. At that point safety and efficacy were clearly documented. I was unable to interest local clinicians to treat spasmodic dysphonia, torticollis, childhood spastic disorders (''cerebral palsy''), and painful and debilitating limb muscle contracture following stroke or spinal disease. However, each of these has since been developed by investigators reporting in this volume. The contributions of over 200 clinical investigators rapidly expanded the knowledge base, subjecting the broad range of localized movement and localized tonic disorders to clinical trial, and the reports in this volume are close to definitive in their evaluation of botulinum toxin effectiveness in them. We waited four years after submitting clinical data before approval of this drug by the FDA in December 1989.

The valuable clinical attributes of botulinum toxin include, first, its specificity. This restricts action to motor terminals, avoiding the sensory effects that would occur with drugs such as tetrodotoxin, saxitoxin, local anesthetics, and other general membrane-active drugs. The long duration of action of botulinum toxin is its second most important feature. Once inside, the active part of the molecule is not substantially transported from the nerve terminal. The time from muscle paralysis until full recovery is typically six months.

What can we expect in the future? The development of circulating antibodies that prevent effectiveness of the toxin will be avoided by more potent preparations containing less antigenic toxin protein. We have already demonstrated this effect in animals for two lots that have been utilized for clinical trial. Types B, F, and G are for individuals immunized to the currently used type A. Weakness of adjacent muscles has been reduced or eliminated by concurrent protective antitoxin injection of these muscles in blepharospasm and strabismus. This allows a higher and longer-lasting toxin dose. This drug will become available for clinical trial. Extension of this approach to other anatomical areas, such as protection of pharyngeal muscles with bilateral neck injection for dystonia, might be considered. Prolonging clinical action is the major challenge. Loading a nerve terminal with combined types of toxin to take advantage of several types of nerve terminal receptors or of separate enzymatic effects within the nerve terminal is a rational approach. A combination of type A and type B toxin has not been more effective than either single toxin in our experiments, but there are many combinations to try. Hybrid molecules that combine the specific nerve terminal receptor affinity of botulinum toxins with ribosomal poisons that are transported to the nerve soma and create cell death would be an important and exquisite advance. This approach is being studied in several laboratories. It has long been suspected that botulinum toxin works as an enzyme. The demonstration of its enzymatic effect on synaptic vesicle proteins (synaptobrevin) may provide a basis for further understanding and for extending duration of action.

I want to thank the many basic scientists, clinicians, and others who have contributed to development of botulinum toxin therapeutically: co-workers at Smith-Kettlewell, Dr. Schantz for toxin, Dr. Lamanna for basic science, Dr. Simpson for education, numerous clinicians including authors in this volume for their contribution, the National Eye Institute for the investigative effort, and Dr. Habig and the staff at the FDA for their knowledge and intelligence.

Alan B. Scott, M.D.
Co-Executive Director
Smith-Kettlewell Eye
Research Institute
San Francisco, California

Preface

Muscular spasms and abnormal involuntary movements are among the most troublesome human afflictions. One of the most disabling forms of muscular spasms is dystonia. Dystonia is a neurological syndrome manifested by involuntary sustained contractions (spasms) of muscles producing abnormal movements and postures. Examples of dystonia include blepharospasm (spasms of eyelids causing involuntary eye closure), torticollis (spasms of neck muscles causing twisting movements, abnormal posture, and neck pain), spasmodic dysphonia (spasms of vocal cords causing strained voice), task-specific dystonias (writer's cramps), and oromandibular dystonia (spasms of mouth and jaw muscles causing grinding of teeth and secondary temporomandibular joint syndrome as well as speech, chewing, and swallowing difficulties). Besides dystonia, there are many other causes of muscular spasms, such as hemifacial spasm, tremor, tics, myoclonus, spasticity, and various musculoskeletal spasms.

In the early 1980s, botulinum toxin (BTX) was introduced for the treatment of strabismus (crossed eyes), and its use subsequently expanded to other conditions manifested by involuntary muscle spasms, including blepharospasm and other focal dystonias, hemifacial spasm, spasticity, and tremors. The use of BTX in the treatment of these and other conditions associated with undesirable muscle contractions represents one of the most important advances in neurological therapeutics. The impact of this therapeutic intervention on functioning of patients with involuntary muscle spasms of various origins has been enormous. As a result of BTX therapy, patients with blepharospasm, for example, are now able to read, drive, and watch television; patients with hemifacial spasm are no longer irritated and embarrassed by involuntary facial twitches; patients with oromandibular dystonia are able to chew and no longer experience grinding of their teeth and discomfort associated with temporomandibular joint syndrome; patients with cervical dystonia have less neck pain and are able to control their head position; patients with spasmodic dysphonia are able to speak in public and on the telephone without strain and strangulation; patients with writer's cramp and tremor can again write and type; patients with tics no longer twitch and jerk; and patients with leg spasticity can ambulate better and have less discomfort from spasms. These are just some examples of the way BTX has ameliorated suffering and meaningfully enhanced the lives of many individuals.

The concept for this book was born during the Consensus Development Conference sponsored by the National Institutes of Health and the Food and Drug Administration in November 1990. Because of many new developments in the field of neurotoxins and in the clinical use of BTX, the editors saw a need for a thorough review and an update of this topic. We were fortunate in being able to obtain contributions from leading authorities on the topic of neurotoxins and their therapeutic applications. The contributors were encouraged not only to review their area of expertise, but to offer suggestions for future directions in research. Some views expressed by the authors, therefore, may be considered controversial, but the reader should have no difficulty differentiating such opinions from hard data and well-established notions. Many chapters contain original, previously unpublished, information. It is inevitable that in a multiauthored text devoted to a single topic, there will be some overlap. The editors, however, tried to eliminate redundancy and at the same time allowed for different points of view and interpretations.

Because of the demonstrated efficacy and safety of BTX, there is growing interest in this therapy among clinicians. Thus far, this therapy has had its greatest impact in neurology, and has been compared to other major therapeutic breakthroughs, such as the introduction of phenytoin for epilepsy and levodopa for Parkinson's disease. As a result of the expanding role in BTX in the treatment of various disorders, there is an increasing need for information about this novel and effective therapy. This is reflected by growing demands for current reviews and educational programs about BTX and its therapeutic potential.

We believe that this book will be of interest not only to neurologists, but also to ophthalmologists, otolaryngologists, plastic surgeons, physiatrists, speech therapists, dentists, orthopedic surgeons, osteopathic physicians, and many other specialists who care for patients who have muscular spasms and involuntary movements.

Joseph Jankovic
Mark Hallett

Contents

Contributors

Michael Adler, Ph.D. Neurotoxicology Branch, U.S. Army Medical Research Institute of Chemical Defense, Aberdeen Proving Ground, Maryland

Kathy Alderson, M.D. Salt Lake City VA Medical Center and University of Utah, Salt Lake City, Utah

Michael J. Aminoff, M.D. Department of Neurology, University of California at San Francisco, San Francisco, California

Reiner Benecke, M.D. Neurology Clinic, Heinrich Heine University, Düsseldorf, Germany

Alfredo Berardelli, M.D. Department of Neurological Sciences, La Sapienza University, Rome, Italy

Albert W. Biglan, M.D. Department of Ophthalmology, University of Pittsburgh School of Medicine, Pittsburgh, Pennsylvania

Andrew Blitzer, M.D., D.D.S. Department of Otolaryngology, Columbia University College of Physicians and Surgeons, New York, New York

Gary E. Borodic, M.D. Department of Ophthalmology, Harvard Medical School; Oculoplastics Service, Massachusetts Eye and Ear Infirmary; and Boston University School of Medicine, Boston, Massachusetts

Susan Bressman, M.D. Movement Disorder Group, Department of Neurology, The Neurological Institute, Columbia-Presbyterian Medical Center, New York, New York

Mitchell F. Brin, M.D.   Department of Neurology, The Neurological Institute, Columbia University College of Physicians and Surgeons, New York, New York

Alastair Carruthers, M.A., B.M., B.Ch., F.R.C.P.(C), F.R.C.P.(Con.)   Department of Medicine, University of British Columbia, Vancouver, British Columbia, Canada

Jean D. A. Carruthers, M.D., F.R.C.S.(Eng). F.R.C.S.(c)   Department of Ophthalmology, University of British Columbia, Vancouver, British Columbia, Canada

Julie A. Coffield, D.V.M., Ph.D.   Division of Environmental Medicine and Toxicology, Jefferson Medical College, Philadelphia, Pennsylvania

Cynthia L. Comella, M.D.   Department of Neurological Sciences, Rush-Presbyterian-St. Luke's Medical Center, Chicago, Illinois

Robert V. Considine, Ph.D.   Department of Medicine, Jefferson Medical College, Philadelphia, Pennsylvania

Earl S. Consky, M.D., F.R.C.P.(C)   Consultant Neurologist, Toronto, Ontario, Canada

Oscar A. Cruz, M.D.   Department of Ophthalmology, Cardinal Glennon Children's Hospital, St. Louis University School of Medicine, St. Louis, Missouri

Carol Dang*   Smith-Kettlewell Eye Research Institute, San Francisco, California

Bibhuti R. DasGupta, Ph.D.   Department of Food Microbiology and Toxicology, University of Wisconsin, Madison, Wisconsin

Sharad S. Deshpande, Ph.D.   Neurotoxicology Branch, U.S. Army Medical Research Institute of Chemical Defense, Aberdeen Proving Ground, Maryland

Günther Deuschl, M.D.   Department of Neurology, University of Freiburg, Freiburg, Germany

Donald T. Donovan, M.D.   Department of Otorhinolaryngology and Communicative Sciences, Baylor College of Medicine, and The Methodist Hospital, Houston, Texas

Richard M. Dubinsky, M.D.   Department of Neurology, University of Kansas Medical Center, Kansas City, Kansas

Jonathan J. Dutton, M.D., Ph.D.   Department of Ophthalmology, Duke University Eye Center, Durham, North Carolina

Present affiliation: BOTOX Quality Assurance, Allergan, Inc., Berkeley, California.

Dennis D. Dykstra, M.D., Ph.D. Departments of Physical Medicine and Rehabilitation, Urologic Surgery, and Pediatrics, University of Minnesota, Minneapolis, Minneapolis, Minnesota

John S. Elston, B.Sc., M.D., F.R.C.S. Oxford Eye Hospital, Radcliffe Infirmary, National Health Service Trust, Oxford, England

Stanley Fahn, M.D. Department of Neurology, The Neurological Institute, Columbia-Presbyterian Medical Center, New York, New York

Robert J. Ferrante, M.S. Department of Neuropathology, Massachusetts General Hospital, Harvard Medical School, Boston, Massachusetts

John T. Flynn, M.D. Department of Ophthalmology, University of Miami School of Medicine, Miami, Florida

Charles N. Ford, M.D., F.A.C.S. Division of Otolaryngology, Department of Head and Neck Surgery, University of Wisconsin Clinical Science Center, Madison, Wisconsin

Mary K. Gentry, B.S. Department of Biological Chemistry, Walter Reed Army Institute of Research, Washington, D.C.

Paul Greene, M.D. Department of Neurology, Columbia-Presbyterian Medical Center, New York, New York

Dallas C. Hack, M.D. Department of Clinical Medicine, U.S. Army Medical Research Institute of Infectious Diseases, Frederick, Maryland

Mark Hallett, M.D. National Institute of Neurological Disorders and Stroke, National Institutes of Health, Bethesda, Maryland

Charles L. Hatheway, Ph.D. Division of Bacterial and Mycotic Diseases, National Center for Infectious Diseases, Centers for Disease Control and Prevention, Atlanta, Georgia

Susan Herman, M.D. Department of Neurology, The Neurological Institute, Columbia-Presbyterian Medical Center, New York, New York

Joseph Jankovic, M.D. Department of Neurology, Baylor College of Medicine, Houston, Texas

Eric A. Johnson, Sc.D. Department of Food Microbiology and Toxicology, Food Research Institute, University of Wisconsin, Madison, Wisconsin

Anthony N. Kalloo, M.D. Gastroenterology Division, Johns Hopkins University and Hospital, Baltimore, Maryland

Barbara Illowsky Karp, M.D.   National Institute of Neurological Disorders and Stroke, National Institutes of Health, Bethesda, Maryland

Sang-Jin Kim, M.D.   Keimyung University, Taegu, South Korea

L. Andrew Koman, M.D.   Department of Orthopedic Surgery, Bowman Gray School of Medicine, Wake Forest University, Winston-Salem, North Carolina

Anthony E. Lang, M.D., F.R.C.P.(C)   Department of Neurology, The Toronto Hospital and University of Toronto, Toronto, Ontario, Canada

Dale J. Lange, M.D.   Department of Neurology, The Neurological Institute, Columbia-Presbyterian Medical Center, New York, New York

Frank J. Lebeda, Ph.D.   Department of Cell Biology and Biochemistry, U.S. Army Medical Research Institute of Infectious Diseases, Frederick, Maryland

Robert S. Lebovics, M.D., F.A.C.S.   Department of Otolaryngology, National Institute on Deafness and Other Communication Disorders, National Institutes of Health, Bethesda, Maryland

E. Löhle, M.D.   Department of Otolaryngology, University of Freiburg, Freiburg, Germany

Christy L. Ludlow, Ph.D.   Division of Intramural Research, Voice and Speech Section, National Institute on Deafness and Other Communication Disorders, National Institutes of Health, Bethesda, Maryland

Elbert H. Magoon, M.D., F.A.C.S.   Department of Pediatric Ophthalmology, Canton Eye Center, Inc., Canton, Ohio

Bruno Mercuri, M.D.   Department of Neurological Sciences, La Sapienza University, Rome, Italy

James F. Mooney III, M.D.   Department of Orthopedic Surgery, Bowman Gray School of Medicine, Wake Forest University, Winston-Salem, North Carolina

Elizabeth Moyer, M.D.   Department of Pharmacology, Athena Neurosciences, Inc., South San Francisco, California

Thomas Murry, Ph.D.   Department of Otolaryngology, University of Tennessee, Memphis College of Medicine, Memphis, Tenneessee

Eric Anthony Nash, M.D.   Division of Intramural Research, National Institute on Deafness and Other Communication Disorders, National Institutes of Health, Bethesda, Maryland

Christopher F. O'Brien, M.D.   Movement Disorders Center, Colorado Neurological Institute, and Department of Neurology, University of Colorado Health Sciences Center, Englewood, Colorado

Richard K. Olney, M.D.   Department of Neurology, University of California at San Francisco, San Francisco, California

Pankaj Jay Pasricha, M.D.   Gastroenterology Division, Department of Medicine, Johns Hopkins University and Hospital, Baltimore, Maryland

L. Bruce Pearce, Ph.D.   Department of Pharmacology, Boston University School of Medicine, Boston, Massachusetts

W. Poewe, M.D.   Department of Neurology, Universitätsklinikum Rudolf Virchow, Free University of Berlin, Berlin, Germany

Alberto Priori, M.D.   Department of Neurological Sciences, La Sapienza University, Rome, Italy

Seth L. Pullman, M.D., F.R.C.P.(C)   Department of Neurology, The Neurological Institute, Columbia-Presbyterian Medical Center, New York, New York

Karen Rhew, M.D.   Voice and Speech Section, National Institute on Deafness and Other Communication Disorders, National Institutes of Health, Bethesda, Maryland

Arthur L. Rosenbaum, M.D.   Department of Ophthalmology, Jules Stein Eye Institute, Los Angeles, California

David B. Rosenfield, M.D.   Speech Motor Control Laboratory, Stuttering Center, Department of Neurology, Baylor College of Medicine, Houston, Texas

Genji Sakaguchi, D.V.M., Ph.D.   Japan Food Research Laboratories, Osaka Branch, Osaka, Japan

Ira Sanders, M.D.   Department of Otolaryngology, Mount Sinai Medical Center, New York, New York

Edward J. Schantz, Ph.D.   Department of Food Microbiology and Toxicology, University of Wisconsin, Madison, Wisconsin

Kenneth Schwartz, P.A.   Department of Neurology, Baylor College of Medicine, Houston, Texas

Paulette E. Setler, Ph.D.   Executive Vice President of Research and Development, Athena Neurosciences, Inc., South San Francisco, California

Christopher M. Shaari, M.D.   Department of Otolaryngology, Mount Sinai Medical Center, New York, New York

Robert E. Sheridan, Ph.D. Neurotoxicology Branch, U.S. Army Medical Research Institute of Chemical Defense, Aberdeen Proving Ground, Maryland

Tomoko Shimizu, Ph.D. Department of Vaccine Production, Chiba Serum Institute, Ichikawa-shi, Chiba, Japan

Lance L. Simpson, Ph.D. Division of Environmental Medicine and Toxicology, Department of Medicine, Jefferson Medical College, Philadelphia, Pennsylvania

Beth Paterson Smith, Ph.D. Department of Orthopedic Surgery, Bowman Gray School of Medicine, Wake Forest University, Winston-Salem, North Carolina

Sheila V. Stager, Ph.D. Voice and Speech Section, National Institute on Deafness and Other Communication Disorders, National Institutes of Health, Bethesda, Maryland

Celia Stewart, M.S., C.C.C.-S.L.P. Departments of Neurology and Otolaryngology, Columbia University College of Physicians and Surgeons, New York, New York

Michael R. Swenson, M.D. Department of Neurosciences, University of California, San Diego Medical Center, San Diego, California

Camilo Toro, M.D. Human Motor Control Section, National Institute of Neurological Disorders and Stroke, National Institutes of Health, Bethesda, Maryland

Joseph King Ching Tsui, M.D. Neurodegenerative Disorders Centre, University of British Columbia, Vancouver, British Columbia, Canada

Jörg Wissel, M.D. Department of Neurology, Universitätsklinikum Rudolf Virchow, Free University of Berlin, Berlin, Germany

Gayle E. Woodson, M.D. Department of Otolaryngology, University of Tennessee, Memphis College of Medicine, Memphis, Tennessee

Petra Zwirner, M.D. Ear, Nose, and Throat Department, Division of Phoniatry and Pedaudiology, Georg August University, Göttingen, Göttingen, Germany

Historical Perspective

It is an interesting fact that some of the toxins and poisons that have caused sickness and death and were considered by warring nations as chemical or biological warfare agents have now become important in medical research and as drugs for human treatment. Botulinum toxin, particularly type A, was considered one of these agents. In 1989 this toxin was licensed by the Food and Drug Administration (FDA) as an orphan drug for the treatment of certain involuntary muscle movements. The following is a brief account of my work on botulinum toxin and collaboration with Alan Scott that led to the use of botulinum toxin type A as a drug for human treatment.

My first real encounter with botulinum toxin came in 1944 during World War II, when I was assigned as a young Army officer to the highly secret program initiated by the National Academy of Sciences. The laboratory work was placed at Camp Detrick (later named Fort Detrick) near Frederick, Maryland. I was assigned to investigations with bacteriologists and physicians to study the nature of some toxins and a means of protecting against them. At Fort Detrick we had very good facilities for work with pathogenic organisms and for the production and purification of the toxins they produce. Purification of botulinum toxin was one of our first objectives. Actually, attempts at the purification of type A toxin were made in the 1920s by Dr. Herman Sommer at the Hooper Foundation, University of California, San Francisco. California had several outbreaks of type A foodborne botulism at the time, and during study of toxin formation Dr. Sommer found that type A toxin could be precipitated from the spent culture fluid of the organism in a highly concentrated form by simply adjusting the pH to 3.5 with acid. This mud-like precipitate was the starting material for much of the experimental work at Fort Detrick involving further purification and the action of the toxin in animals exposed to the toxin by inhalation, by injection, and by mouth.

Although much of the work was done on type A toxin, considerable work was also done on types B, C, D, and E. Toxoids were developed for the five types for immunization of persons working with the toxins. After the end of the war, in 1946, the toxin was obtained in crystalline form, which stimulated much scientific interest in this toxin because of its extremely high toxicity and possible enzymatic action. This toxin was found to be a high-molecular-weight protein ($\sim$900,000 daltons) made up of toxic units ($\sim$150,000 daltons) bound to several nontoxic proteins that are important in stabilization of the toxic unit. The botulinum toxins are unique in this respect.

After the war the National Academy recommended the continuation of many of the studies carried on at Fort Detrick, and I continued work with several toxins, particularly type A botulinum toxin. The important advantage at Fort Detrick was the facilities for the production and purification of large amounts of various toxins such as crystalline type A toxin, saxitoxin, and staphylococcal enterotoxins in lots of many grams at one time. Because I produced large quantities of these toxins, small amounts were made available to research organizations interested in their nature and structure. Through the years I furnished these toxins to researchers in many countries throughout the world, as well as to the FDA, to the Public Health Service, and to many of the contributors to this book. I feel that making the type A crystalline toxin available to these researchers greatly increased our knowledge of botulinum toxin through their publications.

The use of type A toxin for the treatment of many spastic muscle disorders came about through a fortunate set of circumstances in the late 1960s. Dr. Alan B. Scott, a surgeon at the Smith-Kettlewell Eye Research Foundation in San Francisco, called me and asked if any of my toxins would be useful to reduce or paralyze hyperactive muscles in some monkeys he had in experiments. What he was looking for was an alternative to human surgery for strabismus by injecting something into the muscle pulling the eye out of alignment that would reduce the activity, rather than cutting away part of the muscle as is done in surgery. I had on hand two purified toxins that produce flaccid paralysis in animals and that I thought might be useful in his experiments. One was botulinum toxin type A and the other was saxitoxin isolated from poisonous clams and certain dinoflagellates. On the basis of our knowledge of the toxin action in weakening muscles in human botulism, I gave him some of my crystalline toxin for tests. After a short time Dr. Scott sent me the results of the tests on monkeys showing with photographs that the injection of a small amount of the toxin into the active muscle corrected the condition. We were both very pleased with the results since it appeared that I might have the substance he needed. Further experiments proved that the type A toxin was the substance that should be used, and we began our collaboration. However, in 1972, the laboratories at Fort Detrick were closed, and I accepted a professorship in the Department of Food Microbiology and Toxicology at the University of Wisconsin, where I continued the collaboration with Dr. Scott and where most of the studies on the preparation and characterization of the toxins for human treatment were carried out.

After several years of successful tests with different batches of the toxin, Dr. Scott applied to the FDA for an IND permit that allowed the treatment of human volunteers starting about 1978. Because the toxin had to be injected into human muscle, there were many considerations to be addressed regarding toxin for the volunteer work and for licensure by the FDA as a drug for human treatment. No protocols existed for a protein drug of this type, and new ones had to be written. I felt, of course, that purity and good toxic activity were essential. The protocols and criteria that I set down for type A toxin for human treatment were as follows: I chose the Hall strain of *Clostridium botulinum* type A because it consistently produced 10^6 or more LD_{50} per milliliter in a simplified medium of hydrolyzed casein, yeast extract, and dextrose. Although there are different methods of purifying the toxin, I chose a purification procedure not exposing the toxin to enzymes or synthetic substances that might contaminate the final toxin preparation and cause undue reactions in a patient. Also, the crystalline toxin must have a sharp absorption peak at 278 nm, a 260 nm/278 nm absorption ratio of less the 0.6, and a specific toxicity of 3×10^7 mouse LD_{50} per milligram. To ensure long stability, the toxin must be stored in the mother liquor of the second crystallization at 4°C or less. With suggestions from my colleagues at the FDA and discussions with Dr. Scott I decided to prepare sufficient crystalline botulinum toxin (about 200 mg) to carry on extensive studies and to draw up protocols that I thought would be the most satisfactory description of the toxin for treatment by injection. The preparation of this quantity of toxin required several 16-liter cultures of the organism combined into one batch for purification and crystallization that yielded 150 mg on the second crystallization and was designated batch 79-11 (prepared November 1979). One hundred milligrams was sent to Dr. Scott for the volunteer work and 50 mg was kept in my laboratory for storage and reference. This particular batch served as the stock supply for preparing toxin for dispensing to physicians for the volunteer work, and after about 10 years of human treatment by Dr. Scott and other physicians, it was licensed by the FDA as an orphan drug in December 1989 for strabismus and certain dystonias.

The preparation of the toxin for dispensing to the medical profession presented some problems because the toxin had to be diluted over one million times down to concentrations of a nanogram or less. Such great dilution of the toxin required the addition of another protein such as gelatin, bovine serum albumin, and in this case human serum albumin to protect the toxin from rapid detoxification. Under the circumstances at that time, Dr. Scott felt that the toxin should be dried with the albumin and enough sodium chloride to meet body fluids. It was finally dissolved in a solution containing 5 mg human serum albumin and 9 mg of sodium chloride per milliliter and 0.1 ml was dried by lyophilization in small vials for dispensing. Drying the toxin under these conditions resulted in considerable loss in toxicity (as much as 90%), and it became necessary to add sufficient toxin to the solution so that 100 U survived the drying process. Although Scott and I were aware of the possibility that the inactivated toxin might cause trouble because it had to be injected along with the active toxin and possibly be sufficient to cause antibody formation, there was no proof of such action at that time. Early experiments by me, and more recently by Goodnough and Johnson (1992), however, have shown that lyophilization of the toxin without sodium chloride and with HSA at pH 6.2–6.8 greatly reduces the amount of inactivated toxin formed on drying. Further research is in progress in our laboratory at the Food Research Institute to improve the quality and stability of the toxin for dispensing to the medical profession.

A good reliable assay for the toxin is paramount in medical treatment. Two different assays have been used for botulinum toxin in foods: the important one based on paralysis and death in a mouse due to blockage of acetylcholine release to muscle and the other based on the immunological properties of the toxin. The latter method measures inactivated as well as active toxin and of course cannot be used to evaluate the toxin for medical use because only active paralytic toxin is effective in treatment. Although the FDA has mouse assay procedures for the toxin in foods, I felt that the biological evaluation of the toxin for human treatment, as well as in foods, should be based on a reference standard toxin preparation for the mouse assay so that results from different laboratories could be made comparable. About 1974 the FDA provided me with funds for the establishment of a reference standard based on purified crystalline type A toxin, which was evaluated and successfully used as FDA laboratories and several commercial laboratories throughout the United States. This work was carried on by Don Kautter at the FDA laboratories in cooperation with me at the Food Research Laboratories and published in 1978 (*Journal of the Association of Official Analytical Chemists*) with the hope of increasing the accuracy of the mouse assay for botulinum toxins.

In 1985 Eric A. Johnson from the Harvard Medical School joined the Department of Food Microbiology and Toxicology to study various pathogenic organisms causing food-borne disease, in particular clostridia and their toxins. He has contributed to the quality of the toxin through evaluation by gel electrophoresis and also improved the quality of the toxin that is dried for dispensing to physicians. His work should greatly reduce the presence of inactive toxin being injected in patients treated with the toxin, which may be a factor causing them to become refractory to treatment. He has now taken over the research on the toxin for human treatment in our laboratory.

As I look back on my 50 years of work with botulinum toxin and the 20 or more in collaboration with Dr. Scott, I feel lucky to have had the opportunity to prepare and characterize toxin for human treatment. The ingenuity of Dr. Scott in devising a means for testing a substance for its effect on a muscle of a live animal and applying it to human muscle was absolutely essential to all that was accomplished with the toxin. Most of us working with botulinum toxin knew of course that it weakened muscle tissue in animals and in humans with botulism, but we never had an animal model to test it. The possible use of toxin for weakening a muscle was first suggested to me by Dr. Vernon Brooks, a physiologist to whom I furnished toxin for his studies and with whom I occasionally discussed the action of the toxin. He had shown in his publications that acetylcholine was formed at the nerve endings and paralysis resulted because the toxin blocked its release to the muscle. He suggested in the 1950s that the toxin would be good to reduce the activity of a hyperactive muscle.

My work with the toxin has also involved many people who have given me suggestions and help, and I take this opportunity to thank them. I thank Dr. Daniel Drachman, a neurophysiologist at Johns Hopkins University, to whom I furnished toxin for many years, and who suggested to Dr. Scott that I might have some toxins to test in his monkeys. We had many helpful discussions on the effects of the toxin on the nervous system. Much help also came from Dr. Carl Lamanna at the FDA, who first crystallized botulinum toxin at Fort Detrick in 1946 and was the first to show that the type A toxin is composed of toxic units bound to nontoxic proteins some of which are hemolytic. He later made suggestions on FDA requirements for drugs that might apply to the toxin and recommended in 1982 that the toxin be classed as an orphan drug to come under the Orphan Drug Act that became effective in 1983. At the Department of Food Microbiology and Toxicology much credit goes to my colleague and co-worker Eric Johnson, who has taken over the work on the toxin for human treatment. Also, I want to include the work on the toxin of Dr. Sugiyama and Dr. DasGupta and their associates on the structure of the toxin. In particular, I must give credit to Professor Emeritus E. M. Foster, who was department head when I came to the University of Wisconsin in 1972. He became interested in the possible use of botulinum toxin as a drug for human treatment and recommended and made arrangements through the necessary university channels for financial support and for use of university facilities for the toxin work.

My greatest reward in all of my work is that the toxin is giving thousands of people relief from pain and suffering and enabling them to live a more normal life.

Edward J. Schantz, Ph.D.
Professor Emeritus
Department of Food Microbiology
  and Toxicology
University of Wisconsin
Madison, Wisconsin

BASIC SCIENCE

1

The Site and Mechanism of Action of Botulinum Neurotoxin

Julie A. Coffield, Robert V. Considine, and Lance L. Simpson
Jefferson Medical College, Philadelphia, Pennsylvania

INTRODUCTION

Focal dystonias and related neurological problems are characterized by inappropriate and excessive efferent activity in motor neurons. The pathological mechanisms that underlie this excessive activity have not been definitively established. Several possible etiologies have been considered, including (1) central nervous system lesions that produce an overflow of excitatory activity, (2) excessive transmitter release at motor nerve endings, (3) defective transmitter metabolism, and (4) defective receptor function. There is a belief that a central nervous system lesion is the most likely explanation, but decisive evidence to support this belief is not yet available.

In spite of the limitations in our understanding of dystonias and related problems, one important point does emerge. No matter which of the various defects may be involved, each can be corrected by diminishing or abolishing the release of acetylcholine at motor nerve endings. It is precisely this premise that accounts for the introduction of botulinum neurotoxin as a therapeutic agent.

The true value of the toxin as a medicinal agent can best be appreciated by seeking to envision an ideal drug. A rational approach to the treatment of dystonias would be to administer a drug that possesses at least four properties. These are

A highly specific site of action, this being motor nerve endings.

A very sustained duration of action, with initial durations of weeks or even months.

A very high potency of action, with the implication that the low doses needed to produce a therapeutic outcome would not trigger immune responses, allergic responses, or related phenomena.

A highly selective mechanism of action, meaning that therapeutic responses could be evoked at doses unlikely to evoke adverse side effects.

When taken collectively, these four criteria are very stringent. They greatly limit the number of pharmacological agents that can be considered as authentic candidates for study. For example, there are many toxins that act presynaptically (e.g., phospholipase A_2 neurotoxins) and postsynaptically (e.g., curare) to block neuromuscular transmission, but most of these toxins have notable limitations. Phospholipase A_2 neurotoxins, for instance, are not as potent as one would like, and curare has an unacceptably short duration of action. By contrast, botulinum neurotoxin is the most potent pharmacological agent known, and it has a substantial duration of action.

In addition to meeting the four criteria listed above, botulinum neurotoxin has one further advantage, especially in comparison with surgical intervention. The administration of botulinum neurotoxin can be titrated to achieve a maximal therapeutic outcome that is tailored to each patient and to each neurological problem.

Because of its many apparent advantages, botulinum neurotoxin has come to be regarded as the pharmacological intervention of choice for the treatment of several dystonias. Indeed, the favorable results obtained in certain conditions (e.g., blepharospasm, strabismus), combined with an emerging body of positive results in numerous other conditions (see later chapters in this book), suggest that botulinum neurotoxin will ultimately have wide clinical utility. This promising status implies a strong need to develop a sound understanding of the structure and biological activity of the toxin.

NEUROTOXIN ORIGIN AND STRUCTURE

Botulinum neurotoxin is produced by the gram-negative, rod-shaped anaerobic bacterium *Clostridium botulinum*. The neurotoxin is synthesized in seven different serotypes designated A, B, C, D, E, F, and G, and the bacteria that produce these serotypes are given the same designations (1,2). Two other clostridial organisms are also capable of producing the neurotoxin. *Clostridium butyricum* produces a serotype similar but not identical to *Clostridium botulinum* type E (3–6), and *Clostridium baratii* produces a toxin that is similar to *Clostridium botulinum* type F (7).

The location of the genes that encode the various neurotoxins has been determined. The genetic information for botulinum neurotoxin types A, B, E, and F is found in the bacterial genome. The information encoding serotypes C and D is found in phage particles, and the information for type G is in a plasmid (8).

All of the botulinum toxins are synthesized as single-chain polypeptides with molecular weights of approximately 150,000. These single-chain molecules are activated by a selective process of proteolysis known as nicking. In some cases the bacteria themselves possess the proteolytic enzymes that process the toxins, but in other cases the toxins must be exposed to exogenous trypsin-like enzymes. Posttranslational processing of the toxins increases their potency one to two orders of magnitude.

Conversion from the inactive form to the active form involves at least two events. The 150,000-dalton single-chain molecule is nicked by a proteolytic enzyme to give a dichain molecule comprising a 100,000-dalton heavy chain linked by a disulfide bond to a 50,000-dalton light chain (9). Evidence suggests that nicking is essential but not sufficient to give full activation of the neurotoxin. An additional event must occur beyond conversion from a single-chain to a dichain molecule. The possibility that the amino-terminus of either the heavy chain or the light chain is modified has been experimentally discounted. An alteration in the carboxy-terminus of the heavy chain and a change in the three-dimensional structure of the holotoxin are possibilities that remain to be evaluated.

Through traditional protein chemistry and the techniques of molecular biology the complete amino acid sequences of most of the neurotoxins have been determined. Primary structures have been deduced for botulinum neurotoxin type A (10), type B (11), type C (12), type D (13), and type E (14,15). Comparison of the sequences indicates that there is significant homology among the neurotoxins, particularly within the N-terminal of the heavy chain. In addition, the light chains of all the neurotoxins possess a histidine motif characteristic of zinc metalloendopeptidases (10). The implications of this observation with respect to the intracellular actions of the toxin are discussed below.

MODEL OF TOXIN ACTION

Overview

Botulinum neurotoxin acts selectively on peripheral cholinergic nerve endings to inhibit acetylcholine release (1,8,16). Although the toxin is most potent at the neuromuscular junction, its ability to inhibit cholinergic transmission is not limited to motor nerve endings. The toxin is also capable of inhibiting transmitter release from pre- and post-ganglionic cholinergic nerve endings of the autonomic nervous system.

Botulinum neurotoxin does not ordinarily penetrate the blood-brain barrier, and thus it does not block the release of acetylcholine or any other transmitter in the central nervous system of intact organisms. However, the toxin does produce concentration-dependent blockade of exocytosis from isolated synaptosomal preparations. When adequate concentrations of toxin are used, stimulus-evoked release of most neurotransmitters is blocked.

The study of many different bacterial toxins has led to the development of a general model to account for their mechanism of action. According to this model the toxins proceed through three sequential steps that include binding, internalization, and intracellular poisoning. The mechanism by which botulinum neurotoxin selectively inhibits acetylcholine release can also be described by this model. The susceptibility of cholinergic cells to the neurotoxin is dependent on the ability of these cells to bind and internalize the toxin, as well as the presence of an appropriate intracellular target.

Binding

The poisoning process begins with the high-affinity binding of botulinum neurotoxin to specific receptors on the cell surface. Dose-response studies indicate that effective binding occurs at picomolar concentrations or less, which reinforces the belief that the toxin is one of the most potent biological substances known (8). The highly selective nature of the binding has been demonstrated in autoradiographic studies of the neuromuscular junction, in which labeled toxin was associated mainly with the presynaptic nerve terminal membrane (17,18). Labeled toxin did not bind to the nerve fiber trunk or in the postsynaptic region.

Work on electron-microscopic autoradiographic localization of toxin binding has demonstrated different densities of binding sites for serotypes A and B, and it has also demonstrated that the receptors for the two serotypes are not the same. This is in keeping with numerous observations showing that the seven serotypes do not share the same receptor. Each serotype of botulinum neurotoxin appears to have its own unique receptor.

Structure-function analyses suggest that the tissue-targeting domain of the toxin molecule is found mainly in the heavy chain (19,20). Although the existence of distinct receptors for each of the botulinum neurotoxin serotypes is supported by a variety of ligand binding studies (21–28), the exact nature of these toxin-specific binding sites is still under investigation. One significant outcome of this work has been the determination that sialic acid residues are essential components of the binding sites for all serotypes. Gangliosides, which are sialic acid–containing glycosphingolipids, were initially implicated in early work on toxin-binding sites (29,30), but this concept has been replaced by the view that sialoglycoproteins are more likely candidates for toxin-specific receptors. Studies using lectins from *Limax flavus* and *Triticum vulgaris* that have affinity for sialic acid moieties confirmed the importance of sialic acid residues at the toxin-binding site (31). The lectins delayed the onset of toxin-induced neuromuscular blockade at the murine neuromuscular junction and inhibited toxin binding to synaptic membrane preparations. The effect of the lectins was similar for all serotypes of botulinum toxin, and thus the lectins are now recognized as universal antagonists of toxin binding.

Internalization

The second step in the poisoning process requires internalization of bound toxin into the target cell. Internalization can be separated into two distinct events, each of which can be manipulated experimentally to inhibit toxin action. First, the toxin crosses the plasma membrane by receptor-mediated endocytosis and becomes entrapped in endosomes. Second, the toxin exits the endosome to reach the cytosol, where it exerts its effects. The exact nature of botulinum toxin translocation from the endosome to the cytosol has not been determined; however, studies of diphtheria toxin and related substances suggest that translocation could be a pH-dependent process (32,33). The proton pump within endosomal membranes is known to produce a decrease in intraluminal pH. The amino-terminus of the heavy chain of botulinum neurotoxin possesses a ''pH sensor'' that triggers a conformational change in the molecule in response to a pH of 5.5 or lower. This conformational change exposes hydrophobic regions in the toxin molecule that insert into the endosomal membrane and initiate translocation of the toxin to the cytosol. Once the toxin molecule reaches the cytosol, the stage is set for the final step of intracellular poisoning to take place.

Universal antagonism of the internalization step can be achieved in several ways. Endocytosis of receptor-bound toxin is an energy-dependent process and can be diminished by experimentally lowering temperature (34,35). At experimentally lowered temperatures the bound toxin remains on the cell surface and is susceptible to neutralizing antibodies, significantly antagonizing onset of toxicity. In addition, drugs that neutralize endosomal pH and/or inhibit the endosomal proton pump have proved to be effective antagonists of toxin activity, supporting the pH-dependence of translocation for botulinum toxin. For example, methylamine hydrochloride and ammonium chloride, lysosomotropic drugs that neutralize endosomal pH, markedly delay the onset of toxicity (36). Similarly, bafilomycin, a microbial agent that selectively inhibits the proton pump of vacuoles, greatly antagonizes toxin action (37).

Intracellular Poisoning

The final step in neurotoxin action involves modification of an intracellular substrate that governs exocytosis. Structure-function analyses have demonstrated that the poisoning domain of the toxin molecule is located in the light chain. Because of the remarkable potency of the toxin molecule, investigators have long believed that it may be an enzyme. Indeed, recent work has revealed that botulinum neurotoxin contains a histidine-rich sequence common to zinc endopeptidases (10) and furthermore that the light chain expresses high-affinity binding for zinc (38). The metalloprotease-like characteristics of botulinum neurotoxin suggest that some widely distributed polypeptide substrate mediating transmitter release serves as a target for intracellular poisoning.

The precise mechanism of intracellular action of botulinum neurotoxin is still unknown, but recent biochemical studies and a large body of electrophysiological work suggest that at least two targets may exist. Moreover, these studies indicate that the seven serotypes of botulinum neurotoxin can be separated into two functional classes that act at two distinct sites. Details of this work are discussed below. The electrophysiological studies will be considered first, followed by an analysis of the biochemical data.

Electrophysiology

As previously stated, botulinum neurotoxin acts selectively on peripheral cholinergic nerve endings to inhibit acetylcholine release. There are many steps in the transmitter release process that could serve as potential targets for botulinum neurotoxin, although many of these sites have been ruled out by direct investigation (for review, see Refs. 8,16,39,40). For example, presynaptic electrophysiological correlates of nerve function such as action potential propagation, nerve terminal depolarization, and sodium, potassium, or calcium ion channels are not affected by the toxin. In addition, the responsiveness of the postsynaptic cell is not altered by the toxin. These results have narrowed the focus of research to substrates found in the microenvironment of the nerve terminal, such as synaptic vesicles and the plasma membrane.

Several different preparations, including the neuromuscular junction, brain synaptosomes, and permeabilized adrenal cells, have been used to study botulinum neurotoxin activity. Mammalian neuromuscular preparations, especially the isolated phrenic nerve–hemidiaphragm, have been extremely valuable for the electrophysiological analyses of botulinum neurotoxin action (34,41,42). In general, toxin-induced inhibition of stimulus-evoked acetylcholine release has been measured as a progressive decay in twitch amplitude or end plate potential (EPP) amplitude until no response could be evoked, suggesting complete inhibition of transmitter release. Similarly, toxin-induced blockade of spontaneous exocytosis has been measured as a decrease in the frequency of spontaneous miniature end plate potentials (MEPPs).

The seven serotypes of botulinum neurotoxin are similar in size and structure, and all inhibit quantal transmitter release. There is evidence, however, that the serotypes differ in their potency and in their intracellular target site.

Potency. It has been a general observation that serotype A is more potent than the other serotypes in blocking neuromuscular transmission (43–45). For example, serotype A reduces MEPP frequency to less than 1% of control, whereas other serotypes may reduce frequency to less than 10% of control. In addition, serotype A induces sprouting at the neuromuscular junction (46,47), which is not seen with serotype D (48), the only other serotype examined thus far. Sprouting is a nonspecific response to denervation. The fact that sprouting is induced by serotype A but not serotype D may be a reflection of the degree of depression in MEPP frequency caused by serotype A. The extreme decrease in spontaneous transmitter release may also be an indicator of decreased release of presynaptic trophic factors that maintain the integrity of the neuromuscular junction. This in turn may increase the release of postsynaptic trophic factors, stimulating the sprouting process. The presence of synaptically active sprouts is an important clinical consideration when serotype A is used as a therapeutic agent, because the activity of these sprouts may contribute to the need for repeated injections.

Target Sites. Two important conclusions can be drawn from studies on spontaneous transmitter release. First, it appears that the Ca^{2+} sensitivity of botulinum-poisoned terminals is altered. In unpoisoned nerve terminals, the frequency of spontaneous transmitter release is enhanced by techniques that elevate intracellular Ca^{2+} levels, such as increased extracellular Ca^{2+}, K^+ depolarization, or hyperosmotic sucrose solution. When these manipulations are applied to the botulinum serotype A–poisoned nerve terminal, only transient increases in MEPP frequency occur (49,50). Similar results are obtained with the application of a sodium channel activator (51), a calcium ionophore (50,52), or an oxidative phosphorylation inhibitor (53). The inability of moderately elevated Ca^{2+} levels to effectively antagonize botulinum neurotoxin type A suggests that poisoned terminals have been rendered less sensitive to increased Ca^{2+} levels.

A second important conclusion to stem from electrophysiology studies is that the target site for the seven serotypes may not be the same. Black widow spider venom (BWSV), an agent capable of producing an "explosive" increase in spontaneous transmitter release from unpoisoned terminals, is able to antagonize botulinum neurotoxin type A, but it is only minimally effective against botulinum neurotoxin type B (49–51,54,55). The active component of BWSV is α-latrotoxin, and its receptor has recently been identified as a neurexin that has affinity for the synaptic vesicle protein synaptotagmin (56,57). The fact that BWSV is able to antagonize botulinum neurotoxin type A but not type B suggests the existence of at least two different intracellular target sites. These data are further supported by analyses of depolarization-evoked transmitter release.

Stimulus-evoked transmitter release depends on the depolarization of the presynaptic terminal. This depolarization induces an influx of Ca^{2+}, and it is this momentary increase in intracellular Ca^{2+} levels that induces the synchronous release of transmitter quanta that result in an EPP. All serotypes of botulinum neurotoxin significantly decrease the number of evoked transmitter quanta released, resulting in a depressed EPP amplitude and a 90–100% failure to elicit an EPP with a single stimulus. As discussed above, the decrease in evoked release induced by botulinum neurotoxin can be partially antagonized under experimental conditions that elevate intracellular Ca^{2+}, such as high-frequency stimulation and lowered temperature (41,42,44,45). In the case of serotypes A and E, the resultant increased frequency of transmitter release is synchronized, occasionally generating an EPP. However, for serotypes B, D, or F repetitive stimulation induces asynchronous release that rarely produces EPPs.

Qualitatively similar results have been obtained in the presence of certain pharmacological agents. Pretreatment of tissues with aminopyridines, drugs that significantly elevate intracellular Ca^{2+} levels by blocking voltage-gated K^+ channels (58,59), markedly antagonizes poisoning due to serotypes A and E (44,45,60–63). This antagonism is demonstrated by a significant delay in the onset of neuromuscular blockade and a substantial increase in the frequency of synchronous quantal release. These agents are less effective antagonists of serotypes B, C, D, and F (43,45,60).

Biochemistry

The three-step model for botulinum neurotoxin action is well supported by experimental evidence. The toxin binds to nerve cells, undergoes receptor-mediated endocytosis, and escapes the endosome to act in the cytosol. It is the light chain of the toxin that exerts a presumed enzymatic effect in the cytosol of mammalian cells to inhibit exocytosis. Unfortunately, the precise mechanism by which the light chain blocks vesicle release has been difficult to ascertain. This has been due, in part, to an inadequate understanding of the secretory process, which involves, or is regulated by, many different components. The cytoskeleton, energy metabolism, second messengers, and ion channels are all involved in exocytosis. However, none of these components of the secretory process has been unequivocally demonstrated to be a target for neurotoxin action (for review, see Ref. 64).

The most recent hypothesis to be advanced, and the one that appears to hold the greatest promise, is that the neurotoxins are metalloendoproteases that cleave synaptic vesicle proteins. To this end, Schiavo et al. (65) have demonstrated that at least one of the neurotoxins, serotype B, cleaves the synaptic vesicle protein synaptobrevin.

Synaptobrevin is a 19,000-dalton protein that exists in two forms termed synaptobrevin 1 and synaptobrevin 2. In the human genome these two polypeptides are approximately 77% homologous. The proteins are fairly abundant, occurring in all neuronal cells studied as well as other cells with endocrine-type function (66). Based on sequence and biochemical analyses, a four-domain model for synaptobrevin has been proposed (67). The first domain resides in the cytoplasm and consists of a nonconserved amino-terminal dominated by prolines and asparagines. Domain 2 is a highly conserved, highly charged central region located between domain 1 and the vesicle membrane. The transmembrane region is delineated by domain 3, and domain 4 comprises the variable, short carboxy-terminal intravesicular sequence. The role of synaptobrevin in the exocytotic process is at present unknown, but investigators have suggested that it may function in membrane fusion or in vesicle targeting and retrieval (68).

Schiavo et al. (65) observed through electrophoretic techniques that incubation of synaptic vesicles with botulinum neurotoxin type B resulted in a loss of a 19,000-dalton protein. The disappearance of this protein, identified as synaptobrevin by immunodetection, was associated with the appearance of two new fragments of 7,000 daltons and 12,000 daltons. Pretreatment of the neurotoxin with the metal chelator EDTA attenuated the proteolysis of synaptobrevin, a result in keeping with the proposal that the toxin is a metalloendopeptidase. These authors also found that micro-injection of a synthetic peptide that mimics the cleavage site in synaptobrevin antagonized neurotoxin action. They suggested that this peptide acted as a competitive substrate, leading to the preservation of endogenous synaptobrevin.

An important observation as to the specificity of toxin action also emerged from this study. The data indicated that botulinum neurotoxin type B cleaved synaptobrevin, but botulinum neurotoxin type A and type E had no effect. This would suggest the presence of a different but equally important toxin substrate, or a different mechanism of action, for serotypes A and E. Parenthetically, these findings strongly reinforce the belief expressed earlier that the botulinum neurotoxins fall into two groups.

FUTURE DIRECTIONS

Substantial progress has been made in deciphering the structure and function of botulinum neurotoxin. Nevertheless, an at least equally substantial amount of work remains to be done. Two of the remaining tasks apply to the toxin itself. There is a need to identify the substrate or substrates for all seven serotypes of botulinum neurotoxin. This has presumably been done for type B, but there are as yet no clues to the identity of the substrates for the remaining serotypes. A related task is to determine the role of the toxin substrates in exocytosis. This knowledge is essential to developing an understanding of the mechanism by which the toxin blocks transmitter release.

Beyond this, there is work that should be done either to improve the efficacy of botulinum neurotoxin or to find a superior pharmacological agent. For example, botulinum neurotoxin does produce blockade of exocytosis for several weeks to months, but it would be desirable to have an agent that exerts effects for an even longer duration. Perhaps the techniques of molecular biology can be used to engineer a botulinum neurotoxin molecule that is less susceptible to metabolism and elimination. In a similar vein, the small amounts of botulinum neurotoxin that are used in most clinical settings are unlikely to evoke an immune response, but in some situations the amounts given are larger and thus there is a proportionally greater chance of eliciting protective antibodies. In these cases it will be necessary to have (1) substitute serotypes that can replace the ones to which patients are immune, (2) serotypes that are engineered to be less immunogenic, or (3) alternative drugs with little or no prospect of evoking antibody formation.

Clostridial organisms have provided clinicians with an excellent starting point in terms of a medication for the treatment of dystonias. The challenge now is to learn enough about botulinum neurotoxin and about dystonias to design an even better medication.

ACKNOWLEDGMENT

This work was supported in part by NINCDS Grant NS-22153 and by USDOA Contract DAMD17-90-C-0048.

REFERENCES

1. Simpson LL. The origin, structure, and pharmacological activity of botulinum toxin. Pharmacol Rev 1981;33:155–188.
2. Sakaguchi G. *Clostridium botulinum* toxins. Pharmacol Ther 1982;19:165–194.
3. Aureli P, Fenicia L, Pasolini B, Gianfranceschi M, McCroskey LM, Hatheway CL. Two cases of type E infant botulism caused by neurotoxigenic *Clostridium butyricum* in Italy. J Infect Dis 1986;154:207–211.
4. McCroskey LM, Hatheway CL, Fenicia L, Pasolini B, Aureli P. Characterization of an organism that produces type E botulinal toxin but which resembles *Clostridium butyricum* from the feces of an infant with type E botulism. J Clin Microbiol 1986;23:201–202.
5. Gímenez JA, Sugiyama H. Comparison of toxins of *Clostridium butyricum* and *Clostridium botulinum* type E. Infect Immun 1988;56:926–929.
6. Kozaki S, Onimaru J, Kamata Y, Sakaguchi G. Immunological characterization of *Clostridium butyricum* neurotoxin and its trypsin-induced fragment by use of monoclonal antibodies against *Clostridium botulinum* type E neurotoxin. Infect Immun 1991;59:457–459.
7. Hall JD, McCroskey LM, Pincomb BJ, Hatheway CL. Isolation of an organism resembling *Clostridium baratii* which produces type F botulinal toxin from an infant with botulism. J Clin Microbiol 1985;21:654–655.
8. Simpson LL. The actions of clostridial toxins on storage and release of neurotransmitters. In: Harvey A, ed. Natural and synthetic neurotoxins. San Diego: Academic Press, 1993:278–317.
9. DasGupta BR, Sugiyama H. A common subunit structure in *Clostridium botulinum* type A, B and E toxins. Biochem Biophys Res Comm 1972;48:108–112.
10. Binz T, Kurazono H, Wille M, Frevert J, Wernars K, Niemann H. The complete sequence of botulinum neurotoxin type A and comparison with other clostridial neurotoxins. J Biol Chem 1990;265:9153–9158.
11. Whelan SM, Elmore MJ, Bodsworth NJ, Brehm JK, Atkinson T. Molecular cloning of the *Clostridium botulinum* structural gene encoding the type B neurotoxin and determination of its entire nucleotide sequence. Appl Environ Microbiol 1992;58:2345–2354.

12. Hauser D, Eklund MW, Kurazono H, et al. Nucleotide sequence of *Clostridium botulinum* C1 neurotoxin. Nucl Acids res 1990;18:4924.
13. Binz T, Kurazono H, Popoff MR, et al. Nucleotide sequence of the gene encoding *Clostridium botulinum* neurotoxin type D. Nucl Acids Res 1990;18:5556.
14. Poulet S, Hauser D, Quanz M, Niemann H, Popoff MR. Sequences of the botulinal neurotoxin E derived from *Clostridium botulinum* type E (strain Beluga) and *Clostridium butyricum* (strains ATCC 43181 and ATCC 43755). Biochem Biophys Res Comm 1992;183:107–113.
15. Whelan SM, Elmore MJ, Bodsworth NJ, Atkinson T, Minton NP. The complete amino acid sequence of the *Clostridium botulinum* type-E neurotoxin, derived by nucleotide sequence analysis of the encoding gene. Eur J Biochem 1992;204:657–667.
16. Simpson LL. Botulinum neurotoxin and tetanus toxin. San Diego: Academic Press, 1989:1.
17. Black JD, Dolly JO. Interaction of ^{125}I-labeled botulinum neurotoxins with nerve terminals. I. Ultrastructural autoradiographic localization and quantitation of distinct membrane acceptors for types A and B on motor nerves. J Cell Biol 1986;103:521–534.
18. Black JD, Dolly JO. Interaction of ^{125}I-labeled botulinum neurotoxins with nerve terminals. II. Autoradiographic evidence for its uptake into motor nerves by acceptor-mediated endocytosis. J Cell Biol 1986;103:535–544.
19. Bandyopadhyay S, Clark AW, DasGupta BR, Sathyamoorthy V. Role of the heavy and light chains of botulinum neurotoxin in neuromuscular paralysis. J Biol Chem 1987;262:2660–2663.
20. Lomneth R, Suszkiw JB, DasGupta BR. Response of the chick ciliary ganglion–iris neuromuscular preparation to botulinum neurotoxin. Neurosci Lett 1990;113:211–216.
21. Kitamura M. Binding of botulinum neurotoxin to the synaptosome fraction of rat brain. Naunyn-Schmiedebergs Arch Pharmacol 1976;295:171–175.
22. Kozaki S. Interaction of botulinum type A, B and E derivative toxins with synaptosomes of rat brain. Naunyn-Schmiedebergs Arch Pharmacol 1979;308:67–70.
23. Agui T, Syuto B, Oguma K, Iida H, Kubo S. Binding of *Clostridium botulinum* type C neurotoxin to rat brain synaptosomes. J Biochem 1983;94:521–527.
24. Williams RS, Tse CK, Dolly JO, Hambleton P, Melling J. Radioiodination of botulinum neurotoxin type A with retention of biological activity and its binding to brain synaptosomes. Eur J Biochem 1983;131:437–445.
25. Murayama S, Syuto B, Oguma K, Iida H, Kubo S. Comparison of *Clostridium botulinum* toxins type D and C1 in molecular property, antigenicity and binding ability to rat-brain synaptosomes. Eur J Biochem 1984;142:487–492.
26. Evans DM, Williams RS, Shone CC, Hambleton P, Melling J, Dolly JO. Botulinum neurotoxin type B. Its purification, radioiodination and interaction with rat-brain synaptosomal membranes. Eur J Biochem 1986;154:409–416.
27. Park MK, Jung HH, Yang KH. Binding of *Clostridium botulinum* type B toxin to rat brain synaptosome. FEMS Microbiol Lett 1990;60:243–247.
28. Wadsworth JDF, Desai M, Tranter HS, et al. Botulinum type F neurotoxin. Large-scale purification and characterization of its binding to rat cerebrocortical synaptosomes. Biochem J 1990;268:123–128.
29. Simpson LL, Rapport MM. Ganglioside inactivation of botulinum toxin. J Neurochem 1971;18:1341–1343.
30. Simpson LL, Rapport MM. The binding of botulinum toxin to membrane lipids: phospholipids and proteolipid. J Neurochem 1971;18:1761–1767.
31. Bakry N, Kamata Y, Simpson LL. Lectins from *Triticum vulgaris* and *Limax flavus* are universal antagonists of botulinum neurotoxin and tetanus toxin. J Pharmacol Exp Ther 1991;258:830–836.
32. Olsnes S, Sandvig K. Entry of polypeptide toxins into animal cells. In: Pastan I, Willingham MC, eds. Endocytosis. New York: Plenum Press, 1985:195–234.
33. London E. Diphtheria toxin: membrane interaction and membrane translocation. Biochim Biophys Acta 1993;1113:25–51.

34. Simpson LL. Kinetic studies on the interaction between botulinum toxin type A and the cholinergic neuromuscular junction. J Pharmacol Exp Ther 1980;212:16–21.

35. Simpson LL, Kamata Y, Kozaki S. Use of monoclonal antibodies as probes for the structure and biological activity of botulinum neurotoxin. J Pharmacol Exp Ther 1990;255:227–232.

36. Simpson LL. Ammonium chloride and methylamine hydrochloride antagonize clostridial neurotoxins. J Pharmacol Exp Ther 1983;225:546–552.

37. Simpson LL., Coffield JA, Bakry, N. Inhibition of vacuolar ATPase antagonizes the effects of clostridial neurotoxins but not phospholipase A2 neurotoxins. J Pharmacol Exp Ther 1992; in press.

38. Schiavo G, Rossetto O, Santucci A, DasGupta BR, Montecucco C. Botulinum neurotoxins are zinc proteins. J Biol Chem 1992;267:23479–23483.

39. Habermann E, Dreyer F. Clostridial neurotoxins: handling and action at the cellular level. Curr Topics Microbiol Immunol 1986;129:93–179.

40. Wellhöner HH. Tetanus and botulinum neurotoxins. In: Herken H, Hucho F, eds. Handbook of experimental pharmacology. Vol. 102. Selective neurotoxicity. Berlin: Springer-Verlag, 1992:357–417.

41. Dreyer F, Schmitt A. Different effects of botulinum A toxin and tetanus toxin on the transmitter releasing process at the mammalian neuromuscular junction. Neurosci Lett 1981; 26:307–311.

42. Dreyer F, Schmitt A. Transmitter release in tetanus and botulinum A toxin–poisoned mammalian motor endplates and its dependence on nerve stimulation and temperature. Pflugers Arch–Eur J Physiol 1983;399:228–234.

43. Molgó J, DasGupta BR, Thesleff S. Characterization of the actions of botulinum neurotoxin type E at the rat neuromuscular junction. Acta Physiol Scand 1989;137:497–501.

44. Sellin LC, Kauffman JA, DasGupta BR. Comparison of the effects of botulinum neurotoxin types A and E at the rat neuromuscular junction. Med Biol 1983;61:120–125.

45. Sellin LC, Thesleff S, DasGupta BR. Different effects of types A and B botulinum toxin on transmitter release at the rat neuromuscular junction. Acta Physiol Scand 1983;119:127–133.

46. Angaut-Petit D, Molgó J, Comella JX, Faille L, Tabti N. Terminal sprouting in mouse neuromuscular junctions poisoned with botulinum type A toxin: morphological and electrophysiological features. Neuroscience 1990;37:799–808.

47. Thesleff S, Molgó J, Tägerud S. Trophic interrelations at the neuromuscular junction as revealed by the use of botulinal neurotoxins. J Physiol (Eur) 1990;84:167–173.

48. Antony MT, Sayers H, Stolkin C, Tonge DA. Prolonged paralysis, caused by the local injection of botulinum toxin, fails to cause motor nerve terminal sprouting in skeletal muscle of the frog. Quart J Exp Physiol 1981;66:525–532.

49. Cull-Candy SG, Lundh H, Thesleff S. Effects of botulinum toxin on neuromuscular transmission in the rat. J Physiol 1976;260:177–203.

50. Dreyer F, Rosenberg F, Becker C, Bigalke H, Penner R. Differential effects of various secretagogues on quantal transmitter release from mouse motor nerve terminals treated with botulinum A and tetanus toxin. Naun-Schmiedebergs Archiv Pharmacol 1987;335:1–7.

51. Simpson LL. Pharmacological studies on the subcellular site of action of botulinum toxin type A. J Pharmacol Exp Ther 1978;206:661–669.

52. Llados FT, Ross-Canada J, Pappas GD. Ultrastructural and physiological effects of the ionophore A23187 at identified frog neuromuscular junctions. Neuroscience 1992;13: 237–247.

53. Molgó J, Comella JX, Angaut-Petit D, et al. Presynaptic actions of botulinal neurotoxins at vertebrate neuromuscular junctions. J Physiol (Eur) 1990;84:152–166.

54. Pumplin DW, del Castillo J. Release of packets of acetylcholine and synaptic vesicle elicited by brown widow spider venom in frog motor nerve endings poisoned by botulinum toxin. Life Sciences 1975;17:137–141.

55. Kao I, Drachman DB, Price DL. Botulinum toxin: mechanism of presynaptic blockade. Science 1976;193:1256–1258.

56. Petrenko AG, Perin MS, Davletov BA, Ushkaryov YA, Geppert M, Südhof TC. Binding of synaptotagmin to the α-latrotoxin receptor implicates both in synaptic vesicle exocytosis. Nature 1992;353:65–68.

57. Ushkaryov YA, Petrenko AG, Geppert M, Südhof TC. Neurexins: synaptic cell surface proteins related to the α-latrotoxin receptor and laminin. Science 1992;257:50–56.

58. Lundh H, Thesleff S. The mode of action of 4-aminopyridine and guanidine on transmitter release from motor nerve terminals. Eur J Pharmacol 1977;42:411–412.

59. Lundh H. Effects of 4-aminopyridine on neuromuscular transmission. Brain Res 1978; 153:307–318.

60. Kauffman JA, Way JF Jr, Siegel LS, Sellin LC. Comparison of the action of types A and F botulinum toxin at the rat neuromuscular junction. Toxicol Appl Pharmacol 1985;79: 211–217.

61. Simpson LL. A preclinical evaluation of aminopyridines as putative therapeutic agents in the treatment of botulism. Infect Immun 1986;52:858–862.

62. Gansel M, Penner R, Dreyer F. Distinct sites of action of clostridial neurotoxins revealed by double-poisoning of mouse motor nerve terminals. Pflugers Arch–Eur J Physiol 1987; 409:533–539.

63. Molgó J, Siegel LS, Tabti N, Thesleff S. A study of synchronization of quantal transmitter release from mammalian motor endings by the use of botulinal toxins type A and D. J Physiol 1989;411:195–205.

64. Simpson LL, Considine RV, Coffield JA, Jeyapaul J, Bakry N. Bacterial toxins that act on the nervous system. In: Chang LW, ed. Handbook of neurotoxicology. New York: Marcel Dekker, 1993; in press.

65. Schiavo G, Benfenati F, Poulain B, et al. Tetanus and botulinum-B neurotoxins block neurotransmitter release by proteolytic cleavage of synaptobrevin. Nature 1992;359:832–835.

66. Baumert M, Maycox PR, Navone S, DeCamilli S, John R. Synaptobrevin; an integral protein membrane of 18,000 daltons present in small synaptic vesicles of rat brain. EMBO J 1989;8:379–384.

67. Südhof TC, Baumert M, Perin MS, Jahn R. A synaptic vesicle membrane protein is conserved from mammals to Drosophila. Neuron 1989;2:1475–1481.

68. Chin GJ, Goldman SA. Purification of squid synaptic vesicles and characterization of the vesicle-associated proteins synaptobrevin and Rab3A. Brain Res 1992;571:89–96.

2

Structures of Botulinum Neurotoxin, Its Functional Domains, and Perspectives on the Crystalline Type A Toxin

Bibhuti R. DasGupta
University of Wisconsin, Madison, Wisconsin

INTRODUCTION

It was 1895. In the village of Ellezelles, Belgium, 34 members of a music club had eaten some raw salted ham after performing at a funeral. Within the next 20 to 36 hours most of the musicians developed a neuroparalytic syndrome—three died, and 10 others nearly died. Professor E. Van Ermengem isolated the culprit from the food and the victims of food poisoning and named it *Bacillus botulinus*; the anaerobic bacterium was later named *Clostridium botulinum* (1,2). The neurotoxic substance produced by the bacterium became known as botulinum toxin, a protein, and gained notoriety as the most poisonous poison (3). In the New World, 84 years after the discovery of the agent of deadly food poisoning, Dr. Allen B. Scott of San Francisco first reported how to use the most poisonous poison for therapeutic purposes in humans (4,5). Because of this pioneering breakthrough, lauded by Carl Lamanna (6) as "the most imaginative, technically brilliant, and courageous of such applied research," today more people in the United States are exposed to botulinum toxin through deliberate injection by clinicians (7) than by unknowingly ingesting it as a food poison (8).

The proverbial beating of swords into ploughshares was achieved with a body of knowledge mostly accumulated from the pharmacological studies of the toxin (primarily serotype A, see below), which in 1946 became available as a crystallizable preparation (9–11), and with sparse knowledge about the biochemistry of the neurotoxin (NT) (12) and its mechanism of action (13). Another remarkable aspect of this development is the low-grade purity of the NT preparation that was used in the early pharmacological studies (12–15), as well as in the pioneering therapeutic application, and is still being widely used.

Now we know that four primary sequential events lead to the manifestation of the well-known neurotoxicity of botulinum NT: (1) the NT binds to the cholinergic membrane at the neuromuscular junctions, (2) the bound protein reaches inside the nerve endings through the endocytotic/lysosomal vesicle pathway, (3) a segment of the NT penetrates through the endosomal membrane into the cytosol, and then (4) this segment, acting as an enzyme, disrupts the neurotransmitter secretory machinery, resulting in blockage of acetylcholine release and consequent flaccid paralysis. The entire structure of the NT may be regarded in a simple model as a combination of three structural segments designated A-C-B, each with a functional role and joined linearly in that order. Segment B recognizes the NT-specific receptors and allows the NT to bind to the target cells. Segment C forms channels in the endosomal membrane and facilitates penetration of segment A (or A plus segments of C and B) into the cytosol. The enzymatically active segment A causes intracellular injury.

This chapter deals with two primary topics. First, the structural features of the NT and its three segments that now appear directly relevant to the NT's mechanism of action are discussed. A comprehensive review in this area is not presented. The second topic is a critique of the crystalline toxin type A, which contains no more than 20% by weight of the neurotoxin protein, the other 80% of the material being nonneurotoxic macromolecules (16,17) that are yet to be characterized; nevertheless, this is the preparation used clinically (18,19).

THE NEUROTOXIN

Sources of the Neurotoxin

The NT produced by the ubiquitous bacterium *C. botulinum* is found as seven antigenically distinguishable serotypes A, B, C, D, E, F, and G. Certain strains of *C. baratii* and *C. butyricum* have been identified within the past few years that produce NTs similar to classical botulinum NT serotypes F and E, respectively (2,20,21). A minor antigenic relatedness between types E and F has been known (22); with the advent of monoclonal antibodies a common epitope has been detected among types B, C, D, and E (23). One strain of the bacterium produces one serotype, but there may be exceptions to this (20,22). Serotype C at one time had two designations, C1 and C2. The C2 toxin, which ADP-ribosylates nonmuscle actin, is not the NT (2).

Structure of the Neurotoxin

Primary (Covalent) Structure

The neurotoxic protein is synthesized as a single-chain protein (mol. wt. ~150,000). Protease(s) endogenous to the bacterium cleave the single-chain protein within a narrow region inside a disulfide loop located about one-third of the way from the N-terminal to the C-terminal (Fig. 1a). This cleavage is called nicking. The proteolytically processed product—the dichain NT—now contains a light (L) chain (mol. wt. ~50,000) and a heavy (H) chain (mol. wt. ~100,000) that remain linked by an inter-chain disulfide or disulfides and noncovalent bonds. In the absence of the endogenous proteolytic enzymes the single-chain NT remains as such and after isolation from the bacterial culture can be nicked by the exogenous proteases (such as trypsin) into the dichain protein. The proteolytically processed dichain NT is more potent than the single-chain NT. The higher potency is evident whether the assay is mouse lethality, paralysis of neuromuscular junction preparations, or blockage of neurotransmitter release (24–27). This enhancement of biological activity is referred to as activation (28). The type A NT isolated from a 96-hr incubated bacterial culture is found in the dichain form and fully activated (i.e., treatment with trypsin does not activate it further). The type E NT isolated from a 96-hr incubated culture is a single-chain protein, and following controlled trypsinization (nicking) the dichain NT exhibits more than 100-fold activation (12,28). The proteolytic processing at the nicking region involves cleavage of more than a single peptide bond; the result is excision of several amino acid residues. In the cases of type A and type E at least four residues (Gly-Tyr-Asn-Lys) and three residues (Gly-Ile-Arg), respectively, are removed (29,30), as depicted in Fig. 1a.

The complete amino acid sequences of NT serotypes A–F have been deduced on the basis of the corresponding nucleotide sequences (31,32 and references in Ref. 31). The predicted amino acid sequences indicate that the single-chain NTs are made of 1295 to 1251 amino acid residues; they are schematically represented in Fig. 2a. Among these six serotypes type E is the shortest (1251 residues) and type A is the longest (1295 residues). During proteolytic processing of the single-chain NT at the nicking region, additional cleavage at the NT's N-terminal (and hence excision of small peptides) does not occur. Direct amino acid sequence determinations of the NT types A, B, and E have demonstrated that their original N-terminals remain intact. Whether the original C-terminals of the single-chain NT remain in the proteolytically processed NT is yet to be determined.

Alignment of the amino acid sequences (not presented here, but see Refs. 31 and 32 for details) show an overall low homology (~50%), although several short stretches of varying lengths are homologous. This is understandable, because too much homology in sequence would endow the NT serotypes with common antigenic epitopes. Since these proteins do not show serological cross-reactivity (except as mentioned before), their primary and secondary structures are likely to be more dissimilar than similar. The similarity among them is likely to be just enough to conserve the structures required for similar functional properties such as receptor binding, channel formation, and intracellu-

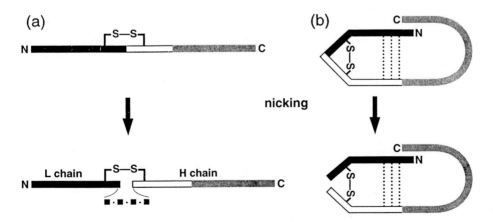

Figure 1 Proteolysis (nicking) converts the single-chain neurotoxin (NT) to dichain NT. Structure of the NT is represented in the straight line (panel a) and folded (panel b) configurations. Cleavages of more than one peptide bond during nicking are depicted by release of four amino acid residues. The light (L) and heavy (H) chains (mol. wt. ~50,000 and ~100,000, respectively) of the dichain (nicked) NT remain linked by a disulfide bond and noncovalent bonds (dotted lines between the L and H chain, see panel b). The two halves of the H chain, the N-terminal and C-terminal halves, are identified as the white and shaded segments, respectively.

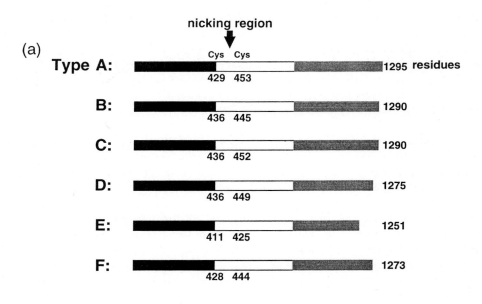

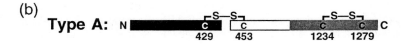

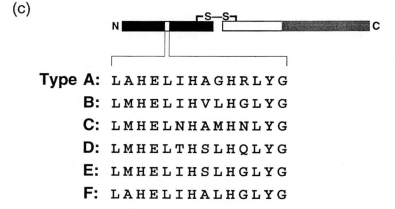

Figure 2 Covalent structures of the neurotoxin (NT) serotypes and a few of their important homologous segments. (a) Total number of amino acid residues, deduced from nucleotide sequences (31,32) present in the single chain NTs before proteolytic processing; also identified are the Cys residues that probably form the interchain disulfide in the dichain NTs. (b) Dichain type A NT and its Cys residues that have been deduced to form inter- and intrachain disulfides. (c) Homologous segment of the L chains of the NTs, containing the sequence His-Glu-Axx-Axx-His-Axx-Axx-His, and the zinc-binding motif.

lar inhibitory action (note below that even some of these properties of the NT serotypes are not identical).

Two Cys residues, the locations of which are conserved among all serotypes and indicated by the residue numbers (e.g., 429 and 453 in type A), flank the nicking region (Fig. 2a). These two Cys residues in the single-chain protein probably form the intrachain disulfide. The length of this disulfide bridge varies from 23 residues (in type A) to 8 residues (in type B). This intrachain disulfide, following nicking of the single-chain NT to the dichain NT, presumably acts as the interchain disulfide between the L and H chain. Evidence for this is inferential; direct chemical proof is yet to come. An intrachain disulfide near the C-terminal of types A and B has been also deduced (see reference in Ref. 33). In the case of Type A, Cys 1234 and Cys 1279 form this intrachain disulfide, as shown in Fig. 2b (33). Type B and E NTs have Cys residues in equivalent locations (31).

Roles of Cys Residues in Biological Activity

Long before the exact number of Cys residues present in type A NT became known (from its amino acid composition and sequences), their importance in the protein's neurotoxicity as free –SH groups and participants of disulfide bond(s) was of obvious interest. On the basis of the simple mouse lethality assay, the free -SH groups were found not essential for toxicity (34), but the integrity of the disulfide bond(s) was found essential (35). These early conclusions have recently been confirmed and refined in the context of the distinct steps of the NT's mechanism of action and the activities of the three functional domains of the NT. It is now known (1) that the productive binding of type A NT with the receptors does not depend on the disulfide bonds (inter- and intrachain) and free -SH groups; (2) that internalization (of the L chain) depends on the integrity of one or both disulfides (experiments could not distinguish between the inter- and intrachains, since selective reductive cleavage of one was not possible); (3) that the L chain's intracellular inhibitory activity does not require a free -SH group (because the L chain was active following alkylation of the free -SH) (36); and (4) that removal of the 32 C-terminal residues of the L chain (which includes Cys 429) does not diminish its intracellular activity (37). Points 2 and 4 together indicate (1) that disulfide bond(s) linking L and H chains, and the Cys 429 on the L chain (see Fig. 2b), have no role in the actual intracellular inhibitory action of the L chain, and (2) that the roles of the interchain disulfide (between Cys 429 and Cys 453) and the participant Cys 429 are to maintain a covalent linkage between the L chain and H chain, after nicking of the single-chain protein—otherwise the L chain, being easily separable from the H chain, might not reach the target cell interior (see below, Fig. 4). These deductions are consistent with the observation that the dichain NT presented to the cytosol of permeabilized cells, bypassing the steps of receptor binding and internalization (by endosomes), shows higher intracellular inhibitory activity after reduction of the interchain disulfide between the L and H chains (27); reduction presumably allows them to separate.

The Zinc-Binding Site of the Neurotoxin

A segment around the midsection of the L chain of all six NT serotypes sequences (Fig. 2c) contains the sequence His-Glu-Axx-Axx-His, which is the zinc-binding motif of Zn endopeptidases. The three proteases thermolysin, *Bacillus cereus* neutral protease, and *Pseudomonas aeruginosa* elastase contain Zn, and their three-dimensional structures, determined by x-ray crystallography, indicate that in each case an atom of Zn^{2+} is bound by a tetrahedral coordination with the two His of the motif His-Glu-Axx-Axx-His, while the Glu residue binds a water molecule acting as the third Zn^{2+} ligand. The fourth ligand is another Glu residue (see Ref. 38 for further references). On the basis of this clue, atomic absorption analysis of type A, B, and E NTs were made; all three NTs contain one Zn atom per molecule of NT (mol. wt. ~150,000). Measurements of Co, Cu, Fe, Mn, and Ni were also made, and none was detected. Additional experiments demonstrated that this peptide segment binds Zn and that two His residues are involved in Zn coordination (38). The possibility that the NTs could be Zn endoproteases was tested, and proteolytic activity has been found (see below, Functional Domains).

Secondary Structures

Analysis of the secondary structural elements (α-helix, β-sheet, β-turn, and random coil) of the NT types A, B, and E revealed that these proteins have highly ordered structures that are dominated by the β-sheets. About 62–72% of the amino acid residues are in the ordered structure at pH 7.2 (21–28% in α-helices plus 41–44% in β sheets), and the rest are in random coils (39). At pH 5.5, which approximates the pH inside the endosomes, the type A NT also retains the highly ordered structure: α-helix 29%, β-sheet 45–49%, and random coils 22–26% (40). The 29% α-helix content of the NT at pH 5.5 compared with 21% at pH 7.2 may reflect the acid-induced conformational change the NT presumably undergoes inside the endosome before channel formation (see below). Analysis of the L and H chains of type A NT following their chromatographic separation gave an interesting insight into their conformational stability (41). The sums of the α-helix, β-sheet, β-turn, and random coil contents of the separated L and H chain, as a weighted mean, were similar to the content of the corresponding structural elements in the NT (see Table 1), e.g., the sum of the α-helix content of the L chain (22%) and the H chain (18.7%), 19.8% as a weighted mean, was similar to the α-helix content of the NT (20%). In other words, the secondary structures of the L and H chains do not change significantly when they are separated. This stability indicates that the two chains, by virtue of their structural integrity, may express their individual biological activities even when physically separated. This notion agrees with two independent experimental observations: (1) The two chains can be separated and then reconjugated to form disulfide-linked NT (mol. wt. 150,000), which is highly active (see references, in Ref. 28). (2) The separated chains, although nonlethal by themselves, are biologically active, i.e., the isolated H chain forms channels in lipid bilayer membranes and binds to the receptor; the isolated L chain presented to the interior of a neuronal or chromaffin cell inhibits secretion of neurotransmitter (see references in Ref. 42).

Table 1 Secondary Structure Elements of Type A Neurotoxin and Its Light (L) and Heavy (H) Chain After Separation

Protein	α-Helix	β-Sheet	β-Turn	Random coil
Neurotoxin (mol. wt. ~150,000)	20.0	37.5	15.2	27.2
L chain (mol. wt. ~50,000)	22.0	27.5	18.7	31.7
H chain (mol. wt. ~100,000)	18.7	40.0	13.0	28.2
Sum of L and H chain (weighted mean)[a]	19.8	35.8	14.9	29.4

These secondary structure elements were obtained from circular dichroism spectra (240–200 nm) of the protein (0.1–0.3 mg/ml) in 10 mM sodium phosphate buffer, pH 8.1, containing 100 mM NaCl, at 23–25°C.
[a]Calculated as (1 × L chain + 2 × H chain)/3 because the H chain is twice the size of the L chain.

Tertiary and Quaternary Structures

A simple model of the folded configuration of the NT has been built based on the results of limited proteolysis (33). Figure 3, which incorporates the ideas presented in Fig. 1b, shows the common narrow regions of the NT serotypes A, B, and E cleaved by various proteases (33). Three of these regions, sites 1, 3, and 4, are highly susceptible. Site 1, the nicking region, is about one-third of the distance from the N-terminus; site 3 is approximately at the middle of the H chain, and site 4 is near the C-terminus. Figure 1b has depicted (1) that following cleavage at site 1, the L chain remains bound to the N-terminal half of the H chain by disulfide and noncovalent bonds (dotted lines between the L and H chains); (2) that noncovalent interactions between the L chain and the C-terminal half of the H chain are virtually absent or extremely weak; and (3) that association between the two halves of the H chain is also absent or very weak. Thus cleavage at site 3 allows the C-terminal half (mol. wt. ~ 50,000) to separate from the rest of the molecule (mol. wt. ~ 100,000) very easily (see references in Ref. 33). The C-terminal half of the H chain (result of cleavage at site 3) has been found completely or extensively digestible by trypsin, chymotrypsin, and pepsin. The N-terminal half of the H chain, on the other hand, survives proteolysis remarkably (reviewed in Ref. 33). Proteolytic digestions of NTs carried out in various laboratories have not reported significant cleavage of the L chain. This suggests (1) that the L chain and the N-terminal half of the H chain probably are individually resistant to proteolysis and/or (2) that the association between these two segments of the NT makes their protease-susceptible sites unavailable for cleavage.

Many observations indicate that the natural foldings of the polypeptides protect the proteins from proteolytic assaults, that limited proteolysis of native proteins is usually restricted to interdomain regions, and that these susceptible regions are flexible hinges on the protein surface. Consistent with this view are the proteolysis-susceptible regions on the NT detected so far. The two halves of the H chain (generated by cleavage at site 3), the N-terminal and C-terminal halves, also retain after separation their channel-forming (43,44) and ganglioside-binding activities (45), respectively. Earlier it was noted that the L chain separated from the H chain retains biological activity. Thus, the three segments of the NT that exhibit biological function after separation, the L chain and the two halves of the H chain, each of ~50,000 mol. wt., represent three domains spaced in the polypeptide backbone by two hinges (indicated in Fig. 3b) and proteolytically susceptible regions. (These segments were referred to as A-C-B above, "Introduction".)

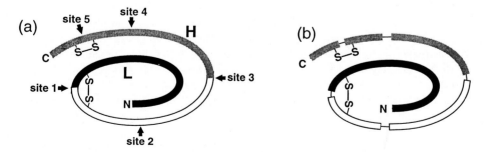

Figure 3 Model of folded configuration of the neurotoxin (NT) based on proteolytic digestions. (a) Sites on NT types A, B, and E cleaved by various proteases (reviewed in Ref. 33). (b) Flexible hinges (the proteolytically susceptible regions) of the NTs, spaced in the polypeptide backbone, are indicated as wasp-waist segments.

The above observations allowed us to build the model in Fig. 3 (33) the salient features of which are as follows: (1) sites 1, 2, 3, and 4 are on the surface and hence accessible to proteolysis, (2) most of the L chain is shielded by the H chain from proteolysis, (3) most of the N-terminal half of the H chain is closely associated with the L chain, (4) the C-terminal half of the H chain is not associated with the rest of the molecule, and (5) the C-terminal segment is highly accessible to receptors on the target cells (see below) and proteolysis, and it allows the NT molecules to associate to form what appear to be "dimers" (see below). The shape of the NT molecule is ellipsoid rather than spherical, so that one of its axes is longer than the others (the reasons are discussed in Ref. 33). The diameters of the NT serotypes A, B, and E, measured by dynamical light scattering, are 100 ± 4, 110 ± 4, and 100 ± 4 Å (46). The diameter of the type A NT, 96 Å (stokes radius = 48 Å), measured many years ago by gel filtration (17), agrees well with the new data. It is not clear yet if this diameter represents the size of the NT monomer (mol. wt. 150,000) or dimer (mol. wt. $2 \times 150,000$).

Three independent lines of evidence indicate that the NT molecules associate to form entities larger than 150,000 (mol. wt. 300,000 and larger): (1) Chromatography of pure type A NT yielded type A NT molecules larger than 150,000 (47). (2) Polyacrylamide gel electrophoresis (without SDS) of pure type A NT demonstrated protein species of mol. wt. 300,000 and larger (33,43,48). The NT without the C-terminal half of the H chain (i.e., after cleavage at site 3) does not associate to form larger-molecular-weight species. (3) Crystals of pure type A NT also indicate dimerization (49).

The pure type of A NT (mol. wt. 150,000) has been crystallized in three different crystal morphologies; all three have the same crystal form and diffract to 3 Å (49). Determination of the three-dimensional structure of botulinum NT at atomic resolution now appears an achievable goal.

Functional Domains

The absolute neurospecificity and extremely high potency of the NT are attributable to its high affinity for specific receptors on the presynaptic membranes and to an enzymatic action, functions of the H and L chains of the NT, respectively (Fig. 4). To explain how the NT at extremely low concentrations can bind specifically to the nerve cells, the proposal of Montecucco (50) deserves reiteration. The NT first binds to the ganglioside-rich lipid membrane, then the lipid-NT complex moves laterally to reach and bind the NT-specific receptor, which is protease-sensitive. Accordingly, any docking of the NT molecule on the membrane results (following the "catch-and-delivery effect") in a productive binding with the NT-specific receptor protein. The lipid-binding step "is actually equivalent to concentrating the NT and its protein receptor in a much smaller volume . . . because the partners of the binding reaction are now restricted to the two-dimensional plane of the plasma membrane rather than in the three-dimensional water phase" (50). The two-step hypothesis agrees with experimental results. Two-dimensional, ordered arrays of NT types A and B form at the interface of a NT solution and phospholipid monolayer containing the ganglioside GT_{1b}. The NT binds the hydrophilic moiety of the ganglioside, and two-dimensional diffusion allows crystals to form (51).

Receptors (also referred to as acceptors) of high affinity have been identified (the K_D values, for example, for type A, B, and E NT range from 0.5 nM to 100 pM; see Refs. 2,15,42 for review). In fact, two receptor species, one with higher affinity and low populations, and another with lower affinity and higher populations, have been identified for type B NT (52). Some NT serotypes do and some do not share the same receptors;

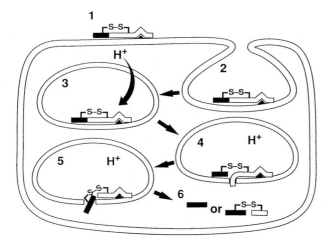

Figure 4 A simple diagrammatic representation of the sequential events that lead to the blockade of neurotransmitter release by the neurotoxin (NT). The NT binds to the receptor (black triangle) on the presynaptic membrane (step 1) via its heavy (H) chain. Endocytosis (step 2) internalizes the NT, which is now inside the endosomes (step 3). The acidic pH inside the endosome (steps 3,4) induces formation of channels in the endosomal membrane by a segment of the H chain (step 4) that allows the light (L) chain to egress from the vesicle (step 5) into the cytosol (step 6), where the L chain acts enzymatically and disrupts the neurotransmitter secretion. This model accommodates the possibility that the single-chain NT, after binding the receptor and internalization, is nicked to the dichain by the endosomal proteases (between steps 3 and 4). The model does not attempt to define the step at which the disulfide bond between the L and H chain is broken.

e.g., types A and E share the same receptor, types A and B do not (53). The densities of the distinct populations of receptor/acceptor (mouse diaphragm) for NT types A and B have been determined; their average numbers are 153 ± 21 and 637 ± 131 per μm^2 of membrane, respectively (54). Black and Dolly (54) considered these densities too high relative to the number of NT molecules needed to induce in vivo paralysis (1 mouse LD_{50} being equivalent to $\sim 1.2 \times 10^{-11}$ g or 8×10^{-17} mol or 5×10^7 molecules of type A NT; at the maximum, 100–1000 molecules are needed to block neurotransmission at each synapse). Thus the receptor/acceptor densities greatly exceed the number of NT molecules needed to block a synaptic transmission, arguing against a "one-hit" model for the NT's mechanism of action. The role of high densities of acceptors therefore appears to be to concentrate the NT on the target membrane surface for the next step—delivery inside the cell via intracellular vesicular compartments.

The ganglioside (GT_{1b})-binding site on type A NT is primarily confined within the C-terminal (50,000 mol. wt.) half of the H chain; the N-terminal half of the H chain did not bind GT_{1b} under any conditions tested, and the L chain exhibited a small degree of binding, which might be nonspecific (45). The demonstrated ganglioside-binding site on type A perhaps can be generalized for the other serotypes. Analogy with tetanus NT, which is very similar to botulinum NT in structure, structure-function relationship, and mechanism of action (2,15,55), further indicates the receptor-binding role of the C-terminal half of the H chain. A protein (mol. wt. ~20,000) expressed by PC12 cells following differentiation with nerve growth factor binds tetanus NT, and the binding is neurospecific. Only the C-terminal half of the H chain of tetanus NT binds to this protein; the remaining segment of the NT, i.e., the L chain and the N-terminal half of the H chain (mol. wt. ~100,000), did not bind (56 & reference 33 therein). These experiments once again demonstrate the role of the C-terminal half of the H chain in receptor binding. A protein(s) that appears to act as the receptor protein for botulinum NT type B has been reported (52,54).

According to the currently held view, when the pH inside the endosomes drops, the NT entrapped within this acidic environment undergoes some conformational change leading to an insertion of a segment of the NT into and across the endosomal membrane (Fig. 4, step 4). This poorly understood process somehow allows the L chain or the L chain and a segment of the H chain to cross the membrane and reach the cytosol. The experimental evidence behind this scenario is low pH–induced channels in lipid bilayers formed by the H chain and the N-terminal half of the H chain. Neurotoxin added to one side of an artificial lipid membrane forms few channels when on both sides the pH is ~7.0 or ~5.0; however, when the pH on the side of the NT is lowered to ~5.0 and kept near 7.0 on the other side, many channels are formed. The channel-forming activity is confined to the N-terminal half (mol. wt. ~50,000) of the H chain (43,44, and references therein). This pH gradient favorable to channel formation mimics the condition of low pH inside the endosome and physiological pH of the cytosol, i.e., outside the endosome. A narrow segment of the N-terminal half of the H chain of type A NT, residues 650–681, has been located that appears to be responsible for channel formation (57). Whether these channels provide a large enough opening for a polypeptide to pass through is not yet known.

Enzymatic activity of NT was recently demonstrated based on the proteolytic cleavage of a neuronal protein (58). Incubation of highly purified small synaptic vesicles (rat cerebral cortex) with the NT serotype B cleaved a single peptide bond (between residues 76 and 77, Gln-Phe) of synaptobrevin-2 (also called VAMP), which is a synaptic vesicle–associated integral membrane protein. Of the two isomers of synaptobrevin, synaptobrevin-1 has Val in the position of Gln; the Val-Phe bond in synaptobrevin-1 was not cleaved. The L chain of tetanus NT also cleaved synaptobrevin-2, and thus by analogy the proteolytic activity of botulinum NT is confined in its L chain. Unlike the type B NT, type A and type E NTs did not show any cleavage (58).

The nonidentical actions of NT types A, B, and E are not surprising; the intracellular inhibitory effects of the type A, B, and E NTs studied in permeabilized chromaffin and PC12 cells also show notable differences. The Ca^{2+}-stimulated secretion of norepinephrine was inhibited most by type E and least by type A (26,27). Long before permeabilized secretory cells were utilized to study the intracellular inhibitory actions of NT, Sellin (53) had proposed, on the basis of other experimental evidence, that various NT serotypes do not follow a single mechanism of action, and that the intracellular site of action of type A is distinct from those of types B, E, and F. (See Note Added in Proof.)

Potential Use of Different Neurotoxin Serotypes and Chimeric Neurotoxins

The different NT serotypes could be used clinically to exploit their nonidentical pharmacological actions rather than only to obviate the immunity that may develop from repeated administration of a single serotype. This idea must have crossed many minds. Further additions to the repertoire of pharmacological differences may be made by generating chimeric neurotoxic molecules, e.g., an NT made of L chain of type E and H chain of type A. The following considerations of the structures and structure-function relationships of the NTs favor the above two ideas. The different paralytic effects (magnitude, rapidity, duration, and recovery/reversal) produced in identical neuromuscular preparations by different NT serotypes (e.g., type A vs. type E, in Refs. 59,60) are probably rooted in the intrinsic structural features of the functional domains of the NT (42) and some of the components of the target neuronal cells. The population of receptors specific for the different NT serotypes present on the neuromuscular junctions of various muscles may not be identical. A therapeutic target area X may be significantly richer in receptors for NT type A than for types B and E, and other target areas Y and Z may have more receptors for NT type B and E, respectively. Experimental knowledge of such differences would indicate that better tools to paralyze muscles at target areas X, Y, and Z could be NT types A, B, and E, respectively. This consideration, based on the function of the H chain, attempts more efficient capturing of the NT and delivery of it inside the target neuronal cells. A corollary of this approach is that a lower amount of administered NT protein also lowers the immunogen load. The actual inhibition of neurotransmitter release could be further manipulated by presenting the target cells' cytosol with an L chain, chosen on the basis of its intracellular inhibitory activity. Thus a chimeric NT can be designed and made from L and H chains from two different NT serotypes, each chosen on the basis of its functional properties. Certain combinations of these two structures could provide therapeutic agents more suitable than the NTs we know of now.

Production of chimeric NT is clearly feasible. The L and H chains of NTs after separation can be reconjugated to generate neurotoxic dichain NT (mol. wt. ~150,000, see references 4–6 in Ref. 61). The chemistry involved in this approach has allowed generation of type A NT that was selectively radiolabeled at either the L or the H chain (one of the separated chains was radiolabeled and then combined with the corresponding nonlabeled chain) (61). More convincing is that the L and H chains of tetanus NT have been combined with H and L chains of botulinum type A NT, and that the chimeric NTs (part tetanus, part botulinum) exhibited predicted biological activities (62,63).

CRYSTALLINE TYPE A TOXIN

The preparation of type A NT that has found rapid and wide acceptance for therapeutic use is the crystallized mixture of type A NT and nonneurotoxic proteins; since 1967 (64) this complex material has hardly received a rigorous analytical scrutiny satisfactory to the standards of modern protein biochemistry. Crystallographic data for the preparation have never been reported.

The following properties of the crystallized toxic preparation are used to judge its purity (19):

1. Around neutral pH it absorbs maximally at 278 nm.
2. The ratio of its absorbance at 260 and 278 nm is 0.6 to 0.55.
3. An absorbance of 1.65 at A_{278} is equivalent to 1 mg protein/ml.
4. Its isoelectric point is 5.6, and at acidic pH it migrates in electric field as a single band.
5. The nitrogen content is 16.2%.*
6. It contains about 0.1% or less RNA.
7. Its specific toxicity is $3 \times 10^7 \pm 20\%$ LD_{50}/mg protein.

The properties listed as items 1, 2, 3, and 5 are not unique features of this protein preparation because these could be parts of general properties of proteins.

---

*This is old data (65), although "the nitrogen content of the toxin was redetermined and found to be 16.08%" (64).

Comments on the Optical Properties

The three aromatic amino acids tryptophan, tyrosine, and phenylalanine, in aqueous solution, absorb light at wavelengths of 250–300 nm in characteristic fashions. Tryptophan, tyrosine, and phenalalanine maximally absorb near 280, 275, and 260 nm, respectively. Thus the absorption profile of a protein in aqueous solution, in the region 250–300 nm, is determined both qualitatively and quantitatively by the absolute number of the three aromatic amino acids and their relative proportion. A protein completely free of nucleic acid (which absorbs maximally near 260 nm) can have significant absorption at 280 and 260 nm, the relative extent of which depends on the characteristic amino acid composition.

The absorption profile of pure type A NT (Fig. 5) shows an absorption maximum at 278.2 nm, a minimum at 249.5 nm, and a steep rise below 250 nm. (Proteins, like many organic compounds, also extensively absorb below 250 nm.) The pure type B and E NTs, prepared in our laboratory, exhibited 278.0 and 277.7 nm as absorption maxima and 249.7 and 250.0 nm as absorption minima, respectively (Table 2). The ratios of the absorption maxima and minima for these type A, B, and E NTs were 0.301, 0.301, and

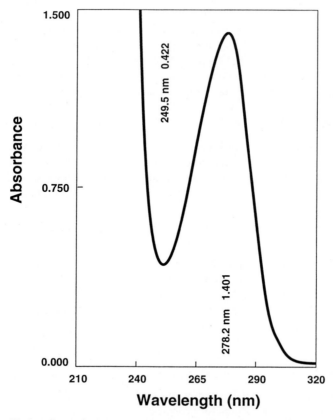

Figure 5 Absorption profile of pure type A neurotoxin (mol. wt. 150,000) in 0.1 M sodium phosphate buffer, pH 7.4, plus 0.05 M NaCl (UVIKON 860 Spectrophotometer, Kontron Instruments).

0.286, respectively. The ratios at A_{260}/A_{278} of the NTs purified by chromatography are invariably below 0.5.

The theoretical molar extinction coefficient of type A NT (mol. wt. 150,000) at 280 nm, calculated from the molar extinction coefficients of tryptophan, tyrosine, and phenylalanine and their known abundance in the protein (15, 74, and 70 residues, respectively, see ref. 3 in 31) is 181,150, which means that 1 mg/ml of the NT has an absorbance of 1.212 at 280 nm (B. R. DasGupta, unpublished data). The large difference between the deduced absorbance of the pure NT, 1.21, and that of the crystalline complex, 1.65, is probably due to the nonneurotoxic components in the complex.

The notion that "the purity of the crystalline toxin cannot be defined strictly in terms of percent purity because of small amounts of undefined material absorbant at 260 nm, most probably nucleic acid material" (19) is not completely right, because as mentioned above any protein with aromatic amino acid residue absorbs at 260 nm even if nucleic acid is entirely absent. Thus the use of the ratio of absorption at 260 and 278 nm has very limited value in judging whether a protein is free from other proteins and nucleic acid. This point is also articulated by the data in the last column in Table 2. Note that any mixture of pure type A, B, and E NT, in any proportion, will have a ratio of absorbance of ~0.50 at 260 and 278 nm.

Electrophoretic Analysis and Criteria for Testing Purity

The electrophoretic migration of the crystallized type A toxin preparation as a single band at acidic pH, an observed fact, has questionable value for judging the purity of the protein preparation. Although it has been known since 1980 (66) that the nonneurotoxic components that form a complex with type A NT can be resolved electrophoretically in the presence of SDS into at least 7 proteins, some of which were partially sequenced recently (67), this author is not aware that the crystalline preparation has been defined as to the exact number of proteins it is composed of and their relative proportion. The basis of the idea that the crystalline toxin (mol. wt. 900,000) "is composed of two molecules of neurotoxin (ca. 150,000 M_r) non-covalently bound to non-toxic proteins" (19) was not described and is not known.

Consideration of the purity of a substance requires a definition of the substance; the more exact the definition of its composition, the more meaningful consideration of its purity becomes. Many biologically active proteins composed of multi-subunits that are homomers and/or heteromers (a few examples are ribosome, ATPase, acetylcholine receptor, hemoglobin, pertussis toxin, and cholera toxin) have been precisely defined.

Table 2 The Ultraviolet Absorption Properties of Botulinum Type A, B and E Neurotoxins

| Neurotoxin | Absorption | | Ratio of absorption | |
	Minimum (a)	Maximum (b)	at a/b	at 260/278 nm
Type A	249.5 nm	278.2 nm	0.301	0.491
Type B	249.7	278.0	0.301	0.495
Type E	250.0	277.7	0.286	0.468

Type A NT in 0.1 M Na-phosphate buffer pH 7.4, plus 0.05 M NaCl.
Type B NT in 0.1 M Na-phosphate buffer pH 8.0, plus 0.05 M NaCl.
Type E NT in 0.1 M Na-phosphate buffer pH 7.4, plus 0.01 M NaCl.

The published literature does not inform us exactly how many different proteins (and nucleic acids) combine in what relative proportion with the NT to form the complex that is eventually crystallized. This understanding needs to be developed rigorously before the issue of purity of the crystallizable complex can become meaningful. If, for example, it can be shown that the crystallized complex is made of NT and, let us say, seven different nonneurotoxic proteins, and all eight proteins combine in certain fixed relative proportion (e.g., 1:1:1:1:1:1:1:1), then the purity of the crystallized complex can be qualified according to the presence of anything in addition to the NT and the hypothetical seven other proteins.

Simple experimental techniques are available to develop this information objectively. Electrophoresis of the complexes of NT and nonneurotoxic proteins in polyacrylamide gel in the presence of SDS resolves the complexes into multiple bands that can be visualized after staining with Coomassie blue or silver (see Ref. 67 for such patterns from type A, B, and E complexes). The total number of different proteins present in a complex and their molecular weights can thus be delineated. Densitometric scanning of the band patterns in such gels provides a dependable quantitative profile of the protein components and thus of their relative proportion in the complex.

Toxin Complex and Crystalline Toxin A, History and Current Status

In the bacterial culture, the NT exists as a large complex made of the NT (mol. wt. ~150,000) and nonneurotoxic protein(s); noncovalent association keeps the proteins together (Fig. 6). The nonneurotoxic protein(s), which seems to be produced by the bacteria simultaneously with the NT, may or may not agglutinate red blood cells, i.e., may or may not have hemagglutinating (Hn) activity. Based on this property these nonneurotoxic proteins have been designated Hn^+ and Hn^- (67).

Attempts made in the mid-1940s to purify the NT from the bacterial culture resulted in the isolation of a complex of the NT and nonneurotoxic proteins, which were crystallized in 1946 by two groups: Lamanna, McElroy, and Eklund (9) and Abrams, Kegeles, and Hottle (11). The molecular weight of this complex is 900,000. Duff et al. (68) modified the earlier protocols for partial purification of the NT (9,10,11) and also obtained a complex that crystallized. This modified protocol, developed in 1957 (68), was used to prepare the crystallized mixture of type A NT and nonneurotoxic proteins that was introduced for therapeutic use (18,19). The mixture of NT, other proteins, and nucleic acid that crystallizes readily was obtained entirely by differential precipitation steps (9,10,11,68) and without the benefit of high resolution achieved by chromatography. Anion-exchange chromatography of the crystalline type A toxin separated the NT from the nonneurotoxic proteins; only about 20% of the protein in the crystalline preparation was found in the NT (16,17).

Thus the preparation may well be called crystalline hemagglutinin rather than crystalline toxin. The alternative name, perhaps frivolous, is more apt simply because the weight of the argument is against the NT content in the preparation. Referring to the crystalline type A botulinum toxin, Lowenthal and Lamanna (69) wrote that "work on the characterization of the type A botulinal toxin was in reality characterization of the toxin-hemagglutinin complex, rather than of toxin alone." The preparation of type C toxin complex that was crystallized (70,71) contains hemagglutination activity, and polyacrylamide gel electrophoresis (without SDS) revealed that it is a mixture of at least three proteins (70).

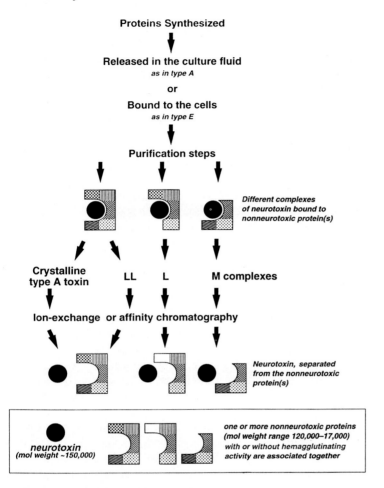

Proteins Synthesized

Released in the culture fluid
as in type A

or

Bound to the cells
as in type E

Purification steps

*Different complexes
of neurotoxin bound to
nonneurotoxic protein(s)*

Crystalline
type A toxin   LL   L   M complexes

Ion-exchange or affinity chromatography

*Neurotoxin, separated
from the nonneurotoxic
protein(s)*

*neurotoxin
(mol weight ~150,000)*

*one or more nonneurotoxic proteins
(mol weight range 120,000–17,000)
with or without hemagglutinating
activity are associated together*

Figure 6 Schematic description of formation of complexes between the neurotoxin (mol. wt. ~150,000) and nonneurotoxic proteins and their eventual separation by chromatography.

The protocol in use since 1957 for isolating type A toxin complex as crystals (68) was modified in 1977 (72). In this improved protocol, one chromatography step was introduced that substituted precipitation of the toxin complex by ethyl alcohol. There were three beneficial results: (1) a twofold greater recovery (33% vs. 17%) of the total toxicity present in the bacterial culture was gained; (2) more effective removals of pigments and nucleic acids (the A_{260}/A_{278} ratio was 0.52) were achieved; and (3) the crystal lots produced were of greater uniformity.

Crystals of the mixture of proteins produced according to the improved procedure (72) and by following Duff et al. (68) contained three antigens (detected by double-diffusion serology with anti–crystalline serum), one of which was the NT (detected by anti–pure NT serum). The minor antigen was eliminated from the crystals produced by either method following recrystallization (72).

Sugii and Sakaguchi (73) had concluded earlier that "the generally accepted notion that type A crystalline toxin consists of two components, neurotoxin and hemagglutinin, will have to be changed.'' They isolated, using chromatography, two kinds of complexes, called L and M (with specific toxicity of 2.5–3.0 × 10^8 and 4.5–5.0 × 10^8 mouse MLD/ mg N, respectively). Both were composed of at least three distinct components, NT, hemagglutinin, and an inert protein. The nonneurotoxic component of M complex contained little or no hemagglutination activity. The nonneurotoxic materials in crystallized toxin and L complex consisted of two distinct antigens and were antigenically identical. The inference was that L complex and crystallized toxin are similar in composition.

The two reports (72,73) indicate that methods using chromatography are available to isolate complexes of NT and nonneurotoxic proteins that in purity are at least equivalent to or better than the crystallizable product produced following the protocol of Duff et al. (68).

Type B NT was also initially isolated as a complex of NT and nonneurotoxic proteins (74); the molecular weight of the large complex was found to be 500,000 (75). Modification of this purification protocol that did not include any chromatographic step yielded a preparation that appeared as a single entity and a large complex (the S_{20W} value was 12.7) by ultracentrifuge analysis (76). Only ion-exchange chromatography could resolve the complex into the NT (initially reported as 165,000 mol. wt.) and the nonneurotoxic proteins (77,78).

Neurotoxin serotypes A and B do not serologically cross-react. Some of the non-neurotoxic proteins associated with type A and type B NTs do cross-react. This has produced a great deal of false data and confusion. Antiserum produced against the complex of type A does not neutralize type B NT (and vice versa) when the assay is mouse lethality. However, the same polyclonal antiserum (i.e., produced against the complex of type A) shows positive reactions in Ouchterlony, ELISA, and RIA assays against a type B NT preparation if it has a detectable amount of the nonneurotoxic Hn^+, Hn^- proteins. These problems can be avoided by producing the polyclonal antiserum against the pure NT completely free of the associated nonneurotoxic proteins. Cocrystallization of two or more substances (organic or inorganic) is a common phenomenon, and it is not peculiar to proteins. Repeated recrystallization of such a mixture using the same or different solvents often generates purer crystallized material, generally at the cost of yield, but also often produces a mixture whose composition remains constant, and thus further selective enrichment of one component cannot be attained by the same approach (azeotropic mixtures and eutectic compositions present analogous situations).

Attempts to improve the quality of the material in the crystallized complex of type A NT by recrystallization appear to have reached the point of diminishing returns. This was recognized as early as 1946, when Lamanna and colleagues (10) wrote: ''Amorphous, crystalline, and recrystallized materials have been determined to have the same toxicity within the limits of errors of mouse titration.'' When the ratio of absorption at 260 and 278 nm was used as a parameter of purity (and as an indicator of the presence of nucleic acid) it was close to 0.6 and near 0.55 at the end of the first and second recrystallization steps, respectively. The third crystallization reduced the ratio only slightly, with a considerable loss of the material (19). The purity of the crystallizable proteins is likely to improve if separation techniques different from the ones currently used (19,68) are employed to break out of the ''constant composition deadlock.'' Introduction of a simple chromatographic step, as mentioned above (72), in the old protocol (68) of preparation of the type A NT complex has indeed reduced the A_{260}/A_{278} ratio to 0.52 and increased the yield of the final product by a factor of 2.

Detoxification of Crystalline Type A Toxin and pH

A recent carefully conducted study (79) found that the freeze-dried crystalline type A toxin (used clinically), which is stable for months under refrigeration, was 43.9% detoxified (statistically significant) after reconstitution for clinical use (50 ng toxin, 500 μg human serum albumin, and 900 μg NaCl at pH 7.3) and storage at 6°C for 12 hr but was not detoxified for the first 6 hr. The authors of this study, noting that the toxin preparation is more stable in solution at pH 6.2 than at pH 7.3, suggested, justifiably, that the reconstituted toxin be maintained at pH 6.2 rather than at pH 7.3. The time-dependent inactivation of the toxin preparations above pH 7.0 was observed by the early workers* and probably for this reason, in many of the past studies with crystalline type A toxin the pH was maintained strictly below 7.0.

One likely reason for the pH- and time-dependent inactivation of the toxin preparations is the possible presence of traces of protease(s) whose activity is suppressed at acidic pH and is high near pH 7.3. This reasoning is favored by the following considerations: (1) The pH- and time-dependent inactivations of toxicity were observed primarily when the neurotoxic preparations were not chromatographically purified. (2) After chromatographic purification, the type A complex could be exposed to pH above 7.0 without notable loss of toxicity (73,80). (3) The pure NT is stable for months at pH 7.9 and 4°C (81). The postulated pH-dependent inactivating agent, probably a protease, therefore appears to be separable from the NT if chromatographic steps are employed.

The rationale for clinical use of the impure type A NT (about 80% of protein in the crystallized complex is nonneurotoxic protein) is that the nonneurotoxic proteins "bound to the neurotoxin apparently play an important role in maintaining the toxic shape of the neurotoxin" (19). If this is so, why then does the diluted crystallized preparation need to be fortified by adding gelatin or serum albumin to maintain neurotoxicity, as is commonly done (18,19)? Does this suggest that the pure NT (mol. wt. ~150,000), separated from the nonneurotoxic proteins, may also be fortified from detoxification with some other clinically acceptable stablizing agent(s)? Such a preparation concocted with a known concentration of the pure NT and a defined added entity (for storage) could have a precisely determined composition.

Progress in this direction is not evident from publications, perhaps because of the assertion that "an important point regarding the use of purified neurotoxin besides its instability is the fact that it cannot be prepared with constant composition and activity" (18). This is not true, and this prevailing view needs rectification. The NT (mol. wt. ~150,000) isolated from the complex by ion-exchange chromatography, first reported in 1966 (16) and now routinely prepared in various laboratories (73,48), has stable activity;

---

*(a) "The toxin . . . is extremely sensitive to pH values above 6.5 to 7.0 at room temperature" (10). (b) ". . . above pH 7.0 the toxin was rapidly destroyed" (11). (c) "Rapid inactivation takes place in solutions above pH 7.0" (82). (d) During purification of the toxin the pH was not allowed to go above 6.5 (9). (e) The highest pH attained during purification of the toxin by Duff et al. (68) was 6.8. (f) Chromatography of the crystalline toxin on DEAE-cellulose was attempted at pH 6.5, and its fluorescence was studied at pH 6.8 (83). (g) Standardization of the crystalline toxin's mouse lethality was done in solutions of pH 6.2 (84). (h) The toxicity of a batch of crystallized type A toxin was found stable at pH 8.0 and 9.0 at 5°C for over 2 months (85). The method used to isolate the toxin appears different from that of Duff et al. (68), but the exact details were not given (85).

Williams et al. (81) have found that the homogeneous preparation of type A NT, stored at 4°C in 0.15 M TRIS-HCl buffer, pH 7.9, is stable for several months. The pure preparations of NT types A and E at very low concentrations (such as 1×10^{-10} M and lower) in physiological buffers, with and without added gelatin or serum albumin, are highly active (25,48,59,73,86). The effect of long-term storage on the pure NTs at high dilutions is not apparent in the published literature. The NT has constant physicochemical composition. Amino acid analysis of multiple batches of type A NT gave reproducible composition (87), and the same is true for type B and type E NTs (see refs. in 88). The amino acid compositions of the L and H chains after separation also show constancy; the sum of the amino acid contents of the two subunits equals the amino acid content of the NT (88). Table 3 shows (1) that the total number of the amino acid residues of the L and H chain of type A, within experimental error, is equal to that of the NT, and (2) that the amino acid composition determined empirically from acid hydrolysis of the protein matches, within experimental error, the composition derived from the amino acid sequence of the NT predicted from nucleotide sequence. Furthermore, those segments of the

Table 3 Number of Amino Acid Residues in Type A Neurotoxin (NT) and the Separated Light (L) and Heavy (H) Chains Determined by Amino Acid Analysis, and Comparison with the Amino Acid Residues of the NT Predicted from Nucleic Acid Sequence

	From amino acid analysis (Ref. 88)				From sequence (Ref. 31)
	L	H	H+L	NT	NT[a]
Asp	65	149	214[c]	200	78
Asn[b]	—	—	—	—	137
Glu	39	79	118	114	76
Gln[b]	—	—	—	—	39
Ser	28	55	83	79	84
Gly	30	37	67	64	64
His	6	6	12[d]	14	13
Arg	15	30	45	43	43
Thr	33	39	72	75	71
Ala	20	35	55	53	54
Pro	20	21	41[c]	44	38
Tyr	25	49	74	71	74
Val	26	40	66[c]	70	72
Met	7	17	24[c]	22	23
Ile	30	82	112	111	119
Leu	40	76	116[d]	104	113
Phe	34	37	71	68	70
Lys	39	63	102	100	103
Cys	4	6	10	10	9
Trp	4	16	20[d]	17	15

[a]The NT sequence, predicted from the nucleotide sequence, gives the amino acid composition of the single-chain protein before nicking. After nicking, 10 residues are excised (Krieglstein, DasGupta, and Henschen, to be published); subtraction of Thr-Lys-Ser-Leu-Asp-Lys-Gly-Tyr-Asn-Lys from this column makes agreement between this and the preceding column closer.

[b]Asn and Gln were determined as Asp and Glu after acid hydrolysis.

[c,d]Deviations between the sum of amino acid residues of H and L, and the parent NT: >5 and <10%,[c] >10%,[d] all others <5%.

NT that have been analyzed for amino acid sequence (based on direct protein sequencing) match with the sequence predicted from the nucleotide sequence (not shown in the table). Also, the sum of the contents of secondary structure elements (α-helix, β-sheet, etc.) of the separated L and H chains equals the content of such elements of the parent molecule; thus the structural domains of the L and H chains are stable.

Toxicity Assays

In a very well conceived plan, the mouse lethality assay of the crystallized type A toxin was rigorously evaluated (84). Using one standardized toxin preparation, assays carried out in 11 independent laboratories according to a single prescribed protocol gave an average value of 0.043 ng toxin equivalent to 1 mouse LD_{50} (the highest and lowest values were 0.075 and 0.032 ng, respectively; standard deviation was 0.012). Thus, 1 ng toxin is equivalent to 23.2 LD_{50}. This has been regarded as the recommended standardized potency of the toxin preparation and assay procedure (19), yet this same publication (19) defined 1 ng as equaling 30 mouse LD_{50} without accounting for the difference between the values of 23.2 and 30 LD_{50} per ng toxin.

The range in mouse lethality results noted in the 11-laboratory study was thought to be due to variation in the response of mice to toxin in each laboratory (84). In this context, consideration of the importance of correct placement of the inoculum during intraperitoneal injection appears relevant. Studies with substances other than botulinum toxin have revealed a 14% (89), 10–20% (90), and 12% (91) error in the placement of intraperitoneal injection of mice with a one-person procedure of injection. All or part of the misplaced inoculum was injected into the lumen of the stomach, the small bowel, or the uterine horn, or was injected subcutaneously, retroperitoneally, or intravascularly. The incidence of error was consistently reduced to 1.2% with a two-person procedure of injection (91).

The assertion that "the only means of evaluating the potency of acetylcholine-blocking power of the toxin is an animal assay [and that] there is no known . . . biological or immunological test available that can replace the mouse test for toxicity evaluation" (19) seems to preclude exploitation of an important alternative approach that actually monitors muscle paralysis, i.e., assessing the immediate postsynaptic effect of poisoning within 3 hr rather than recording the number of mice dying up to 72 hr.

Nerve-muscle preparations used for electrophysiological studies of neuromuscular junctions are useful for assaying the paralyzing effects of botulinum NT. Besides the classic phrenic nerve–hemidiaphragm (14), the plantar nerves–lumbrical muscles of the hind paw of the mouse (86) and the chick ciliary ganglion–iris muscle preparation (59) have been tested for their response to type A and E NTs. Some of these data, including the comparative response of phrenic nerve–hemidiaphragm preparations from various animal species to type E NT, are summarized in Table 4. In these nerve-muscle preparations the relationship between paralysis time (the time elapsed from addition of NT to tissue bath to loss of neurogenic response) and NT concentration (within a certain range) was linear or approximately linear. For example, when the crystalline type A toxin and rat phrenic nerve–hemidiaphragm were used, a plot on logarithmic coordinates of toxin concentration (3×10^{-9} to 1×10^{-11} M) versus paralysis time (80–300 min) yielded a straight line (14). Paralysis time (36–145 min) of mouse plantar nerve–lumbrical muscle was approximately linearly dependent on the concentration range of pure type A NT (1×10^{-9} to 1×10^{-11} M). The chick ciliary ganglion–iris preparation also exhibited muscle paralysis

Table 4 Paralysis of Nerve-Muscle Preparations by Various Concentrations of Type A and E Neurotoxins

Toxin	Toxin Concentration (M)	Paralysis time (min)	Species and tissue	Reference
Crystalline type A toxin	3×10^{-9}–1×10^{-11}	80–300[a]	Rat phrenic nerve–hemidiaphragm	(14)
Pure type A neurotoxin	1×10^{-9}–1×10^{-11}	36–145[b]	Mouse plantar nerve–lumbrical muscle	(85)
Pure type A neurotoxin	1×10^{-7}–1×10^{-9}	24–80[c]	Chick-iris	(59)
Pure type E neurotoxin[d]	3.4×10^{-10}–3.4×10^{-11}	44–89[b]	Mouse plantar nerve–lumbrical muscle	(85)
Pure type E neurotoxin[d]	1×10^{-11}–1×10^{-13}	80–320[a]	Mouse phrenic nerve–hemidiaphragm	(25)
Pure type E neurotoxin[d]	1×10^{-11}	75 ± 7[a]	Mouse phrenic nerve–hemidiaphragm	(25)
Pure type E neurotoxin[d]	1×10^{-11}	104 ± 10[a]	Rat phrenic nerve–hemidiaphragm	(25)
Pure type E neurotoxin[d]	1×10^{-11}	97 ± 10[a]	Hamster phrenic nerve–hemidiaphragm	(25)
Pure type E neurotoxin[d]	1×10^{-11}	101 ± 8[a]	Guinea pig phrenic nerve–hemidiaphragm	(25)

[a]Time to reach 90% paralysis.
[b]Time to reach complete paralysis.
[c]Time to reach 50% paralysis.
[d]In all cases type E is dichain (after trypsinization).

in a dose- and time-dependent fashion within a range of 1–100 nM type A NT and 0.5–100 nM type E NT concentrations.

Looking Ahead

A recent opinion (19) considering the production and purification of botulinum toxins for clinical use, in accordance with appropriate standards of quality, safety, and good manufacturing practice, is notable: "These restrictions required culturing in simplified medium without the use of animal meat products and purification by procedures not involving synthetic solvents or resins [and] avoided exposures to substances such as added enzymes or columns of synthetic resins, used in some methods, that could contaminate the preparation and be carried into the final injected preparations . . . We do not recommend the use of methods of purification involving enzymes, various exchangers, or synthetic solvents because of the chance of contamination."

This view, on the side of caution (for safety), appears to contain the following contradictions. Toxin production (68) starts with a medium containing animal meat products—beef infusion and chopped meat; before crystallization, the toxin is precipitated with ethyl alcohol, a synthetic solvent. The toxin is filtered for sterility and stored in the presence of human serum albumin (19). Chromatography at present is a highly dependable and reliable technique that yields pure products with extraordinary reproducibility. If one assumes that column resins may somehow be a possible source of contamination, the same degree of possibility should then be applicable to the filters used for sterile filtering the toxin because "something" may leach out of the filter material.

The recommended extremely conservative guidelines only perpetuate the technology of 1946 (10), slightly modified in 1957 (68), and merely discourage the use of improved-quality crystallized type A toxin (72) and investigation of the clinical use of the pure NTs (mol. wt. 150,000) and chimeric toxins, because their production will require chromatography. The recommendations from the investigators in England (92), are prudent and more forward-looking. Interestingly, the quality of the toxin prepared in England with modern protein chemistry techniques does not rely on its optical properties (see ref. 48 and 11 in 92), presumably because of the fallacies discussed earlier.

Secure information on the structure of the NTs (mol. wt. ~150,000), the biological activities of the different segments of the NT molecule, the structure-function relationship, and the mechanism of action of the NT is rapidly emerging. It is hoped that more imaginative and courageous scientists and clinicians will team up to further exploit the new information to provide supportive insight into the clinical application of the NT and refinements in the regimen and response.

NOTE ADDED IN PROOF

The neuronal proteins (and some of their cleavage sites) proteolytically cleaved by botulinum neurotoxin serotypes A, C, D, E, and F, which were identified after this chapter was written, are as follows: neurotoxin serotypes A and E cut SNAP25 (soluble NSF attachment protein of mol. wt. 25,000), serotype C cuts syntaxin, serotypes D and F cut VAMP isoform 2. Unlike serotype B, which cuts VAMP between Gln 76–Phe 77, type D cuts VAMP between Ala 67–Asp 68 as well as between Lsy 59–Leu 60, and type F cuts VAMP between Gln 58–Lys 59. In contrast to VAMP (vesicle-associated membrane protein), syntaxin is a protein embedded on the acceptor membrane and SNAP is cytoplasmic protein that associates transiently with membranes (93–95). A diagram on p. 488 of Ref. 95 illustrates the relative positions of these proteins involved in docking of the vesicle with presynaptic membrane.

ACKNOWLEDGMENT

This work was supported in part by the National Institutes of Health (grant NS17742) and the College of Agriculture and Life Sciences and the Department of Food Microbiology and Toxicology, University of Wisconsin, Madison, Wisconsin.

REFERENCES

1. Dolman CE. Botulism as a world problem. In: Lewis KH, Cassel K Jr, eds. Botulism, proceedings of a symposium. U.S. Public Health Service Publication No. 999-FP-1. Cincinnati: Public Health Service, 1964:5–30.
2. Nieman H. Molecular biology of clostridial neurotoxins. In: Alouf J, Freer J, eds. Sourcebook of bacterial protein toxins. New York: Academic Press, 1991:303–348.
3. Lamanna C. The most poisonous poison. Science 1959;130:763–772.
4. Scott AB. Botulinum toxin injection into extraocular muscles as an alternative to strabismus surgery. Ophthalmology 1980;87:1044–1049.
5. Scott AB. Botulinum toxin injection of eye muscles to correct strabismus. Trans Am Ophthalmol Soc 1981;79:734–770.
6. Lamanna C. Microbial toxins in foods and feeds. In: Pohland AE, Dowell VR Jr, Richard JL, eds. Cellular and molecular modes of action. New York: Plenum Press, 1990;19–36.
7. Brin MF, Blitzer A, Stewart C, Pine Z, Borg-Stein J, Miller J, Viswanath NS, Rosenfield

DB. Disorders with excessive muscle contraction: candidates for treatment with intramuscular botulinum toxin (''Botox''). In: DasGupta BR, ed. Botulinum and tetanus neurotoxins: neuromuscular and biomedical aspects. New York: Plenum Press, 1993;559–576.

8. Morbidity and Mortality Weekly Report. Waltham, Massachusetts: Massachusetts Medical Society, December 25, 1992.

9. Lamanna C, McElroy OE, Eklund HW. The purification and crystallization of *Clostridium botulinum* type A toxin. Science 1946;103:613–614.

10. Lamanna C, Eklund HW, McElroy OE. Botulinum toxin (type A); including a study of shaking with chloroform as a step in the isolation procedure. J Bacteriol 1946:52:1–13.

11. Abrams A, Kegeles G, Hottle GA. The purification of toxin from *Clostridium botulinum* type A. J Biol Chem 1946;164:63–79.

12. DasGupta BR, Sugiyama H. Biochemistry and pharmacology of botulinum and tetanus neurotoxins. In: Bernheimer AW, ed. Perspectives in toxinology. New York: John Wiley, 1977:87–119.

13. Simpson LL. The origin, structure and pharmacological activity of botulinum toxin. Pharmacol Rev 1981;33:155–188.

14. Simpson LL. Kinetic studies on the interaction between botulinum toxin type A and the cholinergic neuromuscular junction. J Pharmacol Exp Ther 1980;212:16–21.

15. Habermann E, Dreyer F. Clostridial neurotoxins: handling and action at the cellular and molecular level. Curr Topics Microbiol Immunol 1986;129:93–179.

16. DasGupta BR, Boroff DA, Rothstein E. Chromatographic fractionation of crystalline toxin of *Clostridium botulinum* type A. Biochem Biophys Res Commun 1966;22:750–756.

17. DasGupta BR, Boroff DA. Separation of toxin and hemagglutinin from crystalline toxin of *Clostridium botulinium* type A by anion exchange chromatography and determination of their dimensions by gel filtration. J Biol Chem 1968;243:1065–1072.

18. Schantz EJ, Scott AB. Use of crystalline type A botulinum toxin in medical research. In: Lewis GE, ed. Biomedical aspects of botulism. New York: Academic Press, 1981:143–150.

19. Schantz EJ, Johnson EA. Properties and use of botulinum toxin and other microbial neurotoxins in medicine. Microbiol Rev 1992;56:80–99.

20. Hatheway CL. Toxigenic clostridia. Clin Microbiol Rev 1990;3:66–98.

21. Gimenez JA, Gimenez MA, DasGupta BR. Characterization of the neurotoxin isolated from a *Clostridium baratii* strain implicated in infant botulism. Infect Immun 1992;60:518–522.

22. Sugiyama H. *Clostridium botulinum* neurotoxin. Microbiol Rev 1980;44:419–448.

23. Tsuzuki K, Yokosawa N, Syuto B, Ohishi I, Fujii N, Kimura K, Oguma K. Establishment of a monoclonal antibody recognizing an antigenic site common to *Clostridium botulinum* type B, C_1, D and E toxins and tetanus toxin. Infect Immun 1988;56:898–902.

24. DasGupta BR, Sugiyama H. A common subunit structure in *Clostridium botulinum* type A, B and E toxins. Biochem Biophys Res Commun 1972;48:108–112.

25. Simpson LL, DasGupta BR. Botulinum neurotoxin type E: studies on mechanism of action and on structure-activity relationships. J Pharmacol Exp Ther 1983;224:135–140.

26. Bittner MA, DasGupta BR, Holz RW. Isolated light chains of botulinum neurotoxins inhibit exocytosis. Studies in digitonin-permeabilized chromaffin cells. J Biol Chem 1989; 264:10354–10360.

27. Lomneth R, Martin TJF, DasGupta BR. Botulinum neurotoxin light chain inhibits norepinephrine secretion in PC12 cells at an intracellular membranous or cytoskeletal site. J Neurochem 1991;57:1413–1421.

28. DasGupta BR. The structure of botulinum neurotoxin. In: Simpson LL, ed. Botulinum neurotoxin and tetanus toxin. New York: Academic Press, 1989:53–67.

29. DasGupta BR, DeKleva ML. Botulinum neurotoxin type A; sequence of amino acids at the N-terminus and around the nicking site. Biochimie 1990;72:661–664.

30. Gimenez JA, DasGupta BR. Botulinum neurotoxin type E fragmented with endoproteinase Lys-C reveals the site trypsin nicks and homology with tetanus neurotoxin. Biochimie 1990;72:213–217.

31. Whelan SM, Elmore MJ, Bodsworth NJ, Brehm JK, Atkinson T, Minton NP. Molecular cloning of the *Clostridium botulinum* structural gene encoding the type B neurotoxin and determination of its entire nucleotide sequence. Appl Environ Microbiol 1992;58:2345–2354.

32. East AK, Richardson PT, Allaway D, Collins MD, Roberts TA, Thompson DE. Sequence of the gene encoding type F neurotoxin of *Clostridium botulinum*. FEMS Microbiol Lett 1992;96:225–230.

33. Gimenez JA, DasGupta BR. Botulinum type A neurotoxin digested with pepsin yields 132, 97, 72, 45, 42 and 18 kDa fragments. J Protein Chem 1993;12:351–363.

34. Knox JN, Brown WP, Spero L. The role of sulfhydryl groups in the activity of type A botulinum toxin. Biochim Biophys Acta 1970;214:350–354.

35. Sugiyama H, DasGupta BR, Yang KH. Disulfide-toxicity relationship of botulinal toxin types A, E and F. Proc Soc Exp Biol Med 1973;143:589–591.

36. Ashton AC, dePaiva AM, Poulain B, Tauc L, Dolly JO. Factors underlying the characteristic inhibition of the neuronal release of transmitters by tetanus and various botulinum toxins. In: DasGupta BR, ed. Botulinum and tetanus neurotoxins: neurotransmission and biomedical aspects. New York: Plenum Press, 1993:191–213.

37. Kurazono H, Mochida S, Binz T, Eisel U, Quanz M, Grebenstein O, Wernars K, Poulain B, Tauc L, Niemann H. Minimum essential domains specifying toxicity of the light chains of tetanus toxin and botulinum neurotoxin type A. J Biol Chem 1992;267:14721–14729.

38. Schiavo G, Rossetto O, Santucci A, DasGupta BR, Montecucco C. Botulinum neurotoxins are zinc proteins. J Biol Chem 1992;267:23479–23483.

39. Singh BR, DasGupta BR. Molecular topography and secondary structure comparisons of botulinum neurotoxin types A, B and E. Mol Cell Biochem 1989;86:87–95.

40. Singh BR, Fuller MP, DasGupta BR. Botulinum neurotoxin type A: structure and interaction with the micellar concentration of SDS determined by FT-IR spectroscopy. J Protein Chem 1991;10:637–649.

41. Singh BR, DasGupta BR. Structure of heavy and light chain subunits of type A botulinum neurotoxin analyzed by circular dichroism and fluorescence measurements. Mol Cell Biochem 1989;85:67–73.

42. DasGupta BR. Structure and biological activity of botulinum neurotoxin. J Physiol (Paris) 1990;84:220–228.

43. Shone CC, Hambleton P, Melling J. A 50 kDa fragment from the NH_2-terminus of the heavy subunit of *Clostridium botulinum* type A neurotoxin forms channels in lipid vesicles. Eur J Biochem 1987;167:175–180.

44. Blaustein RO, Germann WJ, Finkelstein A, DasGupta BR. The N-terminal half of the heavy chain of botulinum type A neurotoxin forms channels in planar phospholipid bilayers. FEBS Lett 1987;226:115–120.

45. Schengrund C-L, DasGupta BR, Ringler NJ. Binding of botulinum and tetanus neurotoxins to ganglioside GTlb and derivatives thereof. J Neurochem 1991;57:1024–1032.

46. Stevens RC. Low resolution model of botulinum neurotoxin type A. In: DasGupta BR, ed. Botulinum and tetanus neurotoxins: neurotransmission and biomedical aspects. New York: Plenum Press, 1993:393–395.

47. DasGupta BR, Boroff DA, Cheong K. Cation-exchange chromatography of *Clostridium botulinum* type A toxin on amberlite IRC-50 resin at pH 5.55. Biochim Biophys Acta 1968;168:522–531.

48. Tse CK, Dolly JO, Hambleton P, Wray D, Melling J. Preparation and characterization of homogenous neurotoxin type A from *Clostridium botulinum*. Its inhibitory action on neuronal release of acetylcholine in the absence and presence of β-bungaro toxin. Eur J Biochem 1982;122:493–500.

49. Stevens RC, Evenson ML, Tepp W, DasGupta BR. Crystallization and preliminary X-ray analysis of botulinum neurotoxin type A. J Mol Biol 1991;222:877–880.

50. Montecucco C. How do tetanus and botulinum toxins bind to neuronal membranes? Trends Biochem Sci 1986;11:314–317.

51. Morgan DG, DasGupta BR, Stubbs G, Robinson JP. Two-dimensional crystals of botulinum toxin, serotype B. In: Bailey GW, ed. Proceedings of the 47th Annual Meeting of the Electron Microscopy Society of America. San Francisco: San Francisco Press, 1989:1034–1035.

52. Evans DM, Williams RS, Shone CC, Hambleton P, Melling J, Dolly JO. Botulinum neurotoxin type B; its purification, radioiodination and interaction with rat-brain synaptosomal membranes. Eur J Biochem 1986;154:409–416.

53. Sellin LC. Botulinum toxin and the blockade of transmitter release. Asia Pacific J Pharmacol 1987;2:203–222.

54. Black JD, Dolly JO. Interaction of ^{125}I-labeled botulinum neurotoxins with nerve terminals. I. Ultrastructural autoradiographic localization and quantitation of distinct membrane acceptors for types A and B on motor nerves. J Cell Biol 1986;103:521–534.

55. Simpson LL, ed. Botulinum neurotoxin and tetanus toxin. San Diego: Academic Press, 1989.

56. Schiavo G, Rossetto O, Ferrari G, Montecucco C. The neurospecific binding of tetanus toxin is mediated by a 20 kDa protein and by acidic lipids. In: DasGupta BR, ed. Botulinum and tetanus neurotoxins: neurotransmission and biomedical aspects. New York: Plenum Press, 1993:221–230.

57. Montal MS, Blewitt R, Tomich JM, Montal M. Identification of an ion channel–forming motif in the primary structure of tetanus and botulinum neurotoxins. FEBS Lett 1992;313: 12–18.

58. Schiavo G, Benfenati F, Poulain B, Rossetto O, deLaureto PP, DasGupta BR, Montecucco C. Tetanus and botulinum-B neurotoxins block neurotransmitter release by proteolytic cleavage of synaptobrevin. Nature 1992;359:832–835.

59. Lomneth R, Suszkiw JB, DasGupta BR. Response of the chick ciliary ganglion–iris neuromuscular preparation to botulinum neurotoxin. Neurosci Lett 1990;113:211–216.

60. Sellin LC, Kauffman JA, DasGupta BR. Comparison of the effects of botulinum neurotoxin types A and E at the rat neuromuscular junction. Med Biol 1983;61:120–125.

61. Dekleva ML, DasGupta BR, Sathyamoorthy V. Botulinum neurotoxin type A radiolabeled at either the light or the heavy chain. Arch Biochem Biophys 1989;274:235–240.

62. Weller U, Dauzenroth M-E, Gansel M, Dreyer F. Cooperative action of the light chain of tetanus toxin and the heavy chain of botulinum toxin type A on transmitter release of mammalian motor endplates. Neurosci Lett 1991;122:132–134.

63. Poulain B, Mochida S, Weller U, Hogy B, Habermann E, Wadsworth JDF, Shone CC, Dolly JO, Tauc L. Heterologous combinations of heavy and light chains from botulinum neurotoxin A and tetanus toxin inhibit neuro-transmitter release in Aplysia. J Biol Chem 1991;266: 9580–9585.

64. Stefanye D, Schantz EJ, Spero L. Amino acid composition of crystalline botulinum toxin type A. J Bacteriol 1967;94:277–278.

65. Schantz EJ. Purification and characterization of *C. botulinum* toxins. In: Lewis KH, Cassel K Jr, eds. Botulism. Proceedings of a symposium. U.S. Public Health Service Publication No. 999-FP-1. Cincinnati: Public Health Service, 1964:91–104.

66. DasGupta BR. Electrophoretic analysis of *Clostridium botulinum* type A and B hemagglutinins. Can J Microbiol 1980;26:992–997.

67. Somers E, DasGupta BR. *Clostridium botulinum* types A, B, C_1 and E produce proteins with or without hemagglutinating activity: Do they share common amino acid sequences and genes? J Protein Chem 1991;10:415–425.

68. Duff JT, Wright GG, Klerer J, Moore DE, Bibler RH. Studies on immunity of toxins of *Clostridium botulinum*. I. A simplified procedure for isolation of type A toxin. J Bacteriol 1957;73:42–47.

69. Lowenthal JP, Lamanna C. Characterization of botulinal hemagglutinin. Am J Hygiene 1953;57:46–59.

70. Syuto B, Kubo S. Purification and crystallization of *Clostridium botulinum* type C toxin. Jap J Vet Res 1972;20:19–30.

71. Syuto B, Kubo S. *Clostridium botulinum* type C toxin. Mol Cell Biochem 1982;48:25–32.

72. Sugiyama H, Moberg LJ, Messer SL. Improved procedure for crystallization of *Clostridium botulinum* type A toxic complexes. Appl Environ Microbiol 1977;33:963–966.
73. Sugii S, Sakaguchii G. Molecular construction of *Clostridium botulinum* type A toxins. Infect Immun 1975;12:1262–1270.
74. Lamanna C, Glassman HN. The isolation of type B botulinum toxin. J Bacteriol 1947;54: 575–584.
75. Wagman J, Bateman JB. The behavior of the botulinus toxins in the ultracentrifuge. Arch Biochem Biophys 1951;31:424–430.
76. Duff JT, Klerer J, Bibler RH, Moore DE, Gottfried C, Wright GG. Studies on immunity to toxins of *C. botulinum*: II, Production and purification of type B toxin for toxoid. J Bacteriol 1957;73:597–601.
77. DasGupta BR, Boroff DA, Cheong K. Isolation of chromatographically pure toxin of *Clostridium botulinum* type B. Biochem Biophys Res Commun 1968;32:1057–1063.
78. Beers WH, Reich E. Isolation and characterization of *Clostridium botulinum* type B toxin. J Biol Chem 1969;244:4473–4479.
79. Gartlau MG, Hoffman HT. Crystalline preparation of botulinum toxin type A (BoTox): degradation in potency with storage. Otolaryngology—Head and Neck Surgery 1993; 108:135–140.
80. DasGupta BR, Berry LJ, Boroff DA. Purification of *Clostridium botulinum* type A toxin. Biochim Biophys Acta 1970;214:343–349.
81. Williams RS, Tse CK, Dolly JO, Hambleton P, Melling J. Radioiodination of botulinum neurotoxin type A with retention of biological activity and its binding to brain synaptosomes. Eur J Biochem 1983;131:437–445.
82. Putnam FW, Lamanna C, Sharp DG. Physiochemical properties of crystalline *Clostridium botulinum* type A toxin. J Biol Chem 1948;176:401–412.
83. Schantz EJ, Stefanye D, Spero L. Observations on the fluorescence and toxicity of botulinum toxin. J Biol Chem 1960;235:3489–3491.
84. Schantz EJ, Kautter DA. Standardized assay for *Clostridium botulinum* toxins. J Assoc Off Anal Chem 1978;61:96–99.
85. Spero L. The alkaline inactivation of botulinum toxin. Arch Biochem Biophys 1958;73: 484–491.
86. Clark AW, Bandyopadhyay S, DasGupta BR. The plantar nerves–lumbrical muscles: a useful nerve-muscle preparation for assaying the effects of botulinum neurotoxin. J Neurosci Meth 1987;19:285–295.
87. DasGupta BR, Sathyamoorthy V. Purification and amino acid composition of type A botulinum neurotoxin. Toxicon 1984;22:415–424.
88. Sathyamoorthy V, DasGupta BR. Separation, purification, partial characterization and comparison of the heavy and light chains of botulinum neurotoxin types A, B and E. J Biol Chem 1985;260:10461–10466.
89. Steward JP, Ornellas EP, Beernink KD, Northway WH. Errors related to different techniques of intraperitoneal injection in mice. Appl Microbiol 1968;16:1418–1419.
90. Miner NA, Koehler J, Greenaway L. Intraperitoneal injection of mice. Appl Microbiol 1969;17:250–251.
91. Avioli V, Rossi E. Errors related to different techniques of intraperitoneal injection in mice. Appl Microbiol 1970;19:704–705.
92. Melling J, Hambleton P, Shone LL. *Clostridium botulinum* toxins: nature and preparation for clinical use. Eye 1988;2:16–23.
93. Huttner WB. Snappy exocytoxins. Nature 1993;365:104–105.
94. DeCamilli P. Exocytosis goes with a SNAP. Nature 1993;364:387–388.
95. Barinaga M. Secrets of secretion revealed. Science 1993;260:487–489.

3

Preparation and Characterization of Botulinum Toxin Type A for Human Treatment

Edward J. Schantz and Eric A. Johnson
University of Wisconsin, Madison, Wisconsin

INTRODUCTION

The treatment of many hyperactive muscle disorders by injection of botulinum toxin (BTX) directly into a specific muscle has brought relief to thousands of people and has opened a new field of study on the application of the toxin to nerve and muscle tissue in the human body. During the past 23 years of developmental work on the use of the toxin for human treatment, selective procedures for the production, purification, and dispensing of the toxin have been developed to make it suitable for injection. In December 1989 the U.S. Food and Drug Administration (FDA) licensed botulinum toxin type A (BTX-A) (batch #79-11) as an orphan drug for the treatment of several dystonias and movement disorders.

The purpose of this paper is to describe (1) the essential points of production, purification and characterization of the type A toxin, (2) the specifications used to define the quality of the toxin that was produced at our laboratory at the University of Wisconsin for human treatment, and (3) the use of other serological types of toxin and their application to human treatment. It is important also to bring out developments during the past 23 or more years of research and experimentation that took place between Alan B. Scott and E. J. Schantz and later, in 1985, E.A. Johnson on type A toxin and its application to human treatment. We also propose improvements for attaining and maintaining the highest quality toxin for human treatment. The clinical work using type A toxin was first reported by Scott during the 1980s (1,2), and the properties of the toxin in relation to its use for human treatment were reported by Schantz and Scott in 1981 (3) and later by Schantz and Johnson in 1992 (4).

DEVELOPMENTS LEADING TO THE USE OF BOTULINUM TOXIN TYPE A

Type A is one of seven immunologically distinct types (A through G) of BTX composing a family of similar neurotoxins that produce paralysis by blockage of the release of acetylcholine at the myoneural junction. Because of the apparent high toxicity of type A toxin and its involvement in many outbreaks of food-borne botulism in the United States, it became the first to be investigated to any extent chemically and pharmacologically (3) and as a result was the first to be suggested for human treatment. The first reported attempt at purification of the type A toxin was carried out at the Hooper Foundation, University of California, San Francisco, in 1928 by Snipe and Sommer (5), who found that 90% or more of the toxin produced in deep culture broth could be precipitated by adjusting the pH of the spent culture to 3.5 with acid. This light brown, mud-like precipitate was the source of toxin for many pharmacological investigations and was even considered as a possible biological warfare agent against our troops during World War II. It was therefore investigated at Fort Detrick, Maryland, where it was isolated in crystalline form and many of its chemical, physical, and biological properties were determined (6,7). The Fort Detrick laboratory also furnished crystalline type A toxin to many research laboratories throughout the world that also contributed much to the knowledge of the structure and action of the toxin.

Although BTX had been studied for many years, investigations leading specifically to the use of BTX-A for the treatment of involuntary hyperactive muscle disorders came about through the collaborative work of Scott at Smith-Kettlewell Eye Research Institute in San Francisco and Schantz, who carried out research on several microbial toxins including BTXs from 1944 to 1971 at Fort Detrick, Maryland, and later from 1972 to the present at the Food Research Institute at the University of Wisconsin. The work was initiated by Dr. Scott, who had been searching for a substance to inactivate a hyperactive muscle in experimental rhesus monkeys in which he surgically produced a condition similar to strabismus. The object of his research was to find an alternative to surgery for human strabismus. Among several purified toxins Schantz had on hand, BTX-A was chosen for tests in Scott's monkeys because of its long paralyzing action in animals and in survivors of human cases of botulism. Several trials with the toxin brought about alignment of the eyes in the monkeys and encouraged further experimentation. Preparation of different batches of toxin was carried out to supply toxin for the monkey experiments, and improved results were obtained as Scott developed his technique for treatment. After about 10 years of experimentation, the U.S. Food and Drug Administration approved Scott's investigational new drug application for clinical tests on human volunteers.

For the human trials, particular attention had to be paid to the quality of the toxin (3). Although no protocols were available for the preparation of a protein drug of this type for injection, the use of the toxin for human experimentation clearly indicated that purity and toxicity (paralyzing activity) were important factors if FDA licensure was to be obtained. For these trials, a batch of about 200 mg of recrystallized toxin (batch 79-11) was prepared in November 1979 according to a standard procedure established by Schantz for toxin preparation and purification, with the following specifications on chemical, physical, and biological properties to define quality for this batch and all subsequent batches:

1. Production of toxin with the Hall strain of type A *Clostridium botulinum* in a simplified medium of 2% hydrolyzed casein, 1% yeast extract, and 0.5% dextrose (designated the production medium) containing no animal meat products

2. Purification by repeated precipitation and crystallization methods under conditions not exceeding pH 6.8 and not exposing the toxin to any synthetic organic solvents, resins, or protein substances that might be carried over in trace amounts into the final crystalline toxin (3,4)
3. A maximum ultraviolet (UV) absorbance at 278 nm of the toxin dissolved in sodium phosphate buffer at pH 6.8
4. A 260/278 nm absorption ratio of 0.6 or less
5. A specific toxicity of 3×10^7 mouse $LD_{50} \pm 20\%$ per milligram of protein
6. A characteristic banding pattern on gel electrophoresis

To obtain 200 mg of recrystallized toxin for the human trials it was necessary to culture several 16-L batches of type A *C. botulinum*, combine the acid precipitates from the spent cultures, and purify, crystallize and recrystallize the toxin to make up batch 79-11. One hundred mg of this batch (79-11) was sent to Scott's laboratory in San Francisco, and the remainder was retained in Schantz's laboratory at the Food Research Institute as a backup supply and for further research. This batch supplied all of the toxin for the volunteer trials, and on the basis of the quality of the toxin and the success attained in human treatment, it was recommended by Dr. Carl Lamanna of the FDA in 1982 that it be considered as an orphan drug. The Orphan Drug Law was enacted in 1983. The toxin was licensed by the FDA in December 1989 as an orphan drug for the treatment of strabismus, hemifacial spasm, and blepharospasm. It has also come into use for treatment of many other dystonias including spasmodic torticollis, spasmodic dysphonia, writer's and musician's cramps, and similar involuntary hyperactive muscle disorders, as described in various chapters of this book.

The production of toxin in workable quantities in the simplified medium as specified above required cultures of at least 12 or 16 L. Cultures of this size require a step-up inoculum for rapid growth and good toxin production. For this purpose we use 500 ml of the simplified medium at pH 7.3–7.4 inoculated with type A Hall strain of *C. botulinum* and incubated at 37°C. When in the log phase of growth (about 16 hours) it was used as the inoculum for the large cultures. The 12- to 16-L cultures incubated at 37°C attained their maximum growth in 16 to 20 hr, and lysis of the cells began shortly after and was complete in 48 to 72 hr. An estimate of the toxin produced in the cultures was made from the mouse assay using the factor of 3×10^7 mouse LD_{50} (U*) equivalent to 1 mg of toxin per milliliter. A 16-L spent culture at an assay of 10^6 U/ml contains 530 mg of toxin.

The purification of the toxin for human treatment was carried out by simple precipitation and crystallization procedures to avoid contamination, as indicated in the specifications. The type A toxin in the carboys was precipitated by adjustment of the pH to 3.5 with acid. After the precipitate was washed with water and the toxin extracted with 1 M salt solution at pH 6.5–6.8, it was reprecipitated at pH 3.7. To remove much of the nucleic acid and some other impurities, the toxin was extracted from this precipitate with 0.05 M phosphate buffer at pH 6.8 and reprecipitated with 15% grain alcohol at $-5°C$. For crystallization the toxin was dissolved in sodium phosphate buffer at pH 6.8 and allowed to crystallize after addition of 0.9 M ammonium sulfate solution over a week or two at 4°C. All toxin for human treatment was recrystallized and stored in the mother liquor at 4°C or frozen.

---

*We have used the capital letter U to designate one mouse LD_{50} or 0.033 ng of purified toxin.

The amount of crystalline toxin expressed in milligrams is obtained from the absorbance at 278 nm using the extinction coefficient of 1.65 per milligram of toxin per milliliter in a 1-cm light path. In this manner of calculation the amount of crystalline toxin from 16 L of spent culture is 85 mg, about a 16% yield, and after recrystallization 42 mg, or an 8% yield.

Purity of the crystalline toxin has been based to the largest extent on the 260/278 nm absorbance ratio, which indicates the relation of nucleic acid impurities to toxin. The ratio indicates the presence of nucleic acids, which have a large solution absorptivity at 260 nm. A ratio of 0.6 or less indicates that the amount of nucleic acid in a crystalline preparation is less than 0.1%. Nucleic acid was removed by careful ethanol precipitation and crystallization rather than by adding RNases as is done in some procedures. Analytical gel electrophoresis has been used to compare independently produced batches, and good similarity has been observed. Only slight differences have been observed, and minor bands have been detected in older batches of toxin. The significance of these observations is not known but is under investigation.

The crystalline toxin stored as a suspension in the mother liquor (0.05 M sodium phosphate buffer at pH 6.8 and 0.9 M ammonium sulfate) of the second crystallization is very stable at 4°C or less for many years and constitutes a reserve supply of toxin (3). For dispensing and treatment by Scott's method,* portions of the crystals were drawn from the bulk supply, dissolved in 0.85% sodium chloride solution containing 0.5% human serum albumin (HSA), and diluted to a workable concentration for injection, usually 100 ng/ml. The purpose of the HSA is to stabilize the toxin on such great dilution. One-tenth milliliter of this solution or 10 ng was placed in small serum bottles and dried by lyophilization. However, mouse assays for toxicity in this medium showed a loss of 80–90% in our laboratory, and Scott reported a similar result. To compensate for this loss it was necessary for Scott to increase the concentration of toxin to 25 ng per vial to recover 100 U. The quantity of toxin required to obtain 100 U in this procedure varies for different batches of toxin. Scott's procedure also included filtration for sterility before drying. Subjecting toxin to filtration in our laboratory showed no loss of toxicity, indicating that loss occurs during formulation and drying. The dried formulation when dissolved in 1 ml of water approximated that of body fluids having a pH of 7.3 and a sodium chloride concentration of 85%. Other formulations were investigated at our laboratory and full recovery of toxicity was obtained in solutions at pH 6.2 and 6.8 containing HSA or bovine serum albumin (8). Although this formulation diverges from the composition of body fluids, it may be preferred to prevent loss of toxicity and possible formation of a toxoid.

Stability of the toxin is very important for reliability in dispensing and dosage. Because of the poor stability of the isolated neurotoxin separated from the protective nontoxic proteins, it was decided by Scott and Schantz that only the crystalline toxin should be used in compounding for medical use. Pure neurotoxin can be kept for several weeks in the cold (4°C) but is more prone to inactivation on dilution, formulation, and drying.

The crystalline type A toxin is a unique compound protein with a molecular weight of 900,000 Mr, composed of only natural amino acids (9), that possesses one or more neurotoxic molecules of 150,000 Mr noncovalently bound to several nontoxic protein molecules that play an important role in the stabilization of the neurotoxic properties. The structure of the toxin and other properties are given in other chapters of this volume.

Type A toxin is soluble in dilute aqueous salt solutions at pH 4–6.8. At pH above 7 the

---

*The method used by Allergan to produce Botox® is proprietary and may differ.

stabilizing nontoxic proteins dissociate from the neurotoxin, resulting in gradual loss of toxicity, particularly as the pH and temperature rise. Although the crystalline toxin is most stable below pH 7, it can be readily destroyed in solution when heated above 40°C. Toxin in foods is completely destroyed when heated to boiling and even when heated at 80°C for 1 min (10). In general, the best conditions for stability of the toxin in solution are pH 4.2–6.8 and at temperature below 20°C. It can be frozen and stored for months or years in phosphate buffers at pH 6.2–6.8 or in citrate buffers at pH 5.5. It is very stable for periods of years in acetate buffer at pH 4.2 even at 20°C but cannot be frozen, as this causes complete detoxification, and acetate buffer is not practical for use in many cases. The crystalline toxin is easily inactivated in solution by shaking, which produces bubbles that cause surface denaturation. Loss of toxicity readily occurs in dilutions of high-magnitude such as those of a million or more, which are necessary for human treatment. These were important considerations employed for the storage of the toxin and necessary for the development of a formulation for dispensing and use by physicians.

USE OF TYPES OF BOTULINUM TOXIN OTHER THAN TYPE A

The seven known types of BTX (A through G) that cause paralysis by blockage of acetylcholine at the myoneural junction have been isolated and characterized (11). Although type A is the only type licensed by the FDA for treatment of dystonias, it is proposed that types other than A will be used clinically, particularly in patients who develop antibodies or become refractory to type A (12–15). Use of types B and F for human treatment has already been investigated (16,17). Types A, B, and E have been most commonly involved in human botulism (4,11) and type F has been implicated in at least two outbreaks of food poisoning (18). Toxins produced by nonproteolytic strains of *C. botulinum* types B, E, and F must be treated with a proteolytic enzyme to activate them or change the structure of a poorly toxic molecule to one of full toxicity (11). Treatment of type E toxin in spent culture increases the toxicity of the molecule over 100-fold. Toxins produced by proteolytic strains of *C. botulinum* types A, B, and F are activated in spent culture by proteolytic enzymes produced in the culture. It has not been confirmed that types C1, D, and G cause human botulism, but they may act similarly to type A on injection into humans. The different toxin types are differentiated by their distinctive serological specificities, but some cross-reaction can occur. Types E and F show some cross-reactivity (19), and C1 and D can also cross-react (20). Evidence is accumulating that the different types bind to different receptors and have slightly different modes of action (21–23), and could complement type A in clinical applications.

All toxin types in culture fluids consist of the neurotoxin associated with nontoxic proteins that contribute to stability of the neurotoxin. All of the neurotoxins except type G have been isolated, and the fully activated neurotoxins all have a specific toxicity ranging from to 1×10^7 to slightly more than 10^8 mouse LD_{50}/mg protein (11). The complete amino acid sequences for types A through E have been established (24–29). The toxins may act somewhat differently in humans, and in human food-borne botulism serotypes A, B, and E show some differences in severity. Less severe forms of botulism, in which the course of the illness is milder, have also been reported, particularly for type B (30). Differences in severity have also been observed in infant botulism, in which type A causes many of the severe cases requiring the longest hospital treatments (31). These differences in food-borne botulism might be reflected in the value of the toxin types for human treatment.

SAFETY CONSIDERATIONS FOR WORKING WITH *CLOSTRIDIUM BOTULINUM* AND ITS NEUROTOXINS

Botulinum toxin is currently produced as a sterile, lyophilized preparation of crystalline BTX-A. Each vial prepared in the United States contains 100 U ($\pm$ 30 U) of toxin with 0.5 mg human serum albumin and 0.9 mg sodium chloride as bulking agents. The product is reconstituted with 0.9% sodium chloride injection and stored under refrigeration. As labeled, the reconstituted product should be used within 4 hours.

Botulinum toxin is used clinically by injection of 1 to 300 mouse units. Physicians who work with these relatively low quantities of toxin probably do not require immunization with botulinum toxoid. For safety reasons, personnel who work with relatively large quantities of toxin should be immunized by a schedule of injections of pentavalent toxoid available from the Centers for Disease Control (CDC), Atlanta, Georgia. Botulinum toxin is not flammable or volatile; however, mists or aerosols can form that can result in dangerous exposure. Spills can be inactivated by exposure to 0.5% sodium hypochlorite, and solutions of toxin are readily destroyed by heating to boiling or by autoclaving at 121°C for 20 min.

The minimum toxin quantity to cause human food poisoning is not known but has been estimated to be about 3500 mouse intraperitoneal doses of type B toxin (32). The dose necessary to cause severe botulism by food poisoning in humans was estimated to be 0.1 to 1 μg (3000 to 30,000 mouse LD_{50}) (33). Since the toxin causing food poisoning is ingested, the dose necessary for intoxication by injection may be lower. On the basis of studies with adult primates, the lethal dose on injection in humans has been estimated as approximately 1 ng (30–40 U)/kg of body weight (34).

ASSAY PROCEDURES FOR BIOLOGICAL STANDARDIZATION AND CONTROL

The determination of the paralyzing activity (toxicity) of BTX is most important for proper dispensing and dosage. The toxic and immunological properties of the BTX molecule are separate and distinct entities, and analytical methods based on both are in use in some cases. The usual quantal test (35) with mice measures only the toxic or paralyzing action, which is most important in medical treatment. This test is not type-specific and can be used for any of the seven serological types of toxin. Tests based on the immunological properties of the toxin molecule measure the inactive or detoxified molecules as well as active or toxic molecules for any one type and of course do not give a true measure of the paralyzing action. It is essential therefore that assessment of the medical value of the toxin be based on its paralyzing action in an animal, preferably on the mouse test (35).

Mouse assays for the quantitative determination of BTX activity from various laboratories involved in assays in foods have shown a wide range of results. Twofold differences are common, but differences as high as four- and fivefold have been reported (35). The variation appeared to be due mainly to differences in the strains of mice used, but the conditions under which the mice are housed and variations in the techniques used by the assayers also are important. In an attempt to obtain more accurate and precise results from the mouse assay, a reference standard for BTX-A was developed at the Food Research Institute, and a standardized assay for its use was undertaken by the FDA Division of Microbiology in 1975 (35). The purpose of the reference standard was to provide the assayer at a particular laboratory with a solution containing a definite amount of toxin that was also supplied to all other laboratories carrying out assays for the toxin. In this way each laboratory can determine the nanograms of toxin equivalent to one mouse LD_{50}, and this factor can be used for comparison with other laboratories. A limit of $\pm 20\%$ for differences between laboratories throughout the world should be established, and this is attainable through the use of a reference standard set down by the FDA, the World Health Organization, or International Association of Biological Standardization (36) similar to the one established by the FDA in 1975 (35).

Because all serotypes of BTX appear to have a similar mode of action in causing botulism by a presynaptic block of the release of acetycholine, it should be allowable to express the concentration of other types as type A equivalents. The justification for such a proposal is that type A toxin is the only type readily available in crystalline form that has been researched to a considerable degree. It is uniform in chemical and physical properties from one preparation to another and uniform in toxicity, with a specific toxicity of $3 \times 10^7 \pm 20\%$ LD_{50}/mg.

Other so-called rapid methods include intraperitoneal injection of 0.5 ml of toxin solution (6) in a mouse or the injection of 0.1 ml into the tail vein of the animal (37). When properly carried out these assays yield results within 1 to 3 hours, but the values obtained have two to three times the variability as those yielded by the quantal assay and are used for estimates only.

DISCUSSION

The use of BTX for human treatment by injection has raised new considerations regarding the methods employed for production and purification. Purity and high toxicity with good stability has been the main concern. Because the toxin is a bacterial product, it is likely that one of the main contaminants would be nucleic acids, and we used the 260/278 nm ratio as a measure of purity of the crystalline toxin. At a ratio of 0.6, we have determined that the amount of nucleic acid absorbing material at 260 nm is less than 0.1%. Recrystallization of the toxin usually brings the ratio well below this value, but on each recrystallization we experience a loss of about 50% of the toxin. We recommend the use of the toxin after the second crystallization until it is known whether there is an advantage in using toxin from repeated crystallizations. A ratio of 0.50 appears to be the lowest attainable, because of absorption of the toxin itself at 260 nm.

Another test to help determine the purity of crystalline type A toxin is analytical gel electrophoresis. In conventional electrophoresis, and also in gel electrophoresis, the type A toxin moves as a single component and batch after batch appears similar (4). On reduction and treatment with sodium dodecyl sulfate, which breaks the disulfide and non-covalent bonds, gel electrophoresis has shown a markedly similar but not identical patterns from one batch to another. These small differences in toxin production by the organism have not been resolved but may be a factor in the 50–90% variations Scott observed during lyophilization of different batches.

At the present time batch 79-11 is about 13 years old and is the only batch approved by the FDA. We have attempted over many years to improve the quality of botulinum toxin, and much has been learned of the biochemical and pharmacological properties of type A toxin that is germane to medical use. Further research, particularly in the area of production, purification, and stabilization of toxin preparations, could result in a better-quality product.

REFERENCES

1. Scott AB. Botulinum toxin injection of eye muscles as an alternative to strabismus surgery. Ophthalmology 1989;87:1044–1049.
2. Scott AB. Botulinum toxin injection of eye muscles to correct strabismus. Trans Am Ophthalmology Soc 1981;79:734–770.
3. Schantz EJ, Scott AB. Use of crystalline type A botulinum toxin in medical research. In: Lewis GE, ed. Biomedical aspects of botulism. New York: Academic Press, 1981:143–150.
4. Schantz EJ, Johnson EA. Properties and use of botulinum toxin and other microbial neurotoxins in medicine. Microbiol Rev 1992;56:80–99.
5. Snipe PT, Sommer H. Studies on botulinus toxin. 3. Acid precipitation of botulinus toxin. J Infect Dis 1928;43:152–160.
6. Lamanna C, Carr CJ. The botulinal, tetanal, and enterostaphylococcal toxins: A review. Clin Pharmacol Ther 1967;8:286–332.
7. Schantz EJ. Purification and characterization of *C. botulinum* toxins. In: Lewis KH, Cassel K Jr, eds. Botulism. Proceedings of a symposium. Cincinnati: Public Health Service, 1964: 91–104.
8. Goodnough MC, Johnson EA. Stabilization of botulinum toxin type A during lyophilization. Appl Environ Microbiol 1992;58: 3426-3428.
9. Buehler HJ, Schantz EJ, Lamanna C. The elemental and amino composition of *Clostridium botulinum* A toxin. J Biol Chem 1947;169:295–302.
10. Woodburn M, Somers E, Rodriguez J, Schantz EJ. Heat inactivation of botulinum toxins A, B, E, and F in some foods and buffers. J Food Sci 1979;44:1658–1661.
11. Sugiyama H. *Clostridium botulinum* neurotoxin. Microbiol Rev 1980;44:419–448.
12. Scott AB. Clostridial toxins as therapeutic agents. In: Simpson LL, ed. Botulinum neurotoxin and tetanus toxin. San Diego: Academic Press, 1989:399–412.
13. Hambleton P, Cohen HE, Palmer BJ, Melling J. Antitoxins and botulinum toxin treatment. Br Med J 1992;304:959–960.
14. Jankovic J, Brin MF. Therapeutic uses of botulinum toxin. N Engl J Med 1991;324: 1186–1193.
15. Jankovic J, Schwartz KS. Clinical correlates of response to botulinum toxin injections. Arch Neurol 1991;48:1253–1256.
16. Ludlow CL, Hallett J, Rhew K, et al. Therapeutic use of type F botulinum toxin. N Engl J Med 1992;326:349–350.
17. Borodic G, Ferrante R, Smith K. Botulinum toxin type B as an alternative to botulinum A toxin: a histologic study. Ophthalmol Plast Reconstr Surg (in press).
18. Green J, Spear H, Brinson RR. Human botulism (type F)—a rare type. Am J Med 1983; 75:893–895.
19. Yang KH, Sugiyama H. Purification and properties of *Clostridium botulinum* type F toxin. Appl Microbiol 1975;29:598–603.
20. Oguma K, Syuto B, Kubo S, Iida H. Analysis of antigenic structure of *Clostridium botulinum* type C1 and D toxins by monoclonal antibodies. In: Macario AJL, de Macario EC, eds. Monoclonal antibodies against bacteria. Vol. 2. New York: Academic Press, 1985:159–189.
21. Gansel M, Penner R, Dreyer F. Distinct sites of action of clostridial neurotoxins revealed by double-poisoning of mouse motor terminals. Pflugers Arch–Eur J Physiol 1987;409:404–416.
22. Kozaki S. Interaction of botulinum type A, B, and E derivative toxins with synaptosomes of rat brain. Naunyn-Schniedbergs Arch Pharmacol 1979;308:67–70.
23. DasGupta BR. Structure and biological activity of botulinum neurotoxin. J Physiol (Paris) 1990:84:220–228.
24. Binz T, Kurazono H, Wille M, Frevert J, Wernars K, Niemann H. The complete sequence of botulinum neurotoxin type A and comparison with other clostridial neurotoxins. J Biol Chem 1990;265:9153–9158.

25. Thompson DE, Brehm JK, Oultram JD, Swinfield, Shone CC, Atkinson T, Melling J, Minton NP. The complete amino acid sequence of the *Clostridium botulinum* type A neurotoxin, deduced by nucleotide sequence analysis of the encoding gene. Eur J Biochem 1990;189: 73–81.
26. Whelan SM, Elmore MJ, Bodsworth NJ, Brehm JK, Atkinson T, Minton NP. Molecular cloning of the *Clostridium botulinum* structural gene encoding the type B neurotoxin and determination of the entire nucleotide sequence. Appl Environ Microbiol 1992;58:2345–2354.
27. Hauser D, Eklund MW, Kurazono H, Binz T, Niemann H, Gill DM, Boquet P, Popoff MR. Nucleotide sequence of the *Clostridium botulinum* C1 neurotoxin. Nucl Acids Res 1990;18:4924.
28. Binz T, Jurazono H, Popoff MR, Eklund MW, Sakaguchi G, Kozaki S, Krieglstein K, Henschen A, Gill DM, Niemann H. Nucleotide sequence of the gene encoding *Clostridium botulinum* neurotoxin type D. Nucl Acids Res 1990;18:5556.
29. Whelan SM, Elmore MJ, Bodsworth NJ, Atkinson T, Minton NP. The complete amino acid sequence of the *Clostridium botulinum* type E neurotoxin, deduced by nucleotide sequence analysis of the encoding gene. Eur J Biochem 1992;204:657–667.
30. Cruz-Martinez A, Anciones B, Ferrer MT, Tejedor D, Prez Conde MC, Bescansa E. Electrophysiologic study in benign botulism. Muscle Nerve 1985;6:448–452.
31. Arnon SS. Infant botulism. In: Feigin RD, Cherry JD, eds. Textbook of pediatric infectious diseases. 3d ed. Philadelphia: W.B. Saunders, 1992:1095–1102.
32. Meyer KF, Eddie B. Perspectives concerning botulism. Z Hyg Infektionskr 1951;133: 255–263.
33. Schantz EJ, Sugiyama H. Toxic proteins produced by *Clostridium botulinum*. J Agr Food Chem 1974;22:26–30.
34. Gill DM. Bacterial toxins: a table of lethal amounts. Microbiol Rev 1982;46:86–94.
35. Schantz EJ, Kautter DA. Standardized assay for *Clostridium botulinum* toxins. J Assoc Off Anal Chem 1978;61:96–99.
36. Cockburn WC, Hobson B, Lightbown JW, Lyng J, Magrath D. The international contribution to the standardization of biological substances. II. Biological standards and the World Health Organization 1947–1990. General Considerations. Biologicals 1991;19:257–264.
37. Boroff DA, Fleck U. Statistical analysis of a rapid in vivo method for the titration of the toxin of *Clostridium botulinum*. J Bacteriol 1966;92:1580–1581.

4

Theoretical Analyses of the Functional Regions of the Heavy Chain of Botulinum Neurotoxin

Frank J. Lebeda and Dallas C. Hack
U.S. Army Medical Research Institute of Infectious Diseases, Frederick, Maryland

Mary K. Gentry
Walter Reed Army Institute of Research, Washington, D.C.

INTRODUCTION

Background and Rationale

The peptide neurotoxin from *Clostridium botulinum* (botulinum neurotoxin type A; BTX-A) is perhaps the most lethal substance known. On the other hand, its extraordinary selectivity has been exploited in its use as a pharmacological research tool and as an exquisitely potent drug in the treatment of a variety of dystonias and other neurological disorders (1). A number of clinical reports of BTX-A administration (1–3) have emphasized that BTX-A is safe and efficacious in the treatment of some of these conditions, while there is an occasional appearance of relatively benign toxin-induced symptoms. Several studies, however, have noted a low incidence of more serious complications (e.g., mild choking on fluids, distal muscle weakness) (2,4,5), and some patients may need to be considered at risk if subjected to this therapy. The occurrence of these symptoms in some patients suggests that the toxin is already internalized within the peripheral cholinergic nerve endings and is no longer susceptible to nonpenetrating neutralizing antibodies. This situation will become more complex if serotypes other than the now commonly used BTX-A enter the clinical arena. Thus, there is a need to consider a novel therapeutic approach in dealing with the internalized toxin and these adverse reactions. To achieve this goal, a detailed knowledge of the toxin's mechanism of action is required.

At present, seven immunologically distinct serotypes (A–G) have been identified and are the subjects of several extensive reviews (6–9). The primary toxic effect of all the BTX serotypes (excluding the C2 and C3 serotypes [10]) is flaccid paralysis. The toxin prevents the release of acetylcholine in the periphery, thereby blocking neurally induced muscle contraction (11,12). The toxin also inhibits the release or exocytosis of other neurally active substances in cholinergic and noncholinergic systems, but at concentrations that are higher than those required to exert effects at peripheral cholinergic synapses.

Like diphtheria toxin (DTX), which inhibits protein synthesis (13), the clostridial neurotoxins (including tetanus toxin [TeTX]) block neurochemical transmission by a series of reactions that is related to their tripartite primary structure. The C-terminal half of the heavy (H) chain binds to ectoacceptors that are predominantly located on the target site, peripheral cholinergic nerve terminals (Fig. 1; step 1), whereupon the entire toxin molecule is internalized by an endocytotic process (step 2). Under low pH conditions the N-terminal half of the H chain is induced to insert into the endocytotic vesicular membrane and form ionic channels. The translocation (step 3) of the toxic light (L) chains from the endocytotic vesicles into the cytoplasmic compartment also occurs under low pH conditions and may depend on the formation and function of the H chain–induced ionic channels. Although the heavy chains of TeTX and DTX are capable of forming functional ionic channels in artificial membranes (14–20), studies with DTX indicate that hydro-

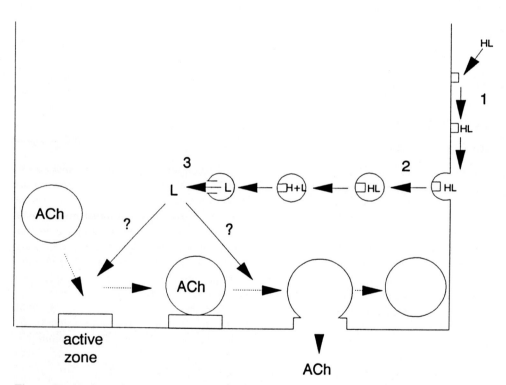

Figure 1   A schematic summary of vesicular release of acetylcholine (ACh) and the hypothetical mechanism of action of botulinum toxin (BTX). The rectangular box represents a cholinergic presynaptic terminal. With depolarizing stimuli, vesicles filled with ACh move toward the active zones and release their contents. The single-chain toxin (HL) binds to ectoacceptors (small squares; step 1) and undergoes endocytosis (step 2), whereupon it separates into heavy (H) and light (L) chains. A decrease in pH in the endocytotic compartment initiates (1) the insertion of the H chain into the endocytotic membrane and the formation of ionic channels and (2) the translocation of the L chain into the cytoplasm (step 3). The final, toxic effect of the L chain is not, as yet, clearly defined, but it is known to differ among the BTX serotypes.

phobic segments of its L chain can also interact with the membrane (21) and take part in the translocation process. Finally, the L chain of BTX exerts the toxic effect, which may be related to its zinc-dependent metalloprotease activity with synaptobrevin-2, a vesicular-associated protein acting as a substrate for some of the serotypes (22). The function of synaptobrevin-2 with regard to vesicular transmitter release is currently not well understood.

If a process in the above multireaction scheme is common to all serotypes, it is possible that a *single* treatment drug could be found and developed for clinical use. From biochemical studies, it appears that at least two different serotype binding sites exist (7,23), which suggests that the ectoacceptor recognition site on the C-terminal halves of the H chains differs among the toxin serotypes. A portion of the present study used a sequence-alignment analysis to determine whether any differences among the primary structures of the serotypes could be detected in this region of the H chain. From electrophysiological data, the mechanism of the neuromuscular blockade is also known to vary among the serotypes (24), and this is discussed by our group in chapter 5.

In contrast to the initial and final steps of the cellular intoxication mechanism, the intermediate L chain translocation (step 3) process, which may involve the H chain–induced ionic channels, is not as well characterized. This is the step that may yield information on a function that the BTX serotypes may have in common. If it is assumed that the ionic channels formed by the toxin H chains play a key role in the L chain translocation, a detailed knowledge of the structure and function of the N-terminal region of the H chains will be of value in understanding the biophysical and pharmacological properties of these ionic channels. In conjunction with the known biophysical properties of toxin-induced channels, our calculations predict that all the BTX serotypes examined have four transmembrane segments located in the N-terminal halves of the H chains that, in turn, could participate in channel formation.

Objectives

A strategy to discover and develop new pharmacological countermeasures against BTX forms the basic thrust of the present research. This study's short-term goal is to identify the amino acid sequences within the H chains of the various serotypes that are involved in the transmembrane regions that make up the toxin-induced ionic channels. Our long-term objective is to identify and develop *single* pharmaceuticals that could be used as pharmacological toxin-induced channel blockers or other medical products for clinical care applications that can counteract the *various* BTX serotypes, rather than develop one for each serotype.

METHODS

Sequence Alignments

Amino acid sequences of the BTX-A, B, C1, D, E, and F serotypes and TeTX were obtained from the National Biomedical Research Foundation (NBRF) data base at the Advanced Scientific Computing Laboratory (National Cancer Institute, Frederick, Maryland). Peptide search, comparison, and analysis software on that facility's mainframe system included FASTA (25), the Sequence Analysis Software Package (Genetics Computer Group, Inc.) (26), the IDEAS package (27), and the programs supported by the Protein Identification Resource (NBRF; Georgetown University Medical Center, Washington, D.C.). Programs on personal microcomputers included the sequence-alignment program MACAW (Center for Biotechnology Information) (28) and the MacVector analysis package (IBI, New Haven, Connecticut).

Transmembrane Segment Calculations

The Kyte-Doolittle hydropathic index (29) was calculated using the authors' program and amino acid hydropathy scale (i.e., the free energy of transfer of an amino acid from a nonpolar medium to water). This index was calculated as a sum of hydrophobicity values of short peptide segments contained within a consecutively moving window. A second program (GES) was written by us to calculate this free energy of transfer using the amino acid polarity scale, window size, and method described by Engleman et al. (30).

Analysis of peptide amphipathicity was performed with the MOMENT program, which uses a consensus scale for the free energy of transfer and a Fourier transform calculation to determine the sequence hydrophobic moment (31–34). Multimeric transmembrane segments were defined on the basis of values for the hydrophobic moment and the hydrophobicity of the sequence of amino acids within a window. The values of the window size (N) for each of these algorithms were selected on the basis of their accuracy in predicting the amino acids within the four transmembrane segments of DTX (35).

RESULTS

Sequence Alignments

Blocks of similar sequences within the toxins examined in this study were determined with MACAW (29) using a modified PAM-120 matrix (36). Regions of amino acid similarity are represented as the larger blocks in Fig. 2. Gaps were automatically inserted by this program to optimize the alignment, and the residue positions are displayed as relative locations on the H chain. The relative amino acid positions for the channel-forming region range from 139 to 229 for BTX-A (see Fig. 3 and ''Hydropathic Analyses'' and ''Hydrophobic Moment Analysis,'' below). While the ectoacceptor-recognition sites are not, as yet, clearly defined, it is notable that a large region of dissimilar sequences among the serotypes occurs in the C-terminals of the H chains (relative positions: 687–843). From our initial analysis it is anticipated that the experimentally observed differences among the BTX serotype binding properties will be related to the different sequences occurring within this range.

Hydropathic Analyses

Our approach in localizing channel-forming regions was to use several different computer-assisted calculations to determine free energies of peptide insertion into biological membranes. We assumed that channels are composed of amphipathic sequences that contain both hydrophobic and hydrophilic amino acid residues (32,33,37). The KD algorithm and amino acid hydrophobicity scale developed by Kyte and Doolittle (29) were used in this portion of the study to obtain an initial estimate of the number of possible transmembrane segments in clostridial toxin H chains. The horizontal bars in Fig. 3 show the extent of the two calculated hydrophobic regions in the N-terminal half of the BTX-A H chain that are long enough to span a biological membrane as either an α-helix or a β-strand. Transmembrane β-strands require at least 10 amino acid residues, while trans-

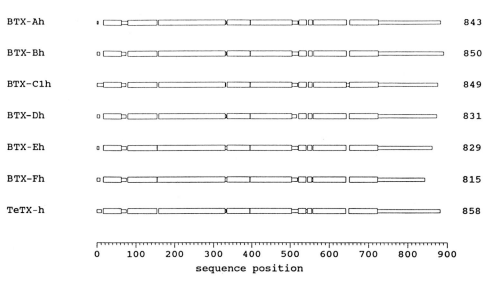

Figure 2 A schematic alignment of the primary structures of the heavy (H) chains of BTX-A, B, C1, D, E, and F and TTX. The larger rectangles represent regions of similar amino acid sequences. The N-terminal end is on the left and the C-terminal end of the H chain is on the right. Gaps were optimally inserted by MACAW. The residue positions are relative to their location on the H chain.

membrane α-helices need about 20 residues (38). The output from the GES program (Fig. 3) indicates that there were also two predicted membrane insertion regions having a sufficient number of amino acids. Although the detected hydrophobic segments were predicted to be transmembrane regions, neither the KD nor the GES algorithm can determine whether they are α-helices or β-strands. From the MACAW (Fig. 2) and the transmembrane segment analyses (Fig. 3), similar results were obtained with the other serotypes examined, and this is consistent with the idea that these ionic channels have similar properties.

Hydrophobic Moment Analysis

Using the Eisenberg algorithm and consensus scale, two regions in the BTX-A H chain were predicted by the MOMENT program to be amphipathic. Because of extensive length of the second segment, it is suggested that it could represent three separate regions. Thus, a total of four transmembrane segments could form in this portion of the H chain. It should be noted here that the MOMENT analysis was quantitatively more accurate than the KD or GES programs when searching for the four putative transmembrane α-helices of DTX (see "Methods," above) and was thus operationally defined as the best algorithm in the present search for the transmembrane segments in the BTX serotypes.

Although the low values of the sequence hydrophobic moment for BTX could not be categorized as strongly reflecting either amphipathic α-helices or β-strands in these regions, an α-helical arrangement for these segments was tentatively assumed. One possible configuration of these amphipathic regions was visualized by the helical wheel display (39). Plots shown in Fig. 4 illustrate the relative orientation of hydrophobic (boxed) and hydrophilic (unboxed) residues within the regions identified in the MOMENT

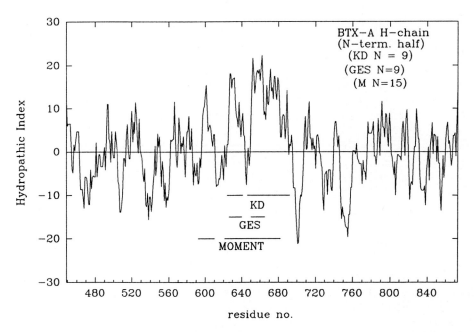

Figure 3 The Kyte-Doolittle hydropathic analysis is shown in this raw data plot for BTX-A. Two hydrophobic regions that are of sufficient length to span a biological membrane are indicated by the horizontal lines labeled KD. Regions calculated as being transmembrane by GES and MOMENT (M) are also shown as horizontal lines. Each calculation was done with an optimal window size (N; see "Methods"). The regions identified by the MOMENT algorithm are of sufficient length to comprise four transmembrane segments (see text). In contrast to Figs. 2 and 5, the numbers on the abscissa refer to the absolute amino acid positions along the N-terminal half of the H chain. Positive and negative numbers on the ordinate represent the calculated hydrophobic and hydrophilic values, respectively, for the residues in a given window.

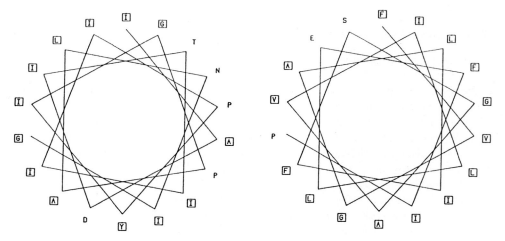

Figure 4 Helical wheel plots of BTX-A show the relative orientation and clustering of the hydrophobic (boxed) and hydrophilic (unboxed) residues in two of the regions shown in the longer region identified by MOMENT in Fig. 3.

analysis. The hydrophilic residues tended to be clustered within one quarter of a possible α-helical conformation, an orientation that will be referred to below (see "Discussion").

Additional Sequence Alignments

A result from another set of sequence comparisons is illustrated in Fig. 5. Amino acid residues in the predicted amphipathic regions of BTX-A, C1, and D and TeTX are similar to those in the putative transmembrane S2 and S3 segments of voltage-gated potassium channels in vertebrate and invertebrate neurons (40). The apparent similarity between peptide toxins and voltage-gated potassium channels in this region lends plausible indirect evidence in support of our assumption (see "Sequence Alignments," above) that the predicted amphipathic regions in these toxins are involved in the formation of ionic channels.

DISCUSSION

The main goals of this study were to examine the ectoacceptor-recognition region (C-terminal half) and to localize the amino acid residues involved in the formation of ionic channels (N-terminal half) within the H chains of various BTX serotypes and TeTX.

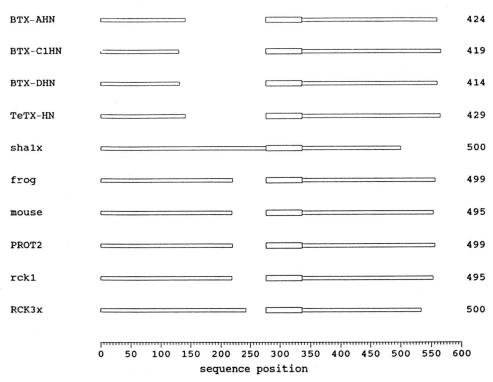

Figure 5 Sequences of amino acid residues in the hydrophobic regions of BTX-A, C1, and D and TeTX are similar to those of transmembrane segments S2 and S3 of peptides forming voltage-gated potassium channels from a variety of species. Only the N-terminal halves of the H chains (HN) are illustrated. As in Fig. 2, the residue positions are relative to their location on the H chain.

Single large regions within the C-terminal halves were not similar according to our alignment analysis. This is consistent with the findings of others that the BTX-A and B serotypes do not compete with the same ectoacceptor (23). It is of interest that two different lectins have been reported to prevent six different BTX serotypes, as well as TeTX, from binding to rat brain membranes (41). These authors suggested that while the serotype ectoacceptors may not be identical, they may share certain structural features, such as being sialoglycoproteins. Thus, a lectin may qualify as a universal antagonist acting extracellularly against all the toxin serotypes—a result that may be clinically relevant in protecting individuals before BTX exposure.

Unlike the region of dissimilarity in the C-terminal halves, the amino acid sequences in the N-terminal halves of the H chains of these serotypes were similar and were predicted to have four segments (Fig. 2). Experiments with TeTX H chain fragments (42) showed that the N-terminal portion of the H chain is involved in a pH-dependent translocation process, and according to Binz et al. (43), this region includes the amphipathic segments as defined by our analyses.

The schematic diagrams in Fig. 6 may be used as a starting point in portraying the formation of ionic channels by toxin H chains. If only a relatively short portion of the H chain traverses the membrane to form two antiparallel segments, it would be expected that both the N- and the C-terminals would remain on the *cis* side of the membrane (Fig. 6a–c). The steps for binding (Fig. 6a), insertion (Fig. 6b), and alignment (Fig. 6c) are shown from a view lateral to the membrane (parallel lines). Further details in the alignment process are illustrated in the view normal to the membrane (Fig. 6d). Shaded areas that correspond to the hydrophilic residues depicted in the helical wheel plots (Fig. 4) are aligned toward the hydrophilic residues located within the opposite region. From the biophysical evidence the concentration-response relation for DTX and BTX is a power function (15,18), a result suggesting that there must be at least two toxin molecules involved in producing a conducting channel. The dimeric arrangement in Fig. 6e is based

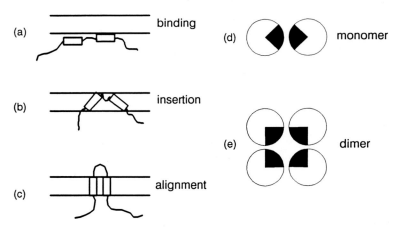

Figure 6 In this hypothetical scheme, two amphipathic regions (rectangles) are shown to bind (a), insert (b), and align (c), themselves starting on the *cis* side of the membrane (parallel lines in panels a–c). The resulting transmembrane topology predicts that both the N- and the C-terminals of the toxin H chain are located on the *cis* side. The top view (d) shows how the hydrophilic residues (shaded areas) could be aligned. (e) A dimer forms a membrane-embedded, predominantly hydrophobic structure whose center is surrounded by the side chains of the hydrophilic residues.

on the hypothesized topology of peptides that form voltage- (44,45) and agonist-gated channels (46,47). These segments are depicted as having residues with hydrophilic side chains that line an aqueous core, interleaved between residues with hydrophobic side chains that face toward the lipid environment (48). This arrangement is consistent with the predicted orientation of tetramers of synthetic fragments of the TeTX H chain that form functional ionic channels (49).

Finally, the alignments of voltage-gated potassium and toxin-induced channels shown in Fig. 5 raise the question of whether their pharmacological properties are similar. Indeed, tetra-alkylammonium derivatives have been demonstrated to block anthrax-induced channels (50) in a manner similar to tetraethylammonium, a well-known blocker of neuronal potassium channels.

From these similarities in primary structures and predicted transmembrane segments, we hypothesize that the BTX-induced ionic channels represent regions of similar amino acid sequences that are common to all of the BTX serotypes and that these structures could be focal points in the future development of therapeutic drugs. Rather than developing drugs that are unique for each serotype (because of their different antigenic, binding, and toxic properties), it is proposed that a *single* drug could be developed that would block the ionic channels formed by the *various* BTX serotypes. If functional toxin-induced channels are necessary for the translocation of the L chain, this single drug may be an effective therapy against the clinical complications produced by all of the BTX serotypes.

ACKNOWLEDGMENTS

Staff support and allocation of computer time were generously provided by the National Cancer Institute's Advanced Scientific Computing Laboratory of the Frederick Cancer Research Facility. Portions of this paper have appeared in previous publications (51,52).

REFERENCES

1. Brin MF et al. Assessment: the clinical usefulness of botulinum toxin-A in treating neurologic disorders. Neurology 1990;40:1332–1336.
2. Ludlow CL, Naunton RF, Sedory SE, Schulz GM, Hallett M. Effects of botulinum toxin injections on speech in adductor spasmodic dysphonia. Neurology 1988;38:1220–1225.
3. Jankovic J, Schwartz K. Botulinum toxin injections for cervical dystonia. Neurology 1990;40:277–280.
4. Brin MF, Fahn S, Moskowitz C, Friedman A, Shale HM, Greene PE, Blitzer A, List T, Lange D, Lovelace RE, McMahon D. Localized injections of botulinum toxin for the treatment of focal dystonia and hemifacial spasm. Mov Disord 1987;4:237–254.
5. Brin MF, Blitzer A, Fahn S, Gould W, Lovelace RE. Adductor laryngeal dystonia (spastic dysphonia): treatment with local injections of botulinum toxin (botox). Mov Disord 1989; 4:287–296.
6. Simpson LL. The origin, structure, and pharmacological activity of botulinum toxin. Pharmacol Rev 1981;33:155–188.
7. Habermann E, Dreyer F. Clostridial neurotoxins: handling and action at the cellular and molecular level. Curr Top Microbiol Immunol 1986;29:93–179.
8. Middlebrook JL. Cell surface receptors for protein toxins. In: Simpson LL, ed. Botulinum neurotoxin and tetanus toxin. San Diego: Academic Press, 1989:95–119.
9. Niemann H. Molecular biology of clostridial neurotoxins. In: Alouf JE, Freer JH, eds. Sourcebook of bacterial protein toxins. London: Academic Press, 1991:303–348.

10. Aktories K, Hall A. Botulinum ADP-ribosyltransferase C3: a new tool to study low molecular weight GTP-binding proteins. Trends Pharmacol Sci 1989;10:415–418.

11. Dickson EC, Shevky E. Botulism. Studies on the manner in which Clostridium botulinum acts upon the body. The effect upon the voluntary nervous system. J Exp Med 1923;38:327–346.

12. Guyton AC, MacDonald MA. Physiology of botulinum toxin. Arch Neurol Psychiat 1947;57:578–592.

13. Collier RJ. Structure and activity of diphtheria toxin. In: Hayaishi D, Ueda K, eds. ADP-ribosylation reactions. New York: Academic Press, 1982:575–592.

14. Donovan JJ, Simon MI, Draper RK, Montal M. Diphtheria toxin forms transmembrane channels in planar lipid bilayers. Proc Natl Acad Sci USA 1981;78:172–176.

15. Kagen BL, Finkelstein A, Colombini M. Diphtheria toxin fragment forms large pores in phospholipid bilayer membranes. Proc Natl Acad Sci USA 1981;78:4950–4954.

16. Misler S. Diphtheria toxin fragment channels in lipid bilayer membranes. Selective sieves or discarded wrappers? Biophys J 1984;45:107–109.

17. Hoch DH, Romero-Mira M, Ehrlich BE, Finkelstein A, DasGupta BR, Simpson LL. Channels formed by botulinum, tetanus, and diphtheria toxins in planar lipid bilayers: relevance to translocation of proteins across membranes. Proc Natl Acad Sci USA 1985;82:1692–1696.

18. Donovan JJ, Middlebrook JL. Ion-conducting channels produced by botulinum toxin in planar lipid membranes. Biochemistry 1986;25:2872–2876.

19. Blaustein RO, Germann WJ, Finkelstein A, DasGupta BR. The N-terminal half of the heavy chain of botulinum type A neurotoxin forms channels in planar phospholipid bilayers. FEBS Lett 1987;226:115–120.

20. Shone CC, Hambleton P, Melling J. A 50-kDa fragment from the NH_2-terminus of the heavy subunit of Clostridium botulinum type A neurotoxin forms channels in lipid vesicles. Eur J Biochem 1987;167:175–180.

21. Montecucco C, Sciavo G, Tomasi M. pH-dependence of the phospholipid interaction of diphtheria-toxin fragments. Biochem J 1985;231:123–128.

22. Schiavo G, Benfenati F, Poulain B, Rossetto O, Polverino de Laureto P, DasGupta BR, Montecucco C. Tetanus and botulinum-B neurotoxins block neurotransmitter release by proteolytic cleavage of synaptobrevin. Nature 1992;359:832–835.

23. Dolly JO, Ashton AC, Evans DM, Richardson PJ, Black JD, Melling J. Molecular action of botulinum neurotoxins: role of acceptors in targeting to cholinergic nerves and in the inhibition of the release of several neurotransmitters. In: Dowdall MJ, ed. Cellular and molecular basis of cholinergic function. Chichester, England: Ellis Horwood, 1987:517–533.

24. Molgo J, Comella JX, Angaut-Petit D, Pecot-Dechavassine M, Tabti N, Faille L, Mallart A, Thesleff S. Presynaptic actions of botulinal neurotoxins at vertebrate neuromuscular junctions. J Physiol (Paris) 1990;84:152–166.

25. Lipman DJ, Pearson WR. Rapid and sensitive protein similarity searches. Science 1985;227:1435–1441.

26. Devereux J, Haeberli P, Smithies O. A comprehensive set of sequence analysis programs for the VAX. Nucl Acids Res 1984;12:387–395.

27. Kanehisa M, Fickett JW, Goad WB. A relational database system for the maintenance and verification of the Los Alamos Sequence Library. Nucl Acids Res 1984;12:149–158.

28. Schuler GD, Altschul SF, Lipman DJ. A workbench for multiple alignment construction and analysis. Proteins Struct Funct Gen 1990;8:180–190.

29. Kyte J, Doolittle RF. A simple method for displaying the hydropathic character of a protein. J Mol Biol 1982;157:105–132.

30. Engleman DM, Steitz TA, Goldman D. Identifying nonpolar transbilayer helices in amino acid sequences of membrane proteins. Annu Rev Biophys Chem 1986;15:321–353.

31. Eisenberg D, Weiss RM, Terwilliger TC, Wilcox W. Hydrophobic moments and protein structure. Faraday Symp Chem Soc 1982;17:109–120.

32. Eisenberg D, Schwarz E, Komaromy M, Wall R. Analysis of membrane and surface protein sequences with the hydrophobic moment plot. J Mol Biol 1984;179:125–142.

33. Eisenberg D, Weiss R, Terwilliger TC. Hydrophobic moments and protein structure. Proc Natl Acad Sci USA 1984;81:140–144.

34. Eisenberg D, Wesson M, Wilcox W. Hydrophobic moments as tools for analyzing protein sequences and structures. In: Fasman GD, ed. Prediction of protein structure nd the principles of protein conformation. New York: Plenum Press, 1989:635–646.

35. Choe S, Bennett MJ, Fujii G, Curmi PMG, Kanantardjieff KA, Collier RJ, Eisenberg D. The crystal structure of diphtheria toxin. Nature 1992;357:216–222.

36. Dayhoff MO, Schwartz RM, Orcutt BC. A model of evolutionary change in proteins. In: Dayhoff MO, ed. Atlas of protein sequence and structure. Vol. 5, Suppl. 3. Washington, D.C.: National Biomedical Research Foundation, 1978:345–352.

37. Finer-Moore J, Stroud R. Amphipathic analysis and possible formation of the ion channel in an acetylcholine receptor. Proc Natl Acad Sci USA 1984;81:155–159.

38. Jähnig F. Structure prediction for membrane proteins. In: Fasman GD, ed. Prediction of protein structure and the principles of protein conformation. New York: Plenum Press, 1989:707–717.

39. Schiffer M, Edmundsen AB. Use of helical wheels to represent the structures of proteins and to identify segments with helical potentials. Biophys J 1967;7:121–135.

40. Temple BL, Papazian DM, Schwarz TL, Jan YN, Jan LY. Sequence of a probable potassium channel component encoded at *Shaker* locus of *Drosophila*. Science 1987;237:770–775.

41. Bakry N, Kamata Y, Simpson LL. Lectins from Triticum vulgaris and Limax flavus are universal antagonists of botulinum neurotoxin and tetanus toxin. J Pharmacol Exp Ther 1991;258:830–836.

42. Rao JK, Boquet P. Interaction of tetanus toxin with lipid vesicles at low pH. J Biol Chem 1965;260:6827–6835.

43. Binz T, Kurazono H, Wille M, Frevert J, Wernars K, Niemann H. The complete sequence of botulinum neurotoxin type A and comparison with other clostridial neurotoxins. J Biol Chem 1990;265:9153–9158.

44. Oiki S, Danho W, Montal M. Channel protein engineering: synthetic 22-mer peptide from the primary structure of the voltage-sensitive sodium channel forms ionic channels in lipid bilayers. Proc Natl Acad Sci USA 1988;85:2393–2397.

45. Hartmann HA, Kirsch GE, Drewe JA, Taglialatela M, Joho RH, Brown AM. Exchange of conduction pathways between two related K^+ channels. Science 1991;251:942–944.

46. Montal M, Montal MS, Tomich JM. Synporins—synthetic proteins that emulate the pore structure of biological ionic channels. Proc Natl Acad Sci USA 1990;87:6929–6933.

47. Galzi J-L, Revah F, Bessis A, Changeux J-P. Functional architecture of the nicotinic acetylcholine receptor: from electric organ to brain. Ann Rev Pharmacol 1991;31:37–72.

48. Sansom MSP. The biophysics of peptide models of ion channels. Prog Biophys Mol Biol 1991;55:139–235.

49. Montal MS, Blewitt R, Tomich JM, Montal M. Identification of an ion channel–forming motif in the primary structure of tetanus and botulinum neurotoxins. FEBS Lett 1992;313:12–18.

50. Blaustein RO, Finkelstein A. Voltage-dependent block of anthrax toxin channels in planar phospholipid bilayer membranes by symmetric tetraalkylammonium ions. J Gen Physiol 1990;96:905–919.

51. Lebeda FJ, Hack DC, Gentry MK. Thermodynamic analyses of transmembrane channel formation by botulinum toxin. In: Kamely D, Sasmor R, eds. Army science: new frontiers. The Woodlands, Texas: Borg Biomedical Services, 1993:45–56.

52. Lebeda FJ, Hack DC, Gentry MK. Amphipathic regions in channel-forming bacterial toxins. In: Gopalakrishnakone P, Tan CK, eds. Recent advances in toxinology research. Vol. 3. Singapore: National University of Singapore, 1993:531–543.

5

Evaluation of Captopril and Other Potential Therapeutic Compounds in Antagonizing Botulinum Toxin–Induced Muscle Paralysis

Michael Adler, Sharad S. Deshpande, and Robert E. Sheridan
U.S. Army Medical Research Institute of Chemical Defense,
Aberdeen Proving Ground, Maryland

Frank J. Lebeda
U.S. Army Medical Research Institute of Infectious Diseases, Frederick, Maryland

INTRODUCTION

Background

The botulinum neurotoxins (BTXs) are a family of seven immunologically distinct proteins produced by toxigenic strains of the anaerobic bacterium, *Clostridium botulinum* (1). These toxins, designated A, B, C1, D, E, F, and G, are the most lethal substances known. For all clostridial neurotoxins, toxicity is produced in three stages: binding to ectoacceptors on the surface of motor nerve endings, internalization of the toxin-receptor complex into the cytoplasm, and inhibition of impulse-evoked transmitter secretion (1,2).

In addition to being a public health problem, the BTXs have been employed as tools for elucidating the regulation of transmitter release, and one serotype, BTX-A, has been employed clinically for the treatment of focal dystonias and strabismus (3). Although the therapeutic use of BTX-A has proven to be safe and effective, the potential risk of systemic toxicity from localized injection cannot be entirely dismissed (3). In the past, food-borne botulism, the most frequent cause of the disease, was fatal in over 70% of patients (4). In recent years, deaths from BTX exposure have become less frequent because of improvements in diagnosis and supportive care and the use of the equine trivalent antitoxin (4,5). Botulism is still very difficult to treat, however, and the disease can require weeks to months of hospitalization (5).

Existing pharmacological therapies aimed at restoring transmitter release with agents such as guanidine or the aminopyridines are only marginally effective in the treatment of botulism (6). Therapies targeted more specifically at reversing the effects of BTX have not hitherto been successful because of the elusive nature of the actual mechanism of BTX action on the release process. A promising new development that may shed light on the mechanism of action of the clostridial toxins was the recent finding that the toxic light chain possesses a zinc-binding motif (7). This suggests that the BTXs may be metalloendopeptidases that act by cleaving essential proteins involved in transmitter exocytosis. In a recent study, BTX-B and tetanus toxin have·been shown to degrade the synaptic vesicle protein synaptobrevin 2 (8).

Focus of Current Study

This chapter will explore two novel approaches for treatment of BTX toxicity. First, results with the proton ionophore nigericin, a compound that interferes with BTX internalization, will be described. Second, studies with the zinc protease inhibitor captopril, a compound that inhibits the toxic mechanism of BTX, will be presented.

METHODS

Animals and Preparation

Male Sprague-Dawley rats (180–200 g) and CD-1 mice (20–30 g) were used in these experiments. Diaphragm muscles were rapidly removed from animals sacrificed by decapitation after being rendered unconscious in a CO_2 chamber. Hemidiaphragms with phrenic nerves were suspended in a tissue chamber for recording contractions in response to nerve stimulation (0.3-msec pulses at 0.1 Hz). The intensity of stimuli was adjusted to four times the threshold to evoke maximal muscle contraction. Tensions were recorded using a strain gauge (Grass FT-03) and a chart recorder (Gould, Model 2800). The protocol for experiments on compounds that alter intravesicular pH was as follows: Mouse hemidiaphragm muscles with phrenic nerves were kept at 4°C for 1 hour in a solution containing the desired concentration of BTX-A or BTX-B. This procedure permitted binding of toxin without internalization. Excess toxin was removed by three rinses with cold physiological solution. The muscles were then mounted in tissue baths for recording contractions at 36°C, and compounds under investigation were added to the bath. In the remaining experiments with rat or mouse diaphragms, the desired concentration of toxin was added to the bath at 32°C or 36°C after an initial 15-min stabilization period. In experiments where drug pretreatment was required, the muscles were exposed to the drug for 30 to 60 min before addition of BTX-A or BTX-B.

Drugs and Solutions

The bathing solution had the following composition (in mM): NaCl 135; KCl 5.0; $CaCl_2$ 1.8; $MgCl_2$ 2.0; $Na_2 HPO_4$ 1.0; $NaHCO_3$ 15; and glucose 6 (pH 7.3 when equilibrated with 95% O_2 + 5% CO_2). Botulinum toxins A and B were obtained from Wako Chemicals USA, Inc., Richmond, Virginia). Captopril, FCCP, CCCP, and NBD-Cl obtained from Sigma Chemical Co. (Saint Louis, Missouri). Monensin and nigericin were supplied by Calbiochem (San Diego, California).

Data Analysis

Statistical analysis between the means of values obtained for various treatments was performed using paired or unpaired *t*-tests as appropriate. Probability values of 0.05 or less were considered significant.

RESULTS AND DISCUSSION

Botulinum Toxin Translocation

Currently, the only approved therapeutic agent that is targeted specifically for BTX intoxication is the trivalent equine antitoxin. This preparation contains antibodies for the three clostridial toxins (A, B, and E) most commonly associated with human outbreaks of botulism (4). The utility of this preparation is limited, however, since BTX is susceptible to the antitoxin only before completion of the internalization reaction (1). The approach described below defines the principles for the next generation of therapeutic agents, those intended to delay the rate of internalization as well as those designed to antagonize the toxic mechanism of BTX.

Internalization of BTX into cholinergic motor nerve terminals is thought to involve endocytosis of the BXT-ectoacceptor complex, acidification of the resulting endocytotic vesicle, dissociation of the light and heavy polypeptide chains, and release of the light chain into the cytosol (1). A schematic diagram showing the acidification process of the BTX-containing endocytotic vesicle and three possible sites for modifying the acidification is shown in Fig. 1. Acidification occurs by active pumping of H^+ from the cytosol to the vesicle interior, which is coupled to the hydrolysis of adenosine triphosphate (ATP) to adenosine diphosphate (ADP) and inorganic phosphate. Acidification is thought to pro-

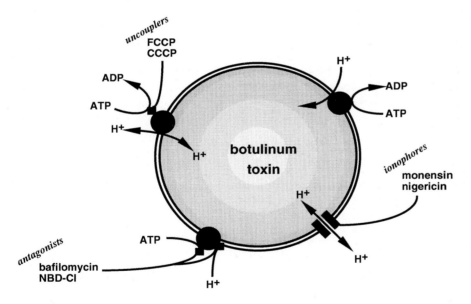

Figure 1 Potential sites for pharmacologic intervention in the acidification of endocytotic vesicles. Following binding of botulinum toxin (BTX) to surface ectoacceptors, the toxin is confined to endocytotic vesicles until subsequent processing results in the escape of the toxic light chain into the cytoplasm. During this confined period, BTX is unable to inhibit transmitter release. The schematic diagram shows constitutive proteins of endocytotic vesicles that are responsible for Cl^- conductance and acidification via the vesicular H^+ ATPase. Also shown are three sites for modifying the H^+ gradient. Collapse of the H^+ gradient is expected to prevent or markedly delay the onset of toxicity.

mote toxin entry by (a) reducing the disulfide bond between the light and heavy chains, thus permitting their dissociation; (b) facilitating the insertion of the heavy chain into the endocytotic membrane to form transmembrane ion channels; and (c) relaxing the tertiary structure of the light chain (1). The relaxed light chain of BTX may then traverse the channel formed by the heavy chain to gain access to and inhibit the structures in the cytosol that regulate transmitter release. If this mechanism is correct, compounds that deter or eliminate the formation of H^+ gradients would be expected to reduce the rate of accumulation of toxin in the cytosol, thereby reducing the rate of inhibition of transmitter secretion by BTX.

To test this hypothesis, we examined the actions of a number of compounds that interfere with vesicle acidification on nerve-evoked twitch tensions in the mouse phrenic nerve–hemidiaphragm preparation. These compounds included the H^+ ionophores monensin and nigericin, the uncouplers carbonyl cyanide p-(trifluoro methoxy) phenylhydrazone (FCCP) and carbonyl cyanide phenylhydrazone (CCCP), and the antagonists of vesicular H^+ ATPase bafilomycin A_1 and 7 chloro-4-nitrobenz-2-oxa-1,3 diazole (NBD-Cl). The H^+ ionophores deplete vesicular pH gradients but do not block the actions of the vesicular H^+ pump. Uncoupling agents act on the H^+ ATPase to dissociate proton transport from ATP hydrolysis, resulting in the conversion of the pump into a protonophore. Vesicular H^+ ATPase antagonists prevent further acidification of the vesicle but do not collapse existing pH gradients.

Figure 2 shows the action of BTX in the absence and presence of nigericin on the time course of inhibition of twitch tensions. This compound was found to be the most efficacious and least toxic of all those examined. As illustrated, for both serotype A (left panel) and serotype B (right panel), nigericin produced a significant slowing in the rate of inhibition of twitch tensions. Moreover, nigericin appeared to be approximately equipotent in prolonging the time to block for each of these two BTX serotypes. This is of interest, since ideal protective agents should be effective against more than a single serotype.

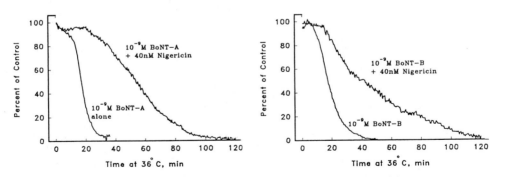

Figure 2 Development of neuromuscular block with botulinum toxin (BTX) and delay elicited by treatment with nigericin. Isolated mouse phrenic nerve–hemidiaphragm preparations were exposed to 1 nM BTX-A (left) or BTX-B (right) for 1 hr at 4°C to equilibrate toxin binding. Paired muscles were washed free of unbound toxin and suspended in 36°C physiological solution with and without nigericin. Single nerve-elicited twitches were recorded at a rate of 0.03 Hz and plotted as the percent of initial peak twitch tension.

Data obtained from a number of such experiments are shown in Fig. 3. In the absence of nigericin, 0.1 and 1.0 nM BTX-A produced a half-time for blockade of twitch tensions of 44.8 and 19 min, respectively. However, when 40 nM nigericin was present, the half-times for blockade were increased to 94.5 and 61 min, respectively. Comparable results were obtained with BTX-B. These two- to threefold prolongations of the time to block are significant and are in the same range as would be expected for a 10-fold decrease in the effective BTX concentration (Fig. 3).

A limitation to the use of agents that alter vesicular pH gradients is their inherent toxicity. Toxicity is difficult to avoid, since proton gradients are utilized in a number of cellular reactions including ATP synthesis and synaptic vesicle filling. The toxicity of four of the compounds used in the present study is summarized in Table 1. The compounds FCCP and NBD-Cl were found to be too toxic to be considered as antidotes for BTX, since they produced spontaneous contracture (rigor) or failure of muscle contraction in response to direct electrical stimulation of the diaphragm. On the other hand, the compounds monensin and nigericin were without effect on directly elicited muscle tensions. However, high concentrations of these ionophores did produce a depression of neuromuscular transmission. Compounds that selectively block H^+ ATPase activity, such as bafilomycin A1, are also of limited utility because of the appearance of neuromuscular toxicity at high concentrations (L.L. Simpson, personal communications). These results suggest that ionophores may be among the most promising of the agents that alter proton gradients, but even for these compounds, the margin of safety may be relatively low.

Captopril

In a recent report (7), it was shown that zinc endopeptidase activity localized in the light chain of BTX-B is specifically targeted toward cleavage of synaptobrevin 2, an integral membrane protein associated with synaptic vesicles (9). The results of a typical experi-

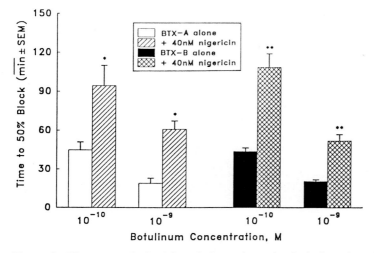

Figure 3 Histograms obtained from 2–5 muscles under the indicated conditions. Botulinum toxin and nigericin additions were similar to those described for Fig. 2. The asterisks indicate levels of significance (* $p \leq 0.05$, ** $p \leq 0.01$).

Table 1 Inherent Toxicity of pH-Altering Drugs

		NMJ toxicity	
Drug	Range	Nerve[a]	Muscle[b]
FCCP	1–10 μM	Yes	Yes
NBD-C1	1–10 μM	Yes	Yes
Monensin	0.1–10 μM	Yes	No
Nigericin	0.05–10 μM	Yes	No

[a]Nerve toxicity is determined by loss of muscle response to nerve stimulation.
[b]Muscle toxicity was generally manifested as a contracture.
NMJ = neuromuscular junction.

ment with a rat diaphragm muscle exposed to BTX-A and one in which the muscle was pretreated with captopril for 45 min before exposure to BTX-A are shown in Fig. 4. Captopril prolonged the time to 50% block from 48 to 88 min; the time to 90% block was lengthened from 135 to 185 min. Since a twofold slowing in the time to block is approximately equivalent to a 10-fold reduction in the effective BTX concentration, the results obtained with captopril are rather striking.

Data from experiments in which muscles were pretreated with captopril before exposure to BTX-A at 32° and 36°C are shown in Table 2. At 32°C, pretreatment of muscles with captopril caused a significant delay in the time to attain 90% inhibition of twitch tensions by BTX-A ($p \leq 0.05$). Raising the temperature to 36°C, however, reduced the apparent efficacy of captopril such that no protection against the action of BTX was apparent. Lowering the BTX to 0.1 nM restored the efficacy of captopril at 36°C, but

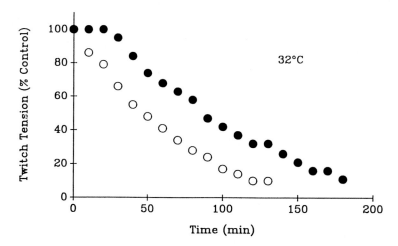

Figure 4 Representative experiment illustrating the effect of captopril on time course of neuromuscular block in the rat diaphragm by botulinum toxin type A (BTX-A) at 32°C. The muscle was pretreated with captopril (1.5 mM) for 45 min before addition of BTX-A (250 pM). Captopril was also present in the bath and throughout the experiment. In the muscle exposed to BTX alone (open circles), the time to 90% block was 135 min. In the captopril-pretreated muscle (filled circles), the time to reach 90% inhibition was delayed by approximately 50 min.

Table 2 Effects of Captopril Pretreatment on the Time-Course of Botulinum Toxin Type A (BTX-A)-Induced Block of Neuromuscular Transmission in Rat Diaphragm[a]

Treatment	Temperature	Number of muscles	Time (min) to block twitch 50% Control	Time (min) to block twitch 90% Control
BTX-A 1×10^{-9}M	32°C	4	96 ± 24	199 ± 36
with captopril	32°C	4	112 ± 19	265 ± 27[b]
BTX-A 1×10^{-9}M	36°C	2	73	151
with captopril	36°C	2	64	145
BTX-A 1×10^{-10}M	36°C	3	122 ± 7	266 ± 23
with captopril	36°C	2	137	325

[a]Values represent the mean ± SE when n ≥ 3, or mean when n < 3.
[b]Significant at $p < 0.05$ with respect to corresponding value for BTX-A alone.

because of the small sample size of this group, statistical comparisons were not attempted. These findings suggest that the metalloprotease activity of BTX is important in its intracellular blocking action. The substrate for BTX-A appears not to be synaptobrevin (8), but some yet unidentified protein that is required for transmitter secretion.

It is likely that the present results underestimate the potential for captopril to antagonize the action of BTX. The highly acid pKa of captopril (3.7) would make it difficult for this compound to penetrate the nerve terminal membrane to gain access to the internalized BTX. To identify better antagonists of BTX, it would be of interest to examine analogues of captopril with higher lipid-solubility or other classes of metalloprotease inhibitors. Alternatively, it would also be of interest to explore enhanced delivery systems for captopril, such as pH-sensitive liposomes (10), which in principle could produce an order of magnitude increase in the rate of drug delivery to the nerve terminal. Thus, the protease inhibitor phosphoramidon has been found to produce significant antagonism of BTX in a mouse nerve-muscle preparation when delivered by liposomes but had little or no effect following conventional bath application (J.O. Dolly, personal communication).

The development of BTX antagonists that can totally arrest muscle paralysis must await elucidation of the three-dimensional structure of the BTXs as well as attainment of a better understanding of the role of synaptic vesicle proteins in transmitter exocytosis.

REFERENCES

1. Simpson LL. The origin, structure and pharmacological activity of botulinum toxin. Pharmacol Rev 1981;33:155–188.
2. Dolly JO, Ashton AC, McInnes C, Wadsworth JDF, Poulain B, Tauc L, Shone CC, Melling J. Clues to the multi-phasic inhibitory action of botulinum neurotoxins on release of transmitters. J Physiol (Paris) 1990;84:237–246.
3. Girlanda P, Vita G, Nicolosi C, Milone S, Messina C. Botulinum toxin therapy: distant effects on neuromuscular transmission and autonomic nervous system. J Neurol Neurosurg Psychiat 1992;55:844–845.
4. Tacket CO, Shandera WX, Mann JM, Hargrett NT, Blake PA. Equine antitoxin use and other factors that predict outcome in type A foodborne botulism. Am J Med 1984;76:794–798.
5. Black RE, Gunn RA. Hypersensitivity reactions associated with botulinal antitoxin. Am J Med 1980;69:567–570.

6. Simpson LL. Molecular pharmacology of botulinum toxin and tetanus toxin. Annu Rev Pharmacol Toxicol 1986;26:427–453.

7. Schiavo G, Poulain B, Rossetto O, Benfenati F, Tauc L, Montecucco C. Tetanus toxin is a zinc protein and its inhibition of neurotransmitter release and protease activity depend on zinc. EMBO J 1992;11:3577–3583.

8. Schiavo G, Bonfenati F, Poulain B, Rossetto O, de Laureto PP, DasGupta BR, Montecucco C. Tetanus and botulinum-B neurotoxins block neurotransmitter release by proteolytic cleavage of synaptobrevin. Nature 1992;359:832–835.

9. De Camilli P, Jahn R. Pathways to regulated exocytosis in neurons. Annu Rev Physiol 1990;52:625–645.

10. Chu C-J, Dijkstra J, Lai M-Z, Hong K, Szoka FC. Efficiency of cytoplasmic delivery by pH-sensitive liposomes to cells in culture. Pharmaceutic Res 1990;7:824–834.

6

Botulinum Toxin Type B: Experimental and Clinical Experience

Elizabeth Moyer and Paulette E. Setler
Athena Neurosciences, Inc., South San Francisco, California

INTRODUCTION

Botulinum toxins BTXs (types A, B, C1, D, E, F, and G) are among the most potent toxins known. The toxins have been studied since the turn of the century, initially to gain an understanding of botulism, a form of food poisoning. Later, they were studied as something of a curiosity, because of the uniquely long-lasting and specific muscle paralysis induced by minute amounts of the toxins. Today, that "curiosity" is beginning to be exploited in the treatment of movement disorders such as blepharospasm and torticollis.

The type B toxin is possibly the first BTX ever discovered, having been identified as the causative agent in a 1895 outbreak of botulism (1). In this incident, which took place in Ellezelles, Belgium, three musicians died. The cause of death appeared to be a neuroparalytic toxin produced by an anaerobic, spore-forming bacterium. When these bacteria were cultured, the culture medium was found to cause botulism-like toxicity in a variety of experimental animals, by various routes of administration. It was later found that this toxicity was not prevented by protective antisera produced against toxin from bacteria isolated from a different incident of botulism, in Germany. Similarly, antisera protective against the Belgian toxin were not protective against the German toxin, although the bacteria that yielded the two toxins, and the toxicity they produced, were similar (2). Although both cultures were later lost, it is believed that the second type of *Clostridium botulinum* was a strain of what we today call type A (3). Thus began a long list of publications related to the bacteria and their toxins: there are far more publications related to BTXs in the following years than there have been documented cases of human botulism.

STRUCTURE OF BOTULINUM TOXIN TYPE B

Toxin–Nontoxic Protein Complex

As isolated from the bacterial culture medium, type B toxin (like type A toxin) is found combined with nontoxin proteins. In the case of type B toxin, stable complexes of two different sizes are formed. These complexes have sedimentation coefficients of 16 and 12 S, and are called L (large) and M (medium), respectively. (The uncomplexed, pure toxin protein is sometimes called the S, or small, form.) The M complex contains nontoxin proteins that reportedly do not have hemagglutinin activity (4). The larger of the two types of complex (L form, about 450–500 kD) contains other protein(s), in addition to these nontoxin proteins, that do have hemagglutinin activity. These toxin–nontoxin protein complexes are not held together by covalent bonds and can reversibly dissociate, releasing the toxin protein, depending on the pH and ionic strength of the solution. Both pH greater than 8 and low ionic strength favor dissociation of the complex. There is some antigenic cross-reactivity and sequence homology between the hemagglutinins of the type A and B toxins (5). However, neutralization of type B hemagglutinin activity with a type A antitoxin prepared against a type A toxin–hemagglutinin complex does not neutralize the type B toxin (6). Formation of an association complex with the nontoxin proteins appears to stabilize the activity of BTXs, perhaps by helping to maintain a necessary secondary or tertiary structure (7). It is presumably for this reason that the only currently commercially available BTX for clinical use, type A, is formulated in the form of a toxin–hemagglutinin-containing nontoxin protein complex, rather than as a formulation of the pure toxin.

Toxin

The type B toxin is synthesized by the bacteria as a single protein chain that has low activity until proteolytically cleaved. This cleavage—"nicking"—occurs endogenously by the action of bacterially produced protease(s) (8,9). Strains that activate most of the produced toxin are termed "proteolytic," such as the strains "Beans" and "Okra." Full activation of the toxin can also be achieved artificially by trypsinization: the bacterial nicking protease and trypsin cleave at or very near the same site. The amount of endogenous activation varies according to the *C. botulinum* type B strain and the fermentation conditions. Even under the best conditions, using the proteolytic strains, both nicked and unnicked toxin may be produced (10).

The nicked toxin has a molecular weight of about 150,000 kD and is composed of a heavy and light chain, held together by a disulfide bond and noncovalent bonding. Reduction of the disulfide bond causes a separation of the chains and loss of toxicity (11): neither chain by itself is toxic. The molecular weights of the two chains are about 100,000 and 50,000 kD, respectively (12). The nicking site is one-third of the length of the single chain, and the light chain is formed from the amino-terminal portion. The amino-terminal sequences of the unnicked type B are identical to the amino-terminus of the light chain of the nicked toxin (13). Whether this proteolytic cleavage termed "nicking" is sufficient to activate the toxin remains controversial (14).

Until very recently, only limited structural information about the type B toxin was available. Most of this information was derived by inference from antigenicity studies (although there was a limited amount of sequence data obtained from fragments of the toxin). The antigenicity data suggested significant differences between the various types of BTX in terms of their amino acid sequences. The antigenic differences are so significant and reproducible, in fact, that the botulinum bacteria are primarily classified by the antigenic specificity of the toxins they produce, with additional subdivision by group and by strain. Assignment to group is based on slight differences in culture characteristics (proteolytic ability, heat resistance of spores, optimal temperature for growth). Various type B bacterial strains within these groups have been described, primarily on the basis of the first source of culture. Some amino acid sequence differences between type B toxin produced by different strains of type B *C. botulinum* (15,16) have been reported, and even, in some cases (depending on the strain), antigenic differences (17). However, neutralizing type B antitoxin raised against one strain of type B bacterial toxin is protective against type B toxin produced from a variety of strains of type B bacteria (18).

The structure of the type B toxin is loosely related to that of tetanus toxin, also produced by bacteria of the genus *Clostridium*. The general size and subunit structure of the two classes of toxin are similar, and some aspects of mechanism of action also appear to be comparable. Antipeptide antibody binding studies indicate some limited sequence homology exists between various BTXs and tetanus toxin, particularly in specific regions of the purified (possibly partially unfolded) proteins (19). However, human and mouse polyclonal antibodies that neutralize tetanus toxicity do not cross-react with the BTXs. This implies that the homologous sequences in the primary structure of tetanus and botulinum toxins are generally short amino acid segments that are either not accessible or not immunogenic in the native conformation state of the molecules. The functional implications of the sequence homology are not yet understood but may be of great interest in understanding the mechanism of action of the various toxins.

Recently, two groups (20,21) have reported sequence information about the type B toxin, from two different type B strains. Comparable information was already available for the other types of BTX and for tetanus toxin. A comparison of the type B sequence with the sequence of these other toxins indicates that the heavy chain of type B toxin produced by the Danish strain has a sequence homology of 48% to the heavy chain of type A toxin and 35% homology to the equivalent portion of the tetanus toxin sequence. A hydrophilicity plot comparison of various strains of BTX types and of tetanus toxin suggests that for all of them, there is a conserved hydrophobic region in the heavy chain. This region may be important for translocation of the toxin across the extracellular membrane (see below). In contrast, the portion of the toxins that has previously been hypothesized to be most important to receptor binding, the heavy chain carboxyl-terminal end, is one of the regions of most divergent sequence. The sequence difference in this portion of the toxins could explain the specificity of receptor binding reported for the various types of clostridial toxins.

The light chain of the type B toxin produced by the Danish and Okra strains have 31–32% homology to the light chain of type A toxin as reported by these two groups (20,21). Surprisingly, the type B toxin was also found to have a 50–52% homology to the equivalent portion of the tetanus toxin sequence. The light chains of type A, C1, and D BTXs have a lower (roughly 30%) homology to the equivalent portion of the tetanus toxin. Analysis of the light chain sequences of the various types of BTX and of tetanus toxin also indicates a highly conserved region that contains a histidine-rich sequence. This sequence is typical of the active site of metalloproteinases, and it is tempting to assume that such activity could have some role in the intracellular action of the toxins.

PHARMACOLOGY AND TOXICOLOGY OF BOTULINUM TOXIN TYPE B

Mode of Action

Botulinum toxins, including type B toxin, probably act through a three-step process: extracellular binding onto the neuron, internalization, and intracellular poisoning (22). Binding appears to occur as a result of an interaction with specific acceptors on the surface of the presynaptic motor nerve terminal membrane (23). Using radiolabeled toxins and various in vitro/ex vivo models, distinct acceptor sites on the presynaptic terminal for some of the toxins have been found. Using rat cerebrocortical synaptosomes, sites specific for types A, B, E, and F have been reported: the sites are saturable, and toxins of one type bind weakly, if at all, to the acceptors of another type (24). In studies using mouse hemidiaphragms, type B toxin was not found to affect type A binding at all. (However, Black and Dolly reported that a large excess of type A toxin slightly reduced type B toxin binding to mouse hemidiaphragms in vitro [25]). Evaluating binding affinities with rat brain synaptosomes, Evans et al. found that there are two populations of acceptors for type B toxin: a smaller number of high-affinity sites (K_D = 0.3–0.5 nM; B_{max} about 30–60 fmol/mg protein), and a larger number of low-affinity sites (K_D = 16–21 nM; B_{max} > > 3000 fmol/mg protein) (26). In mouse hemidiaphragms, the total density of acceptors for type B toxin (627 ± 21% sites/μm^2) is approximately four times that of acceptors for type A toxin (152 ± 20% sites/μm^2) by electron microscope autoradiography (25).

Binding of the various BTXs to neurons is mediated by the carbonyl end of their heavy chain (27). Both the single-chain unnicked toxin and the heavy chain of type B toxin bind to rat brain synaptosomes, and the heavy chain is a potent inhibitor of the binding of the single chain, whereas the light chain is much less effective (28). Preincubation with the heavy chain of type B toxin antagonizes the in vitro paralysis of mouse hemidiaphragm induced by the active type B dichain (29).

Botulinum toxin binding to the presynaptic nerve membrane may involve both membrane determinants containing sialic acid (probably gangliosides) and one or more proteins (acceptor/receptor proteins) on the neuronal surface membrane (30). The acceptors for BTXs have not yet been isolated or characterized, and the evidence for this double receptor hypothesis is indirect, particularly for the role of gangliosides. Gangliosides, but not other membrane lipids, inactivate BTX in vitro and in vivo (31). Certain lectins with affinity for sialic acid–containing sugars reduce the binding of BTXs to brain membranes and reduce the neuromuscular blocking activity of the toxins (32). The specific gangliosides involved may differ between the various types of BTX. Type A toxin binds avidly to GQ_{1b} gangliosides, whereas type B toxin binds less efficiently to GQ_{1b} ganglioside (33), and more efficiently to GD_{1a} and GT_{1b} gangliosides than type A toxin (34). The results of these studies are highly dependent on the pH and ionic strength of the medium, however. Less is known about the protein component of BTX binding to neurons. It is presumed that there is such a component, and that it has functional significance, by analogy to other, better-characterized receptors. Also, toxin binding to synaptosomal membranes is affected by pretreatment of the membranes with either neuraminidase (attacking the sialic acid residues of the gangliosides) or proteases (35). This combination of neuronal-specific phospholipid and receptor protein requirements may help explain the very specific neuronal affinity of the botulinum toxins.

Binding of the toxin to its acceptor is neither sufficient nor, under experimental conditions, necessary to cause paralysis. Intracellular toxicity of the toxins can be observed using methods that bypass the binding step. Such methods include intracellular injection of the toxin into *Aplysia* ganglia (36), or using permeabilized cells (37). Similarly, there appears to be a time lag between in vitro binding of the toxin, when toxin antibody is protective, and subsequent paralysis (38).

A number of studies, including the histological studies cited above, have shown that the toxin is internalized after binding to the cell surface. For example, in vitro kinetic studies using mouse hemidiaphragm and antibodies to BTX revealed that after a while, toxin bound to the cell surface became inaccessible to the antibodies. The toxin is therefore presumably internalized (thus inaccessible) before the onset of paralysis (39). More direct evidence was provided by electron microscopy autoradiography, which showed that the toxin appeared to be internalized, in vacuole-like structures (25).

The internalization process is not completely understood, but, like binding, seems to require the presence of the heavy chain of the toxin. After binding, the toxin/receptor complex is taken into an endosome by an active, temperature-dependent process, and the toxin then somehow enters into the cytosol. The endosome has a lower pH than the extracellular milieu, and the lower pH appears to induce a conformational change in the toxin. As a result of the conformational change, hydrophobic domains are exposed that interact more extensively with lipids, as demonstrated using a liposome model system (40). It is hypothesized that the highly conserved hydrophobic region of the heavy chain inserts into the neuronal membrane and forms a channel, allowing some or all of the toxin molecule into the cell. At least in the case of the type B toxin, using a planar lipid bilayer model, it appears that at acidic pH, the heavy chain is capable of forming channels (41).

Inhibition of neurotransmitter secretion is probably caused by a site on the light chain (42). The mechanism by which intracellular poisoning is achieved is unknown for BTX-B, but it is generally believed to involve enzymatic activity and not mass action or receptor occupancy effects. This hypothesis is attractive for two reasons. First, since the paralysis induced by minuscule amounts of the toxin lasts for weeks or months, it seems likely that the toxin must act on an intracellular component by some means that is only slowly reversed. Such changes would most likely be catalyzed by an enzyme. Second, an enzymatic mechanism seems likely by extrapolation from the more clearly understood mechanism of action of other bacterial toxins, such as ricin and diphtheria toxin. These toxins have dichain structures and apparent structure/function activities generally similar to those of BTXs. The heavy chains of ricin and diphtheria toxin are also involved in binding and internalization, and the light chain is the portion with intracellular activity. In these cases, the activity has been demonstrated to be enzymatic (43). Botulinum toxins types C1 and D have been shown to ADP-ribosylate a membrane protein in mouse synaptosomes (44), but until recently there was no convincing evidence that enzymatic activity was associated with the other BTX serotypes, including type B. As noted above, there is some recently discovered homology between a segment of the amino acid sequence in the central core of the light chain of the various BTXs and zinc-dependent metalloproteinases. This sequence contains a histidine-rich motif that for the metalloproteases represents a zinc-binding site and part of the active site of the protease. Initial experiments using type A toxin mutants in which the histidine site has been affected have not shown any effect of the mutations on the effectiveness of BTX in *Aplysia* neurons (45). These results therefore do not support the hypothesis that this putative metalloprotease active site is important to BTX intracellular activity. At the same time, chelating agents such as 1,10-phenanthroline, which are capable of stripping zinc, iron, and calcium from proteins, are capable of inactivating BTXs including type B toxin (46).

All of the BTX serotypes prevent both spontaneous and evoked quantal release of acetylcholine from the presynaptic neuromuscular junction. However, the intracellular mechanism by which this effect is achieved appears to be different. A series of studies has been performed that emphasizes these differences, in synaptosomal preparations, in phrenic nerve–hemidiaphragms, and also in a double-poisoning experiment using types A and B toxins on a triangularis sterni nerve-muscle preparation (47). These studies all suggest differences between the toxins in terms of the response to pharmacologic manipulation of calcium ion movement, or to microtubule-dissociating drugs.

The most frequently studied difference between the toxins is reversibility of acetylcholine release inhibition by the aminopyridines. These agents increase impulse-evoked Ca^{2+} influx by blocking presynaptic potassium channels. As a result, neurotransmitter release can take place. Aminopyridines reverse the poisoning induced by types A and E (48), but the effect is greatest with type A toxin. The poisoning induced by B, D, and F is not reversible by aminopyridines. An increase in extracellular calcium or use of a Ca^{2+} ionophore, A23187 (49), or guanidine more effectively reverses the effects of type A than of type B, C, or E toxins (50). When synaptosomes were preincubated with microtubule-dissociating drugs, there was a reduction of type B (but not of type A) toxin inhibition of neurotransmitter release. This effect did not appear to be related to prevention of binding or internalization of the toxin (49). The most probable explanation for these differences is that the toxins act at different steps in the process that results in neurotransmitter release.

Comparative Muscle Paralytic Efficacy

Relatively few studies have been reported evaluating the in vivo muscle paralytic potency of BTX types other than type A. Usually, these studies have been performed using rats, a species apparently particularly resistant to type B toxin (see below), or rat tissues. In a study by Burgen et al. using a rat in vitro phrenic nerve–diaphragm preparation, when the toxin was added to the perfusate of the in vitro system, it took amounts of type B toxin ''. . . about 500 times greater than the amount of type A toxin required to produce a similar rate of paralysis. When, however, the phrenic nerve–diaphragm preparation was obtained from young guinea-pigs (150–200 g.) typical neuromuscular block followed the addition of 2000 units/ml. of either type A or type B toxin. There were no marked differences in the latent period or rate of paralysis between types A and B toxins on this preparation. The guinea pig is known to be susceptible to type B toxin. . .'' (51).

Another study, by Sellin et al. (52), found that it required 1200 mouse LD_{50} of type B toxin to prevent measurable evoked potentials in a rat ex vivo nerve-muscle preparation. The difference between these two studies in terms of the effective dose for type B toxin–induced paralysis may be that Sellin et al. administered the toxin subcutaneously, above the tibialis anterior muscle in vivo, then later removed the extensor digitorum longus muscle to measure in vitro electrophysiological effects, while Burgen et al. added the toxin to the perfusate of their in vitro preparation.

In rats, no toxin studied has been found to be as potent as type A. Type E (53) and F (54) toxins have also been studied with the same model, and it was found that the dose and duration of the paralysis induced in rats was less than with type A. Unfortunately, given the species-specificity of the various toxin types, rodent studies must be considered inconclusive with respect to predicting the relative clinical potency of the various types of BTX.

For this reason, we have undertaken to study the paralytic efficacy of BTX-B in normal nonhuman primates. In these studies, the toxin was injected into three muscles: the trapezius, the abductor pollicis brevis (APB) muscle of the thumb, and the extensor digitorum brevis (EDB) muscle of the foot. Doses injected into muscles ranged from 5 to 80 U/muscle (1 U is the dose equivalent to a mouse intraperitoneal LD_{50} dose). Efficacy in these studies was measured electrophysiologically, by a decrease in the peak amplitude of the evoked compound muscle action potential. Botulinum toxin type B was found to paralyze injected muscles effectively. At 2 weeks after the initial injection, there was a reduction of maximal muscle electromyographic (EMG) amplitude of 80% or more in the APB and EDB muscles injected at all of the doses tested, in all subjects. A similar reduction of maximal trapezius muscle EMG amplitude was observed after 2 weeks in 10 of 11 animals injected with doses greater than or equal to 80 U/muscle. Muscles paralyzed by BTX-B recovered over time. All of the muscles injected with doses in the estimated therapeutic range had evoked compound muscle action potentials that could be measured by approximately 3 months after the last injection. This result is in contrast to results obtained in the same animals 2 weeks after the initial injection, when several muscles had no measurable evoked compound muscle action potentials. On the basis of visual estimates of the mass of the three muscles tested (the actual mass of the injected muscles was not determined), it appeared that for any given dose, the smaller the muscle mass (abductor pollicis brevis < extensor digitorum brevis < trapezius), the longer the duration of paralysis. Evoked compound muscle action potentials in the injected APB tended to be lower in each animal at each injected dose than in the trapezius, although the dose of BTX-B injected into the APB was one-fourth of the trapezius dose. Similarly, whereas at the end of the study the evoked compound muscle action potentials in the APB and trapezius muscles in the lowest-efficacy dose group were no longer statistically significantly different from baseline values, the evoked compound muscle action potentials of both muscles in the highest-efficacy dose group were significantly less than at baseline.

Reinjection of recovering muscles with a second dose of BTX-B resulted in a decrease in the evoked compound muscle action potentials measured 2 weeks after administration of the second dose. The response of the muscle injected with the second dose of the drug did not indicate a cumulative effect of the doses: reinjected muscles were neither more completely paralyzed nor longer paralyzed than muscles injected with a single dose of the drug.

For type A toxin, histochemical studies have been made, evaluating the changes that occur after injection of the toxin. Duchen (55) performed a series of such studies, injecting the type A toxin into the calf muscles of mice. Typically, the muscles atrophied, as expected from a functional denervation. Also observed was a sprouting of nerve fibers and a formation of new end plates, which occurred more rapidly in the soleus (a slow-twitch red muscle) than in the gastrocnemius (a fast-twitch white muscle). The sprouting was observed to take place preterminally as well as terminally, and collateral sprouting was also observed. Over time, as the muscle recovered function, the number of these collateral sprouts decreased. Similar sprouting after type A toxin injection has been reported in frogs (56), primates (57), and humans (58).

The mechanism by which the type B toxin muscle paralysis is reversed over time is unknown, but it may be assumed to be similar to recovery after type A–induced paralysis. This conclusion is based on results of a study submitted for publication, cited in a recent review article (59). The review article reports that this study was performed in albino rabbits, evaluating histochemical changes (acetylcholinesterase stain, muscle fiber size, and ATPase staining) after injection of either BTX-A or a "crude preparation" of type B toxin." The denervation indicated by histochemical staining and fiber size analysis appeared transient and lasted for about 3 months for both type A and B toxins."

Comparative Toxicity Data

Type B toxin is known to be toxic for humans, as noted in the introduction, when ingested in poorly processed foods. In the United States, most reported cases of botulism have been related to either type A or type B toxin: together they accounted for 91% of the cases of known toxin-type botulism reported to the Centers for Disease Control from 1970 to 1979. Type A toxin is responsible for twice as many cases of food botulism as type B (60). Of the two types of human botulism, type A is considered to be the more severe (61). Human oral toxic doses are difficult to estimate from these oral food poisoning reports, however, and the clinically toxic dose, even by the oral route, is unknown.

Typically, it takes 1 to 2 days for the symptoms of botulism to develop. The highest cranial nerves are affected first, causing medial rectus paresis, ptosis, and sluggish pupillary response to light. They are followed by the lower cranial nerves, then the peripheral motor neurons, finally and often fatally including those that innervate the respiratory muscles. Effects on peripheral muscles are not observed in the absence of ophthalmic changes: in one study of an unusually large outbreak of type B botulism (53 people were hospitalized), all of the patients who later experienced respiratory difficulty or peripheral muscle weakness first demonstrated cranial nerve impairment (62). In some cases, patients have signs of autonomic nervous system dysfunction: constipation, distention of the urinary bladder, and decreased salivation and tearing (63). Blood counts, urinalysis, and clinical chemistry values are normal in botulism, unless there are secondary complications (the most frequent of which is pneumonia associated with respiratory muscle paralysis) (64).

A definitive diagnosis of botulism can be made by electromyography (EMG). In muscles weakened by botulism, the amplitude of the compound muscle action potential is reduced in response to a supramaximal stimulation of the nerve (65). In partially paralyzed muscles, the response to a double stimulus shows an incremental response (66). However, in severely paralyzed muscles, the neuromuscular blockade may be so complete that repetitive stimulation may not be effective (67). Other EMG measurements appear to remain normal in botulism patients: in a report of an extensive EMG study made in a single type B botulism patient, the latency of facial nerve and upper limb motor and sensory conduction velocities remained normal (68).

Within- and between-species toxicity data from various sources for the type B toxin are difficult to compare, for several reasons:

1. Different end points (minimum lethal dose versus LD_{50}); reference species used (in some cases, the data are expressed as mouse lethal units, in other cases, as guinea pig lethal units).
2. Different normalizing units: units per milligram total nitrogen, per absorbance at different wavelengths, per milligram protein measured using different assays. (Interconversions between these units of measure are approximations at best.)
3. Probable differences in the purity of the toxin and/or percentage nicked versus unnicked toxin in the test material.
4. Differences in route of administration: intraperitoneal, subcutaneous, intravenous, oral, even inhaled.

However, as reported even in the earliest studies by van Ermengem, there appears to be species-specificity in terms of the relative sensitivity to type B toxin, with guinea pigs more sensitive to type B toxin than rats or rabbits (69).

Route of administration also appears to make a difference, at least in terms of the amount of the drug required for toxicity by various routes of administration. This should not be surprising, as pointed out in a paper by Lamanna (70):

> Poisoning of an animal by any mode of exposure to a toxin, including inhalation, will depend on the outcome of a sequence of four events: first, the capacity of the toxin to escape destruction inherent in the techniques of application; second, the capacity of the toxin to get to and to remain at the site of deposition where effective systemic absorption can take place; third, the capacity of the toxin after absorption to be transported to the primary site of poisoning; and fourth, the capacity of the toxin to resist specific or nonspecific forces of detoxification on route to the sites of action.

In this paper, for type B toxin, the rapidity of death (presumably inversely proportional to the amount of toxin required for overt toxicity) in rabbits appeared to differ significantly depending on the route of administration. The data, taken from an older article (71), are in Table 1. Note that time to death after injection of the toxin by the intraperitoneal route is significantly longer than after intramuscular injection. Intraperitoneal injection is the route typically used with mice to standardize the relative potency of various preparations of BTXs. Despite differences in the route of administration, the symptoms of poisoning were not apparently different. This is also consistent with toxicity data available for other BTXs.

A great difference in the relative toxicity of type A and type B toxins was also seen in the rat, in the study by Burgen et al. described above, where the LD_{50} (intraperitoneal injection) in 200 g rats of the two toxins were found to be approximately as follows: rat LD_{50}, type A toxin = 25 mouse LD_{50}; rat LD_{50}, type B toxin = 10,000 mouse LD_{50}. Sellin et al., in the comparable study, found that doses of type B toxin of 5000 mouse LD_{50}

Table 1 Order of Rapidity of Death of Rabbits by Various Routes of Injections of Botulinum Toxin Type B

Route	Time of death		
	days	hr	min
Intravenous		2	25
Intra-arterial		2	45
Intramuscular		4	30
Intracerebral		4	35
Intrapulmonary		5	0
Occipital		6	10
Subcutaneous		7	45
Eye anterior chamber		8	15
Intraperitoneal		9	5
Intrasciatic		10	53
Intragastric		33	45
Intrarectal	4	9	0

Source: From Legroux, Levarditi and Jéramec, 1945, as cited in Ref. 70.

caused debilitation or death (in contrast, only 20 mouse LD_{50} units of type A toxin caused similar toxicity). In the Lamanna paper, data were also given comparing the sensitivities of guinea pigs to different types BTX administered by various routes, as listed in Table 2. The doses in this table are expressed in mouse intraperitoneal units, in which one unit is the mouse LD_{50} dose by that route of administration. Whereas for BTX-A and BTX-B toxicity by the various routes is of the same order of magnitude, the type E toxin appeared to be much less toxic. Although no information about the bacterial source strains, level of purification, or pretreatment was provided, the difference is presumably due—at least in part—to the amount of nicking in the tested toxins. Type A toxin is always nicked by the organisms, type B may be (depending on whether the source strain was proteolytic or not), and type E toxin is not nicked endogenously.

In another report, using type B toxin crudely purified from a nonproteolytic strain (the toxin was therefore presumably mostly in an unnicked form), another comparison of route of administration versus test species was made (72). The results are summarized in Table 3. The data from this study suggest that the relative oral potency of this toxin preparation may have been much greater than for the toxin preparation cited by Lamanna. This may reflect the amount of nicking of the toxin (by the oral route, the toxin may have become activated in the gastrointestinal tract, while less activation occurred after parenteral administration).

No primate toxicity data for type B toxin were found in the literature, other than a single-animal, single-dose report. In this study, it was reported that for rhesus monkeys, oral administration of 100 guinea pig minimum lethal dose (least amount that will kill a 350 g guinea pig in 96 hours after subcutaneous injection) was lethal within 24 hours.

As part of our studies evaluating the effects of BTX-B in normal nonhuman primates, we also evaluated the potential toxicity of doses 10 to 20 times those that effectively paralyzed muscles. In these studies, the toxin was injected intramuscularly, in doses divided over five different muscles: the trapezius, abductor pollicis brevis, extensor digitorum brevis, gluteus maximus, and biceps femoris. Doses in this phase of the study ranged from total body doses of 120 to 480 U/kg total body weight. Toxicity was evaluated by clinical observations, clinical chemistries, ophthalmoscopic evaluations, electrocardiograms, and electrophysiological measurements: changes in peak evoked compound muscle action potential of muscles not injected with the drug (expected to be reduced if system weakening was caused by the drug), nerve conduction velocities of peripheral motor and sensory nerves (expected to change as a result of distal myelinopathies and axonopathies), and somatosensory evoked potentials to evaluate potential dysfunction

Table 2   Toxicity of Botulinum Toxins for the Guinea Pig by Various Routes

Type	Mouse intraperitoneal (ip) units		
	ip	oral	respiratory
A	5.2	840	141
B	4.8	413	350
E	78.0	456,000	778

Source: From M.A. Cardella and J.V. Jemski, personal communication, as cited in Ref. 70.

Table 3 Relative Susceptibility of Mice, Guinea Pigs, and Rabbits to Type B Toxin Administered Subcutaneously, or Orally, as Multiples of Number of Guinea Pig Minimum Lethal Subcutaneous Doses

Species	Route of administration	
	Subcutaneous	Oral
Mice	0.2	2
Guinea pigs	1	2
Rabbits	20	100

Source: Based on data from Ref. 72.

in the central nervous system. No signs of toxicity were observed, even after injection of a total of 480 U/kg, either when administered in a single dosing or when administered as two separate doses of 240 U/kg given 11 weeks apart. Specifically, there were no signs of autonomic nervous system deficits, ophthalmic changes, difficulty in swallowing, or inability to maintain normal posture, even at the highest dose tested. Electrocardiographic changes initially observed in a preliminary segment of the study were found to be the result of the ketamine and pentobarbital anesthesia regimen, rather than related to the toxin itself. The EMG studies also did not indicate any central or peripheral neuropathy or systemic muscle weakness, even at the highest doses tested. In one of the test groups, a dose of 240 U/kg was reinjected into the same animals less than 3 months after an initial dose of 240 U/kg. Again, in these animals, no signs of toxicity were observed, according to the measures listed above.

CLINICAL USES OF BOTULINUM TOXIN TYPE B

The relative clinical value of BTX-A and BTX-B in the treatment of cervical dystonia, or other movement disorders, is currently unknown. The structural and pharmacologic differences between the types of toxin, summarized above, suggest that they might not be therapeutically equivalent. Such differences, if real, are likely to be demonstrated only after injection into dystonic muscles. However, even assuming no specific therapeutic benefit of one toxin type over the other, type B toxin could still be useful for this indication. Because the two toxins are antigenically different (antibodies to type A do not block the effects of type B toxin, and vice versa, in animals or in vitro models), the two toxins could be used together, or in rotation, thus reducing antigenic presentation of either toxin. This, in turn, could delay, reduce, or prevent the development of resistance to toxin therapy. In those patients who have already developed resistance to botulinum toxin type A, the type B toxin could provide the best treatment available.

While our studies in nonhuman primates suggest that BTX-B may be effective and have an excellent therapeutic index, the actual effectiveness of this drug can be judged only after use in dystonia patients. The extrapolation of these results from normal nonhuman primates to dystonic humans assumes no major difference in terms of sensitivity to this specific serotype of the toxin, and no unique difference in muscle responsiveness associated with dystonia as opposed to normal muscles.

SUMMARY

The type B botulinum toxin has many biochemical and biological similarities to other serotypes of BTX. At the same time, there are some indications that the type B toxin may have some unique properties that could have beneficial clinical implications. Most obvious of these is that its amino acid sequence is sufficiently different from those of other serotypes that type A–resistant patients may respond to type B. The mechanistic differences in the mode of action of the various types of BTX have not yet been intensively studied under conditions that will allow prediction of clinical benefit (if any) to dystonia patients. Most of these studies to date have been performed in normal rodents or using in vitro/ex vivo models, which, because of interspecies differences in sensitivity to various types of the toxin, may not be directly applicable. Preliminary data from our laboratory, however, suggests that type B toxin effectively paralyzes nonhuman primate muscle after intramuscular injection and is possibly less likely to cause systemic toxicity than type A toxin.

REFERENCES

1. Van Ermengem E. A new anaerobic bacillus and its relation to botulism. Rev Infect Dis 1979;1:701–719. (An abridged translation of the original publication, Ueber einen neuen anaeroben Bacillus and seine Beziehungen zum Botulismus. Z Hyg Infecktionskr 1897;26:1–56.

2. Sakaguchi G. *Clostridium botulinum* toxins. Pharmacol Ther 1983;19:165–194.

3. Dolman CE, Murakami L. *Clostridium botulinum* Type F with recent observations on other types. J Infect Dis 1961;109:107–128.

4. Kozki S, Sakaguchi S, Sakaguchi G. Purification and some properties of progenitor toxins of Clostridium botulinum Type B. Infect Immun 1974;10:750–765.

5. Somers E, DasGupta BR. Clostridium botulinum Types A, B, C1 and E produce proteins with or without hemagglutinating activity: do they share common amino acid sequences and genes? J Protein Chem 1991;10:415–425.

6. Lamanna C, Lowenthal JP. The lack of identity between hemagglutinin and the toxin of Type A botulinum organism. J Bacteriol 1951;61:751–752.

7. Sugii S, Ohishi I, Sakaguchi G. Correlation between oral toxicity and in vitro stability of *Clostridium botulinum* type A and B toxins of different molecular sizes. Infect Immun 1977;16:910–914.

8. DasGupta BR. Activation of Clostridium botulinum Type B toxin by an endogenous enzyme. J Bacteriol 1971;108:1051–1057.

9. Tjaberg TB. Proteases of Clostridium botulinum. III. Isolation and characterization of proteases from Clostridium botulinum Types A, B, C, D, and F. Acta Vet Scand 1973;14:538–559.

10. DasGupta BR, Sugiyama H. Molecular form of neurotoxins in proteolytic Clostridium botulinum Type B cultures. Infect Immun 1976;14:680–686.

11. Sugiyama H, DasGupta BR, Yang KH. Disulfide-toxicity relationship of botulinal toxin Types A, E, and F. Proc Soc Biol Med 1973;143:589–591.

12. DasGupta BR, Sugiyama H. Comparative sizes of Type A and B botulinum neurotoxins. Toxicon 1977;15:357–363.

13. Schmidt JJ, Sathyamoorthy V, DasGupta B. Partial amino acid sequences of botulinum neurotoxins B and E. Arch Biochem Biophys 1985;238:544–548.

14. DasGupta BR. The structure of botulinum neurotoxin. In: Simpson LL, ed. *Botulinum neurotoxin and tetanus toxin*. San Diego: Academic Press, 1989:53–67.

15. DasGupta BR, Datta A. Botulinum neurotoxin type B (strain 657): partial sequence and similarity with tetanus toxin. Biochemie 1988;70:811–817.

16. Binz T, Kurazono H, Wille M, Frevert J, Wernars K, Niemann H. The complete sequence of Botulinum neurotoxin Type A and comparison with other clostridial neurotoxins. J Biol Chem 1990;265:9153–9158.

17. Hatheway CL, McCroskey LM, Lombard GL, Dowell VR. Atypical toxin variant of *Clostridium botulinum* type B associated with infant botulism. J Clin Microbiol 1981;14: 607–611.

18. Sakaguchi G. Clostridium botulinum toxins. Pharmacol Ther 1983;19:165-194.

19. Halpern JL, Smith LA, Seamon KB, Groover KA, Habig WH. Sequence homology between tetanus and botulinum toxins detected by an antipeptide antibody. Infect Immun 1989;57: 18–22.

20. Whelan SM, Elmore MJ, Bodsworth NJ, Brehm JK, Atkinson T, Minton N. Molecular cloning of the *Clostridium botulinum* structural gene encoding the Type B neurotoxin and determination of its entire nucleotide sequence. Appl Environ Microbiol 1992;58:2345–2354.

21. Kurazono H, Mochida S, Bintz T, Eisel U, Quantz M, Grebenstein O, Wernars K, Poulain B, Haberman H. Minimal essential domains specifying toxicity of the light chains of tetanus toxin and botulinum neurotoxin Type A. J Biol Chem 1992;267:14721–14729.

22. Simpson LL. Kinetic studies on the interaction between botulinum toxin type A and the cholinergic neuromuscular junction. J Pharmacol Exp Ther 1980;224:135–140.

23. Dolly JO, Black JD, Williams RS, Melling J. Acceptors for botulinum neurotoxin reside on motor nerve terminals and mediate its internalization. Nature 1984;307:457–460.

24. Wadsworth DF, Desai M, Tranter HS, King HJ, Hambleton P, Melling J, Dolly JO, Shone CC. Botulinum type F neurotoxin. Large-scale purification and characterization of its binding to rat cerebrocortical synaptosomes. Biochem J 1990;268:123–128.

25. Black JD, Dolly JO. Interaction of ^{125}I-labeled botulinum neurotoxins with nerve terminals. I. Ultrastructural audioradiographic localization and quantitation of distinct membrane acceptors for types A and B on motor nerves. J Cell Biol 1986;103:521–534.

26. Evans DM, Williams RS, Shone CC, Hambleton P, Melling J, Dolly JO. Botulinum neurotoxin type B. Its purification, radioiodination and interaction with rat-brain synaptosomal membranes. Eur J Biochem 1986;154:409–416.

27. Poulain B, Tauc L, Maisey EA, Wadsworth JDF, Mohan PM, Dolly JO. Neurotransmitter release is blocked intracellularly by botulinum neurotoxin, and this requires uptake of both toxin polypeptides by a process mediated by the larger chain. Proc Natl Acad Sci USA 1988;85:4090–4094.

28. Kozaki S. Interaction of botulinum toxin Type A, B, and E derivative toxins with synaptosomes of rat brain. Naunyn-Schmiedebergs Arch Pharmacol 1979;308:67–70.

29. Bandyopadhyay S, Clark AW, DasGupta BR, Sathyamoorthy V. Role of the heavy and light chains of botulinum neurotoxin in neuromuscular paralysis. J Biol Chem 1987;262:2660–2663.

30. Montecucco C. How do tetanus and botulinum toxins bind to neuronal membranes? Trends Biochem Sci 1986;11:314–317.

31. Simpson LL, Rapport MM. The binding of botulinum toxin to membrane lipids: sphingolipids, steroids and fatty acids. J Neurochem 1971;18:1751–1759.

32. Bakry N, Kamata Y, Simpson LL. Lectins from *Triticum vulgaris* and *Limax flavus* are universal antagonists of botulinum neurotoxin and tetanus toxin. J Pharmacol Exp Ther 1991;258:830–836.

33. Schengrund C-L, DasGupta BR, Ringler NJ. Binding of botulinum and tetanus neurotoxins to ganglioside GT 1b and derivatives thereof. J Neurochem 1991;57:1024–1032.

34. Kozaki S, Ogasawara J, Shimote Y, Kamata Y, Sakaguchi G. Antigenic structure of Clostridium botulinum Type B neurotoxin and its interaction with gangliosides, cerebroside and free fatty acids. Infect Immun 1987;55:3051–3056.

35. Shone CC, Hambleton P. Toxigenic clostridia. In: Minton NP, Clarke DJ, Eds. *Clostridia*. New York: Plenum Press, 1989:265–292.

36. Maisey EA, Wadsworth JDF, Poulain B, Shone CC, Melling J, Gibbs P, Tauc L, Dolly JO. Involvement of the constituent chains of botulinum neurotoxins A and B in the blockade of neurotransmitter release. Eur J Biochem 1988;177:683–691.

37. Stecher B, Weller U, Habermann E, Gratzl M, Ahnert-Hilger G. The light chain but not the heavy chain of botulinum A toxin inhibits exocytosis from permeabilized adrenal chromaffin cells. FEBS Lett 1989;255:391–394.

38. Simpson LL. The interaction between divalent cations and botulinum toxin Type A in the paralysis of the rat phrenic nerve–hemidiaphragm preparations. Neuropharmacology 1973;12:165–176.

39. Simpson LL. Kinetic studies on the interaction of botulinum toxin type A and the cholinergic neuromuscular junction. J Pharmacol Exp Ther 1980;212:16–21.

40. Montecucco C, Shiavo G, DasGupta, B. Effect of pH on the interaction of botulinum neurotoxins A, B, and E with liposomes. Biochem J 1989;259:47–53.

41. Hoch DH, Romero-Mira M, Ehrlich BE, Finkelstein A, DasGupta BR, Simpson LL. Channels formed by botulinum, tetanus, and diptheria toxins in planar lipid bilayers: relevance to translocation of proteins across membranes. Proc Natl Acad Sci USA 1985;82:1692–1696.

42. Bittner MA, DasGupta BR, Holtz RW. Isolated light chains of botulinum neurotoxins inhibit exocytosis. Studies in digitonin-permeabilized chromaffin cells. J Biol Chem 1989;264: 10354–10360.

43. Simpson LL. Targeting drugs and toxins to the brain: magic bullets. Int Rev Neurobiol 1988;30:123–147.

44. Ashton AC, Edwards K, Dolly JO. Lack of detectable ADP-ribosylation in synaptosomes associated with inhibition of transmitter release by botulinum neurotoxins A and B. Biochem Soc Trans 1988;16:883–884.

45. Niemann H, Bintz T, Grebenstein O, Kurazono H, Thierer J, Mochida S, Poulain B, Lauc L. Clostridial neurotoxins: from toxins to therapeutic tools? Behring Inst Mitt 1991;89:153–162.

46. Bhattacharyya SD, Sugiyama H. Inactivation of botulinum and tetanus toxins by chelators. Infect Immun 1989;57:3053–3057.

47. Gansel M, Penner R, Dreyer F. Distinct sites of action of clostridial neurotoxins revealed by double-poisoning of mouse motor nerve terminals. Pflugers Arch 1987;409:533–539.

48. Molgo J, DasGupta BR, Thesleff S. Characterization of the actions of botulinum neurotoxin type E at the rat neuromuscular junction. Acta Physiol Scand 1989;137:497–501.

49. Ashton AC, Dolly JO. Microtubule-dissociating drugs and A23187 reveal differences in the inhibition of synaptosomal transmitter release by botulinum neurotoxins types A and B. J Neurochem 1991;56:827–835.

50. Simpson LL. Use of pharmacologic antagonists to deduce communalities of biologic activity among clostridial neurotoxins. J Pharmacol Exp Ther 1988;245:867–872.

51. Burgen ASV, Dickens F, Zatman LJ. The action of botulinum toxin on the neuro-muscular junction. J Physiol 1949;109:10–24.

52. Sellin LC, Thesleff S, DasGupta BR. Different effects of types A and B botulinum toxin on transmitter release at the rat neuromuscular junction. Acta Physiol Scand 1983;119:127–133.

53. Sellin LC, Kauffman JA, DasGupta BR. Comparison of the effects of botulinum neurotoxins types A and E at the rat neuromuscular junction. Med Biol 1983;61:120–125.

54. Kauffman JA, Way JF, Siegel LS, Sellin LC. Comparison of the action of types A and F botulinum toxin at the rat neuromuscular junction. Toxicol Appl Pharmacol 1985;79:211–217.

55. Duchen LW. An electron microscopic study of the changes induced by botulinum toxin in the motor end plates of slow and fast skeletal muscle fibres of the mouse. J Neurol Sci 1971;14:47–60.

56. Diaz J, Molgó J, Pécot-Dechavassine M. Sprouting of frog motor nerve terminals after long-term paralysis by botulinum type A toxin. Neurosci Lett 1989;96:127–132.

57. Spencer RF, McNeer KW. Botulinum toxin paralysis of adult monkey extraocular muscle. Arch Ophthalmol 1987;105:1703–1711.

58. Alderson K, Holds JB, Anderson RL. Botulinum-induced alterations of nerve-muscle interactions in the human orbicularis oculi following treatment for blepharospasm. Neurology 1991;41:1800–1805.

59. Schantz EJ, Johnson EA. Properties and use of botulinum toxin and other microbial neurotoxins in medicine. Microbiol Rev 1992;56:80–99.

60. Tacket CO, Rogawski MA. Botulism. In: Simpson LL, ed. *Botulinum neurotoxin and tetanus toxin*. San Diego: Academic Press, 1989:351–378.

61. Hughes JM, Blumenthal JR, Merson MH, Lombard GL, Dowell VR, Gangarosa EJ. Clinical features of types A and B food-borne botulism. Ann Intern Med 1981;95:442–445.

62. Terranova W, Palumbo JN, Bremen JG. Ocular findings in botulism Type B. JAMA 1979;241:475–477.

63. Long SS, Gajewski JL, Brown LW, Gilligan PH. Clinical, laboratory and environmental features of infant botulism in southeastern Pennsylvania. Pediatrics 1985;75:935–941.

64. Donadio JM, Gangarosa EJ, Faich GA. Diagnosis and treatment of botulism. J Infect Dis 1971;124:108–112.

65. Cherington M. Electrophysiologic methods as an aid in diagnosis of botulism: a review. Muscle Nerve 1982;6:528–529.

66. Pickett J, Berg B, Chaplin E, Brunstetter-Shafer M-A. Syndrome of botulism in infancy: clinical and electrophysiological studies. N Engl J Med 1976;295:770–772.

67. Jablecki CK. Electrodiagnostic evaluation of patients with myasthenia gravis and related disorders. Neurol Clin 1985;3:557–572.

68. Martinez AC, Anciones B, Ferrer MT, Diez Tejedor E, Perez Conde MC, Bescansa E. Electrophysiologic study in benign human botulism type B. Muscle Nerve 1985;8:580–585.

69. Wright GP. The neurotoxins of *Clostridium botulinum* and *Clostridium tetani*. Pharmacol Rev 1955;7:413–464.

70. Lamanna C. Immunological aspects of airborne infections: some general considerations of response to inhalation of toxins. Bacteriol Rev 1961;25:323–330.

71. Legroux R, Levaditi JC, Jéramec C. Influence de voies d'introduction de la toxine sur le botulisme expérimentale du lapin. Ann Inst. Pasteur 1945;71:490–493.

72. Gunnison JB, Meyer KF. Susceptibility of monkeys, goats, and small animals to oral administration of botulinum toxin, types B, C, and D. J Infect Dis 1930;46:335–340.

7

Production and Properties of Type F Toxin

Tomoko Shimizu
Chiba Serum Institute, Ichikawa-shi, Chiba, Japan

Genji Sakaguchi
Japan Food Research Laboratories, Osaka Branch, Osaka, Japan

INTRODUCTION

Clostridium botulinum toxin is classified into seven types, A through G, based on the antigenicity of the toxic component. Therapy for strabismus was initiated with type A crystalline toxin (1), which has been used since then to treat various kinds of dystonia. In October 1987, the authors became aware of a patient in the United States who developed an unusual form of dystonia of the back of the tongue resulting in marked difficulty speaking. He was looking for botulinum toxin of a type other than types A–E, since he had received a pentavalent (A–E) botulinum vaccine years before when he was participating in studies on botulism. We decided to formulate type F toxin. Later, we became aware that there were a considerable number of patients who were not responding to type A toxin because of the development of antibodies. It was thought that they might also benefit from treatment with botulinum toxin of a type other than type A. Formulation was finished in December 1988, and all necessary assays were completed in March 1989. Therapeutic trials with type F were initiated in the United States at the beginning of 1991.

Following are the protocols of production and the properties of formulated type F toxin. Clinical trials have been reported by Ludlow et al. (2) and are updated in chapter 19.

TOXIN PRODUCTION

Clostridium botulinum type F strain Langeland (the type F prototype strain, proteolytic) was used (3). Tubes of a suspension of about 1000 viable spores/ml in 0.05 M acetate buffer, pH 5.0, were kept frozen. One of the tubes was thawed and inoculated into the medium for toxin production (1000 spores/5 L). The medium for toxin production consisted of glucose (1.0%), yeast extract (1.0%, Oriental Yeast, Osaka), peptone (2.0%, Mikuni Sangyo Co., Tokyo), and 0.025% sodium thioglycolate with pH 7.0, and was dispensed into two 5-L flat-bottomed spherical flasks. The culture was incubated for 4 days at 30°C. The toxicity of the culture reached about 100,000 mouse ip LD_{50}/ml.

PURIFICATION OF TYPE F PROGENITOR TOXIN

Step 1: Acid Precipitation

The whole culture, pH 5.6, was acidified to pH 4.0 by adding 3N sulfuric acid and allowed to stand overnight in a refrigerator (3). The clear supernatant fluid was removed by siphoning. The precipitate in the bottom fluid was packed by centrifugation at 6000 rpm for 10 min. The packed precipitate was resuspended in 0.2 M phosphate buffer, pH 6.0 (0.08 volume of the culture).

Step 2: Ammonium Sulfate Fractionation

A 0.25 volume of a saturated ammonium sulfate solution was added to the suspension. The precipitate formed in 30 min at room temperature (mostly nontoxic material) was removed by centrifugation. The toxin in the supernatant was precipitated at 70% saturation of ammonium sulfate. The precipitate formed was dissolved in 0.1 M acetate buffer, pH 4.5 (0.004 volume of the culture).

Step 3: The Second Acid Precipitation by Dialysis

The above solution was dialyzed against 0.05 M acetate buffer, pH 4.5. The toxin was precipitated in the dialysis casing. The precipitated toxin was collected by centrifugation and washed with 0.2 M sodium chloride–0.05 M acetate buffer, pH 4.5. The washed precipitate, containing most of the toxic activity, was dissolved in 0.5 M sodium chloride–0.05 M acetate buffer, pH 4.5. The residual precipitate was extracted three times with the same buffer. All the extracts were combined and clarified by centrifugation.

Step 4: Protamine Treatment

An equal quantity of 0.5 M sodium chloride–0.05 M citrate buffer, pH 4.5, was added to the extract. A 2.0% water solution of protamine sulfate (salmon sperm origin, Seikagaku Kogyo Co., Tokyo) was added to the extract until the A_{260}/A_{280} ratio of the supernatant became 1.0 or lower.

Step 5: SP-Sephadex Chromatography

The above solution was diluted with distilled water to lower the sodium chloride concentration to 0.2 M and adjusted to pH 4.2 with 1 M acetic acid. The diluted toxin solution was applied to a column of SP-Sephadex C-50 (Pharmacia Fine Chemicals, Uppsala, Sweden) equilibrated with 0.1 M sodium chloride–0.05 M acetate buffer, pH 4.2. Type F progenitor toxin was adsorbed onto the column, which was eluted by linear gradient increase in sodium chloride concentration from 0.1 M to 0.6 M in 1000 ml of the buffer. The toxin fractions eluted were collected, pooled, and concentrated to a small volume by ultrafiltration through Amicon PM-30 membrane (Amicon Co., Lexington, Massachusetts).

Step 6: Gel Filtration on Sephadex G-200

The concentrated toxin was applied onto a column (2.5 × 100 cm) of Sephadex G-200 (Pharmacia Fine Chemicals) equilibrated with 0.2 M sodium chloride–0.1 M acetate buffer, pH 6.0. Type F toxin was eluted in the void volume.

Step 7: Re–Gel Filtration on Sephadex G-200

The eluted toxin described above was concentrated by ultrafiltration and subjected to re–gel filtration under the same conditions. The purified type F toxin, with a molecular weight of about 300,000, contained approximately 1×10^8 mouse ip LD_{50}/mg protein nitrogen. From a 10-L culture, about 10 mg of purified type F progenitor toxin was obtained.

CHARACTERIZATION OF TYPE F PROGENITOR TOXIN

The purified toxin (4) appeared to be homogeneous, with a molecular weight of about 300,000 (a molecular weight of 235,000 was reported by us, but the value was corrected by DasGupta et al. [5]), and was dissociated into two components, toxic and nontoxic, of the same molecular sizes upon exposure to pH 7.5–8. The maximum absorption of the progenitor toxin was at 278 nm and the minimum at 250 nm, with an A_{278}/A_{250} ratio of 2.86. In the agar gel diffusion test with anti–purified type F toxin rabbit serum, purified type F toxin formed two distinct precipitation lines, as was the case with M toxin of any other type. It was also confirmed that type F derivative toxin (dissociated toxic component) was much more labile than was the progenitor toxin (the toxin complex), particularly at pH below 5.

These results show that *C. botulinum* type F produces M toxin only as a progenitor toxin, which is composed of one molecule each of the toxic component and the nontoxic component of the same molecular weights of about 150,000.

PREPARATION OF BULK MATERIAL

The purified toxin, kept for some period in a frozen state, was tested for toxic potency and specific activity by the mouse intraperitoneal inoculation test. The results indicate that the toxin was so diluted as to contain about 10^5 mouse ip LD_{50}/ml. The protein concentration was 50 μg/ml. The specific toxicity was found to be 1.25×10^7/mg N. To this dilution, human serum albumin (HSA) was added as a stabilizer at a concentration of 2.5 mg/ml. We adopted an HSA product of Japanese Red Cross, which met the Minimum Requirements of Biological Products (6) and proved to be free from AIDS and hepatitis viruses. The solution was filtered through a membrane of 0.22-μm pore size (Sterimax, Japan Millipore Ltd., Tokyo). During the sterility test, the filtrate was kept in a refrigerator for 2 weeks. The loss of potency by the filtration was less than 30% (Table 1).

PREPARATION OF FINAL PRODUCT

The bulk material was diluted with a sterilized HSA solution just before the freeze-drying process. Bottling was done as quickly as possible, and mild conditions were selected for the freezing and drying schedule. The process was finished within 2 days. In our system,

Table 1 Recoveries of Toxic Potency During Steps of Production of Type F and A Toxins

Steps	Type F lot 1 (LD$_{50}$/ml) (%)	Type A lot 1 (LD$_{50}$/ml) (%)	Type A lot 2 (LD$_{50}$/ml) (%)	Type A lot 3 (LD$_{50}$/ml) (%)
Bulk material	1,100 (100)	400 (100)	500 (100)	90 (100)
Final bulk	994 (90)	330 (83)	370 (74)	84 (93)
Final product	837 (76)	303 (76)	358 (72)	100 (111)

handling 500 to 1500 vials as one lot is convenient for production of botulinum toxin, without being accompanied by any significant loss of potency, as shown in Table 1.

PROPERTIES OF FINAL PRODUCT

The ingredients of a vial of freeze-dried botulinum toxin type F were botulinum toxin type F, 2000 units (2 μg of protein); human serum albumin, 6000 μg without any preservative; and attached solvent, 10 ml of normal saline.

For assay of the final product of type F toxin, we applied the addendum of Minimum Requirements of Biological Products for freeze-dried crystallized type A botulinum toxin put forward by the National Institute of Health, Tokyo. Tests of the product were made in regard to the following items:

1. Color and appearance of the freeze-dried cake and reconstituted solution
2. Moisture content
3. The time required for reconstitution
4. pH
5. Osmotic pressure
6. Protein content
7. Albumin content
8. Sterility
9. Freedom from abnormal toxicity
10. Pyrogenicity
11. Potency
12. Neutralization with Type F antitoxin

The detailed methods for testing are described in Minimum Requirement for Biological Products (6).

We tried to compare the results with those for type A toxin (Table 2). (1) In appearance the freeze-dried cakes were like thin white disks, some of which had a few cracks. The cakes were about 25 mm in diameter and 5 mm in thickness. (2) The moisture content of the products was less than 3%. (3) When 10 or 20 ml of the attached solvent was introduced into a vial, the content was completely dissolved to a transparent and colorless solution within 10 seconds. (4) The pH of the reconstituted solution was 5.8. (5) Its osmotic pressure was isotonic to physiological saline. (6) The protein content of the reconstituted solution was 6 mg/ml. Almost all of this was HSA added as a stabilizer. The

Table 2 Properties of Type F and A Toxins

Test item	Type F toxin	Type A toxin
Material toxin		
Molecular size	10S (200–300 kD)	19S (500–900 kD)
Form	Amorphous	Crystalline
Specific toxicity	10^7 LD_{50}/mg N	10^8 LD_{50}/mg N
Final product		
1. Appearance	White cake with cracks in a 20-ml vial. After reconstitution, colorless and transparent	White cake with cracks in a 10-ml vial. After reconstitution, colorless and transparent
2. Moisture content (%)	0.8–1.5	0.7–1.6
3. Time for reconstitution (sec)	7–10	7–10
4. pH	5.8	5.5–6.0
5. Osmotic pressure (mOsm/kg H_2O)	275	260–280
6. Protein content (mg protein/vial)	6	6–7.5
Toxin protein content (μg/vial)	2	0.02
7. Albumin content (%)	94–99	97–99
8. Sterility test	Pass (no growth of organisms)	Pass (no growth of organisms)
9. Test for freedom from abnormal toxicity	Pass (354 g→390 g, 366 g→408 g, 366g→D)	Pass (367 g→414 g, 355 g→380 g, 356 g→D)
10. Pyrogen test	Pass (0.75°C)	Pass (1.10°C)
11. Potency test (units/vial)	2400	293
12. Neutralization test	1/63L + = 80 units	1/63L + = 15 units

amount of HSA introduced into each vial was 6 to 8 mg. (7) In thin-layer electrophoresis, only a single peak of albumin was observed. (8) Sterility was checked at every step of the preparation processes, because no preservative at all was used throughout the processes. (9) To check for abnormal toxicity, two or three guinea pigs, weighing 300–400 g, were used. It was necessary to add less than a 1/50 portion of botulinum antitoxin type F to the inoculum (5 ml); otherwise the inoculated animals would certainly die on the day after inoculation. We observed a little weight loss just after the inoculation, but the animals restored their body weights very soon, within 5 days, provided that they were given type F antitoxin with the type F toxin preparation. (10) The pyrogen test also was made with type F toxin containing type F antitoxin. No pyrogen response was observed in any rabbit. (11) The potency test is the most important for this product. No other method is available to detect such a small amount of toxin, in the nanogram range, other than the mouse inoculation tests. We repeated the mouse intraperitoneal inoculation test more than 10 times before determining the toxic potency. Female mice of the ddy strain, 4 weeks old, weighing 16 to 20 g, were used. The average of the titers was 2400 mouse ip LD_{50} per vial. We decided to label the vials as containing 2000 U/vial. (12) The toxin was neutralized specifically with botulinum antitoxin type F. One-sixty-third unit of International Standard Botulinum Antitoxin Type F neutralized 80 units of the type F toxin prepared. The larger the amount of the toxin neutralized with a constant test level of antitoxin, the smaller the amount of toxoid contained by the toxin preparation. For testing type A toxin, we adopted 1/63 L + level of antitoxin because this level of type A antitoxin neutralizes approximately 1 ng or 25 mouse ip LD_{50} of crystalline type A toxin. Since a unit of type A antitoxin and one of type F antitoxin are not comparable to each other, further tests will be necessary to select an adequate test level of type F antitoxin. The larger the amount of toxoid injected, the larger the amount of antibody produced by the patient. The antitoxin produced by the patient would hinder the efficacy of the toxin. This should be prevented. According to our experiences, horses respond significantly more weakly to type F toxin than to type A toxin. This is the reason why 10,000 IU each of types A, B, and E antitoxins but only 4000 IU of type F antitoxin was required for each vial of our botulinum tetravalent antitoxin for therapy, in Minimum Requirements of Biological Products (6).

STABILITY OF TYPE F TOXIN

It is believed that a freeze-dried biological product is stable for a long period of time, such as 10 years or more. In fact, freeze-dried botulinum antitoxin is effective for more than 10 years. During storage, toxins of biological origin, even highly purified ones, gradually lose their activities and change into toxoid. We have repeated the potency tests of the product after keeping it in a refrigerator below 4°C for more than 3 years. In the type F toxin preparation, we have found no change in potency or any other item checked during these years from the time of its production. We found a decrease in potency to half of its original value in 2½ years with the first lot of crystalline type A toxin. With the second and the subsequent lots of type A toxin and type F toxin, the initial toxicities have been maintained for more than 3 years.

Once the toxin is reconstituted, the solution is unstable because it does not contain any preservative. The reconstituted solution, therefore, must be used within 3 hr. In 1–2 hr from the reconstitution of type F toxin, we sometimes noticed fine fluffs in the solution. Such fluffs had no relation with the potency of type F toxin.

REFERENCES

1. Schantz EJ, Scott AB. Use of crystalline type A botulinum toxin in medical research. In: Lewis GE, ed. Biomedical aspects of botulism. New York: Academic Press, 1981:143–148.
2. Ludlow CL, Hallett M, Rhew K, Cole R, Shimizu T, Sakaguchi G. Therapeutic use of type F botulinum toxin. N Engl J Med 1992;326:349–350.
3. Ohishi I, Sakaguchi G. Purification of *Clostridium botulinum* type F progenitor toxin. Appl Microbiol 1974;28:923–928.
4. Ohishi I, Sakaguchi G. Molecular construction of *Clostridium botulinum* type F progenitor toxin. Appl Microbiol 1975;29:444–447.
5. DasGupta BR, Sugiyama H. Single chain and dichain forms of neurotoxin in type F *Clostridium botulinum* culture. Toxicon 1977;15:466–471.
6. Association of Biologicals Manufacturers of Japan. Minimum Requirements of Biological Products (English version). 1986.

8

Immunogenicity of the Neurotoxins of *Clostridium botulinum*

Charles L. Hatheway
National Center for Infectious Diseases, Centers for Disease Control and Prevention, Atlanta, Georgia

Carol Dang*
Smith-Kettlewell Eye Research Institute, San Francisco, California

INTRODUCTION

The immunologic aspects of the botulinum neurotoxin (BTX) molecule are of particular interest when the toxin is used for therapeutic purposes, because an immune response of a patient under treatment can well render the toxin useless. This chapter will cover the immunologic studies pertaining to development and use of toxoids for active immunization of humans, since the results of these studies indicate the degree and effectiveness of the immune response when it is evoked purposely. Means of assessing the immune response will be covered, and details for determining neutralizing antibody levels in serum by the mouse bioassay will be presented. Finally, we present our findings of evidence of immune response in patients under treatment with BTX.

IMMUNOGENICITY OF BACTERIAL PROTEIN TOXINS

Behring and Kitasato reported in 1890 that animals injected with sublethal amounts of purified diphtheria and tetanus toxins developed an immunity to the diseases caused by the organisms and their toxins. The immunity was mediated by a component of the blood as well as of the extravascular fluid; it could be conferred on nonimmunized animals by transfusion (1). The discovery of "antitoxins," later recognized as specific antibody proteins of the blood, immediately opened the way for effective treatment by serotherapy.

Present affiliation: Allergan, Inc., Berkeley, California.

ANTITOXINS AGAINST BOTULINUM NEUROTOXINS

After van Ermengem established in 1897 that botulism is caused by a bacterial toxin (2), Kempner (3) succeeded in producing an antiserum to BTX in goats by administering increasing doses of toxic cultures and subsequently injecting concentrated toxin recovered from cultures by precipitation. Leuchs (4) discovered that there were differences between strains of organisms that caused different outbreaks of botulism, and that the antitoxins that neutralized their toxins were serologically distinct. In 1919, the designations of type A and B toxins and their corresponding antitoxins were established on the basis of studies by Burke (5). Types C, D, E, F, and G followed in sequence as strains were discovered whose toxins could not be neutralized with the existing antitoxins (6). Antitoxins generally are more stable than toxins, and they are therefore used as standards by which to define the toxins as well as other antitoxin reagents. International standards for *Clostridium botulinum* antitoxins were established in 1963 for types A, B, C, D, E (7), and F (8) and were made available through the World Health Organization. These serve as reference reagents for qualitative and quantitative standardization of botulinum toxins and antitoxins throughout the world. Diagnostic antitoxins that are satisfactory for specific identification of the toxins, but less precise quantitatively, are available in the United States from the Centers for Disease Control and Prevention (CDC). Therapeutic antitoxins of equine origin for treatment of botulism in humans are also available from the CDC.

In general, there are no cross-neutralizations of BTXs by antitoxins of heterologous types. Exceptions to this are minor cross-reactivities between types C and D (9) and between types E and F (10,11).

ACTIVE IMMUNIZATION OF HUMANS
WITH BOTULINUM TOXOIDS

Development of Toxoids at Fort Detrick

Since humans can be effectively protected from tetanus and diphtheria by active immunization, it follows by analogy that the same protection against botulism can be attained. Since botulism is such a rare disease, it has not been necessary to consider widespread immunization. Laboratory workers who handle the toxins or the organisms that produce them are an obvious group with an increased risk of intoxication by BTX. Consideration of the potential use of BTX as a biological warfare weapon prompted the military establishment to develop means of protecting troops against this threat. The U.S. Army Biological Laboratories at Fort Detrick, Maryland, developed a pentavalent botulinum toxoid for protecting humans against toxin types A, B, C, D, and E (12,13). This product has been made available through the CDC under an investigational new drug (IND) exemption by the U.S. Food and Drug Administration, since its limited use has not generated the volume of safety and efficacy data necessary for a "licensed product." The experience of immunization of experimental animals and humans with monovalent and polyvalent toxoids should be helpful in assessing the immunity problems that might arise from the therapeutic use of BTX.

Preparation of Botulinum Toxoids

Toxins from well-characterized strains of *C. botulinum* of each of the first five toxin types were partially purified, inactivated with formaldehyde, standardized, and combined with aluminum phosphate gel, which served as an immunizing adjuvant. The pentavalent

Table 1 Antigen Content of Botulinum Toxoids Used for Human Immunization[a]

Type	Purity LD$_{50}$/mg N[b]	Antigen concentration LD$_{50}$/ml	Antigen concentration mg protein[c]/ml	Single human dose LD$_{50}$	Single human dose mg protein
A	1.75×10^8	6×10^5	0.02125	3×10^5	0.0106
B	1.75×10^8	4×10^5	0.01428	2×10^5	0.0072
C	7.50×10^6	5×10^4	0.04167	2.5×10^4	0.0208
D	2.50×10^8	2×10^5	0.00500	1×10^5	0.0025
E	2.5×10^7	1×10^5	0.02500	5×10^4	0.0125

[a]LD$_{50}$ refers to biological activity before inactivation with formaldehyde.
[b]N = Nitrogen as determined by Kjeldahl method.
[c]Protein calculated as $6.25 \times$ N.

product was prepared by combining monovalent toxoids of the individual toxin types. The purity and composition of the toxoid antigens are listed in Table 1. The activity of each toxoid is expressed as mouse lethality before inactivation with formaldehyde. Before combining with adjuvant and testing for immunogenicity, each fluid toxoid is tested for innocuity (lack of toxicity). A satisfactory test requires the subcutaneous injection of 20–40 human doses in guinea pigs without causing adverse effects.

Immunogenicity Testing of Botulinum Toxoids in Animals

Standards for immunogenicity of pentavalent botulinum toxoid are contained in the protocols included in the approved IND application held by the CDC for the toxoid. Immunogenicity of monovalent and pentavalent toxoid preparations is evaluated by subcutaneous injection of guinea pigs (300–400 g) with single doses of 1 ml. Thirty days later, serum samples are obtained from immunized animals for determining the level of toxin-neutralizing antibodies, using mouse protection tests (described below). Levels are expressed as antitoxin units (IU) per milliliter. A minimum response of guinea pigs, determined by neutralizing antibodies, must be attained for each component of the vaccine. In addition, groups of immunized guinea pigs are challenged by intraperitoneal inoculation with 10^5 mouse LD$_{50}$ of each of the types of the corresponding toxins (for type A toxin, this is 2×10^4 guinea pig lethal doses). At least 50% of the guinea pigs must survive challenge with each of the toxins.

The relationship between serum antitoxin titer and level of resistance to challenge is shown in Fig. 1 (13). For all types, guinea pigs showing even the minimum demonstrable level of antitoxin had more than 50% survival of challenge with 10^5 mouse median lethal doses of toxin. At higher serum antitoxin levels (generally requiring more than one injection of toxoid), animals were resistant to challenges as high as 10^7 to 10^8 mouse LD$_{50}$.

Immunization of Humans with Botulinum Toxoids

Based on observations in animal studies, immunization trials with the toxoids were performed with humans, and the satisfactory dose (Table 1) and injection schedule in use today were established. The full immunization course consists of an initial series of three deep subcutaneous injections of 0.5 ml at 0, 2, and 12 weeks, and a booster at 1 year after the initial rejection (13). Subsequent boosters are scheduled at 2-year intervals.

Evaluation of pentavalent toxoid preparations and of the immunization schedule showed that the large majority of human recipients had measurable titers of neutralizing

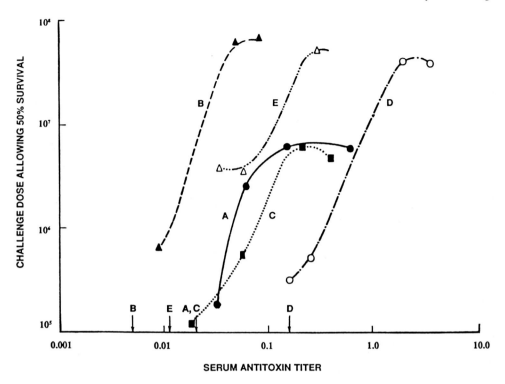

Figure 1 Resistance to intraperitoneal challenge as a function of serum antitoxin titer in guinea pigs. (From Ref. 13; used with permission of the author.)

antibodies to each of the five types of toxin after the third injection (12 weeks), and essentially all had satisfactory titers for each type after the 1-year booster (13). For type A toxin the titers were less than 0.02–0.30 IU/ml after the initial series, and 0.03–6.40 IU/ml after the booster at 1 year.

Since 1975, the CDC has been evaluating serum levels of type A, B, and E antitoxins in toxoid recipients who are due for subsequent 2-year boosters. This is to avoid giving unnecessary boosters. Boosters are given only if serum antitoxin levels are less than 0.25 IU/ml for any of the toxin types. The antigenicity of the toxoids as observed through these titer evaluations has been quite satisfactory. Two different lots have been distributed during this period. Some recipients who have had a history of multiple boosters before the evaluation policy was established have maintained adequate titers for 10 years or more after their last booster. Studies reported by Siegel (14,15) on antitoxin levels in recipients of the currently distributed pentavalent toxoid show strong responses to type A, B, and E components. The type A postbooster titers (5.74–51.6 IU/ml) were usually several times higher than the type B titers (1.26–18.2 IU/ml) (15). The type E titers were often higher (0.61–10.0 IU/ml) than the type B titers, but in view of the lower toxin-neutralizing potency of the type E unit (7), the protection against type E toxin was actually lower in every case. Despite the reported cross-immunity to type F toxin induced by type E antitoxin (10,11), no neutralization of type F toxin was demonstrable in any of the recipients' sera.

TESTING FOR ANTIBODIES TO BOTULINUM TOXIN

Antibodies to any antigen can be demonstrated by one or more of a variety of serologic reactions. Unfortunately, antibodies produced against a given antigen can be directed against a variety of components in the antigen preparation, or against different epitopes of a highly purified single protein. In consideration of immunity against a toxin, only those antibodies that effectively neutralize the biologic activity of the toxin are relevant. Two methods for detecting antibodies against botulinum neurotoxin will be described: the mouse bioassay and the enzyme immunosorbent assay (ELISA).

Mouse Bioassay

The standard method for detecting and quantitating botulinum antitoxins has been the mouse protection bioassay. This assay tests the ability of increasing dilutions of the serum to inactivate the lethality of a test dose of the neurotoxin. Mouse protective end points are determined for the test serum, and also for the standard antitoxin of known unitage, which is titrated simultaneously. The results can be assumed to correlate with level of immunity in the subject from whom the blood sample was obtained, and the specificity of the protection is defined by the test toxin used in the assay. Details for performing the assay and calculating the results in terms of international units (IU) per milliliter are presented below.

Enzyme-Linked Immunosorbent Assay

Antibody-detection assays generally are derived by modifying antigen-detecting assays. A number of in vitro assay methods have been proposed for detecting and quantitating BTXs. Among these, the ELISA has become the method of choice (16). Tests for toxin involve coating the wells of a microtiter plate with a capture antibody, adding test samples to the coated wells, and then using a second antibody to detect the toxin bound by the capture antibody. The second antibody is detected by a specific anti-antibody conjugated to an enzyme such as alkaline phosphatase that catalyzes a chromogenic reaction. The intensity of the color in the well of each microtiter plate well is proportional to the amount of antigen captured by the first antibody.

The toxin ELISAs still present a number of problems. Systems employing polyclonal antibody reagents lack specificity, e.g., cross-reactions usually occur between types A and B toxins (17,18). The reaction intensity does not correlate well with biological activity of the toxin samples. Use of monoclonal antibodies (in particular, ones that neutralize biological activity) improves specificity, but lowers sensitivity; the minimum detectable level is increased, and the reaction intensity, or sensitivity (absorbance:mouse LD) varies for toxins derived from different strains. Using a monoclonal antibody–based *amplified* ELISA, Shone et al. (19) found that while the sensitivity was equivalent to that of the bioassay, not all type A toxins were detectable.

Tests for antibodies are performed by coating the microtiter plate wells with BTX, which serves as the capture antigen. This may be accomplished by direct absorption of the antigen to the plastic surface (14,20), or by mediating the adsorption by means of a specific antibody adsorbed to the surface. Antibodies in the test sample that recognize epitopes on the capture antigen are detected by an appropriate anti-antibody conjugated to an enzyme; for human antibodies, conjugates such as goat anti–human IgG/alkaline phosphatase or rabbit anti-human IgG/peroxidase may be used.

In attempting to detect antibodies that neutralize the biological activity of BTX by ELISA, the problems are more difficult than with the toxin assay. The antibodies in the serum samples of interest are unavoidably polyclonal. Evaluating the immune status of a person or an animal by testing serum samples would necessitate restricting the serologic epitopes of the toxin antigen to only those that are recognized by antibodies that can neutralize biologic activity. It is difficult to ascertain how this can be done. Even if a highly purified toxin with very high specific activity is used as the capture antigen, it is likely that denaturation of toxin molecules takes place during storage or in the process of adsorption onto the plastic surface of the microtiter plate. Direct adsorption of a protein to the wells is usually carried out at an alkaline pH, a condition under which BTXs are readily inactivated. Epitopes not accessible on biologically active molecules are likely to be exposed and recognized by antibodies produced by the immune system of the donor of the test sample. The interaction of irrelevant antibodies and epitopes probably is the reason for much of the sensitivity of in vitro assays. This would appear to be borne out by the lower intensity of reaction when monoclonal antibodies with neutralizing activity are used (16,19).

Shone et al. (20) used purified type A or type B toxins as the capture antigen, and while they generally found correlation of the ELISA reaction with protective potency among high-titered samples, the reactions with low-titered samples were barely above background. Siegel (14) tested sera from botulinum toxoid recipients by both mouse protection assays and ELISA for antitoxins of types A and B, also using purified toxins as the capture antigens. The correlation of ELISA results with mouse protection was especially poor for samples from recipients early in the immunization series. Overall, her conclusion was that ELISA results "cannot be extrapolated to toxin-neutralizing antibody levels."

Rubin et al. (21) tested serum samples from two infants who had botulism due to intestinal colonization with *C. botulinum* (infant botulism) for antibodies to BTX, using an ELISA method. They found moderately elevated titers 30 and 60 days after the onset of illness. At the CDC, we also have found that infants with botulism develop antibodies to crude toxin preparations detectable by ELISA, but only one of the ten we have been able to test adequately showed mouse protection (C.L. Hatheway, unpublished data).

PROTOCOL FOR PERFORMING THE MOUSE BIOASSAY FOR BOTULINUM ANTITOXIN

The mouse protection assay detects and quantitates the neutralization of biologic activity of BTXs by specific antibodies. The procedures described in this section are those used in the CDC laboratory for determining botulinum antitoxin levels in human toxoid recipients, as well as in therapeutic-antitoxin recipients (botulism patients), and in serum of animals immunized for the purpose of preparing special antitoxin reagents. They have also been used to determine the immune status of patients treated therapeutically with toxin.

Materials

Standard Antitoxins

International standards for *C. botulinum* antitoxins, types A, B, C, D, E, and F, have been available from the World Health Organization (WHO), through Staten Seruminstitute, Copenhagen, Denmark. These are carefully reconstituted with 50% aqueous glycerol to contain 25 IU/ml and are stored in a freezer at $-20°C$. One international unit of antitoxin was originally established as that amount of the antitoxic serum that would neutralize 10^4 mouse LD_{50} of toxin, for types A, B, C, and D; for type E, 1 IU would neutralize only 10^3 LD_{50} (7).

Toxins

1. Stable toxins. Ideally, toxins from the immunizing strains should be used. Those used in the CDC laboratory were derived from the strains used in the manufacture of the toxoids for human immunization. Toxins precipitated from trypticase–yeast extract–glucose cultures by acidification or by adding ammonium sulfate to half-saturation have been found to be stable in the precipitate and usable for more than 10 years. Precipitated toxins may be redissolved in 50% aqueous glycerol and stored at $-20°C$.
2. Culture supernatant toxins. The toxic supernatant from a culture of a strain of the desired type of *C. botulinum* provides a suitable source of toxin as long as the toxin level is at least 100 mouse LD_{50}/ml.
3. Type E toxins employed in the neutralization tests in the CDC laboratory are activated with trypsin before precipitation.

Mice

Eighteen- to 25-g ICR strain mice are satisfactory (22).

Diluent

All dilutions of test sera, antitoxin standards, or toxin are made with gelatin phosphate diluent (0.2% gelatin, 0.4% Na_2HPO_4, adjusted to pH 6.2 with HCl).

Test Procedure

A constant amount of toxin is tested against increasing dilutions of the test serum to determine the highest dilution that will neutralize the toxin (50% end point). Simultaneously, the toxin is tested against increasing dilutions of the antitoxin standard. The end point dilution of the test serum contains the same amount of antitoxin as the standard at its end point dilution. The amount of toxin used in the titrations has been predetermined as the amount that will be neutralized (50% end point) by a prescribed level of standard antitoxin. The prescribed level is considered the minimum amount of toxin that will produce reliable results and thus allow the greatest test sensitivity.

Determining Test Dilution for Each Toxin
The example given is for type A.

1. The test levels for toxin are prescribed as follows (types A through E, Ref. 13; type F, Ref. 23): type A, 0.02 IU/ml; type B, 0.005 IU/ml; type C, 0.02 IU/ml; type D, 0.16 IU/ml; type E, 0.0125 IU/ml; type F, 0.0025 IU/ml.
2. Eight microliters of the stock solution of type A antitoxin standard in 50% glycerol containing 25 IU/ml is added to 10 ml of diluent, making a dilution of 1:1250; this dilution contains 0.02 IU/ml.
3. A series of twofold dilutions of the type A test toxin is made over the range within which the end point is anticipated (e.g., 1:5000, 1:10,000, 1:20,000, 1:40,000, 1:80,000, 1:160,000).
4. One milliliter of the diluted antitoxin is added to 1 ml each of the six dilutions of the type A toxin.

5. The contents of each tube are mixed using a vortex mixer (avoiding formation of any bubbles or froth), then incubated for 1 hr at room temperature.
6. One syringe is filled with 0.8 ml for each toxin-antitoxin mixture; 0.2 ml is injected i.p. into each of four mice.
7. The mice are observed daily for 4 days, and deaths are recorded on the test record sheet.
8. After the final reading, the 50% end point dilution of the test toxin is calculated by the method of Reed and Muench (24). This dilution of toxin is used in tests for determining type A antitoxin levels in test sera. The test toxin dose for each of the other types of antitoxin is determined in an analogous fashion.

Testing Sera for Antitoxin Levels

1. Six dilutions of the test serum are made. Typically, for sera from toxoid recipients, they are 1:1, 1:4, 1:16, 1:64, 1:256, and 1:1024. This is done by adding 1.5 ml of serum to the first empty tube, and 0.5 ml to the second tube, which contains 1.5 ml of diluent. After mixing the second tube, 0.5 ml is transferred to the third tube, which also contains 1.5 ml of diluent. Subsequent transfers are made so that each tube is a 1:4 dilution of the previous one, and each contains 1.5 ml of the test serum dilution (0.5 ml from the sixth tube is removed and discarded after mixing).
2. Six dilutions of the antitoxin standard are made. Usually these are twofold dilutions that bracket the test level. Typically for the type A standard, these dilutions contain 0.08, 0.04, 0.02, 0.01, 0.005, and 0.0025 IU/ml. These dilutions are made by making an initial dilution containing 0.08 IU (1:312.5) and then doubling the dilutions (1.5 ml standard dilution + 1.5 ml diluent) in the tubes for the rest of the series.
3. One and one-half milliliters of toxin at the predetermined test dilution is added to each tube containing 1.5 ml of diluted test serum or antitoxin standard. The tubes are mixed with the vortex mixer (avoiding foaming) and incubated at room temperature for 1 hr.
4. While incubating, 0.8 ml from each tube can be drawn into 1 ml tuberculin syringes with 25-gauge, 5/8-inch needles.
5. One hour after beginning of incubation, 0.2 ml of each mixture is injected into four mice. Usually, eight test sera and the WHO standard are titrated on the same test day.
6. Mouse deaths are recorded for 4 days.
7. At least four mice are injected with 0.1 ml of the test toxin without any test serum. At least 75% of these control mice should die before the end of the fourth day after injection.
8. The 50% end points are calculated by the Reed and Muench method for both the test serum and the standard; the end point for the serum will be a dilution factor and for the standard it will be a unitage (IU/ml).
9. The units per milliliter in the test serum are equal to its end point dilution factor multiplied by the units per milliliter of the standard at its calculated end point.

Example of 50% End Point Calculations According to the Reed and Muench Method

A hypothetical antitoxin titration on a test serum sample is shown. The results are tabulated in Table 2 and calculated as follows:

Table 2 Data for Calculations of 50% End Points in Hypothetical Titration of Type A Antitoxin[a]

Test serum dilution	Mice		Cumulative		% survived
	Dead	Survived	Dead	Survived	
1:1	0	4	0	16	100
1:4	0	4	0	12	100
1:16	0	4	0	8	100
1:64	1	3	1	4	80
1:256	3	1	4	1	20
1:1024	4	0	8	0	0
WHO antitoxin (IU/ml)					
0.08	0	4	0	11	100
0.04	0	4	0	7	100
0.02	1	3	1	3	75
0.01	4	0	5	0	0
0.005	4	0	9	0	0
0.0025	4	0	13	0	0

[a]Data obtained from hypothetical mouse test.
WHO = World Health Organization.

1. Calculation of unitage at 50% end point of the WHO standard:

$$\text{log distance} = \frac{(\% \text{ surv. @ 0.02 IU/ml}) - 50\%}{(\% \text{ surv. @ 0.02 IU/ml}) - (\% \text{ surv. @ 0.01 IU/ml})} \times \text{log dilution factor}$$

$$= \frac{75 - 50}{75 - 0} \times \log 2 = \frac{25}{75} \times 0.301 = 0.001$$

$$\text{distance} = \text{antilog } 0.100 = 1.26$$
$$(\text{distance} = \text{the distance between 0.02 and 0.01})$$

$$50\% \text{ endpoint} = \frac{0.02 \text{ IU/ml}}{1.26} = 0.0159 \text{ IU/ml}$$

2. Calculation of 50% end point dilution of the test serum:

$$\text{log distance} = \frac{(\% \text{ surv. @ 1:64}) - 50\%}{(\% \text{ surv. @ 1:64}) - (\% \text{ surv. @ 1:256})} \times \text{log dilution factor}$$

$$= \frac{80 - 50}{80 - 20} \times \log 4 = \frac{30}{60} \times 0.602 = 0.301$$

$$\text{distance} = \text{antilog } 0.301 = 2.0$$
$$(\text{distance} = \text{the distance between 1:64 and 1:256})$$

$$50\% \text{ endpoint} = \frac{1/64}{2.0} = 1/128 = 1:128$$

3. Calculation of unitage of the test serum: The 1:128 dilution of the test serum contains 0.0159 IU/ml; the undiluted serum contains

$$128 \times 0.0159 \text{ IU/ml} = 2.03 \text{ IU/ml}$$

In summary, it can be seen from the table that the 50% end points are between the 1:64 and the 1:256 dilution of the test serum and between 0.02 and 0.01 IU/ml for the WHO antitoxin standard. The unitage of the standard at the 50% end point is calculated as 0.0159 IU/ml. The end point dilution of the test serum is calculated as 1:128, and thus contains 0.0159 IU/ml. The potency of the undiluted serum is equal to 0.0159 IU/ml multiplied by 128, which is 2.03 IU/ml.

MODIFICATIONS FOR TESTING SERA FROM PATIENTS TREATED WITH BOTULINUM TOXIN

The product used for treatment of the patients may serve as the test toxin in the neutralization tests if other sources of toxin are not readily available. This may be more appropriate in any case, since it is precisely the neutralization of this product that the physician is concerned about.

To increase the sensitivity of the test, a larger volume of patient serum may be tested against the test toxin. For example, when the size of the sample is sufficient, 2 ml of serum is placed in a tube, and 0.5 ml of the test toxin is added. After mixing and incubating, a syringe is filled with 2 ml of the mixture, and 0.5 ml is injected into each of four mice. Twofold dilutions of the serum may be made, and 0.5 ml of the test toxin is added to 2 ml of each dilution of serum: four mice are likewise injected with 0.5 ml of each dilution-toxin mixture in order to obtain the neutralization end point. In such a test, each mouse will receive 0.4 ml of test serum or dilution thereof and 0.1 ml of the toxin. This increases the sensitivity fourfold.

If one is interested only in qualitatively establishing that the patient has neutralizing antibodies, a titration is not necessary, and only the undiluted serum is tested against the toxin. A negative control serum should also be tested, and 100% of the mice should die because of its failure to neutralize the toxin. In general, screening tests may be made on undiluted sera, and only those showing neutralizing potency need to be titrated.

IMMUNE RESPONSE TO THERAPEUTIC INJECTIONS OF BOTULINUM TOXIN

In view of the antigenicity of the BTXs, an immune response to multiple injections, especially in larger doses, may be anticipated. Such a response would be expected to render further treatment with toxin useless. When certain patients who were initially helped by treatment showed no improvement with later injections of toxin, tests for antitoxin were performed on their sera. The tests were performed in the CDC Botulism Laboratory, since it was one of the few places where the mouse bioassay for botulism antitoxins was being used. When it became apparent that there would be a continuing need for these tests, arrangements were made with Dr. Alan Scott of the Smith-Kettlewell Eye Research Institute in San Francisco for performing tests in that facility.

Results of Immune Assessment of Patients

Between October 1984 and February 1988, 198 serum samples from BTX-treated patients were received, mainly from two clinics, and tested at the CDC. The results are shown in

Table 3 Characteristics of Serum Samples from Botulinum Toxin–Treated Patients Tested at the Centers for Disease Control for Botulinum Type A Antitoxin, 1984–1988.

Clinic	No. samples	Results	Titer	IU/ml
A	94	Neg	<1:1	<0.003
B	85	Neg	<1:1	<0.002
	13	Pos	1:1–1:40	0.002–0.101
C	2	Neg	<1:1	<0.002
	1	Pos	1:11	0.017
D	1	Neg	<1:1	<0.002
E	1	Neg	<1:1	<0.002
F	1	Pos	1:20	0.030

Table 3. All 94 samples from the first clinic were negative for neutralizing antibodies according to the mouse bioassay. Of 98 samples received from the second clinic, 13 were positive for neutralizing antibodies; for the 8 samples for which actual end points could be determined, the range of titers was 0.002–0.101 IU/ml. No information on the responsiveness of the patients or on the amount of toxin any of them had received was supplied.

Results of Continued Evaluation of Patients by the Smith-Kettlewell Institute

Tests performed at the Smith-Kettlewell Eye Research Institute employed as the test toxin the type A botulinum toxin (BTX-A) product used to treat patients. The toxin was used at a dilution that would result in the injection of 5 U (5 mouse lethal doses) mixed with 0.4 ml of patient serum into each of four mice. A result was considered negative if three or more mice died, and positive if three or more of the mice survived. When 0.4 ml of the WHO international standard for type A antitoxin was recently titrated at the CDC against 0.1 ml containing 5 U of this toxin product, the neutralizing end point was reached at 0.052 IU/ml. Thus, any serum samples that neutralized this test dose of toxin would have to contain at least 0.052 IU of antitoxin per milliliter.

Between October 1988 and May 1992, 195 serum samples were tested. Of these, 28 were known to be from patients who continued to be responsive to treatment, and all were negative. The remaining 167 serum samples were presumed to be from patients whose treating physician considered their therapeutic response abnormally low or absent. Of these 167 samples, 48 (28.7%) neutralized BTX-A. Three of the positive sera were quantitated: one sample contained 0.052 IU/ml, and two samples contained 0.104 IU/ml.

Complete data on the quantity of BTX injected 1 year before blood drawing were available for 88 patients in this study (Table 4). These patients received from 0 to 2550 U of toxin in that time period. Of these 88, 29 (33%) tested positive. The positive patients received an average of 1051 U, and the negative patients received an average of 301 U. The percent positive ranged from 2.6% of patients receiving less than 500 U or less to 84% of patients receiving 1000 U or more.

Table 4 Serum Samples from Botulinum Toxin–Treated Patients Tested at Smith-Kettlewell Eye Research Institute; Relation Between Toxin Received and Detection of Neutralizing Antibodies

| | Antitoxin test result | | |
Dosage	Positive[a]	Negative	% positive
< 500 U	2	43	4%
500–1000 U	11	13	45%
1000–2000 U	15	3	83%
> 2000 U	1	0	100%
Total	29	59	33%

[a]Positive sera contain 0.052 IU/ml or more of type A antitoxin.

DISCUSSION

In the early work on the botulinum toxoid, the relationship between measurable serum antitoxin levels in guinea pigs and resistance to the toxin was very clear (Fig. 1). At a titer of 0.1 IU/ml of type A antitoxin, guinea pigs resisted a challenge of about 6×10^6 LD_{50} of type A toxin. In those studies, it was also noted that immunized guinea pigs with titers below the detectable limit also had a significant level of protection (25). On the basis of body weight, a human should be able to neutralize about 150 times the amount tolerated by a guinea pig with a similar antitoxin titer.

Neutralization of BTX by specific antitoxin in in vivo and in vitro tests is very efficient. In a series of experiments, 1 IU of type A antitoxin neutralized approximately the same amount of toxin ($1.8–3.5 \times 10^4$ mouse LD_{50}) whether mixed in a tube and then injected immediately or incubated as long as 30 min before being injected into mice (22). Similar results were obtained when the antitoxin was injected separately into mice that were then challenged immediately, or at intervals up to 60 min. Thus, it would seem that the therapeutic efficacy of BTX would be extremely poor in a patient who had circulating antitoxin.

A person who is immunized with toxoid against BTX-A is injected three times with the equivalent of 3.5×10^5 U of toxin combined with an adjuvant. Bioassays performed after the first two injections are generally, if not always, negative. Two weeks after the third injection, one can expect a titer of about 0.05 IU/ml (13). This active immunization results from an exposure to much more antigen than a patient under treatment would probably receive in a lifetime. However, the BTX used for treatment of patients may be more effective antigenically than toxoid. Patients may actually be receiving a mixture of toxin and toxoid, and thus more antigen than is indicated by the measured biologic activity. Repeated injections of small amounts of antigen, or injections at multiple sites, are means sometimes used for enhancing an immune response in experimental animals.

The method we have endorsed for establishing the immune status of patients is the mouse bioassay. Some patients who are not responsive to treatment and are negative by the bioassay may nevertheless have had an immune response. Guinea pigs with minimally detectable antitoxin levels show a high resistance to toxin (13) (Fig. 1). Obviously, protective immunity can be substantial at levels slightly below the detectable limit. Other factors such as concomitant drug therapy and misinjections should be considered when evaluating nonresponsive patients. Further studies are needed to understand better the various factors contributing to response levels in patients.

Our mouse bioassays on serum samples from patients who continued to respond to treatment were negative for toxin-neutralizing antibodies. The 63 patients who tested positive for neutralizing antibodies should be presumed to be untreatable with the toxin. An estimated 3×10^4 to 3×10^6 mouse lethal doses of BTX-A toxin could be neutralized by antibodies in the circulation of those persons. Detection of neutralizing antibodies was correlated with the amount of toxin injected into the patient. Since we did not know the response status of many of the patients we tested, some unresponsive patients whose serum samples tested negative may possibly possess low levels of circulating antibodies that cannot be detected by the bioassay. Continued treatment of patients who have sub-detectable levels of antibodies might serve to boost the antitoxin titers above the minimum demonstrable level.

We have pointed out the shortcomings of the ELISA. The test results may show some correlation with immunity, but at this point in the development of the test, they certainly are not conclusive. It would be worthwhile to test by an ELISA method sera from both responding and nonresponding patients who have received multiple injections of BTX. Reactivity may be seen in the test without any interference with the activity of the toxin for some patients. There may be some threshold intensity of the reaction beyond which immunity to the toxin may be assumed. On the other hand, we may find that any ELISA reactivity is correlated with unresponsiveness. With more experience with the in vitro assay and improvement in its specificity, it may become a reliable means of assessing the immune status of patients.

SUMMARY

Botulinum neurotoxins are immunogenic. Experiments with immunization of animals with botulinum toxoids have shown that the neutralizing potency of sera as determined by mouse bioassay is clearly correlated with protection against challenge with neurotoxin. The biologic activity of the toxin is inactivated by the circulating antibodies. Immunized animals with subdetectable levels of antitoxin can have significant immunity to the toxin. Humans immunized with botulinum toxoid develop high levels of specific antitoxin and can be assumed to possess corresponding immunity to the toxins analogous to that of the experimental animals.

Circulating antitoxin has been detected in patients who have been treated repeatedly with botulinum toxin. This finding should make physicians aware that the choice of toxin dose and placement of toxin must be made most judiciously. Noting the long-lasting immunity in persons actively immunized against botulism, and the strong anamnestic response to boosters, it seems possible that patients who develop an immunity because of treatment with botulinum toxin will not be able to be effectively treated again with toxin of the same type. Efforts should be made to provide the most highly active toxin preparations for this use, to allow injection of the minimum amount of antigen. Some inactive toxin molecules may act as toxoid and contribute to development of neutralizing antibodies. Since there is no cross-neutralization between antitoxins and toxins of differing types, development of toxins of various types for treatment of neuromuscular problems may provide alternative means for continuing treatment after immunity occurs.

At present, the mouse bioassay is the only reliable means of determining the presence of neutralizing antibodies in the serum of humans or animals. The ELISA methods give results that are not well correlated with neutralization of the biological activity of the toxin. Adequate in vitro tests may be developed in the future, but they will have to be evaluated on samples from responding and refractory patients that have also been tested by the bioassay.

REFERENCES

1. Grundbacher FJ. Behring's discovery of diphtheria and tetanus antitoxins. Immunol Today 1992;13:188–190.

2. Van Ermengem E. Ueber einen neuen anaeroben Bacillus and seine Beziehungen zum Botulismus. Z Hyg Infektionskr 1897;26:1–56. (For abridged English translation, see Rev Infect Dis 1979;1:701–719.)

3. Kempner W. Weiterer Beitrag zur Lehre von der Fleischvergiftung. Das Antitoxin des Botulismus. Z Hyg Infektionskr 1897;26:481–500.

4. Leuchs J. Beitraege zur Kenntnis des Toxins und Antitoxins des *Bacillus botulinus*. Z Hyg Infektionskr 1910;65:55–84.

5. Burke GS. Notes on *Bacillus botulinus*. J Bacteriol 1919;4:555–565.

6. Smith LDS, Sugiyama H. Botulism: the organism, its toxins, the disease. Springfield, Illinois: Charles C. Thomas, 1988:23–38.

7. Bowmer EJ. Preparation and assay of the International Standards for *Clostridium botulinum* types A, B, C, D and E antitoxins. Bull WHO 1963;29:701–709.

8. Harrell WK, Green JH, Winn JF. Preparation, evaluation, and use of *C. botulinum* antitoxins. In: Lewis KH, Cassel K Jr, eds. Botulism; proceedings of a symposium. PHS Publ. No. 999 FP-1. Cincinnati: U.S. Public Health Service, 1964:165–174.

9. Shimizu T, Kondo H. Techniques for assaying C1, C2 and D botulinal antitoxins. In: Eklund MW, Dowell VR Jr, eds. Avian botulism. Springfield, Illinois: Charles C. Thomas, 1987:363–369.

10. Dolman CE, Murakami L. *Clostridium botulinum* type F with recent observations on other types. J Infect Dis 1961;109:107–128.

11. Yang KH, Sugiyama H. Purification and properties of *Clostridium botulinum* type F toxin. Appl Microbiol 1975;29:598–603.

12. Fiock MA, Cardella MA, Gearinger NF. Studies on immunity to toxins of *Clostridium botulinum*. IX. Immunologic response of man to purified pentavalent ABCDE botulinum toxoid. J Immunol 1963;90:697–702.

13. Cardella MA. Botulinum toxoids. In: Lewis KH, Cassel K Jr, eds. Botulism: proceedings of a symposium. PHS Publ. No. 999 FP-1. Cincinnati: U.S. Public Health Service, 1964:113–130.

14. Siegel LS. Human response to botulinum pentavalent (ABCDE) toxoid determined by a neutralization test and by an enzyme-linked immunosorbent assay. J Clin Microbiol 1988;26:2351–2356.

15. Siegel LS. Evaluation of neutralizing antibodies to type A, B, E, and F botulinum toxins in sera from human recipients of botulinum pentavalent (ABCDE) toxoid. J Clin Microbiol 1989;27:1906–1908.

16. Notermans S, Nagel J. Assays for botulinum and tetanus toxins. In: Simpson LL, ed. Botulinum neurotoxin and tetanus toxin. San Diego: Academic Press, 1989:319–331.

17. Dezfulian M, Bartlett JG. Detection of *Clostridium botulinum* type A toxin by enzyme-linked immunosorbent assay with antibodies produced in immunologically tolerant animals. J Clin Microbiol 1984;19:645–648.

18. Dezfulian M, Hatheway CL, Yolken RH, Bartlett JG. Enzyme-linked immunosorbent assay for detection of Clostridium botulinum type A and type B toxins in stool samples from infants with botulism. J Clin Microbiol 1984;20:379–383.

19. Shone C, Wilton-Smith P, Appleton N, et al. Monoclonal antibody–based immunoassay for type A *Clostridium botulinum* toxin is comparable to the mouse bioassay. Appl Environ Microbiol 1985;50:63–67.

20. Shone C, Appleton N, Wilton-Smith P, et al. In vitro assays for botulinum toxin and antitoxins. Dev Biol Standard 1986;64:141–145.

21. Rubin LG, Dezfulian M, Yolkin RH. Serum antibody response to *Clostridium botulinum* toxin in infant botulism. J Clin Microbiol 1982;16:770–771.

22. Hatheway CL, Ferreira MC, McCroskey LM. Evaluation of various factors in the mouse toxicity test for identification of botulinal toxin (abstr). Annual Meeting, American Society for Microbiology, Las Vegas, Nevada, 1985.

23. Hatheway CL. Toxoid of *Clostridium botulinum* type F: purification and immunogenicity studies. Appl Environ Microbiol 1976;31:234–242.

24. Reed LJ, Muench H. A simple method of estimating fifty percent endpoints. Am J Hyg 1938;27:493–497.

25. Fiock MA, Devine LF, Gearinger NF, Duff JT, Wright GG, Kadul PJ. Studies on immunity to toxins of *Clostridium botulinum*. VIII. Immunological response of man to purified bivalent AB botulinum toxoid. J Immunol 1962;88:277–283.

9

Systemic Effects of Botulinum Toxin

Dale J. Lange
The Neurological Institute, Columbia-Presbyterian Medical Center, New York, New York

INTRODUCTION

There are several toxins produced by the bacterium *Clostridium botulinum* that are potent and specific blockers of acetylcholine (ACh) release at cholinergic synapses, including the neuromuscular junction. They are among the most lethal toxins known to man. The most lethal of the botulinum toxins is type A. Estimates show that only 0.1 μg of toxin can cause a human death when taken orally (1).

Partial weakness occurs in a normal rat muscle injected with small amounts of botulinum toxin type A (BTX) and is followed by full recovery in 9 months (2). Diluted BTX to partially weaken chronically contracting muscle was first used in overactive eye muscles in children with strabismus, preventing the need for surgery (3). Botulinum toxin in small doses to partially weaken injected muscles is now used in a variety of disorders, as addressed in other chapters in this book (4–15). Despite the potential toxicity of BTX, few untoward effects have been encountered; however, weakness in muscles near the site of injection may occur, and *symptoms* of generalized weakness (16) or weakness in areas remote from the injection site (17) have been reported. This chapter will review the effects of BTX on the nervous system and the various systemic effects reported using small doses of BTX to control overactive muscles from various causes.

BACKGROUND

Botulinum toxin A binds to high-affinity recognition sites on the outside of cholinergic nerve terminals—i.e., those for which ACh is the neurotransmitter. Cholinergic nerve terminals are found in neuromuscular junctions of skeletal muscle as well as the autonomic nervous system. Binding of BTX to the presynaptic terminal decreases the amounts of ACh released after nerve depolarization. The lesser amounts of synaptic ACh result in inefficient neuromuscular transmission and consequent weakness. In autonomic neurons, the effects are less specific because of the dynamic relationship between cholinergic and adrenergic neurons. Patients with cholinergic blockade of the autonomic system show hypotension, nausea, vomiting, intestinal cramps, and pupillary dilatation.

At the neuromuscular junction, ACh is synthesized by the enzyme choline acetyltransferase in the presynaptic terminal from acetyl coenzyme A and choline and stored in vesicles in the presynaptic neuron (Fig. 1). The vesicles release their contents (ACh molecules) into the synapse spontaneously (one at a time) or en masse when a nerve action potential arrives at the synaptic terminal. The ACh molecules traverse the synapse to bind with ACh receptors (AChRs) on the postsynaptic muscle membrane. The ACh-AChR interaction causes ionic channels in the adjacent membrane to open, and the resulting ionic movement produces local depolarization. The ACh in the vesicles released spontaneously produces a small local depolarization of the muscle membrane (miniature end plate potential [MEPP]) that is not propagated beyond the region of the synapse. The many ACh-AChR interactions that occur when many vesicles are released after nerve terminal depolarization result in a large, local depolarization of the postsynaptic muscle membrane (end plate potential [EPP]). If the EPP is sufficiently large (determined by the number of receptors with successful ACh binding), a propagated action potential in the muscle membrane occurs and results in myofibril activation and muscle contraction (18).

Botulinum toxins interfere with cholinergic transmission by irreversibly blocking both the spontaneous release of ACh (MEPPs) as well as the EPP. They do *not* affect the propagation of the nerve action potential. Furthermore, botulinum toxin does not affect the synthesis or storage of ACh. Accordingly, the toxins must affect the release process itself (19).

The inhibition of ACh release is not immediate. Time is required for binding of the toxin to the external membrane, and the toxin is then translocated to the internal milieu, where blockage of ACh release occurs (19). Toxin is also transported in a retrograde fashion, up the axon, because botulinum toxin has been found in the cell body of the motor neuron (20,21).

The specific mechanism by which BTX interferes with ACh release is uncertain. Physiological studies show that EPPs produced by the synchronous release of ACh-containing vesicles are lower in amplitude in the presence of BTX (22). This suggests that the release of vesicles is impeded in the presence of BTX. One study from a patient with type A intoxication estimated that some nerve terminals released only 7 quanta (the physiological equivalent to 7 ACh vesicles) after 100 stimuli were delivered to the presynaptic nerve twig (22). A normal motor nerve releases as many as 60 vesicles per stimulus (23). The fewer the number of quanta released per nerve impulse, the smaller the EPP. The smaller the EPP, the lower the probability that a propagated muscle action potential will occur with successful muscle fiber contraction. In the autonomic nervous system, blockage of ACh release causes failure of transmission in the cholinergic neurons.

A common way to test cholinergic transmission in the neuromuscular system is with repetitive nerve stimulation. Supramaximal stimulation of peripheral nerve results in a maximal contraction of the innervated muscle. The electrophysiological correlate of maximal muscle contraction is the maximal compound muscle action potential (CMAP). The CMAP is the voltage change caused by electrical depolarization of all muscle fibers in the pick-up area of the recording electrode, commonly a surface electrode 1 cm in diameter placed over the motor point of the muscle being activated. This is a summated potential of many muscle fibers under the electrode. Repetitive stimulation of peripheral

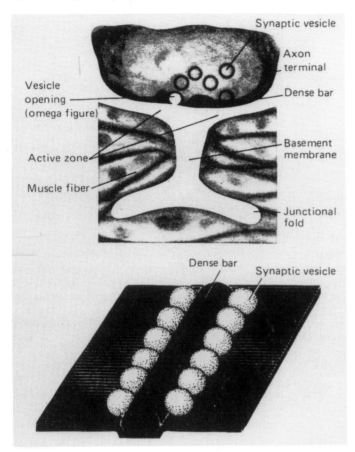

Figure 1 Schematic diagram of one area of vesicle release at a neuromuscular junction. (From Ref. 18.)

nerve produces a decline in the number of ACh-containing vesicles available for release, but the EPP never falls before threshold (Fig. 2). When neuromuscular transmission is impaired or fails (i.e., the EPP fails to reach threshold), individual muscle fibers lying beneath the electrode are not activated, and because there are fewer action potentials to summate, the CMAP is smaller. During repetitive stimulation of nerve at 2 or 3 Hz, failure to replenish ACh-containing vesicles available for immediate release, impairment of vesicle release mechanisms (as in botulism), or a reduced number of postsynaptic binding sites (as in myasthenia gravis) will result in fewer activated muscle fibers and a progressive loss of CMAP amplitude (decremental response) (Fig. 2). When vesicle release is impeded by BTX, the first CMAP amplitude is low, and subsequent CMAPs produced by low rates of stimulation (2–3 Hz) show a progressive decrease or decrement in amplitude. At rapid rates of stimulation (40–50 Hz) larger numbers of vesicles are released (probably because of increased amounts of presynaptic calcium) (18). The increased amount of synaptic ACh causes the EPP in more muscle fibers to exceed threshold and produce a propagated muscle action potential and contraction. The larger numbers of activated muscle fibers is reflected in a progressive increase in the CMAP

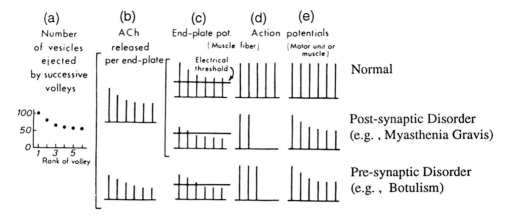

Figure 2 Schematic model to show principles of neuromuscular transmission in diseases of neuromuscular transmission. (a) Depletion of acetylcholine (ACh)-containing vesicles from the presynaptic store during repetitive stimulation of 2–3 Hz. (b) Amount of ACh released in normal persons and in diseases that do not influence ACh release (top), and in diseases that impair release of ACh (bottom). (c) Intrasynaptic recording of end plate potentials from individual neuromuscular junctions in each condition and (d) whether or not an individual propagated muscle fiber contraction is produced by each stimulus. (e) Findings that would be observed in the surface-recorded compound muscle action potential. (Modified from Ref. 41.)

amplitude (an incremental response). Therefore, in the presence of BTX, neuromuscular transmission inefficiency should produce low CMAP amplitudes, decrement during slow rates of repetitive stimulation, and increment during fast rates. These events occur only in the presence of weakness, and therefore have never been observed clinically in patients receiving diluted BTX for dystonia. However, if objective weakness is induced by BTX, these changes should be expected (24).

The surface-recorded CMAP reflects the synchronized electrical activity of many muscle fibers under the electrode. Changes in amplitude occur only when propagated action potentials from large numbers of muscle fibers fail (i.e., are blocked). Weakness is usually present. Repetitive stimulation is abnormal only when large numbers of muscle fibers are blocked. Furthermore, because there is a margin of safety within which neuromuscular transmission can be impaired but not blocked, successful muscle activation can occur in the presence of impaired transmission. Repetitive-stimulation studies obtain normal results in such circumstances. To detect such abnormalities, recording from individual muscle fibers is required.

Fibrillation potentials and positive sharp waves represent propagated action potentials from single muscle fibers and are seen during needle electromyography in botulism (25). However, these are found only after transmission is blocked. Inefficient neuromuscular transmission within the margin of safety (i.e., before transmission block and weakness occurs) is best studied using the technique of single-fiber electromyography (SFEMG). Single-fiber electromyography uses a special needle with the active electrode mounted on the side to prevent recording from damaged muscle fibers. Using this needle and setting the low-frequency (high-pass) filter to 500 Hz allows recording of extracellular action potentials generated by single muscle fibers (26).

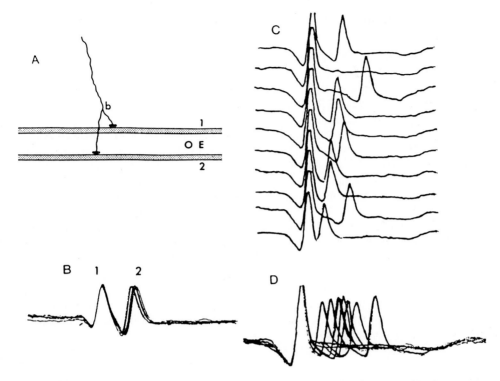

Figure 3 Schematic model of the recording of extracellular muscle action potentials from two muscle fibers innervated by the same motor axon (divided at point b) and therefore belonging to the same motor unit using the single fiber-electron (E). (B) Ten superimposed successive discharges of a fiber pair showing the small amount of jitter found in normal neuromuscular junctions. (C) Ten successive traces from a patient who received botulinum toxin 2 weeks previously, showing increased jitter and blocking. (D) The same traces superimposed showing the classical appearance of abnormal amounts of jitter and blocking (muscle: extensor digitorum communis; Cal 200 μV/div; 0.5 msec/div). (Adapted from Ref. 27.)

When a motor unit (i.e., the motor axon and all muscle fibers it innervates) is activated, all its constituent muscle fibers are activated simultaneously. Therefore, time-linked muscle fibers are considered part of the same motor unit. In SFEMG recordings, the needle is positioned so that two or more time-linked fibers are repeatedly seen on successive oscilloscope traces during voluntary activation of the muscle under study (Fig. 3). The variability in the interval between the two potentials, called jitter, is measured. There is a small amount of jitter in normal muscle, reflecting slight variability in transmission across the synapse (Fig. 3B). As inefficiency increases, jitter increases. Weakness does not occur until blocking of transmission occurs (Fig. 3C).

The packing density of muscle fibers belonging to a motor unit is reflected by the number of time-locked muscle action potentials at one recording site. The average of the number of time-locked potentials at several sites (usually > 20) is called *fiber density*. Anatomical studies show that BTX induces prominent neuronal sprouting with changes in the postsynaptic muscle membrane resembling those seen in denervation (27). Increased fiber density is the physiological correlate of sprouting (26).

CLINICAL FINDINGS ASSOCIATED WITH BOTULINUM TOXIN INJECTION

There are several effects of BTX injection that occur in areas close to the site of injection of diluted toxin. Weakness may occur close to the site of injection. For example, ptosis may occur after injection for blepharospasm (28), and swallowing problems may occur after injection of neck muscles for torticollis (4,8). Such local effects of injection are beyond the scope of this discussion.

Although we have never encountered a patient who received an overdose of BTX, there is potential for such a situation to develop. Miscalculations of dose might occur, or there may be differences in strength of different preparations (7) (although limitations of the total dose per vial make this unlikely). If a patient receives an excessive dose of BTX, there may be a delay of 18 to 36 hours in the onset of symptoms. Initial symptoms would include double or blurred vision, difficulty swallowing, dry mouth, and slurred speech. The patient may complain of nausea, vomiting, and abdominal pain because of autonomic effects. Weakness usually occurs in a descending fashion, involving cranial nerves, then neck, arm, leg, and thoracic muscles, causing shortness of breath. Examination shows orthostatic hypotension and tachycardia, hypohydrosis, ileus, constipation, and urinary retention. Cranial nerve examination shows ptosis, external ophthalmoparesis, and fixed, dilated pupils. Although pupillary abnormalities are frequent and important findings, they are not required for the diagnosis, and their absence should not eliminate the diagnosis from consideration (29). Weakness is accompanied by normal or slightly diminished tendon reflexes. Sensory examination is usually normal, but two patients with sensory loss in the face have been reported (30,31). Respiratory weakness is common and may result in the need for mechanical ventilation.

Generalized fatigue with mild, generalized weakness may occur after patients receive BTX for limb dystonia (16). Some patients refer to these symptoms as ''flu-like.'' We have performed electrodiagnostic evaluation in patients with such symptoms, and they show normal results of nerve conduction studies, normal responses to repetitive stimulation, and normal results of SFEMG studies. Therefore, these symptoms may not be due to BTX-induced neuromuscular transmission inefficiency. The cause of these symptoms remains uncertain. One placebo-controlled study found no difference in frequency of fatigue in the control and placebo groups (32).

One study reported dysphagia lasting for 4 weeks after injection of the tibialis anterior muscle, an observation compatible with a remote effect of BTX (17). Further diagnostic evaluation was refused by that patient.

Allergic reactions to BTX do occur and are one of the three absolute contraindications to the use of the drug (the two others are use in pregnancy, because the effects have not been established, and injecting into sites of infection or inflammation) (33).

SUBCLINICAL EFFECTS ASSOCIATED WITH BOTULINUM TOXIN INJECTION

Even though there are a few generalized signs or symptoms of minor severity that may occur after injection of small amounts of diluted BTX, widespread subclinical effects on neuromuscular transmission can be detected if SFEMG is used to study muscles distant from the site of injection (34–38). The first observation that jitter was increased in muscles distant from the site of injection occurred in a patient receiving small amounts of BTX for blepharospasm. Abnormal jitter in the extensor digitorum communis was ob-

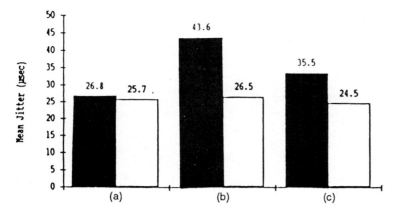

Figure 4 Changes in mean jitter over time in botulinum toxin–treated (filled bars) and placebo-treated (open bars) patients. (a) Mean jitter found in both groups before injection (values for jitter are shown as insert). (b) Two weeks after injection ($p < 0.05$). (c) Twelve weeks after injection ($p > 0.05$) (muscle: extensor digitorum communis; site of injection: neck for torticollis). (From Ref. 35.)

served 2 weeks after the ocular muscles were injected (38). The abnormal jitter usually resolves within 3 months (36), paralleling the duration of the clinical response (8). Repeated injections with high doses of BTX may induce long-lasting changes in motor unit architecture through sprouting induction, and these changes are manifested as increased fiber density (36). In muscle injected directly with diluted BTX, intramuscular nerves show profuse growth of sprouts and enlarging of the motor unit (2,28). The increased fiber density is compatible with similar effects being exerted in distant muscle. The abnormal SFEMG findings affect both arm and leg muscles. We have seen jitter in the tibialis anterior and biceps muscles after injection of the neck muscles for torticollis.

In a double-blind trial, we have shown that increased jitter in distant muscles is the result of the locally injected BTX (34). Patients receiving BTX for torticollis showed increased jitter 2 weeks after injection, but the placebo group showed no change from preinjection jitter values (Fig. 4). The observed jitter is probably due to a presynaptic disorder, because the jitter decreases as the firing rate increases (Fig. 5). Although similar changes in jitter relative to firing rate may be found in postsynaptic disorders, they are more characteristic of presynaptic disease.

The observed magnitude of jitter helps explain why weakness is not seen. The mean jitter for the BTX-treated group was only 42 μsec (normal is < 32 μsec). For weakness to occur, many fibers with blocking are needed. Blocking occurs only when jitter is greatly increased (usually above 100 μsec). Although blocking was seen in patients immediately after BTX injection, it never occurred in more than 20% of the fiber pairs studied. Some studies suggest that there is a dose-response relationship; i.e., as the amount of BTX injected increases, the amount of jitter will increase (36,37).

Antibodies

Antibodies to botulinum toxin are found in some patients after several injections. The antibodies may be responsible for the tolerance to BTX developed by some patients (16,39).

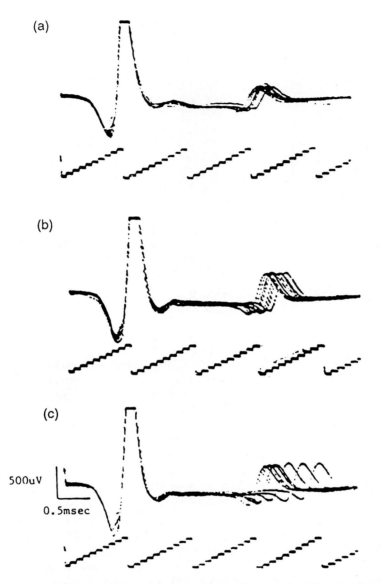

Figure 5 Effects of firing rate on jitter in botulinum toxin–injected patient. Jitter is minimal with fast firing rates (a), increases at moderate firing rates (b), and is maximal at slow firing rates (c) (muscle: extensor digitorum communis). (From Ref. 36.)

Implications of Subclinical Effects of Botulinum Toxin

Patients with disorders of neuromuscular transmission, such as myasthenia gravis, who are clinically without detectable weakness are at risk for worsening weakness when drugs that compromise neuromuscular transmission are given (40). Such drugs include aminoglycosides, penicillamine, quinine, and calcium channel blockers. Botulinum toxin should be included in this list. Furthermore, the combination of such drugs with BTX poses a potential risk for the appearance of clinical weakness in BTX-treated patients. No patient receiving BTX has ever shown objective weakness in distant muscles after injection. However, awareness of possible interactions is essential. Accordingly, the presence of an underlying neuromuscular disease is a relative contraindication to administration of BTX (33).

CONCLUSION

There are few systemic effects of locally injected BTX to control excessive focal muscle contraction, such as dystonia. However, there is good evidence that the toxin does affect neuromuscular transmission in muscles remote from the site of injection, and the possibility of generalized clinical effects therefore exists. It is thus essential for clinicians using BTX as a therapeutic agent to be familiar with all of the systemic effects of BTX.

REFERENCES

1. Simpson LL. The action of botulinal toxin. Rev Infect Dis 1979;1:656–659.
2. Duchen LW, Strich SJ. The effects of botulinum toxin on the pattern of innervation of skeletal muscle in the mouse. Q J Exp Physiol 1968;53:84–89.
3. Scott A. Botulinum toxin injection of eye muscles to correct strabismus. Trans Am Ophthalmol Soc 1981;79:734–770.
4. Blackie JD, Lees AJ. Botulinum toxin treatment in spasmodic torticollis. J Neurol Neurosurg Psychiatry 1990;53:640–643.
5. Lorentz IT, Subramaniam SS, Yiannikas C. Treatment of idiopathic torticollis with botulinum toxin A: a double blind study on 23 patients. Mov Disord 1991;6:145–150.
6. Jankovic J. Botulinum A toxin in the treatment of blepharospasm. Adv Neurol 1988;49:467–472.
7. Stell R, Thompson PD, Marsden CD. Botulinum toxin in spasmodic torticollis. J. Neurol Neurosurg Psychiatry. 1988;51:920–933.
8. Greene P, Kan U, Fahn S, Brin M, Moscowitz C, Flaster E. Double-blind placebo controlled study of botulinum toxin injection for torticollis. Neurology 1990;40:1213–1218.
9. Jankovic J, Ford J. Blepharospasm and orofacial-cervical dystonia: clinical and pharmacological findings in 100 patients. Ann Neurol 1983;13:402–411.
10. Jankovic J, Orman J. Botulinum A toxin for craniocervical dystonia: a double-blind, placebo controlled study. Neurology 1987;37:616–623.
11. Blitzer A, Brin MF, Fahn S, et al. Localized injections of botulinum toxin for the treatment of focal laryngeal dystonia. Laryngoscope 1988;98:193–197.
12. Tsui JK, Eisen A, Mak E, et al. A pilot study on the use of botulinum toxin in spasmodic torticollis. Can J Neurol Sci 1985;12:314–316.
13. Savino PJ, Sergott RC, Bosley TM, et al. Hemifacial spasm treated with botulinum toxin A injection. Arch Ophthalmol 1985;103:1305–1306.
14. Cohen LG, Hallett M, Geller BD, et al. Treatment of focal dystonias of the hand with botulinum toxin injections. J Neurol Neurosurg Psychiat 1989;52:355–363.
15. Jankovic J, Schwartz K, Donovan DT. Botulinum toxin treatment of cranial-cervical dystonia, spasmodic dysphonia, other focal dystonias and hemifacial spasm. J Neurol Neurosurg Psychiat 1990;53:633–639.
16. Brin MF, Fahn S, Moscowitz C, et al. Localized injections of botulinum toxin for treatment of focal dystonia and hemifacial spasm. In: Fahn S, Marsden CD, eds. Dystonia 2. New York: Raven Press, 1988:559–608.
17. Nix WA, Butler IF, Roontga S, Gutmann L, Hopf HC. Persistent unilateral tibialis anterior muscle hypertrophy with complex repetitive discharges and myalgia: report of two unique cases and response to botulinum toxin. Neurology 1992;42:602–606.

18. Gershon MD, Schwartz JH, Kandel ER. Morphology of chemical synapses and patterns of interconnection. In: Kandel ER, Schwartz JH, eds. Principles of neural science. 1st ed. New York: Elsevier, 1983:91.

19. Harvey AL. Presynaptic toxins. In: Smythies JR, Bradley RJ, eds. International review of neurobiology. Vol. 32. San Diego: Academic Press, 1990:201–239.

20. Wiegand H, Erdmann G, Wellhoner HH. I125-labeled botulinum A neurotoxin: pharmacokinetics in cats after intramuscular injection. Naunyn-Schmiedebergs Arch Pharmacol 1976;292:161–165.

21. Black JD, Dolly JO. Interaction of I125-labeled botulinum neurotoxins with nerve terminals. I: Ultrastructural autoradiographic localization and quantitation of distinct membrane receptors for types A and B on motor neurons. J Cell Biol 1986;103:521–534.

22. Lambert EH, Engel AG, Cherington M. End-plate potentials in human botulism. In: Bradley WG, Gardner-Medwin D, Walton JN, eds. Third International Congress on Muscle Disease. Amsterdam: Excerpta Medica, 1974:65.

23. Pickett JB. AAEE case report # 16: botulism. Muscle Nerve 1988;11:1201–1205.

24. Gutman L. Disorders of neuromuscular transmission. In: Joynt RJ, ed. Clinical neurology. Philadelphia: J.B. Lippincott, 1991:14–15.

25. Maselli RA, Burnett ME, Tonsgard JH. In vitro microelectrode study of neuromuscular transmission in a case of botulism. Muscle Nerve 1982;15:273-276.

26. Stalberg E, Thiele B. Single-fiber electromyography. Surrey, England: Miravalle Press, 1979.

27. Alderson K, Holds JB, Anderson RL. Botulinum-induced alteration of nerve-muscle interactions in the human orbicularis oculi following treatment for blepharospasm. Neurology 1991;41:1800–1805.

28. Elston JS. Botulinum toxin treatment of blepharospasm. In: Fahn S, Marsden CD, eds. Dystonia 2. New York: Raven Press, 1988:579–581.

29. Cherrington M. Botulism: ten year experience. Arch Neurol 1974;30:432–437.

30. Castrillo JCM, Real MD, Gonzalez AH, DeBlas G, Alvarez-Cermeno JC. Botulism with sensory symptoms: a second case. J Neurol Neurosurg Psychiat 1991;54:844–845.

31. Goode GB, Sherarn DL. Botulism: a case with associated sensory abnormalities. Arch Neurol 1982;39:55.

32. Lorentz IT, Subramaniam SS, Yiannikas C. Treatment of idiopathic torticollis with botulinum toxin A: a double blind study on 23 patients. Mov Disord 1991;6:145–150.

33. National Institutes of Health Consensus Development Conference Statement. November 12–14, 1990: Clinical use of botulinum toxin. Arch Neurol 1991;48:1294–1298.

34. Lange DJ, Rubin M, Greene PE, et al. Distant effects of locally injected botulinum toxin: a double blind study of single fiber EMG changes. Muscle Nerve 1991;14:672–675.

35. Lange DJ, Brin MF, Warner CL, et al. Distant effects of local injection of botulinum toxin. Muscle Nerve 1987;10:552–555.

36. Lange DJ, Brin MF, Fahn S, et al. Distant effects of locally injected botulinum toxin: incidence and course. In: Fahn S, Marsden CD, eds. Dystonia 2. New York: Raven Press, 1988:609–613.

37. Olney RK, Aminoff MG, Gelb DJ, et al. Neuromuscular effects distant from the site of botulinum neurotoxin injection. Neurology 1988;38:1780–1783.

38. Sanders DB, Massey EW, Buckley EC. Botulinum toxin for blepharospasm: single fiber EMG studies. Neurology 1986;36:545–547.

39. Rosenbaum F, Jankovic J. Task-specific focal dystonia and tremor: categorization of occupational movement disorders. Neurology 1988;38:522–526.

40. Argov Z, Mastaglia FL. Disorders of neuromuscular transmission caused by drugs. N Engl J Med 1979;301:409–413.

41. Desmedt JE. The neuromuscular disorder in myasthenia gravis. In: Desmedt JE, ed. New developments in electromyography and clinical neurophysiology. Basel: Karger, 1973:321.

10

Pharmacology and Histology of the Therapeutic Application of Botulinum Toxin

Gary E. Borodic
Harvard Medical School, Massachusetts Eye and Ear Infirmary, and Boston University School of Medicine, Boston, Massachusetts

Robert J. Ferrante
Massachusetts General Hospital, Harvard Medical School, Boston, Massachusetts

L. Bruce Pearce
Boston University School of Medicine, Boston, Massachusetts

Kathy Alderson
Salt Lake City VA Medical Center and University of Utah, Salt Lake City, Utah

INTRODUCTION

Since the introduction of botulinum toxin (BTX) into therapeutics in 1978 for strabismus (1–3), its use has been expanded to other indications including blepharospasm, adult-onset spasmodic torticollis, spasmodic dysphonia, occupational hand cramps, and jaw dystonia. Application of this therapy to other disorders is on the horizon and is contributing to the driving force for expansion of clinical and basic research (4–12). However, despite the success obtained with BTX for treatment of blepharospasm and other focal and segmental movement disorders, its application is limited by the following properties of the therapy:

1. Need for indefinitely repeating injections when treating chronic disease
2. Untoward spread of toxin to other muscles not targeted for injection
3. Antibody formation with resistance to the therapeutic action of the toxin after repeated injections
4. The consistency of biologic activity contained within the labeled vials
5. Lack of standardization of the injections sites
6. Placement of the therapeutic toxin preparation into the correct anatomical position when access to the muscles is difficult, requiring electromyographic assistance (particularly for treatment of occupational hand disorders)
7. Inadequate understanding of long-term benefits and effects of repeated treatment with the therapeutic preparation
8. Inadequate comprehension of the nature of any permanent microanatomical changes in striated muscle and motor nerve terminals after repeated botulinum toxin injections

9. Inadequate fundamental understanding of the pathophysiology of focal and segmental dystonias

This chapter will address the histologic changes produced by therapeutic injections of botulinum toxin with pertinent clinical data, so that clinical-pathologic correlations can be made. Some of the issues outlined above will be explored.

BIOCHEMICAL CHARACTER AND HISTOLOGIC EFFECTS OF BOTULINUM TOXIN IN STRIATED MUSCLE

Biochemistry and Cellular Physiology

The first apparent histologic effect appears to be clustering of vesicles at the presynaptic membrane, indicating an impairment of release of acetylcholine (13). This finding has been well documented with electron microscopy (13).

The therapeutic actions of BTX are a consequence of the complex structure and function of this molecule and its actions at the nerve terminal. The BTX molecule has a molecular weight of approximately 150,000 daltons, and the active form of the toxin exists as a dichain molecule consisting of a light (M_r approximately 50,000 daltons) and heavy (M_r approximately 100,000 daltons) chain linked by a disulfide bond (14,15). All the neurotoxins produced by *Clostridium botulinum* are immunologically distinct, which suggests significant differences in the amino acid sequences of these toxins. For example, analysis of the partial amino acid sequences of the A and B types has revealed greater homologies between the primary and secondary structure for the light chains than for the heavy chains. The degree of primary structure homology is only 20% for the light chains and 40% for the heavy chains (16). Although they are similar in secondary and tertiary structure, it is believed that differences in the conformation of the neurotoxins at or near the active site may be responsible for the differences in neurotoxicity (17).

Botulinum toxin exists normally in a complex with another protein, hemagglutinin. This accessory protein probably contributes to both conformational stability and resistance to degradation by enzymes. The latter has been shown to be particularly important to the oral toxicity (18) of BTX. While studies have not been reported to support the importance of hemagglutinin to the tissue-reactivity of BTX, it is conceivable that the efficacy of various preparations of the toxin may depend on the stability conferred by this complex formation.

The toxin's effect on neuronal function is apparently limited to the nerve terminal. The toxin, in particular the heavy chain, binds to its membrane receptor, which is apparently localized only at nerve terminals (19). Studies that have examined the binding of radiolabeled toxin molecules suggest that the different serotypes, in particular the type A and B toxins, may bind to different receptor molecules (15,20).

Electrophysiologic studies have demonstrated that botulinum toxins affect different steps in the neurotransmitter release process. Botulinum toxin type B affects synchronization of quantal transmitter release, whereas type A toxin does not (21). Similarly, differences exist with regard to the reversibility of inhibition of calcium-dependent release of neurotransmitter. Introduction of calcium into nerve terminals using a calcium ionophore produces the release of transmitter from synaptosomes poisoned by BTX-A more readily than from those poisoned by BTX-B (22). At the neuromuscular junction, aminopyridine was also more effective at reversal of inhibition produced by BTX-A (23). Ashton and Dolly (22) recently demonstrated that microtubule-dissociating drugs were effective in blocking the inhibitory effects of BTX-B on neurotransmitter release and ineffective against BTX-A. The differences in the toxic and neurophysiologic effects of type A and B toxins are presumably related to the existence of two distinct receptor sites for these species.

The denervation that occurs at the neuromuscular junction is a consequence of irreversible inhibition of normal neurotransmitter release (24,25). The active form of the toxin produces denervation through a three-step process as suggested by Schmitt et al. and Simpson (24,25). The three-step process involves (1) binding of the heavy chain to the membrane receptor molecule; (2) translocation of the toxin into the nerve terminal via receptor-mediated endocytosis; and (3) irreversible inactivation of normal neurotransmitter release, which is thought to be mediated by the presumed enzymatic properties of the light chain of the toxin. Preliminary studies have suggested that the toxin may be a protease, possibly with zinc dependence (26).

Histological Effects on Muscle Fibers

Within 7 to 10 days of injection, collateral axonal sprouting occurs at the terminal axon or occasionally from the distal node of Ranvier (27,28). Within 10 to 14 days, the muscle fibers begin to atrophy. This atrophy continues to develop over a 4 to 6 week period. Figure 1A–C shows the fiber atrophy achieved in an albino rabbit longissimus dorsi muscle 4 weeks after injection of 10 IU of BTX compared with a saline-injected control specimen. Note that there is not only fiber atrophy as indicated by generalized reduction in fiber diameters but also a large degree of *fiber size variability*. Collateral axonal sprouts reestablish proximity to neuromuscular junctions within a period of several months after injection (29). This sprouting phenomenon is of interest and may provide future insight into the changes in physiologic responses after repeated injections into muscle (see below).

During a period of 3 to 4 weeks after injection, there is considerable spread of acetylcholinesterase (AChE) staining activity on the sarcolemma of muscle fibers. This diffuse AChE staining persists until the 12th to 16th week postinjection, after which there is considerable reduction of staining. After 5 months, AChE activity again becomes confined to the neuromuscular junction, the only area the stain reacts with in noninjected muscles. Spread of AChE staining activity is also correlated with spread of AChE receptors on sarcolemma.

Acetylcholine Nicotinic Receptor Density and Distribution in Response to Denervation

Innervation is known to strongly influence protein synthesis in striated muscle and, in particular, the density and distribution of nicotinic acetylcholine receptors (nAChRs) and AChE (30). The nicotinic receptor is the element responsible for transducing the signal carried by acetylcholine (ACh) into end plate potentials and ultimately muscle contraction. Acetylcholinesterase on the other hand is localized at the end plate at high concentrations and serves to rapidly hydrolyze and inactivate ACh that is released into the synaptic space. Dramatic influences on the density and distribution of these critical elements of the neuromuscular junction are observed during development and synaptogenesis and following denervation. Normally, nAChRs are localized, almost exclusively, to the neuromuscular junction (NMJ) end plate regions of striated muscle (31). In mature striated muscle either before synapse formation or following denervation, nAChRs are observed over the entire muscle surface (32,33). Miledi (34) observed that 10 weeks after complete denervation of frog sartorius muscle, marked hypersensitivity to ACh was detectable over

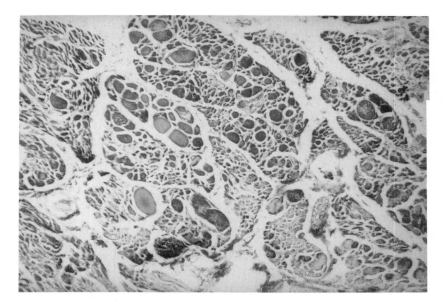

(A)

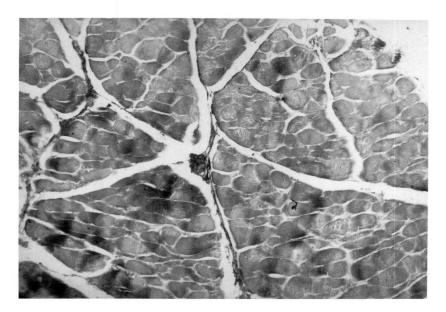

(B)

Figure 1 Dose-dependent muscle fiber responses: muscle fiber atrophy at the injection site (original magnification 4×). (A) Fiber atrophy is seen after botulinum toxin injections is longissimus dorsi of albino rabbit. (B) Saline control. (C) With increasing doses of botulinum toxin, the degree of fiber atrophy at the injection site increases. (Average fiber diameter represented $n = 3200$ for each point.)

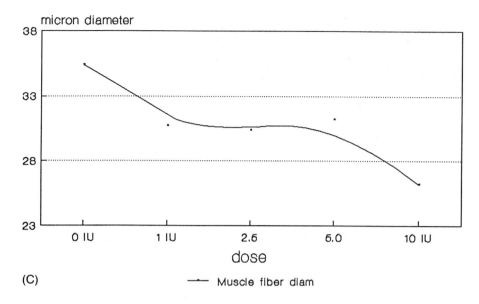

(C)   —•— Muscle fiber diam

the entire muscle surface. This hypersensitivity was still observed after 158 days, despite the marked muscle atrophy evident at this time. Hypersensitivity to ACh was also observed after partial denervation, a condition more germane to BTX treatment. Consistent with these early observations, Goldman and Stape (35) have reported that denervation of rat soleus muscle resulted in unequal distribution of nAChR subunit RNAs in extrajunctional areas of the muscle as compared with normally innervated muscle, where the RNAs were localized below the end plate region of the muscle membrane. These observations are consistent with the fact that normal innervation suppresses extrajunctional nAChR gene expression and that denervation removes this trophic influence. These observations are in agreement with the spread of AChE staining seen following partial denervation with BTX.

Normal reversal of the effects of BTX is associated with nerve terminal sprouting and reestablishment of myoneuronal junctions. The trophic effects of regeneration of these junctions has been studied in animal models (36–38) and human tissue (39).

Muscle Fiber Morphometric Studies and Histochemistry after Injection

The fiber atrophy measured as reduced fiber diameter, and diameter variability on cross-sectional analysis, is a reversible phenomenon with recovery over a 4- to 6-month period. Spread of AChE on human muscle fibers 5 weeks after BTX injection to the orbicularis oculi muscle is seen in Figure 2A. Figure 2B demonstrates the correlation between fiber size (diameter) variability and cholinesterase staining pattern 5 weeks after injection in albino rabbit muscle. Clinically, this correlation is helpful in assessing therapeutic BTX effects in muscle biopsies. These findings are consistent with those found in human muscle after BTX injections (39–41). Seventeen orbicularis oculi muscle specimens taken from patients during ptosis and myectomy surgery were evaluated for cholinesterase staining characteristics and fiber variability (39). Diffuse cholinesterase activity started at weeks 3 to 4, and this staining pattern was maintained through 3 to 4 months after injection (Fig. 3A). In all patients studied after 6 months, cholinesterase staining was confined to the NMJs and could not be distinguished from that seen in controls. It is also

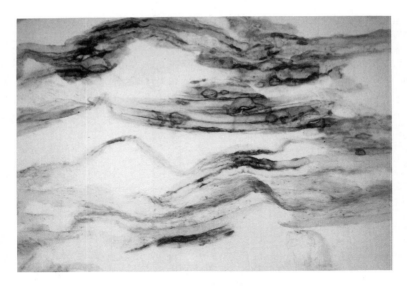

(A)

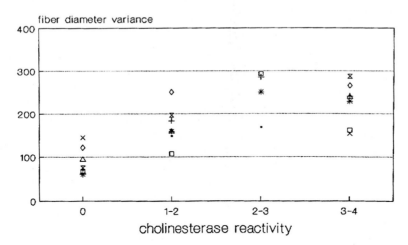

(B)

Figure 2 (A) Acetylcholinesterase staining in human Orbicularis oculi muscle. Spread of acetylcholinesterase is seen on human muscle fibers 5 weeks after injection of botulinum toxin. A similar effect was previously described in animal muscle fibers (see Fig. 6). (B) A direct correlation between fiber size variability and acetylcholinesterase spread characteristics on muscle biopsies evaluated from the animal study.

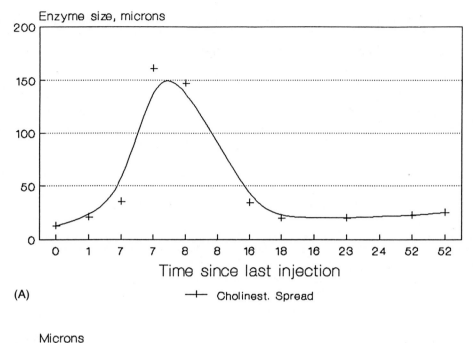

(A)

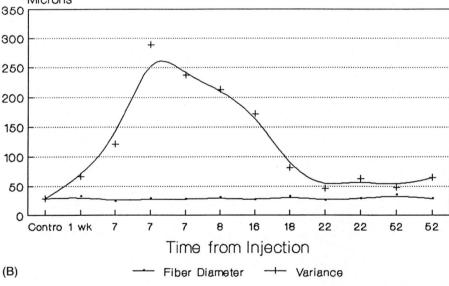

(B)

Figure 3 Cyclic histological changes after botulinum toxin (BTX) injection in human muscle (39). (A) Denervation reflected by cholinesterase spread. (B) Variations in orbicularis oculi muscle fiber size after BTX injection. The duration of action of BTX appears to correlate with fiber variability and chlolinesterase spread characteristics seen in human orbicularis muscle specimens. The results of these specimens were evaluated with respect to the last injection of BTX. The specimens were obtained at the time of ptosis surgery and myectomy surgery in patients being treated by this technique for their diseases. The fiber morphometric response and cholinesterase activity correlate with the clinical duration of action. The time scale on the graphs is in weeks.

of note that fiber size variability appeared to correlate temporally with cholinesterase spread pattern. Fiber size variability appeared to be transient, lasting 3 to 12 weeks after injection (Fig. 3B). Temporal relationships between these histologic changes correlate with the duration of action achieved with therapeutic doses of BTX, which varies between 10 and 16 weeks in most dystonia applications (42).

Another important goal in evaluating human muscle specimens after the injection of BTX is assessing long-term muscle fiber effects. If human orbicularis oculi muscle specimens were not injected within 6 months of biopsy, there was no difference in fiber size or cholinesterase staining pattern compared with the control specimens taken from routine ptosis surgery (39). Chronic denervation and muscle fiber atrophy does not appear to occur with repetitive use of the toxin. However, there appear to be permanent changes within the myoneural junctions, with increased number of preterminal axon sprouts and multiple projections into the myoneural junctions, as will be demonstrated later in this chapter (see below, "Motor Nerve Terminal Morphology Following Botulinum Toxin Type A Injection"). Although changes may be present at the neuromuscular junction with respect to sprouting, there was no substantial residual atrophy after multiple injections of BTX. Such data appear to indicate that the reinnervation process after BTX administration is nearly complete, and that permanent trophic changes within muscle fibers do not occur.

Adenosinetriphosphatase (ATPase) enzyme histochemistry on animal muscle tissues injected with BTX has demonstrated slight alteration in the pattern of muscle fiber types. The number of type I muscle fibers slightly increased after the injection. However, the most significant finding was type grouping (see Figure 4). Fiber size variability was seen

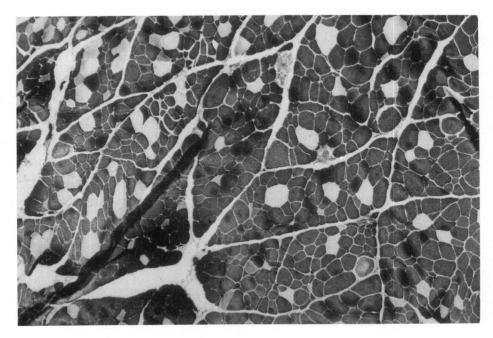

Figure 4   Adenosine triphosphatase stain at pH 9.4. The amount of type I fiber grouping appears to be greater after injection of botulinum toxin in comparison with controls. However, the total number of type I and type II fibers did not seem to be substantially different from that seen in controls. This appearance is consistent with denervation.

in both type 1 and type 2 muscle fibers. Muscle fibers that belong to the same motor unit are morphologically, histochemically, and physiologically similar. Type I fibers are innervated by low-threshold motor neurons, while type 2 fibers are innervated by higher-threshold neurons. They can be differentially identified using ATPase enzyme histo-chemistry. In the normal condition, there is a mosaic-like pattern to the distribution of innervation by each motor unit. Although this pattern varies between different muscle groups, it can be somewhat likened to a checkerboard. The successful reinnervation of denervated muscle from nearby collateral axon sprouts by a different motor unit type will convert the reinnervated muscle fiber to that type. As a consequence, the distribution of muscle fiber types changes. Fiber type grouping is a common occurrence. The altered mosaic pattern of fiber typing in animal muscles injected with BTX, as observed using ATPase enzyme histochemistry, is consistent with that observed in denervation. These changes occur more slowly and are not as dramatic as the spread of AChE activity seen in animal tissues 3 to 5 weeks after BTX injection.

The pattern of oxidative enzyme activity with nicotinamide adenine diaphorase histo-chemistry was also changed in animal muscle treated with BTX. The muscle fibers appeared "moth-eaten," with a focal, irregular loss of enzyme activity. This finding has been associated with an abnormal redistribution of mitochondria within the affected muscle fibers. Neither target nor targetoid fibers were observed. As with the alterations of fiber typing, the dysmorphic changes in oxidative enzyme activity are compatible with a denervative process.

MOTOR NERVE TERMINAL MORPHOLOGY FOLLOWING BOTULINUM TOXIN TYPE A INJECTION

Botulinum toxin blocks neuromuscular transmission and produces functional muscle denervation (27,43,44). The motor axon remains in anatomical contact with the muscle end plate, but because neuromuscular transmission is blocked, the muscle is paralyzed. In rats and other experimental mammals, two morphological changes develop at the NMJs following functional denervation by BTX. In proximal muscles, there is conspicuous motor axon sprouting. In more distal muscles, expansion of the end plate region is more pronounced, through both responses can be seen in any muscle.

Sprouts develop from multiple sites of the preterminal axon (Fig. 5), including the terminal axonal arborization over the end plate region (ultraterminal sprouts), the axon immediately proximal to the end plate (terminal sprouts), and the nodes of Ranvier of preterminal axons (preterminal sprouts). By electron microscopy, the axon sprout follows the inner layer of a basal lamina, either of muscle or of the enveloping Schwann cell (K. Alderson, unpublished data). The sprouts are otherwise nondirected, growing through the muscle, but not generally terminating at muscle end plates (dead ends). There has been mention in the literature of these sprouts terminating at end plates (44). The sprouts decrease in abundance after several months, though the process of sprout loss is not well understood. Expansion of the end plate is more apparent in distal muscles following BTX exposure, with increased branching of the terminal axonal arborization over the end plate and enlargement of the cholinesterase-containing end plate region, from the normal length of 30–60 μm to more than 120 μm (Fig. 6 and Fig. 2A). The end plate region is not always continuous, with cholinesterase-containing regions separated by 5–15 μm. Synaptic vesical antigenicity is present along the extended branches of the axonal arborization (Fig. 7), suggesting that the expanded neuromuscular junction is capable of neuromuscular transmission.

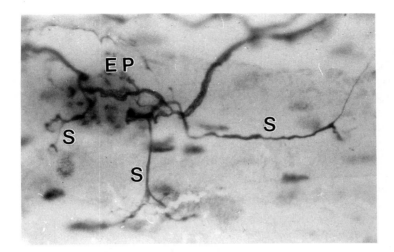

Figure 5 Axonal sprouts in the rat rhomboid muscle 14 days following injection of botulinum toxin type A. Exuberant ultraterminal axonal sprouts (S) arise from the terminal axonal arborization over the end plate (EP) region (silver-cholinesterase, × 500).

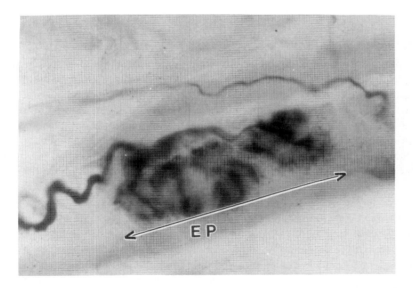

Figure 6 Expansion of the end plate (EP) in the rat soleus muscle 14 days following botulinum toxin injection into the muscle. The diameter of the cholinesterase-containing region has increased from the normal 30–60 μm to, here, 120 μm (arrows). Synaptic vesicle antigenicity is the fuzzy area surrounding the axonal processes over the terminal arborization (SCI, using an antibody to the synaptic vesicle protein synaptophysin). (× 600.)

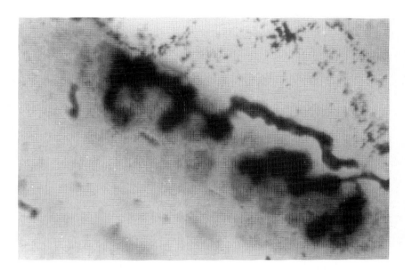

Figure 7 Two cholinesterase-containing end plate regions are separated by a non-cholinesterase-containing muscle membrane. An axonal process extends to the second end plate region. Synaptic vesicle antigenicity surrounds the axonal processes over the terminal arborization (SCI, using an antibody to the synaptic vesicle protein synaptophysin, × 800).

Human Terminal Motor Axon Configuration Following Botulinum Toxin Injection

Some patients with disabling blepharospasm in whom BTX injections or medical therapy is not successful in controlling the spasms elect orbicularis oculi myectomy as treatment (45). Surgical specimens of this muscle were evaluated to study the effect of BTX on terminal motor axons in humans (29,46).

Orbicularis oculi muscle from three groups of patients, age 35–81 years, was evaluated:

1. Nine patients with blepharospasm who had previously received 2 to 19 botulinum toxin type A (BTX-A) injections 5 weeks to 3 years before undergoing orbicularis oculi myectomy as treatment for blepharospasm. Four of the 9 patients failed to achieve sustained responses to repetitive BTX treatment and required an increased dose on subsequent injections. One patient had severe and prolonged paralysis following his second injection, and refused further injections. The other four had continuing response to injections.
2. Two patients with blepharospasm without prior BTX therapy electing orbicularis oculi myectomy.
3. Six ''normal'' patients without blepharospasm having cosmetic blepharoplasty.

Normal Human Orbicularis Oculi Terminal Motor Axons

Terminal motor axon and NMJ morphology in muscle not exposed to BTX, in both ''normals'' and patients with blepharospasm, was identical (Fig. 8) (29,46). Single preterminal axons exit the intramuscular nerve. All axons are myelinated up to the muscle end plate region. There are no unmyelinated axons. Most preterminal axons are unbranched and innervate a single muscle fiber; fewer than 10% of preterminal axons branch

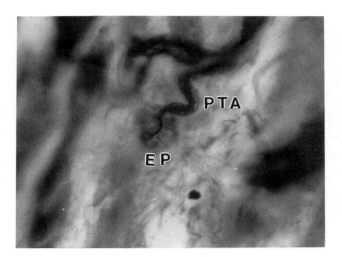

Figure 8 Normal orbicularis oculi muscle terminal motor axons. The preterminal axon (PTA) is myelinated as it leaves the intramuscular nerve, and myelination extends to the muscle end plate (EP) region (× 250, SCI using an antibody to PO).

to innervate more than one muscle fiber. Muscle end plates are not segmented, with a diameter between 6 and 34 μm, mean 20 μm (29). Each muscle fiber contained a single end plate region.

Motor Axons and Neuromuscular Junctions Following Botulinum Toxin Exposure: Sprouts

As expected on the basis of animal data, axonal sprouts develop following BTX injections into human orbicularis oculi (Fig. 9) (46). Preterminal, terminal, and ultraterminal sprouts are present in all BTX-treated muscle, though of greater incidence in muscles having more injections. The sprouts are almost uniformly unmyelinated. Some sprouts clearly end in a small bulbous dilatation, presumed to be the growth cone (Fig. 10).

Alteration of End Plate Size and Arrangement

As in animal muscle, cholinesterase-containing end plate regions expand in the orbicularis oculi following BTX injections (Fig. 2) (29). Segmented end plates form, with cholinesterase-containing regions separated by relatively long areas of non-cholinesterase-containing muscle fiber membrane. Each region of the segmented end plate is innervated by axon processes from the terminal or ultraterminal region of a single axon (Fig. 11). It appears that the axonal sprout can induce the formation of an end plate region on the underlying muscle membrane.

Very small end plates are also present, innervated by thin, unmyelinated axonal processes. End plate diameter ranged from 3 to 65 μm. Though the mean end plate diameter in BTX-treated muscle is about 20 μm, similar to untreated muscle, the preponderance of larger and smaller end plates contributes to a significantly larger standard deviation. The number of end plates in an area of muscle increases, and the number of end plate regions identified on an individual muscle fiber increases, from one in normal muscle to five or more in BTX-treated muscle.

hypothesis that repeated functional denervation in humans allows axonal sprouts to induce formation of new end plates on the functionally denervated muscle fiber, thus forming collateral innervation.

Axonal collaterals form readily in partial denervation associated with loss of motor axons (48–53). The reduction in the number of motor axons is readily appreciable as decreased density of axons in the intramuscular nerve in experimental partial denervation and in human denervating disease, such as amyotrophic lateral sclerosis or peripheral neuropathy. It is unlikely that there is a significant loss of motor axons following BTX injection, as the morphology and density of axons in the intramuscular nerve is normal, whereas a reduction would be expected if collateral sprouting developed because of a partial denervation from loss of axons.

Small end plates innervated by collaterals could represent either end plates on atrophic fibers or end plates formed under the influence of BTX. The presence of multiple end plates on a single muscle fiber, as well as segmented end plates, suggests that sprouts can induce the formation of new end plates on muscles ''functionally denervated'' by BTX. Two end plates on one muscle fiber, each innervated by different axons, can be induced and maintained experimentally in mammals by implanting a motor axon 5 mm from an end plate functionally denervated by BTX (47). The arrangement of the orbicularis oculi, with widely scattered regions of end plates and sprouts developing from motor axons in each region, may facilitate the development and persistence of multiple end plates, so that a single muscle fiber can be innervated at separate sites by collaterals from more than one axon.

Although evaluation of sprouting is subjective, ranking of patients by the relative abundance of unmyelinated axons and noncollateral sprouts is justified, as sprouting clearly varied among patients. Since the relative abundance of sprouts increases with the total number of injections, the effect of botulinum injection on sprouting from terminal motor axons may be cumulative.

Long-Term Muscle Fiber Changes Following Repetitive Botulinum Toxin Injections

Muscle fiber atrophy, as well as gross atrophy of the muscle, develops following BTX administration in both experimental animals and humans (39,54,55). The atrophy reverses readily in experimental animals. After several months, the histological appearance of the muscle returns to ''normal.'' To determine if muscle fiber atrophy persists in humans, the histological appearance of the same muscles described above was studied and compared with normal orbicularis oculi muscle and muscle from patients with blepharospasm not previously treated with BTX injection. Mean fiber diameters and variance were not different from controls if specimens were taken from patients who had not been injected within 4 months of the biopsy (39,54). There are no long-term, persistent changes in orbicularis muscle fiber appearance following BTX injections, and BTX-induced muscle fiber atrophy in humans is reversible (Fig. 14).

The Maintenance of Altered Neuromuscular Interactions Following Botulinum Toxin Injection

The normal NMJ is not static but is constantly remodeled. Axonal sprouts spontaneously grow from the terminal axonal arborization, and other axonal processes retract. Overall, the area of neuromuscular contact remains relatively constant. In muscles treated with

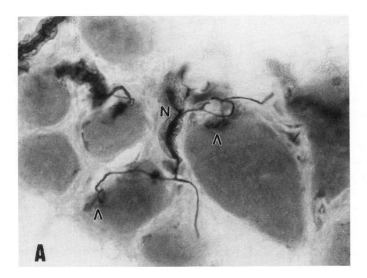

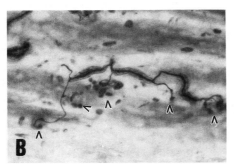

BTX, in contrast, the potential sites of neuromuscular contact seem to increase. There are more end plates on muscle fibers, and many of the end plates are larger than normal. Why these synapses are not remodeled is not known. Investigation of the persistence of these synapses may have implications for understanding abnormal synapse maintenance in disease.

In summary, BTX injection into the human orbicularis oculi muscle produces axonal sprouts, variation in the size of end plates, with expansion of some end plates and the apparent formation of new and smaller end plates, and reorganization of muscular innervation. Repeated and long-standing functional denervation allows axonal sprouts to induce the formation of nascent end plates on the functionally denervated muscle fibers, thus producing axonal collaterals. The number of muscle fibers innervated by a single preterminal axon increases. A single muscle fiber may be innervated by more than one preterminal axon (Table 1). Muscle fibers do not remain atrophic despite more persisting changes in the motor axon terminals.

Morphological abnormalities of terminal motor axons and NMJs increase with the number of injections or the severity of the paralysis, and seem to be persistent. These observations may have implications for understanding the stability of the NMJ and may have clinical relevance as well.

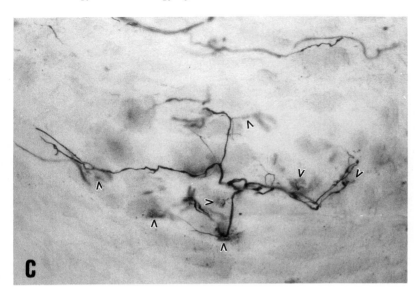

Figure 12 Axonal collaterals. (A) Terminal innervation = at least 2. Unmyelinated collaterals originate at nodes of Ranvier (N) of a preterminal axon and from the terminal axon, and extend to end plates on adjacent muscle fibers in a patient receiving nine injections ($\times$ 500, SCI using an antibody to PO). (B) Terminal innervation = 5 in a patient receiving 2 injections. Unmyelinated and myelinated collaterals (arrowheads) extend from nodes and from the terminal axon ($\times$ 200, SCI using an antibody to PO). (C) Terminal innervation = 7 in a patient with 18 injections. ($\times$ 200, silver-cholinesterase.)

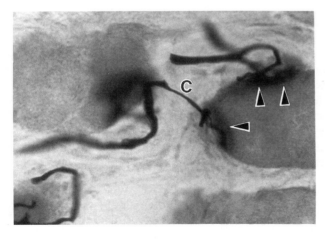

Figure 13 Dual innervation of muscle fibers. An ultraterminal collateral (C) extends to an end plate on a muscle fiber also innervated by another preterminal axon ($\times$ 600, silver-cholinesterase).

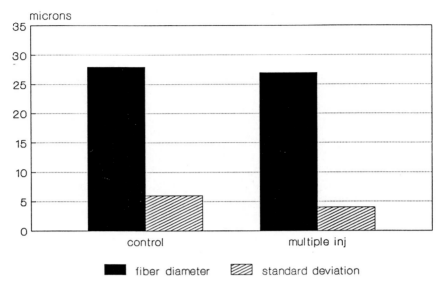

Figure 14 Muscle fiber size and variance after repeated injections. Long-term muscle fiber atrophy does not occur after repeated injections but does occur within 3–12 weeks and is reversible.

DIFFUSION OF BIOLOGICAL ACTIVITY FROM THERAPEUTIC INJECTION SITES: CLINICAL SIGNIFICANCE

Strabismus

"Strabismus" is an ophthalmic term that describes pathological misalignment of the eye. Therapy with BTX had been advocated by Scott (1–3) as an alternative to conventional extrocular muscle surgery because of the greater simplicity of the procedure. Unfortunately, therapy offered by the toxin injection is temporary, and the injection needs to be repeated in a majority of cases to maintain ocular alignment. The ability of the clinician to target the desired muscle exactly is limited by BTX diffusion away from the site of injection. Treatment usually involves injection of the medial rectus or lateral rectus muscles (horizontal rectus muscles) to treat horizontal deviations of the eyes. Diffusion of BTX into the vertical rectus muscles resulting in complications is common (1–3). Induced vertical deviation of the eye when horizontal deviations are being treated is clearly a limiting factor, occurring in approximately 15% of cases (3). Ptosis from intraorbital

Table 1 Summary: Morphology of Botulinum Toxin-Induced Sprouts In Humans

"Nondirected" sprouts following muscle or Schwann cell basal lamina
Expansion of muscle end plate regions
Increased number of end plates on a single muscle fiber
Increased number of end plates in regions of muscle
Axonal collaterals
Increased number of muscle fibers innervated by a single motor axon
More than one axon innervating a single muscle fiber with no loss of motor axons and normal
   muscle histochemistry

injections of BTX into extraocular muscles with diffusion into the levator palpebrae superioris muscle is also very common (see below).

Blepharospasm and Meige Syndrome

Over the past 12 years, BTX therapy has expanded to treatment of focal and segmental dystonias (4–11). In these conditions, neurologic imaging and even postmortem examination usually do not reveal structural lesions within the brain.

The first dystonia for which BTX therapeutic technology was used was benign essential blepharospasm and Meige syndrome (4). This form of neurologic blepharospasm is associated with blinding involuntary eyelid closure that leads to debilitation and desperation. In the past, therapy had included the use of neuroleptic medications, which were usually ineffective (56). Surgical therapy involving transection of the facial nerve or removal of the orbicularis oculi muscle in surgical stripping procedures (57,58) was tried, but in many patients this approach is only partially effective, and it is occasionally associated with undesirable complications.

Botulinum toxin has become the only consistent therapy for neurologic forms of blepharospasm. The eyelids are injected with small quantities of BTX (15–75 IU), producing an effective weakening of the protagonist muscle of eyelid closure, the orbicularis oculi. This muscle must be injected every 3 months in the case of essential blepharospasm and Meige syndrome and every 5 months in blepharospasm associated with hemifacial spasm and aberrant regeneration of the seventh cranial nerve (60).

As BTX therapy for this disease has proven to be effective (4,5,7), it has also been limited by several complications, including ptosis, exposure keratopathy, diplopia (double vision), and epiphora (tearing). Ptosis is defined as a drooping of the upper eyelid causing encroachment of the upper lid on the visual axis and effectively decreasing vision. This complication is generally transient and disappears as the denervative effect of the botulinum toxin wears off. It occurs in approximately 10% of patients treated and is particularly prone to occur when the injections of BTX are made close to the superior sulcus. Although patients already have eyelid disease causing obstruction of vision, visual function is further impaired by the ptosis. Understanding the cause of this complication is important to the effective application of the therapy. The occurrence of ptosis is thought to relate to diffusion of the toxin from the injected orbicularis oculi muscle into the superior orbit, effectively weakening the retractor of the upper eyelid, the levator palpebrae superioris muscle (5). Weakening of the muscular portion of the levator causes dropping of the upper lid margin. Given that the control of upper eyelid movement is primarily a balance between the actions of the orbicularis muscle and those of the levator palpebrae superioris muscle, effective application of BTX for blepharospasm involves confining the biological effect of the toxin to the orbicularis muscle, the protagonist muscle causing the abnormal movement. *The anatomical configuration of the muscles of the upper eyelid allows selective weakening of the orbicularis muscle and, therefore, effective therapy with BTX. The long tendon of the upper eyelid retractor, the levator aponeurosis, extends along the undersurface of the orbicularis muscle into the tarsal plate. In that the muscular portions of the levator palpebrae superioris muscle are remote from its antagonist (the orbicularis muscle), there is less likelihood that the BTX will diffuse into the elevator of the eyelid. This anatomical distance between eyelid orbicularis (pretarsal orbicularis) and levator muscle provides an anatomic explanation for therapeutic success in selectively targeting the orbicularis muscle in treating blepharospasm. This explanation also provides insight into the cause of this complication and a method to guard against its occurrence.*

Another complication associated with therapeutic injections of BTX into the eyelids is diplopia. This occurs less commonly ($< 5\%$ of patients) and is transient, lasting several days to several weeks. Nelson and her co-workers (61) have linked this complication to injections in the lower lid, particularly the inner aspect of the lower lid. The reason for the occurrence of diplopia appears to relate to the anatomical proximity of the inferior oblique muscle to the inner portion of the lower lid. The inferior oblique muscle arises in the very anterior portions of the medial orbit and penetrates the major fascia of the lower lid (capsulopalpebral fascia) very close to the cutaneous surface of the medial lower lid. Injection into the inner aspects of the lower lid brings the toxin within several millimeters of this muscle, so that the toxin can readily diffuse into this region and produce this complication. Avoiding medial lower lid injections reduces the incidence of diplopia (61).

With respect to the issue of efficacy in the treatment of blepharospasm, it appears that diffusion may again play a role. The location of the injection sites used today was empirically derived and was based on apparent efficacy as well as a strategy that limited complications. The need for multiple injection points adds to the discomfort of the application procedure. Initially, therefore, the effects of injecting only electrically deter-mined motor points of the orbicularis oculi muscle were studied (62). The motor points of the orbicularis oculi muscle are essentially in two locations, the outer portion of the upper eyelid and the medial portion of the lower eyelid. The motor point is defined as the area within muscle that has the lowest threshold for contraction in response to external electrical stimulation. Generally, motor points correspond to points of major motor nerve branch penetration into the muscle proper (62). Comparisons of single motor-point injection with multiple-point injections were made in a series of 10 patients by using the multiple-point injection strategy on one eye and the motor-point injection strategy on the other, each eye receiving the same dose. Eight of the 10 patients found that the eye treated by multiple-point injection technique had a substantially better result than the eye treated with single motor-point injection. The other two patients noted no differences between eyes (62). The results of this clinical study suggested several points:

1.   Dose-independent variables are involved in determining efficacy in BTX treatment.
2.   Spreading the toxin throughout the muscle may have increased toxin diffusion throughout most of its innervation zone.
3.   The results tend to negate the opinion that motor points could provide a superior injection location.

Histologic Innervation Zone Analysis of Human Orbicularis Oculi

In an effort to explore the innervation zone, that is, the topographical distribution of NMJs within a muscle, strips of orbicularis oculi muscle taken from the pretarsal portions of the muscle during routine ptosis surgery were analyzed for concentration and distribution of the NMJs using an AChE enzyme histochemistry method (62). Although only the pretarsal portions of the muscle were analyzed in this study, this portion of the muscle is exactly over the lateral motor point of the upper lid. The results indicated that the NMJs were diffusely distributed through the entire upper portion of the orbicularis muscle (Fig. 15). This finding clearly correlates with the large degree of facial nerve projection and ramification into the orbicularis muscle from temporal, zygomatic, and buccal branches. This observation leads to the hypothesis that multiple injection points were preferable because this injection technique tended to cover more of the innervation zone of the orbicularis muscle as compared with a single-point large-dose injection. For orbicularis muscle, this appears to be a plausible explanation for the superiority of the multiple-point

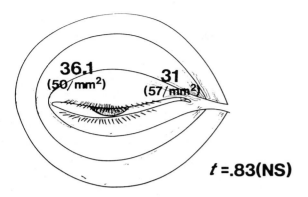

Figure 15 Distribution of the neuromuscular junctions within the upper eyelid orbicularis oculi muscle. Acetylcholinesterase staining can be used to map the distribution of neuromuscular junctions (innervation zone) within a muscle. Neuromuscular junction distribution was determined for the portion of the orbicularis oculi contained in the upper eyelid from specimens taken to debulk the upper eyelid fold during routine ptosis surgery on a patient never injected with botulinum toxin (62). The distribution of the neuromuscular junctions is diffuse within these muscle strips and specifically not concentrated over the electrically determined motor points for this muscle (62). The diffuse distribution of the innervation zone may be the reason that multiple injections into this muscle for the treatment of blepharospasms are superior to single or ''motor point'' injections. Large numbers refer to absolute NMJ counts, and small numbers relate these counts according to surface area. The motor point of the upper lid is directly over the lateral pretarsal orbicularis muscle.

injection technique. It appears that diffusing the toxin along the muscle proper was preferable in this particular anatomical location. This study also disproved the notion that motor point of the muscle corresponds to the innervation zone (distribution area of motor end plates within a given muscle).

Adult-Onset Spasmodic Torticollis

Adult-onset spasmodic torticollis is a segmental dystonia involving cervical muscles. The condition can occasionally be associated with Meige syndrome or other forms of head and neck movement disorders. A thickened protruding sternocleidomastoid muscle is the most characteristic finding in these patients on physical examination. Torticollis has variable expression, the most common pattern being a distorted posture with head rotated to a side of shoulder elevation (type 1, type 2) (6). Another variation involves tilting of the head toward the side of shoulder elevation (type 3) (6). Another variation includes involuntary backward tilting of the head (retrocollis, type 4a) or flexing of the head toward the chest (antecollis, type 4b) (6). Patients often develop pain early in the course of the disease, which is frequently progressive. The disease is often associated with involuntary jerking movements of varying frequency and amplitude.

Past therapy has included the use of neuroleptic medications, various forms of myectomy and denervating surgery, and occasionally biofeedback (63,64). Unfortunately, previous medical therapies have not been satisfactory. Surgical procedures are often associated with inconsistent results and occasionally with disfiguring scarring and further impairment in posture.

The application of BTX to the treatment of this segmental disorder has been a great contribution to neurological medicine. It has proven to be the most efficacious therapy for torticollis and can be maintained over a period of years (6,12,23).

The major complication associated with the use of BTX for spasmodic torticollis has been dysphagia (40). Dysphagia is defined as difficulty in swallowing that can occasionally lead to the misdirection of food into the upper airway. Such misdirection can occasionally cause complete upper airway obstruction, which is a medical emergency possibly leading to death. Upper airway obstruction has occurred in at least one patient involved in the North American clinical studies (40). This patient was immediately and successfully treated by the Heimleich maneuver. Other complications have included weakness of the cervical muscles.

The diffusion model has proven to be important in finding a solution to the dysphagia problem. In retrospective studies, dysphagia appeared to be linked to the dose of BTX injected into the sternocleidomastoid muscle (Fig. 16): data indicated that doses in excess of 100 IU were associated with the complication (Table 2). In prospective data analysis, limiting the dose to the sternocleidomastoid muscle was shown to markedly decrease the incidence of this complication. The complication rate reported initially in our studies was comparable to those noted in other studies, approximately 15% (8,11,40,42). Limiting the sternocleidomastoid dose to less than 100 IU during an injection session reduced the

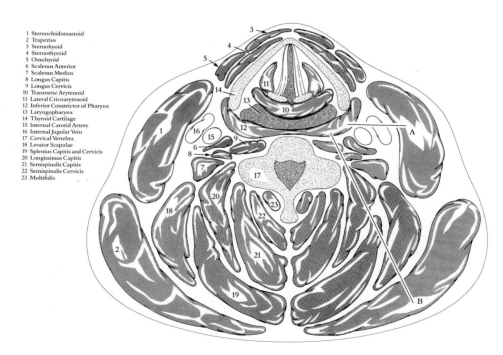

1 Sternocleidomastoid
2 Trapezius
3 Sternohyoid
4 Sternothyroid
5 Omohyoid
6 Scalenus Anterior
7 Scalenus Medius
8 Longus Capitis
9 Longus Cervicis
10 Transverse Arytenoid
11 Lateral Cricoarytenoid
12 Inferior Constrictor of Pharynx
13 Laryngopharynx
14 Thyroid Cartilage
15 Internal Carotid Artery
16 Internal Jugular Vein
17 Cervical Vertebra
18 Levator Scapulae
19 Splenius Capitis and Cervicis
20 Longissimus Capitis
21 Semispinalis Capitis
22 Semispinalis Cervicis
23 Multifidis

Figure 16 Dysphagia and the treatment of adult-onset spasmodic torticollis. Dysphagia can result from diffusion of botulinum toxin into the peripharyngeal musculature. This complication particularly occurs when high doses of botulinum toxin are given to the sternocleidomastoid muscle, which directly overlays the peripharyngeal muscles. This complication occurs as a result of direct spread of biological effect from injected sternocleidomastoid muscle into the deeper structures of the neck. Table 2 outlines the results of the clinical study linking dysphagia to the dose of botulinum toxin given over the sternocleidomastoid muscle.

Table 2 Comparison of Botulinum Toxin Dose and Injection Strategies in Patients Who Later Experienced Dysphagia and Those Who Did Not

	Dysphagia	No dysphagia
Sternocleidomastoid dose		
No. injection	7	42
Median dose	150	100
Interquartile range	10	150
Wilcoxon test	$Z = 2.22$	$p = 0.026$
Total dose		
No. injection	7	42
Median dose	160	150
Interquartile range	25	100
Wilcoxon test	$Z = 0.75$	$p = 0.45$

incidence of this complication to less than 2%. A plausible explanation for these findings is that diffusion of toxin from the sternocleidomastoid muscle into the peripharyngeal musculature resulted in weakening of the muscles involved in the swallowing reflex. The sternocleidomastoid muscle lies directly over the peripharyngeal musculature, while the other muscles usually injected in the treatment of spasmodic torticollis (levator scapulae, posterior scalene, trapezius, splenius capitis, splenius cervicis, and others) are more posterior to and remote from the pharyngeal muscles.

Since it appears that *dysphagia was secondary to toxin jump*, that is, toxin spread and diffusion from the sternocleidomastoid muscle, this complication can be limited by reducing the dose in this muscle (Fig. 16). Such an explanation for the results of these clinical studies suggest a dose-dependent diffusion phenomenon for the sternocleidomastoid muscle.

Efficacy in the treatment of adult-onset spasmodic torticollis may also depend on diffusion of the biological effects of the toxin from the injection sites. As this disease is definitely associated with multiple muscle group involvement in remote areas of the neck, injection of the entire complex of muscles involved with the posture disfigurement is necessary to achieve the most beneficial result.

Table 3 Response Rates, Comparing Multiple-Point and Single-Point Injections

	Single-Point	Multiple-Point	Mean dose, favorable response (IU)	Mean dose, no response (IU)
Pain	15/31	27/31[a]	165.7	147[b]
Posture deformity	13/42	33/44[a]	162.7	148.3[b]
Range of motion	15/39	33/44[a]	156.4	144.3[b]
Activity	13/39	29/38[a]	187.9	145.6[c]
Hypertrophy	27/39	34/44	161.4	154.6[b]
Tremor	4/17	9/17	163.5	146.9[b]

[a] $p < 0.002$, chi-square.
[b] Not statistically significant (Wilcoxon's test).
[c] $p = 0.04$.

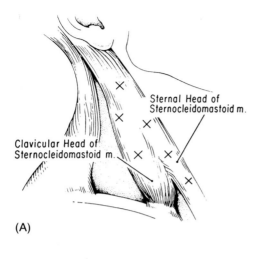

(A)

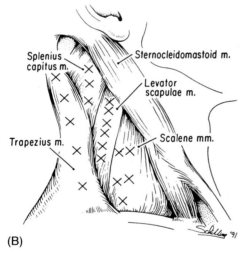

(B)

Figure 17 Efficacy and injection technique in the treatment of spasmodic torticollis. In clinical studies, the method of administration is as important to the beneficial results as is the dose of botulinum toxin administered. Figure 17 depicts two types of injection strategy to large dystonic anterior and posterior cervical muscles. The strategy of multiple-point injection per muscle (A,B) produces a superior clinical benefit compared with single injection points per muscle (C,D) or injection points just along a single area. An interpretation of these clinical results is that the multiple-point injection strategy allows a more homogeneous diffusion of the biologic effect of the toxin in the targeted muscles (Table 3).

Given the superior clinical results obtained with multiple-point injections in treating blepharospasm, a study was designed to test multiple-point versus single-point injection per muscle for the treatment of torticollis. By typical efficacy criteria for treatment of spasmodic torticollis—that is, effectiveness with respect to pain, posture deformity, range of motion of the cervical spine, hypertrophy, and activity limitation—better clinical results clearly were achieved in the group receiving multiple-point injections (Table 3, Figure 17). There was no significant difference in the total dose given to each of these

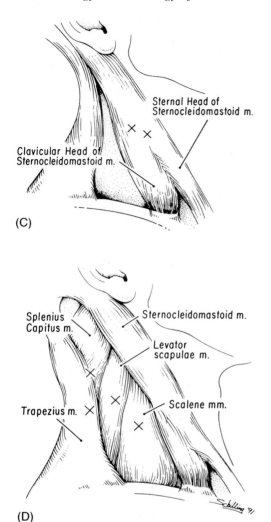

(C)

(D)

groups. These findings suggested that the technique of administration within individual large muscles was important to efficacy. It is unknown whether the innervation zone in these muscles is diffusely spread throughout the muscle rather than focally distributed. However, the results of the clinical study tend to suggest a diffuse innervation of most muscles involved with the syndrome. Two of us (G. E. Borodic, R. J. Ferrante) have recently shown that the albino rabbit longissimus dorsi, a very large paraspinal muscle, contains a diffuse innervation zone with periodic bands of NMJs approximately distributed at each spinal nerve root level.

A Depiction of the Diffusion Denervation Field in a Patient

An excellent example of the denervation field produced by a point injection of BTX is the regional depression of the vertical furrowing lines produced by the contraction of the corrugator muscles. These lines are associated with aging. An application demonstrating the denervation field is direct injection of the frontalis muscle in patients with expres-

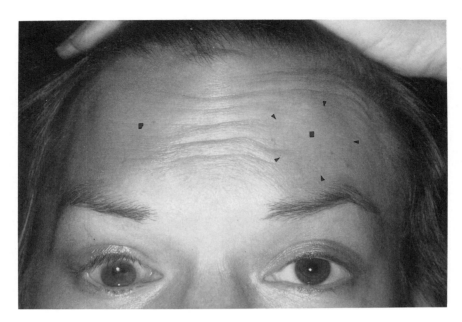

Figure 18 Depiction of denervation field in a patient. The forehead creases are generated by attachments of the frontalis muscle to the skin dermis. This patient was injected along the forehead. Note that the creases are blunted over a circular area after a point injection of botulinum toxin. The blunting of these creases indicates the field of effect of botulinum toxin in this clinical situation.

sionistic overcorrection after ptosis surgery by frontalis sling procedure (65). For instance, the patient shown in Fig. 18 had undergone a frontalis sling to correct total ptosis, using a tendon graft taken from her leg. During the high-amplitude facial movements naturally occurring with emotional expression, the upper lid would become overcorrected. The contractility of this patient's frontalis muscle was reduced on both sides, for symmetry, with point injections of BTX (Fig. 18). This resulted in the blunting of the transverse creases of the forehead over a circular area. The transverse creases are generally produced by the insertion of the frontalis muscle into the dermis of the forehead skin. With high-amplitude contractions and high tone in the muscles, these creases are accentuated. The circular area of blunting of creases indicates decreased tone in the frontalis muscle over a defined region within this muscle. Of note, this patient was injected with 10 IU to each location, and each injection has produced a denervation field of approximately 15 mm radius.

The denervation field is a phenomenon that may vary within various muscle fiber arrangements, after repetitive injections, and with different preparations of the toxin. Further evaluations with respect to these variables are currently under way.

Histologic Determination of the Denervation Field and Botulinum Toxin Activity at Therapeutic Doses

Muscle fiber size, fiber size variability, and AChE staining characteristics were used to assess muscle fiber response and diffusion of biologic activity from a point injection within a long muscle, in an attempt to further define the denervation field scientifically.

The albino rabbit longissimus dorsi muscle was chosen because of its length, generally parallel fiber orientation, diffuse innervation zone, and easy accessibility for muscle biopsy and injection. Subsequent to these studies, a diffuse periodic distribution of NMJs evenly down the length of this muscle was found that further validates this model. Longissimus dorsi muscles in 2- to 3-kg albino rabbits were injected at a point along the middorsal spine (40). At the injection point, a tattoo was applied over the skin and muscle with India ink. In addition to the tattoo, the injection point was anatomically placed at the dorsal eminence of the right levator scapulae to insure reproducible localization of the injection site even if the tattoo faded or tissue plane sliding made identification of the injection point difficult.

Botulinum toxin type A (Oculinum; Oculinum Inc.) was diluted at various concentrations used for clinical study. Control injections were made with 0.9% sodium chloride diluent.

After injection, 5 weeks were allowed to elapse to provide an adequate interval for optimum muscle fiber atrophy and AChE spread (40). Dissection was made over the dorsal spine, removing the latissimus dorsi muscle and exposing the longissimus dorsi muscle down its entire length to the caudal end of the lumbar spine. Biopsy samples were taken at 15-mm intervals and frozen with liquid nitrogen (Fig. 19A). Statistical variations in fiber diameter were compared with F ratio analysis. Fiber diameter and diameter variance analysis were done in each specimen beginning at the injection site and at 15-mm intervals to 45 mm from the injection point.

The intensity of AChE staining was estimated using reference photographs representing gradations of spread and intensity of staining (Fig. 19 B–E). These gradations were rated 0–4. The spread and intensity of AChE staining activity for each biopsy was matched to the closest reference photograph. Four biopsies were developed from each muscle, including controls, and two or three animals were used for each dose determination in the histochemical analysis as well as the analysis of fiber diameter variability and size.

The muscle fiber average diameter was determined from summation of counts on four biopsies taken at 15-mm intervals over a linear distance of 4.5 cm from the injection site. The average muscle fiber diameter through the entire muscle (four biopsies) appeared to correlate to the dose of BTX administered. The average muscle fiber diameter after a 10-IU injection was 26.7 μm (s = 14.8) (n = 1600), at 5 IU, 31.7 μm (s = 14.6) (n = 1600), at 2.5 IU, 30.4 μm (s = 14.0) (n = 1600), and at 1 IU, 30.7 μm (s = 11.1) (n = 2400). Control fiber diameter was 35.4 μm (s = 9.2) (n = 1600).

Fiber size variability also correlated directly with the dose administered at the injection site and through the entire muscle (Fig. 20).

The field of biologic activity within the injected muscle was assessed morphologically by measuring fiber size variability and histochemically by means of AChE staining characteristic. The diffusion of biologic activity within the injected muscle correlated with the dose administered. Fiber size variability at 1 IU became insignificant in comparison with controls at 15 mm from the injection point (F ratio <1.4 based on 200 fiber counts per specimen). At 2.5, 5, and 10 IU the biologic effect reflected by fiber size variability was sustained throughout a 45-mm length along the muscle strip (Fig. 21). Fiber size variation was significantly different from controls at all higher doses down the entire muscle strip (F ratio > 1.4). Spread and intensity of AChE staining confirmed that the biological effect substantially diminished at 15 mm for the 1-IU dose. The AChE activity suggested that higher doses (2.5–10 IU) produced a biological effect throughout the 45-mm length of the muscle strip (Fig. 22).

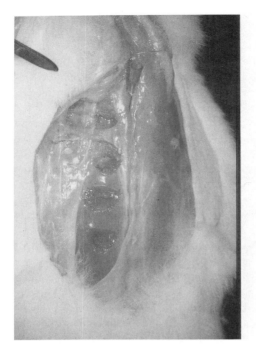

(A)

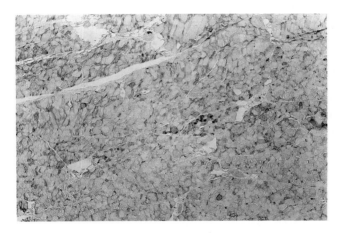

(B)

Figure 19 Animal model for quantization of botulinum toxin diffusion. (A) Animal model for evaluating diffusion of botulinum toxin down longissimus dorsi muscle involves taking multiple biopsies along this muscle. The contralateral muscle is also used for assessment of extramuscular spread. Other contiguous muscles can also be used. (B–E) Diffusion down the longissimus dorsi muscle can be monitored using the acetylcholinesterase staining characteristic. Note that at the injection site after 1.25 IU of botulinum toxin, there is diffuse spread of cholinesterase. Over 45 mm, there is gradual decrease in cholinesterase spreading until the stain become concentrated only at the neuromuscular junctions. The photographs used in this illustration provided reference standards by which tissue at varying distances were used to evaluate diffusion of biologic effect at varying doses (see Figs. 1,2,20,21,22).

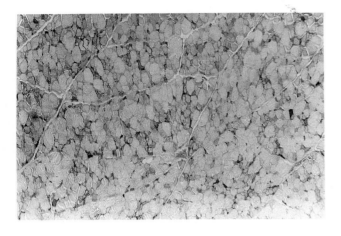

(C)

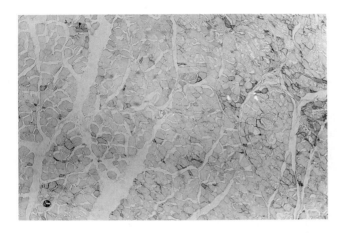

(D)

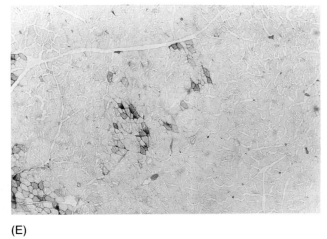

(E)

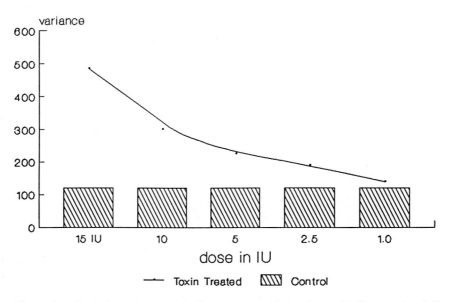

Figure 20 Dose-dependent muscle fiber responses. Fiber size variability correlated directly with the dose at the injection site, as did the average fiber diameter throughout the muscle.

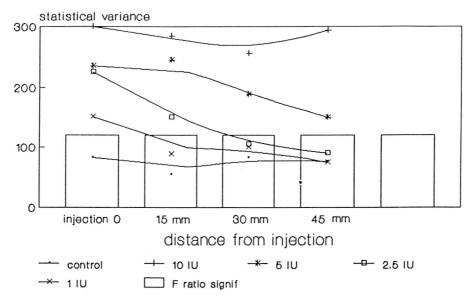

Figure 21 Dose-dependent diffusion. The biological effect within longissimus dorsi muscle appears to be dose-related. The larger the dose the more homogeneous the effect is throughout the muscle strip evaluated. Fiber variations were compared using F ratios.

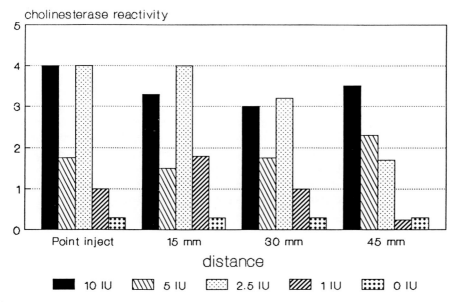

Figure 22 Dose-dependent diffusion: Acetylcholinesterase staining characteristic suggested that higher dose produced a biological effect throughout the entire strip, whereas the smaller dose produced a gradient down the length of the strip studied.

In order to assess extramuscular diffusion properties of BTX-A, fiber diameter variations and fiber diameter size were determined on the contralateral longissimus dorsi muscle at 45 mm from the injection site at each dose. Fiber size variation was significantly greater in the injected muscle at 45 mm than at an extramuscular site 45 mm from the point of injection for 10 IU (F = 2.5, $p < 0.01$) and 5 IU (F = 1.7, $p < 0.01$). For 2.5 IU and 1 IU the differences in fiber size variation between the intramuscular and extramuscular sites were not significant. These data indicated that linear spread of biologic effect may be greater within the injected muscle than in a remote muscle at an equivalent distance from the point of injection of BTX, although the biologic effect did spread to contiguous muscles when larger doses were used.

The AChE activity and the fiber variability pattern confirmed the presence of a dose-dependent field of action for BTX-A.

Diffusion of toxin away from targeted muscles ("toxin jump") appears to cause complications (40). It is therefore useful to attempt to quantify diffusion of biologic activity from a point injection at various doses used in clinical practice. The findings indicate that the degree of fiber atrophy and fiber size variability as well as intensity of AChE staining at the point of injection are directly related to the dose administered. Furthermore, the diffusion of biologic effects from the point of injection within the longissimus dorsi muscle is dose-dependent. Animals given 2.5–10 IU showed substantial diffusion of the toxin's biological effects over a linear distance of 45 mm within this individual large muscle. In contrast, animals given 1 IU demonstrated a graduated biological effect inversely related to the distance from the point injection. There appeared to be collapse of biological effect as indicated by fiber size variation and AChE staining characteristics between 15 and 30 mm from the point of injection of 1 IU within the injected muscle.

The biological effect in contiguous muscles was evaluated in the longissimus dorsi muscle contralateral to the injection. At lower doses, the toxin's activity did not spread to 45 mm on a muscle remote from the injected muscle. In a previous study (40), the biological activity of BTX has been shown to cross fascial planes and cause histochemical changes in noninjected muscles within lesser distances (<2 cm.). The explanation for the extension of biological effect to a greater distance within the injected longissimus muscle than in extramuscular locations may be that the toxin's activity diffuses to a greater degree within an individual muscle. Alternatively, the linear distance over which chemodenervation occurs may be exaggerated in muscles with very long parallel muscle fibers, such as the longissimus dorsi. At higher doses there appeared to be dissemination of biological activity down the contralateral muscle, although not to the same degree as in the injected muscle.

Containment of biological activity within a targeted area of the body is a desirable goal for BTX injection therapy, and these data offer insight into the intensity and diffusion of biological activity within the injected muscle and at muscles remote from the injection site. Diffusion of biological activity within the muscle appears to be a function of dose and can be graduated. The denervation field can be defined as a linear distance from the point of injection over which BTX causes a denervation effect. The degree of denervation as indicated by fiber size atrophy and fiber size variation is at any distance from the point of infection a function of dose. The size of the denervation field is also a function of dose, as indicated by the homogeneous effects the larger injection doses produced down the long muscle strip. As denervation field size and degree of neurogenic fiber atrophy are both dose-dependent, larger doses of BTX can be expected to produce more weakness and fiber atrophy but with greater spread of the toxin from the injection sites. As complications in clinical practice are often related to undesirable toxin spread, the field of denervation must be considered in the clinical use of BTX.

Since, in clinical practice, muscle atrophy has been noted to occur qualitatively after injection on gross inspection, it is of interest to quantitate the degree of muscle fiber atrophy in this experimental model. From cross-sectional muscle fiber diameter changes after BTX injection, it appears that fiber atrophy of 25% was possible. This analysis is consistent with clinical observations, particularly in the sternocleidomastoid muscles of patients treated for torticollis.

Because the diffusion of biological activity away from a point of injection is dose-related and measurable, it may be possible to calculate in clinical protocols reasonable diffusion fields from a site of a given dose of BTX. Diffusion fields can be established within injected muscles, within contiguous muscles, and within muscles of various fiber orientations. The results of this study underscore the importance of the clinician's being knowledgeable about the anatomical distances between important muscles within the area being injected as well as the action of muscle groups in which BTX is administered. Such information may provide a scientific approach to determining distances between injection sites at various doses. Furthermore, the minimum dose necessary to produce a homogeneous denervation effect down a long muscle would be ideal if just that muscle were being targeted for injection. Doses in excess of the minimum dose for homogeneous denervation would be more prone to spread outside the fascial planes of the muscle and into contiguous muscle groups, potentially causing complications.

Sensitization after Repetitive Botulinum Toxin Injections

According to the literature (66–68), the incidence of sensitization appears to be approximately 3–5% over several years of repeated injections for cervical dystonia (torticollis), and sensitization is found in approximately 30% of patients who lose beneficial response to therapy (67). Sensitization has occurred with both Botox and Dysport. When present, neutralizing antibodies have generally rendered the therapy ineffective.

Previous authors, however, have not demonstrated antibody formation with lower-dose application for the treatment of blepharospasm and Meige syndrome and have argued that at the doses typically used for these indications, it is unlikely that antibodies can form (69,70). In contrast to these reports, the following case demonstrates that antibody-mediated resistance can be associated with treatment failure for low-dose applications such as treatment of blepharospasm.

Case Report

A 57-year-old magazine managing editor presented with visual loss secondary to blepharospasm. The problem gradually developed over several years and became disabling particularly during driving and conversation. Shortly after the onset of involuntary blepharospasm, involuntary lower facial grimacing was noted. The patient's son had developed involuntary hand tremor at the age of 19 years.

Initial therapy included injection of 30 IU (total dose) of BTX-A. There was minimal improvement. Another injection of 60 IU to each eye, was administered with improvement in symptoms. Repeated injections at 3-month intervals involved doses ranging from 50 to 100 IU. After each injection there was some subjective improvement and decreased orbicularis contractility on physical examination. After eight beneficial injections, no benefit was achieved with an additional six injections at 3-month intervals. Orbicularis muscle contractility was not weakened with subsequent injections.

A limited therapeutic myectomy procedure demonstrated no evidence of fiber atrophy or spread of AChE staining activity from the NMJ on the sarcolemma 4 weeks after the last injection (Fig. 23). Figure 2 shows a typical AChE staining response in orbicularis oculi muscle after 5 weeks. A supramaximal quantity of BTX (200 IU) was injected into the patient's eyelids and produced no benefit or orbicularis weakness. A serum specimen was obtained for mouse antibody bioassay.

The patient's serum was tested for neutralizing BTX antibodies. Two samples containing patient plasma were tested, one with BTX-A, and the other with BTX-B. One milliliter of patient plasma was mixed with 1 ml of buffer (30 mM phosphate buffer, pH 6.2, containing 0.2% human serum albumin) and 25.7 IU of either BTX-A or BTX-B. Two control samples with buffer only plus toxin were simultaneously run for each of the toxin serotypes. These mixtures were allowed to incubate at room temperature for 1 hour before analysis for biological activity. A mouse bioassay was used to determine the levels of BTX in any sample. A 0.2-ml (2.57 IU toxin) aliquot of each of the mixtures was injected into five mice. Following injection the animals were monitored for 5 days, and the total deaths in each group were determined.

To provide an estimate of the amount of antitoxin present in the patient plasma, a series of dilutions of plasma were examined. Probit analysis of titration data is shown in Table 4 and indicates that the LD_{50} was at the 1:3.96 dilution. At this dilution there was enough antitoxin present in the diluted plasma to neutralize 1.57 IU of BTX-A. On the basis of these calculations, 1 ml of this patient's plasma contained enough antitoxin to neutralize

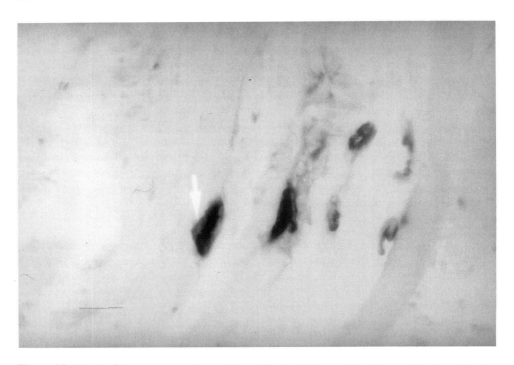

Figure 23 Lack of tissue response in a patient with circulating anti–botulinum A toxin antibody: This orbicularis oculi biopsy was stained for acetylcholinesterase in a region injected with botulinum toxin 5 weeks before the procedure. Note that the acetylcholinesterase activity remains confined to a neuromuscular junction and is not diffusely staining (see Figs. 2,19,22). This patient subsequently was found to have developed botulinum A toxin antibodies (see Table 4).

31.1 IU of BTX-A. Expressed in terms of international units of antitoxin, this is 0.0003 IU/ml of plasma.

Titration of the amount of antibody in plasma was accomplished by examining the neutralizing properties of seven dilutions of patient plasma: 1:1, 1:2, 1:4, 1:8, and 1:16. One milliliter of each dilution was incubated for 1 hr with an equal volume of buffer containing 25.7 IU of BTX-A. Five mice were injected with 0.2 ml of each test dilution. The mice were monitored for 5 days and the mortality with each dilution was determined. The dilution at which 50% death occurred was determined by probit analysis. At the

Table 4 Toxin vs Serum or Buffer

	Percent Mortality	
Conditions	Test 1	Test 2
BTX-A + serum	0	0
BTX-A + buffer	100	80
BTX-B + serum	100	100
BTX-B + buffer	80	100

LD_{50}, there was sufficient antitoxin present to neutralize 3 IU of BTX-A, and 1 IU remained. Estimations of the antibody titers in the patient plasma were determined on this basis.

Presented in Table 4 are the results from two tests in which patient plasma was diluted 1:1 with buffer containing 20 IU of either BTX-A or BTX-B. These results show that patient plasma inactivated only samples containing BTX-A, whereas samples containing BTX-B were unaffected. The controls indicate that these results cannot be accounted for on the basis of low BTX activity. This test indicates only that there was at least enough antitoxin present in 1 ml of patient plasma to neutralize 4 IU of BTX-A.

This case report demonstrates immunologically mediated resistance causing a poor response after repeated injections in a patient who received relatively small amounts of therapeutic BTX. The presence of neutralizing antibody specific for BTX-A was demonstrated. Furthermore, tissue resistance to BTX injection was demonstrated with muscle biopsy using AChE staining. The true incidence of circulating antibodies in patients with various diseases treated with BTX is still an open question. There is also a need for a conventional assay to measure circulating antibodies.

Biological Activity of Preparations and Immunological Considerations

When BTX is prepared from ammonium sulfate crystals with other inert proteins, the preparation is known as the botulinum toxin protein complex (41). Botox is a BTX protein complex. Further protein purification can be used, removing inert proteins from the BTX protein complex and yielding higher grade of neurotoxin per quantity of protein. An index useful in evaluating the relative purity of a biologically active protein preparation is specific activity. Specific activity is defined as the ratio of biologic activity (IU using the standard mouse assay) to the quantity of protein present in the preparation as determined photometrically (71,72). The specific activity of the first preparation used in clinical studies was 2.5 IU/ng protein in the preparation. Some initial efforts have been made to ensure that reasonably pure protein preparations are used clinically. The batches used to prepare the pharmaceutical material are required to demonstrate greater than 1,000,000 LD_{50}/ml before dilution and lyophilization. However, the specific activity of the final preparation can be influenced by each step of the pharmacological preparation process. The potential significance of specific activity in clinical practice is unknown, but it may have a bearing on the immunogenicity of the final therapeutic agent. The antigenicity of BTX preparations is clearly an issue requiring further careful studies.

Toxic Dose of Botulinum Toxin in Man

One international unit is the LD_{50} dose for a 20- to 30-g white mouse. Over the past decade this unitage has been adapted to clinical application for the treatment of regional movement disorders. It has been estimated that approximately 3000 IU are needed to produce BTX intoxication in man (73).

SUMMARY

1. Diffusion of therapeutic botulinum toxin from points of intramuscular injection appears to be a dose-dependent phenomenon. Intensity of the denervative effect is also dose-dependent.

2. Diffusion of the denervative effect outside the muscles targeted for injection ("toxin jump") is responsible for side effects associated with the clinical use of botulinum toxin.

3. Limiting the dose of BTX in critical anatomical areas can be helpful in preventing complications (e.g., limiting the sternocleidomastoid muscle dose to prevent dysphagia in patients treated for spasmodic torticollis patients).

4. Multiple-point injections within targeted muscles have produced the most desirable clinical effects in patients with blepharospasm and adult-onset spasmodic torticollis. This injection approach may be more beneficial because it diffuses the biologic effect of the toxin more evenly throughout the innervation zone of the muscle.

5. Muscle fiber size variability and spread of AChE on muscle fibers are consistent histologic markers for therapeutic BTX effect. A dose-dependent gradient of biological activity can be demonstrated both within muscles injected and within adjacent muscles.

6. Long-term, repetitive treatments with therapeutic injections do not seem to produce permanent denervative effects as assessed through fiber size variation and cholinesterase staining characteristics in human muscle specimens.

7. Sprouting appears to cause changes in terminal axonal projections into muscle fibers, so that more fibers are innervated by a terminal axon.

8. Sensitization to BTX-A may occur after repetitive injections and can be an explanation for poor responses after such injections.

ACKNOWLEDGMENTS

We would like to thank Carolyn Driscoll for assistance in the preparation of this manuscript and Dr. Charles Hatheway for assistance developing the botulinum toxin antibody bioassay. Dr. Alderson would like to thank Drs. Richard Anderson and John Holds, who performed the orbicularis oculi myectomy, and Drs. Cheryl Harris and Jonathan Nebeker for assistance with muscle histochemistry.

REFERENCES

1. Scott AB. Botulinum toxin injections to eye muscles to correct strabismus. J Am Ophthalmol Soc 1981;79:734–770.
2. Scott AB, Magoon EH, McNeer KW, Stager DR. Botulinum treatment of strabismus in children. Trans Am Ophthalmol Soc 1990;87:174–180; discussion 180–184.
3. Scott AB. Strabismus injection treatment. In: NIH consensus development conference on clinical use of botulinum toxin, November 12–14, 1990. 117–118.
4. Scott AB, Kennedy EG, Stubbs HA. Botulinum A toxin injection as a treatment for blepharospasm. Arch Ophthalmol 1985;103:347–350.
5. Borodic GE, Cozzolino D. Blepharospasm and its treatment, with emphasis on the use of botulinum toxin. Plast Reconstr Surg 1989;83:546–554.
6. Borodic GE, Mills L, Joseph M. Botulinum A toxin for the treatment of adult-onset spasmodic torticollis. Plast Reconstr Surg 1991;87:285–289.
7. Borodic GE, Cozzolino D, Townsend DJ. Dose-response relationships in patients treated with botulinum toxin for more than three years (abstr). Sixth International Meeting of the Benign Essential Blepharospasm Research Foundation: 1988, August 25–27; Cambridge, MA. Ear Nose Throat J 1988;67:914.
8. Jankovic J, Orman J. Botulinum toxin for cranial cervical dystonia: a double blind placebo controlled study. Neurology 1987;37:616–623.

9. Blitzer A, Brin MF, Greene PE, Fahn S. Botulinum toxin injection for the treatment of oromandibular dystonia. Ann Otol Rhinol Largyngol 1989;98:93–97.

10. Fletcher NA, Quinn N. Dystonic syndromes. Curr Opin Neurol Neurosurg 1989;2:330–333.

11. Gelb DJ, Lowenstein DH, Arminoff MJ. Controlled trial of botulinum toxin injections in the treatment of spasmodic torticollis. Neurology 1989;39:80–84.

12. Borodic GE, Pearce LB, Joseph M. Cranial cervical dystonias, multiple vs single injection strategies. A clinical study. Head Neck 1992;14:33–37.

13. Kao I, Drachman D, Price DL. Botulinum toxin: mechanism of presynaptic blockade. Science 1976;193:1256.

14. Tse CK, Dolly JO, Hambleton P, Wray D, Melling J. Preparation and characterization of homogeneous neurotoxin type A from Clostridium botulinum. Its inhibitory action on neuronal release of acetylcholine in the absence and presence of bungarotoxin. Eur J Biochem 1982;122:493–500.

15. Evans DM, Williams RS, Stone CC, Hambleton P, Melling J, Dolly JO. Botulinum neurotoxin type B: its purification, radioiodination and interaction with rat brain synaptosomal membranes. Eur J Biochem 1986;154:409–416.

16. Dasgupta BR. Structure and biological activity of botulinum neurotoxin. J Physiol (Paris) 1990;84:220–228.

17. Singh BR, Dasgupta BR. Molecular topography and secondary structure comparisons of botulinum neurotoxin types A, B and E. Mol Cell Biochem 1989;86:87–95.

18. Sakaguchi G, Ohishi I, Kozaki S. Purification and oral toxicities of Clostridium botulinum progenitor toxins. In: Biomedical aspects of botulinum toxin. Academic Press, 1981:21–33.

19. Black JD, Dolly JO. Selective location of acceptors for botulinum neurotoxin A in the central and peripheral nervous systems. J Cell Biol 1986;103:521–534.

20. Williams RS, Tse CK, Dolly JO, Hambelton P, Melling J. Radioiodination of botulinum neurotoxin type A with retention of biologic activity and its binding to brain synaptosomes. Eur J Biochem 1983;131:437–445.

21. Molgo J, Comella JX, Angaut-Petit D, Pecot-Dechavassine M, Tabit N, Faille L, Mallart A, Thesleff S. Presynaptic actions of botulinal neurotoxins at the vertebrate neuromuscular junctions. J Physiol (Paris) 1990;84:152–166.

22. Ashton AC, Dolly JO. Microtubule-dissociating drugs and A23187 reveal differences in the inhibition of synaptosomal transmitter release by botulinum neurotoxins types A and B. J Neurochem 1991;56:827–835.

23. Gansel M, Penner R, Dreyer F. Distinct sites of action of clostridial neurotoxins revealed by double-poisoning of mouse motor nerver terminals. Eur J Physiol 1987;409:533–539.

24. Schmitt A, Dreyer F, John C. At least three sequential steps are involved in tetanus toxin–induced block of neuromuscular transmission. Naunyn-Schmiedebergs Arch Pharmacol 1981;317:326–330.

25. Simpson LL. The origin, structure, and pharmacological activity of botulinum toxin. Pharmacol Rev 1981;33:155–188.

26. DasGupta BR, ed. Proceedings of the International Conference on Botulinum and Tetanus Neurotoxins. Madison, Wisconsin, May 1992.

27. Duchen LW. Changes in motor innervation and cholinesterase localization induced by botulinum toxin in skeletal muscle of mouse: differences between fast and slow muscles. J Neurol Neurosurg Psychiat 1970;33:40–54.

28. Duchen LW. Histologic differences between soleus and gastrocnemius muscles in the mouse after local injection of botulinum toxin. J Physiol (Lond) 1969;204:17–18.

29. Aldersen K, Holds JB, Andersen RL. Botulinum induced alteration of nerve muscle interactions in human orbicularis oculi following treatment for blepharospasm. Neurology 1991;41:1800–1805.

30. Schuetze SM, Role LW. Developmental regulation of nicotinic acetylcholine receptors. Annu Rev Neurosci 1987;10:403–457.

31. Fertuke HC, Salpeter MM. Localization of acetylcholine receptors by I 125a bungarotoxin binding at mouse neuromuscular junction. Proc Natl Acad Sci USA 1974;71:1376–1378.
32. Bevan S, Steinbach JH. The distribution of bungarotoxin binding sites on mammalian skeletal muscle developing in vivo. J Physiol 1977;267:195–215.
33. Fambrough DM. Acetylcholine receptor: revised estimates of extrajunctional receptor density in denervated rat diaphragm. J Gen Physiol 1974;64:468–472.
34. Miledi R. The acetylcholine sensitivity of from muscle fibers after complete and partial denervation. J Physiol 1960;151:1–23.
35. Goldman D, Staple J. Spatial and temporal expression of acetylcholine receptor RNAs in innervated and denervated rat soleus muscle. Neuron 1989;3:219–228.
36. Pestronk A, Drachman DB, Griffin JW. Effect of botulinum toxin on trophic regulation of acetylcholine receptors. Nature 1976;264:787–789.
37. Yee WC, Pestronk A. Mechanisms of postsynaptic plasticity: remodeling of the junctional acetylcholine receptor cluster induced by motor nerve terminal outgrowth. J Neurosci 1987;7:2019–2024.
38. Angaut-Petit D, Molgo J, Comella JX, Faille L, Tabti N. Terminal sprouting in mouse neuromuscular junctions poisoned with botulinum type A toxin: morphological and electro-physiological features. Neuroscience 1990;37:799–808.
39. Borodic GE, Ferrante R. Histologic effects of repeated botulinum toxin over many years in human orbicularis oculi muscle. J Clin Neuro-Ophthalmol 1992;12:121–127.
40. Borodic GE, Joseph M, Fay L, Cozzolino D, Ferrante R. Botulinum A toxin for the treatment of spasmodic torticollis. Dysphagia and regional toxin spread. Head Neck 1990;12:392–398.
41. Borodic GE, Pearce LB, Johnson EJ, Schantz E. Clinical and scientific aspects of botulinum toxin. Ophthalmol Clin N Am 1991;43:491–503.
42. Jankovic J, Brin M. Therapeutic uses of botulinum toxin. N Engl J Med 1991;324:1194.
43. Kao I, Drachman DB. Motor nerve sprouting and acetylcholine receptors. Science 1978;193:1256.
44. Duchen LW, Stritch SJ. The effects of botulinum toxin on the pattern of innervation of skeletal muscle in the mouse. Q J Exp Physiol 1968;53:84–89.
45. Gillum WN, Anderson RL. Blepharospasm surgery: an anatomical approach. Arch Ophthalmol 1981;99:1056–1062.
46. Holds JB, Alderson K, Fogg SG, Anderson RL. Terminal nerve and motor end plate changes in human orbicularis muscle following botulinum A toxin injection. Invest Ophthalmol Vis Sci 1990;31:178–181.
47. Wohlfart G. Collateral sprouts from residual motor nerves in amyotrophic lateral sclerosis. Neurology 1957;7:124–134.
48. Alderson K, Yee WC, Pestronk A. Reorganization of intrinsic components in the distal motor axon during outgrowth. J Neurocytol 1989;18:541–552.
49. Duchen LW, Tonge DA. The effects of implantation of an extra nerve on axonal sprouting usually induced by botulinum toxin in skeletal muscle of the mouse. J Anat 1977;124:205–215.
50. Edds MV. Collateral regeneration of residual motor axons in partially denervated muscles. J Exp Zool 1950;113:517–551.
51. Hoffman H. Local reinnervation in partially denervated muscle. A histophysiological study. Aust J Exp Biol 1950;28:383–397.
52. Hopkins WG, Brown MC, Keynes RJ. Nerve growth from nodes of Ranvier in inactive animals. Brain Res 1981;222:125–128.
53. Brown MC, Holland RL, Hopkins WG. Motor nerve sprouting. Annu Rev Neurosci 1981;4:17–42.
54. Harris CP, Alderson K, Nebeker J, Holds JB, Anderson RL. Histology of human orbicularis muscle treated with botulinum toxin. Arch Ophthalmol 1991;109:393–395.
55. Spencer RF, McNeer KW. Botulinum toxin paralysis of adult monkey extraocular muscles. Arch Ophthalmol 1987;105:1703–1711.

56. Jankovic J, Ford J. Blepharospasm and oro-facial dystonia. Pharmacologic findings in 100 patients. Ann Neurol 1979;36:635.

57. Frueh BR, Callahan A, Dortzbach RR et al. The effects of differential section of the seventh nerve on patients with blepharospasm. Trans Am Acad Ophthalmol Otolaryngol 1976;81:595.

58. Callahan A. Surgical correction of intractable blepharospasm, technical improvement. Am J Ophthalmol 1965;60:788.

59. Janetta PJ, Abbasy M, Maroon JC, Ramos FM, Albin MS. Etiology and differential micro-surgical treatment of hemifacial spasm. J Neurosurg 1977;47:321.

60. Borodic GE, Metson R, Townsend D, McKenna M, Pearce LB. Botulinum toxin for aberrant facial nerve regeneration. Dose response relationships. Plast Reconstr Surg 1991;

61. Frueh BR, Nelson CC, Kapustiak JF, Musch DC. The effects of omitting the lower eyelid in blepharospasm treatment. Am J Ophthalmol 1988;106:45–47.

62. Borodic GE, Weigner A, Ferrante R, Young R. Orbicularis oculi innervation zone and implications for botulinum A toxin therapy for blepharospasm. Ophthalm Plast Reconstr Surg 1991;7:54–59.

63. Bertrand C, Molina-Negro P, Martinez SN. Technical aspects of selective peripheral denerva-tion for spasmodic torticollis. Appl Neurophysiol 1982;45:326–330.

64. Bertrand C, Molina-Negro P, Bouvier G, Gorczyca W. Observations and results in 131 cases of spasmodic torticollis after selective denervation. Appl Neurophysiol 1987;50:319–323.

65. Borodic GE. Botulinum A toxin application for expressionistic ptosis overcorrection after frontalis sling procedures. Ophthalm Plast Reconstr Surg 1992;8:137–142.

66. Tsui JK, Wong NLM, Wong E, Calne DB. Production of circulating antibodies to botulinum-A toxin in patients receiving repeated injections for dystonia (abstr). Ann Neurol 1988;23:181.

67. Jankovic J, Schwartz K. Clinical correlates of response to botulinum toxin injections. Arch Neurol 1991;48:1253–1256.

68. Hambleton P, Cohen HE, Palmer BJ, Melling J. Antitoxins and botulinum toxin treatment. Br Med J 1992;304:959–960.

69. Biglan AW, Gonnering R, Lockhart LB, Rabin B. Fuerste FH. Absence of antibody produc-tion in patients treated with botulinum A toxin. Am J Ophthalmol 1986;101:232–235.

70. Gonnering RS. Negative antibody response to long-term treatment of facial spasms with botulinum toxin. Am J Ophthalmol 1988;105:313–315.

71. Cardella MA. Botulinum toxoids. In: Lewis KH, Cassel K Jr, eds. Botulism: proceedings of a symposium. PHS Publication No. 999-FPI. Washington, D.C., Government Printing Office, 1964:113–130.

72. Hatheway CH, Snyder JD, Seals JE, Edell TA, Lewis GE Jr. Antitoxin levels in botulism patients with trivalent equine botulism antitoxin to toxin types A,B, and E. J Infect Dis 1984;150:407–412.

73. Scott AB, Suzuki D. Systemic toxicity of botulinum toxin by intramuscular injection in the monkey. Mov Disord 1988;3:333–335.

11

Assessment of the Biological Activity of Botulinum Toxin

Christopher M. Shaari and Ira Sanders
Mount Sinai Medical Center, New York, New York

INTRODUCTION

Since botulinum toxin (BTX) was first introduced in 1981 to treat strabismus, almost every clinical study of the toxin has attempted to manipulate injection parameters to produce the most effective paralysis with minimal side effects. Clinical observation has empirically guided the injection protocol. For example, when treating blepharospasm, Scott (1) noted that smaller doses of toxin injected into the orbicularis oculi muscle decreased spread to the levator palpebrae muscle, and hence decreased the incidence of ptosis. Others noted that injecting the toxin at multiple sites into the thyroarytenoid and sternocleidomastoid muscles seemed to increase effectiveness and decrease side effects (2–4).

Until 1990, there were no animal models to test these clinical observations. At that time, Borodic et al. (5) provided histological information about how BTX spreads from the injection site. The authors stained injected latissimus dorsi muscles of rabbits for acetylcholinesterase, which appeared more diffuse in the region of chemical denervation. Using this indirect method of tracing, they demonstrated that a diffusion gradient crossing fascia and bone spread a distance of 30–45 mm from the injection point, thus providing histological evidence of toxin spread.

In a second study published in 1991, Shaari et al. (6) reported a method to quantify muscle paralysis in a rat model, and they subsequently showed that fascia reduced the spread of toxin by only 19%. Using the same animal model to quantify paralysis, the authors explored the effects on paralysis when other injection parameters were changed, including (1) the location of injection, (2) the dose, and (3) the volume of injection (7). The methods and results are described therein.

METHODS

Our animal model is based on the observation that prolonged electrical stimulation of the nerve to a muscle causes depletion of glycogen within muscle fibers (8). Botulinum toxin blocks neuromuscular transmission at the motor end plate and, therefore, preserves glycogen in those areas of a muscle into which it is introduced. Thus, from the presence of glycogen in cross-sections of injected muscle the area of effective BTX action could be inferred.

The rat tibialis anterior (TA) muscle was chosen because of its large size and surgical accessibility, the simple longitudinal arrangement of muscle fibers in its midsection, its homogeneous content of type II (fast-twitch) muscle fibers, and the presence of motor end plates (MEPs) that are restricted to a band about midway down the muscle fibers (8,9).

In this experiment, three reference terms were used: midbelly, MEP band, and superior protuberance of the tibia. The midbelly was grossly determined to be the widest part of the muscle and was identified as being 0.5 cm superior to the superior protuberance of the tibia. In the dose and volume experiments described below, this midbelly was chosen as the injection site. Only after performing the location experiment did we realize that our midbelly was about 0.5 cm superior to the MEP band, and that the MEP band thus corresponded to the superior protuberance of the tibia.

General Methods

Thirty-one male Sprague-Dawley rats (350–400/g) were used in total. After ketamine anesthesia (50 mg/ml, 0.4 ml IP) the leg to be operated on was immobilized, shaved, and sterilized with hexachlorophene. By microsurgical technique, the midbelly of the TA muscle was exposed. Depending on the experiment, BTX was either injected to a depth of 3 mm into the muscle or dripped onto the midbelly of the muscle, and the wound was sutured closed. Lyophilized botulinum toxin type A (BTX-A) (Oculinum, Oculinum Inc., Berkeley, California) was used in all experiments, and was reconstituted with normal saline immediately before use.

Twenty-four hours later the animal was anesthetized and the TA muscle was reexposed. A 1-cm portion of the common peroneal nerve was isolated and placed across bipolar electrodes. Ten minutes of electrical stimulation was given using biphasic pulses at 3 mAmp and 20 Hz. The TA muscle was immediately excised and quick-frozen in liquid nitrogen. The animals were immediately sacrificed by an overdose of potassium chloride. Eight-micron frozen sections were cut through the midbelly of the muscle, mounted on slides, and stained for glycogen using Periodic Acid Schiff (PAS) reagent (Sigma Chemical Co., Saint Louis, Missouri) Sections were projected on a computerized digital pad (Zeiss Videoplan 2), and area measurements were made of the areas of stained and unstained fibers.

Specific Methods

Controls

To establish basal parameters in normal muscle, the TA muscle was removed from two rats and immediately frozen in liquid nitrogen. Eight-micron frozen sections were prepared and then stained for glycogen with PAS. These specimens were expected to contain maximum amounts of glycogen. In a second control experiment, the common peroneal nerve of two rats was isolated and electrically stimulated (3 mAmp, 20 Hz, 10 min). After stimulation, the muscle was processed in the same manner as normal control. These stimulated muscle specimens were expected to contain the least glycogen.

Changing Injection Location

To study how varying injection site relative to the motor end plate region affected paralysis, we injected toxin in different locations of the TA muscle in five rats. Botulinum toxin was injected at 0.5-cm intervals above and below the midbelly. The dose and volume were kept constant at 0.2 U in 1 μl of saline. We predicted that paralysis would be greatest when toxin was injected near the motor end plate area.

Increasing Injection Dose

To study the effect of increasing dose on muscle paralysis, we injected each of nine rats with increasing doses of toxin, ranging from 0.02 to 20.0 U. These values were chosen because they approximated the doses of toxin used clinically. All injections were made in the midbelly of the muscle, with concentration of toxin kept constant at 1 u/5 μl.

Increasing Injection Volume

To study the effect of increasing the injection volume of a fixed dose of toxin, we injected each of four rats with varying dilutions of 0.2 U of toxin in 1 μl, 10 μl, 25 μl, and 100 μl of saline.

Spread of Toxin Across Fascia

To determine whether muscle fascia prevents the spread of toxin, we exposed the TA muscles on both legs of nine rats. On one side the fascia covering the TA muscle was left intact, while on the opposite side, a 0.5-cm circle of fascia was removed from over the midbelly of the muscle. Equal doses of toxin were placed on the surface of both TA muscles in each rat. The volume administered was kept constant at 10 μl, while the dose of toxin was increased from 0.2 to 10.0 U.

RESULTS

Controls

Tibialis anterior muscles in normal controls showed complete glycogen retention throughout the muscle (Fig. 1). As predicted, these specimens contained the maximum amount of glycogen. Tibialis anterior muscles in normal controls that were stimulated for ten minutes showed almost complete glycogen depletion (Fig. 2). These specimens contained minimum amounts of glycogen.

Changing Location

Injections given closest to the superior tibial protuberance (located 0.5 cm inferior to the "midbelly") produced the greatest area of glycogen retention (32.26 mm^2). The injections placed 0.5 cm inferior or superior to this point produced 50% less paralysis. No paralysis was observed when the injection was given 1 cm inferior to the MEP band. Representative sections are shown in Figs. 3,4,5, and 6. Figure 7 graphically displays the results.

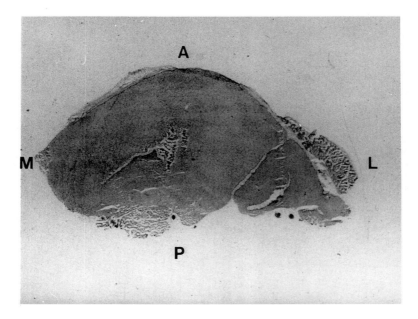

Figure 1 Sections of sham-operated tibialis anterior muscle are shown. The entire muscle stains dark, representing fibers containing glycogen. A = anterior; P = posterior; L = lateral; M = medial. These orientations apply to all muscles shown in the figures.

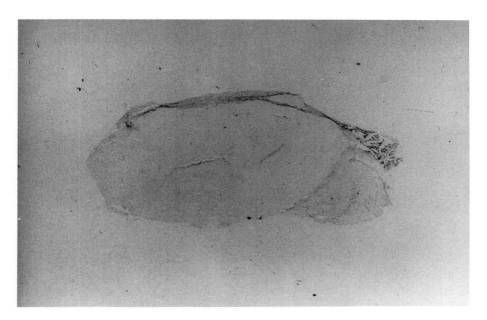

Figure 2 Stimulated normal tibialis anterior muscle. The entire muscle is pale, suggesting that all muscle fibers contracted for sufficient time to deplete their glycogen stores fully.

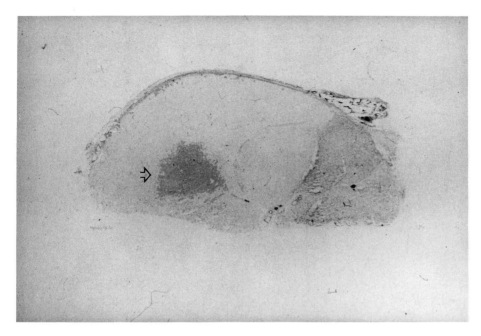

Figure 3 Section of muscle injected with 0.2 U toxin at 1.0 cm superior to the motor end plate band. Arrow points to glycogen-retained fibers, which represent areas of botulinum toxin action. Pale areas are glycogen-depleted, and thus were not paralyzed by the toxin injection.

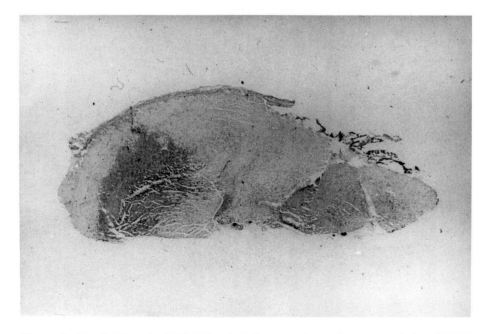

Figure 4 Muscle injected with 0.2 U toxin 0.5 cm superior to the motor end plate (MEP) band. The area of glycogen-retained fibers increased as the injection was given closer to the MEP band.

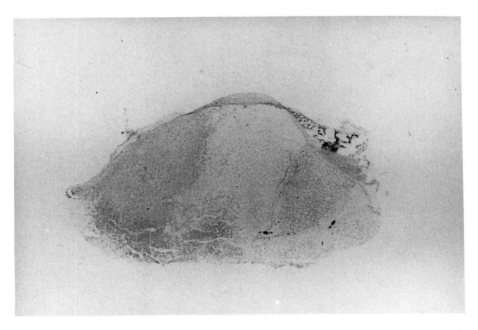

Figure 5 Muscle injected with 0.2 U at the motor end plate band. Area of staining (paralysis) was greatest here.

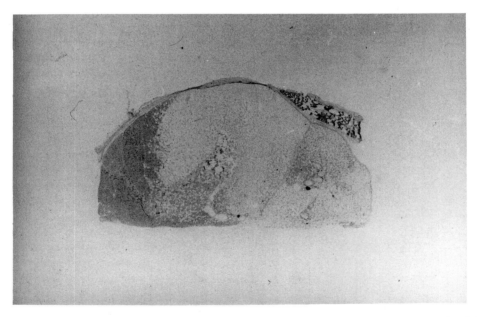

Figure 6 Muscle injected with 0.2 U toxin 0.5 cm inferior to the motor end plate (MEP) band. The area of glycogen-stained fibers decreases as distance from the MEP band increases, and approximates similar doses given 0.5 cm superior to the MEP band.

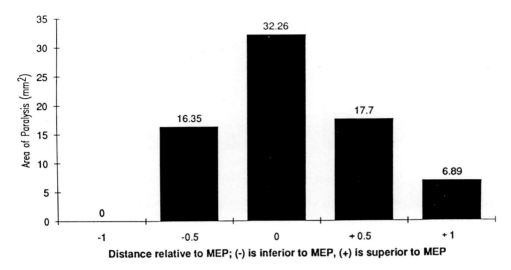

Figure 7 Graphic representation of location versus area of paralysis. Maximum paralysis occurs when toxin is given at the motor end plate (MEP) band. No quantifiable paralysis was measured when the same dose was given 1.0 cm inferior to the MEP band.

Increasing Injection Dose

As the dose of toxin increased so did the area of paralysis (Fig. 8). These measurements represented increasing dose and volume simultaneously. Note that even small subclinical doses of toxin (0.02 u) induced a significant area of paralysis. With doses greater than 5.0 u, the area of paralysis plateaued because of the presence of sufficient toxin to cause complete paralysis. Paralysis doubled with a 20-fold increase in dose.

Increasing Injection Volume

These results demonstrate an increased area of paralysis attributable to an increase in toxin dilution. With a constant dose of 0.2 u, increasing the volume of injection resulted in increasing areas of glycogen retention (Fig. 9). At lower volumes (1.0 and 10.0 µl) the toxin remained localized to the midbelly of the muscle, whereas at higher volumes (25 and 100 µl) there was a tendency for the toxin to diffuse through the muscle and affect a larger area. Paralysis doubled with a 100-fold increase in volume.

Spread of Toxin Across Fascia

All muscles showed a stained band across the entire anterior portion of the muscle (Fig. 10) that represented the area of paralysis. In all dose-matched pairs, the area of paralysis was greater in the muscle without fascia, except for 0.8 U, with which the converse was true. At 0.4 and 4.0 u, the areas were equal. Results are graphically displayed in Fig. 11. The average decrease in paralysis when fascia was intact was 19%.

DISCUSSION

This study had several objectives. Foremost, we wanted to develop a model to quantify muscle paralysis induced by BTX. This objective was clearly achieved. Once the model was established, we sought to provide histologic evidence for the spread of toxin,

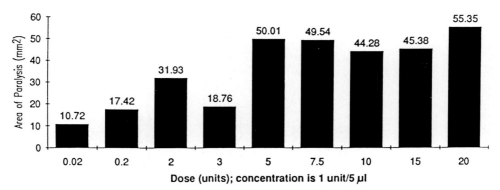

Figure 8 Graphic representation of injection dose versus area of paralysis. Paralysis increases with dose until a maximum of approximately 50 mm^2 is reached, which represents the total cross-sectional area of tibialis anterior muscle.

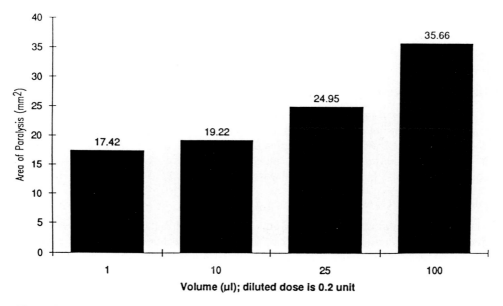

Figure 9 Effect of dilution on paralysis. As injection volume of 0.2 U toxin increased, so did paralysis. This increase in paralysis, however, was more gradual than when proportional increases in dose were used.

including the effects of increasing dose and volume, the effect of fascia as a barrier, and the effect of distance from the MEP band on total area of paralysis. We also sought to correlate these histological findings with clinical observation. To our knowledge this is this first such quantitative study.

In this technique, normal muscle stained completely dark, representing full glycogen retention, whereas neurally stimulated muscle was pale, representing full glycogen depletion. Therefore, the dark-stained areas within the experimental muscles represented the area to which BTX had spread in quantities sufficient to cause complete neuromuscu-

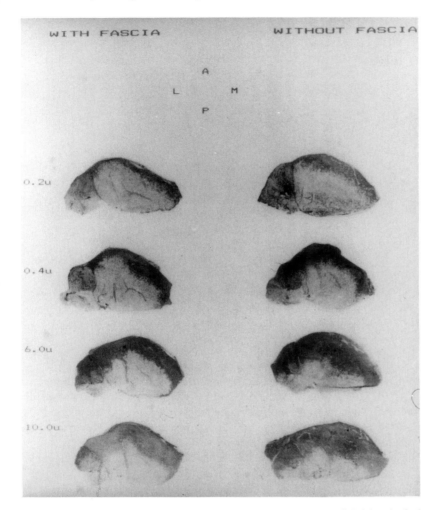

Figure 10 Effect of muscle fascia on toxin spread. The superficial band of glycogen staining corresponds to the limits of botulinum diffusion. The area of paralysis increases with dose and with removal of fascia.

lar blockade. Thus, the method is a physiological tracer of BTX. It is probable that the toxin has diffused farther than the areas shown on the slide. Thus, the stained regions should be considered as demonstrating the minimum extent of BTX-evoked paralysis, and a clinically relevant paralysis may involve considerably more of the muscle.

Several clinically relevant points can be derived from this study. First, we found that toxin injections given only 0.5 cm from the MEP band produced 50% less paralysis than injections made near the MEP band. This finding correlates well with clinical observations. In general, injecting toxin at multiple sites of head and neck muscles increases effectiveness and reduces local side effects. This may be a result of more even distribution of toxin to the scattered neuromuscular junctions that are frequently encountered in muscles of the head and neck (3). Conversely, muscles of the extremities (e.g., the flexor

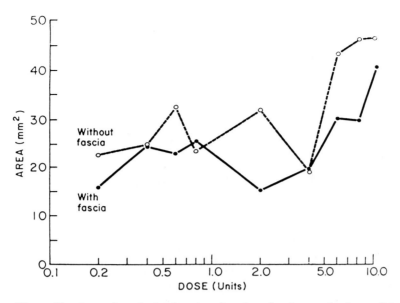

Figure 11 Area of paralysis plotted against dose for the two fascia conditions. Dose is plotted logarithmically. In general, muscles covered with fascia had a smaller area of paralysis than dose-matched muscles without fascia.

digitorum) benefit from injections localized to the midbelly, since this is where the end plates are located (10). For example, the effectiveness of toxin therapy for spasmodic dysphonia is improved when multiple sites of the thyroarytenoid muscle are injected (3). Blackie and Lees (11) showed that the incidence of dysphagia was reduced by nearly 50% when multiple rather than single injection sites were used to treat torticollis. This finding is consistent with other reports (4). Finally, the incidence of ptosis following injections into the upper eyelid for blepharospasm is reduced when smaller aliquots are given throughout the upper eyelid (12,13). This finding may also be related to the volume of the injection bolus (see below).

A second clinical correlation concerns the increased incidence of toxin spread when either dose or volume of injection is increased. Borodic (5) recently demonstrated that dysphagia following sternocleidomastoid muscle injections could be reduced while maintaining clinical efficacy when the total dose injected was decreased by 30%. Others have also noted that dysphagia is a dose-related complication of treating cervical dystonia (4,11) and was reduced when the total dose of toxin was reduced. It is hypothesized that as the total dose of injected toxin is increased, there is more unbound toxin available to spread to surrounding pharyngeal constrictors. Approximately 10% of patients treated for blepharospasm experienced ptosis as a side effect, and the incidence increased with higher injection doses (1,14).

Larger injection volumes may also influence the incidence of side effects. Injections of 0.3-ml aliquots into two separate muscle sites produced less severe and less frequent (15%) dysphagia than did single injections of 0.6 ml into one site (28%) (11). This finding may be attributed to binding of less toxin to the neuromuscular junction, as a result of the larger injection volume. Patrinley (13) recommends that the smallest injection volume and the strongest concentration of toxin should be used to minimize diffusion of toxin to undesirable locations. Unfortunately, if side effects do occur when more concentrated solutions are used, they are usually more disabling. For example, two of 10 patients treated for torticollis developed aspiration and vocal cord paralysis when injected with more concentrated solutions (the same total dose being disolved in one-half the volume (15).

Our study demonstrates histologically what is observed clinically. Our results show the following direct relationships between dose and spread and between volume and spread: (1) fascia reduced the spread of toxin through muscle by only 19%; (2) muscle paralysis doubled with a 20-fold increase in injection dose; and (3) muscle paralysis doubled with a 100-fold increase in injection volume. An unexpected finding was that even small doses of toxin that would normally be considered subclinical (0.02 and 0.2 u) induced significant paralysis if injected near the MEP band. This finding suggests that very small amounts of toxin that may spread beyond the target muscle may indeed be sufficient to weaken neighboring muscles.

Evidently, several parameters particular to each muscle must be optimized to produce effective paralysis while minimizing side effects. Difficulty often arises in predicting these parameters, as is evidenced by conflicting clinical data. For example, although electromyographic guidance to MEPs would seem to be an effective way to localize the end plates and hence increase the effectiveness of injections, several studies have refuted this concept (16–18). Furthermore, some authors have demonstrated that even total dose of toxin is not significantly related to the incidence of side effects (3,16). The only injection technique that clearly seems to be advantageous in producing effective paralysis while minimizing side effects is the use of multiple injection sites in muscles with diffuse innervation zones (e.g., thyroarytenoid, sternocleidomastoid, orbicularis oculi). Conversely, single injection sites can be used for limb muscles with narrow innervation zones confined to the midbelly.

From our data, we can at least extrapolate that the risk of complications is highly and directly related to the distance of injection from the MEPs, but only moderately and directly related to dose and volume of injection. Small deviations of only 0.5 cm from the MEP region reduced paralysis by 50%. The unbound toxin could easily spread through muscle, encountering little resistance to spread at fascial planes (19% reduction). Conversely, a 20-fold and 100-fold increase, respectively, in dose and volume were needed to double muscle paralysis, and these multiples are not realistically encountered in clinical settings.

REFERENCES

1. Scott AB, Kennedy RA, Stubbs MA. Botulinum A toxin injection as a treatment for blepharospasm. Arch Ophthalmol 1985;103:347–350.
2. Jankovic J, Schwartz K, Donovan DT. Botulinum toxin treatment of cranial-cervical dystonia, spasmodic dysphonia, other focal dystonias and hemifacial spasm. J Neurol Neurosurg Psychiatry 1990;53:633–639.
3. Ludlow CL, Naunton RF, Sedory SE, Schulz GM, Hallett M. Effects of botulinum toxin injections on speech in adductor spasmodic dysphonia. Neurology 1988;38:1220–1225.
4. Maurri S, Barontini F. Responsiveness of idiopathic spasmodic torticollis to botulinum A toxin injection. A critical evaluation of five cases. Clin Neurol Neurosurg 1990;92:165–168.
5. Borodic GE, Joseph M, Fay L, Cozzolino D, Ferrante RJ. Botulinum A toxin for the treatment of spasmodic torticollis: dysphagia and regional toxin spread. Head Neck 1990;12:392–398.

6. Shaari CM, George E, Wu BL, Biller HF, Sanders I. Quantifying the spread of botulinum toxin through muscle fascia. Laryngoscope 1991;9:960–964.

7. Shaari CM, Sanders I. Quantifying how location and dose of botulinum toxin injections affect muscle paralysis. Muscle Nerve 1993;16:964–969.

8. Edstrom L, Kugelberg E. Histochemical composition, distribution of fibers and fatigability of single motor units. J Neurol Neurosurg Psychiat 1968;31:424–433.

9. Coers C. Structural organization of the motor nerve endings in mammalian muscle spindles and other striated muscle fibers. Am J Phys Med 1959;38:166–175.

10. Cohen LG, Hallett M, Geller BD, Hochberg F. Treatment of focal dystonias of the hand with botulinum toxin injections. J Neurol Neurosurg Psychiat 1989;52:355–363.

11. Blackie JD, Lees AJ. Botulinum toxin treatment in spasmodic torticollis. J Neurol Neurosurg Psychiat 1990;53:640–643.

12. Shorr N, Seiff SR, Kopelman J. The use of botulinum toxin in blepharospasm. Am J Ophthalmol 1985;99:542–546.

13. Patrinely JR, Whiting AS, Anderson RL. Local side effects of botulinum toxin injections. In: Jankovic J, Tolosa E, eds. Advances in neurology, vol. 49: facial dyskinesias. New York: Raven Press, 1988:439–499.

14. Botulinum toxin therapy of eye muscle disorders, safety and effectiveness. American Academy of Ophthalmology 1989:37–41.

15. Stell R, Thompson PD, Marsden CD. Botulinum toxin in spasmodic torticollis. J Neurol Neurosurg Psychiat 1988;51:920–923.

16. Jankovic J, Schwartz K. Botulinum toxin injections for cervical dystonia. Neurology 1990;40:277–280.

17. Tsui JK, Eisen A, Mak E, Carruthers J, Scott A, Calne DB. A pilot study on the use of botulinum toxin in spasmodic torticollis. Can J Neurol Sci 1985;12:314–316.

18. Gelb DJ, Lowenstein DH, Aminoff MJ. Controlled trial of botulinum toxin injections in the treatment of spasmodic torticollis. Neurology 1989;39:80–84.

DYSTONIA

12

Dystonia

Stanley Fahn
The Neurological Institute, Columbia-Presbyterian Medical Center, New York, New York

INTRODUCTION

The term "dystonia musculorum deformans" was coined by Oppenheim (1911) to describe a syndrome occurring in children that was marked by twisted postures; muscle spasms; bizarre walking with bending and twisting of the torso; rapid, sometimes rhythmic jerking movements; and progression of symptoms leading eventually to sustained fixed postural deformities. Oppenheim created the word "dystonia" to indicate that in this disorder there would be hypotonia on one occasion and tonic muscle spasm on another, usually but not exclusively elicited by volitional movements. Later that year Flatau and Sterling (1911) emphasized that the disorder is probably an inherited disease and suggested the name of progressive torsion spasm. On the basis of the clinical features described by these and other early observers, dystonia is now defined as a syndrome of sustained muscle contractions, frequently causing twisting and repetitive movements, or abnormal postures (Fahn et al., 1987; Fahn, 1988). A number of recent reviews are available to which the reader is referred for more details than are provided in this chapter (Fahn et al., 1987; Fahn and Marsden, 1987; Rothwell and Obeso, 1987; Fahn et al., 1988; Jankovic and Fahn, 1988; Fahn, 1989a; Fahn, 1990).

PHENOMENOLOGY OF DYSTONIC MOVEMENTS

The speed of dystonic movements varies from slow to rapid but is more often the latter. The movements can be so fast that they have the appearance of repetitive myoclonic jerking. The term "myoclonic dystonia" has been applied to such dystonia (Obeso et al., 1983; Kurlan et al., 1988; Quinn et al., 1988), and the rapid jerks may respond to alcohol (Quinn et al., 1988).

Dystonic movements are almost always aggravated during voluntary movement. The appearance of dystonic movements with voluntary movement is referred to as action dystonia. Idiopathic dystonia commonly begins with a specific action dystonia, that is, the abnormal movements appear with a special action and are not present at rest. For example, a child who develops idiopathic dystonia may have the initial symptom in one leg, but only when walking forward. It could be absent when the child runs or walks backward. Other common examples are the task-specific dystonias seen with writing, playing a musical instrument, chewing, and speaking. As the dystonic condition progresses, less specific actions of the affected leg may activate the dystonia, e.g., tapping the floor. With further evolution, actions in other parts of the body can induce dystonic movements of the involved leg, so-called "overflow." With still further worsening, the affected limb can develop dystonic movements while it is at rest. Eventually the leg can have sustained posturing. Thus, dystonia at rest is usually a more severe form than pure action dystonia.

In addition to progression in a specific body part, dystonia often spreads to involve other parts of the body. Most often the spread is to contiguous body parts. As a general rule, the younger the age at onset, the more likely it is that dystonia will spread; childhood onset usually leads to eventual generalized dystonia (Marsden et al., 1976; Fahn, 1986). The severity of dystonia can be quantitated with rating scales for generalized dystonia and the various focal dystonias (Fahn, 1989b).

Dystonic movements tend to increase with fatigue, stress, and emotional states; they tend to be suppressed with relaxation, hypnosis, and sleep (Fish et al., 1991). One of the characteristic and almost unique features of dystonic movements is that they can be diminished by tactile or proprioceptive "sensory tricks." Thus, touching the involved body part or an adjacent one can often reduce the muscle contractions. For example, patients with torticollis will often place a hand on the chin or side of the face to reduce nuchal contractions. Dystonia usually is present throughout the day whenever the affected body part is in use, or in more severe cases at rest, and disappears with deep sleep.

Pain is uncommon in dystonia except in cervical dystonia; 75% of patients with cervical dystonia (spasmodic torticollis) have pain (Chan et al., 1991). Dystonia in most parts of the body rarely is accompanied by pain; when it is, it is not clear whether the pain is due to painful contractions of muscles or some other factor. The high incidence of pain in cervical dystonia appears to be due to muscle contractions, because this pain is usually relieved by injections of botulinum toxin (Greene et al., 1990). It is believed that the posterior cervical muscles are rich in pain fibers, and that continual contractions of these muscles result in pain. Tension headaches are similarly due to chronic nuchal muscle contractions.

Patients with idiopathic torsion dystonia sometimes have rhythmic movements manifested as a tremor (Yanagisawa et al., 1972; Jankovic and Fahn, 1980). There are basically two types of tremor seen in dystonic patients: an accompanying tremor that resembles essential tremor and a tremor that is a rhythmic expression of rapid dystonic movements (Yanagisawa and Goto, 1971). The latter can usually be distinguished from the former by showing that the tremor appears only when the affected body part is placed in a position of opposition to the major direction of pulling by the abnormal dystonic contractions. Dystonic tremor appears to be less regular than essential tremor (Jedynak et al., 1991). Sometimes it is very difficult to distinguish between the two types, however, particularly with writing tremor and cervical tremor. Primary writing tremor can sometimes represent task-specific dystonia or task-specific essential tremor (Cohen et al.,

1987; Rosenbaum and Jankovic, 1988; Elble et al., 1990). A family history of tremor (and stuttering) is increased in idiopathic torsion dystonia (Fletcher et al., 1991a). Although accompanying essential tremor is recognized in patients with dystonia (Lou and Jankovic, 1991), it is uncertain how common this occurrence is. Tics are another type of involuntary movement that appears to occur more commonly in patients with dystonia than in the general population (Shale et al., 1986; Stone and Jankovic, 1991).

EPIDEMIOLOGY

An epidemiological study of dystonia in the population living in Rochester, Minnesota, found the prevalence of generalized idiopathic torsion dystonia to be 3.4 per 100,000 of the population, and that of focal dystonia 30 per 100,000 (Nutt et al., 1988). In a study of dystonia in Israel, Zilber et al. (1984) estimated the prevalence of generalized dystonia among Jews of Eastern European ancestry to be 1/15,000 or 6.8/100,000, which is double the prevalence in the general population of Rochester.

VARIANTS FROM CLASSICAL TORSION DYSTONIA

Some patients who otherwise satisfy the criteria of idiopathic dystonia may be relatively free of dystonic movements and postures in the morning and afflicted severely in the late afternoon, evening, and night. This temporal pattern has been considered a variant of dystonia and referred to as dystonia with marked diurnal variation by Segawa and colleagues (1976). There are three other clinical features that highlight this disorder: many cases have features of parkinsonism, it begins in childhood, and these patients respond remarkably well to low-dosage levodopa. More recently, it has been recognized that exquisite sensitivity to low-dosage levodopa is not always associated with diurnal fluctuation, and the term dopa-responsive dystonia (DRD) has been applied to this particular form of dystonia (Nygaard, 1989; Nygaard et al., 1990). This dystonia is inherited as an autosomal dominant disorder and needs to be recognized because it is so easily treated. Because the additional phenotypic expression of abnormal postural stability, rigidity, and bradykinesia is not seen in classical torsion dystonia, this condition is considered a variant of the classical form (Fahn, 1989c). The phenotype of DRD is not always easily distinguished from juvenile parkinsonism, but features that help in the differential diagnosis are presented in Table 1. Among the important differences is that long-term treatment with levodopa in DRD is not associated with complications (Nygaard et al., 1991), whereas this treatment in juvenile parkinsonism is associated with many complications.

While both DRD and classical idiopathic torsion dystonia, as well as focal dystonias (Waddy et al., 1991), are inherited as autosomal dominant disorders, there is a form of dystonia that is inherited as an X-linked recessive trait. This is present in males from the island of Panay in the Philippines. The disease can begin with either dystonia or parkinsonism; with progression, parkinsonism develops eventually, even in those who had dystonia earlier (Lee et al., 1991).

Dystonia is seen in other disorders as well, and these should be considered as separate entities from the classical type of torsion dystonia (Fahn, 1989c). These variants are the dystonia seen in dystonic tics, paroxysmal dystonia, hypnogenic dystonia, and myoclonic dystonia (Table 2).

Table 1 Differential Features of Juvenile Parkinsonism (PD) and Dopa-Responsive Dystonia (DRD)

	Juvenile PD	DRD
Onset	1st and 2nd decade	1st and 2nd decade
Sex	Predominantly male	Predominantly female
Dystonia	At onset	Throughout
Diurnal	No	Sometimes
Bradykinesia	Present	Present
Pull test	Abnormal	Abnormal
Gait	Abnormal	Abnormal
Dopa-responsive	Yes	Yes
Dopa dosage	Moderate to high	Very low
Complications	Fluctuations	Stable
Dyskinesias	Prominent	Uncommon
Dopa PET scan	Very decreased	Modest decrease
Prognosis	Progressive	Plateaus

PET = positron emission tomography.

CLASSIFICATION OF TORSION DYSTONIA

Torsion dystonia is classified in three ways: by age at onset, by body distribution of abnormal movements, and by etiology (Table 3).

Classification by Age at Onset

Classification by age at onset is useful because this is the most important single factor related to prognosis of idiopathic dystonia. As a general rule, the younger the age at onset, the more likely that the dystonia would become severe and would also spread to involve multiple parts of the body. In contrast, the older the age at onset, the more likely dystonia will remain focal.

Classification by Distribution

Since dystonia usually begins by affecting a single part of the body (*focal dystonia*), and since dystonia can either remain focal or spread to involve other body parts, it is useful to classify dystonia according to its distribution of involvement of body parts.

Table 2 Classification of the Clinical Variants of Dystonia

Classified as idiopathic torsion dystonia	Classified as other dyskinesias
Classical torsion dystonia	Dystonic tics
Paradoxical dystonia	Paroxysmal dystonia
Myoclonic dystonia	Hypnogenic dystonia
Diurnal dystonia	
Dopa-responsive dystonia	
X-Linked dystonia-parkinsonism	

Table 3   Classifications of Dystonia

I.	By age at onset	
	A.	Childhood-onset: 0–12 years
	B.	Adolescent-onset: 13–20 years
	C.	Adult-onset: > 20 years
II.	By distribution	
	A.	Focal
	B.	Segmental
	C.	Multifocal
	D.	Generalized
	E.	Hemidystonia
III.	By etiology	
	A.	Idiopathic
		Sporadic
		Familial
	B.	Symptomatic

Focal dystonia is that in which only a single area of the body is affected. Frequently seen types of focal dystonia tend to have specific labels, such as blepharospasm, torticollis, oromandibular dystonia, spastic dysphonia, writer's cramp, and occupational cramp. If dystonia spreads, it most commonly does so by next affecting a contiguous body part. When dystonia affects two or more contiguous parts of the body, it is referred to as *segmental dystonia*. Segmental cranial dystonia is commonly called Meige syndrome.

Generalized dystonia is defined as a combination of leg involvement and involvement of any other area of the body. The term *multifocal dystonia* fills a gap in the above designations. It applies to the involvement of two or more noncontiguous parts of the body. Dystonia affecting one half of the body is called *hemidystonia*. Almost always, hemidystonia indicates that the dystonia is symptomatic rather than idiopathic (Marsden et al., 1985; Narbona et al., 1984; Pettigrew and Jankovic, 1985).

Adult-onset focal dystonias are much more common than generalized dystonias (Fahn, 1986; Marsden, 1986) (Table 4).

The most common idiopathic focal dystonia is torticollis, followed by dystonias affecting cranial musculature, such as blepharospasm and spastic dysphonia (Table 5). The most common idiopathic segmental dystonia involves the cranial structures (Table 6).

Classification By Etiology and Genetics of Dystonia

The etiologic classification divides dystonia into two major categories: idiopathic (or primary) and symptomatic (or secondary). The idiopathic group consists of familial and nonfamilial (sporadic) types. Although most patients with torsion dystonia have a negative family history for this disorder, the presence of other affected family members allows the family to be investigated with a view to localizing the abnormal gene(s) for dystonia. There is a higher prevalence of dystonia in the Ashkenazi Jewish population. In both Jewish (Bressman et al., 1989) and non-Jewish groups (Zeman and Dyken, 1967), dystonia is inherited as an autosomal dominant disorder, and the gene has been localized to the long arm of chromosome 9 (9q32–34) (Ozelius et al., 1989; Kramer et al., 1990). Because of allelic association with dystonia in the Ashkenazi Jewish population, it is now

Table 4 Distribution of Dystonia by Body Parts

	N	%
Focal	1230	50
Segmental	837	34
Generalized	383	16
	2450	100

possible to use this information to carry out predictive testing in this population. The first use of carrier detection, including prenatal detection, in a family with idiopathic torsion dystonia has been reported, using molecular genetic techniques (de Leon et al., 1991). Accuracy is estimated to be greater than 95%.

The rate of gene expression in the Ashkenazi Jewish population is approximately 30% (Bressman et al., 1989; Risch et al., 1990). Previously it had been proposed by Eldridge (1970) that dystonia in the Ashkenazi Jewish population was inherited as an autosomal recessive disorder. Interestingly, reanalysis of Eldridge's data by segregation analysis has now shown that dystonia in this population was in fact inherited as an autosomal dominant disorder (Pauls and Korczyn, 1990). A detailed analysis compared the clinical course of dystonia in the Jewish and non-Jewish populations with inherited dystonia, and no major difference was found (Burke et al., 1986a). The prevalence of dystonia among Jews of Eastern European ancestry has been estimated to be 1/15,000 (Zilber et al., 1984), while for non-Jews it is 1/200,000 (Zeman and Dyken, 1967). Intrafamilial correlation for age at onset of dystonia is low (Fletcher et al., 1991b).

Dopa-responsive dystonia is also inherited as an autosomal dominant disorder (Nygaard et al., 1990), but its abnormal gene has been excluded from 9q32–34 (Kwiatkowski et al., 1991). Fluorodopa positron emission tomography (PET) scanning reveals a modest reduction of dopa uptake (Sawle et al., 1991). An X-linked recessive form that is characterized by a combination of dystonia and parkinsonism occurs in affected males from the island of Panay in the Philippines (Lee et al., 1976; Fahn and Moskowitz, 1988). Its abnormal gene has been localized near the centromere of the X chromosome (Kupke et al., 1990; Wilhelmsen et al., 1991; Kupke et al., 1992).

Table 5 Distribution of Focal Dystonias at Columbia-Presbyterian Medical Center

Type of dystonia	N	%
Blepharospasm	140	13.9
Oromandibular	31	3.1
Spastic dysphonia	257	25.5
Torticollis	447	44.4
Right arm	96	9.5
Left arm	20	2.0
Trunk	5	0.5
Right leg	4	0.4
Left leg	6	0.6
	1006	100

Table 6 Distribution of Segmental Dystonias at Columbia-Presbyterian Medical Center

Type of dystonia	N	%
Segmental cranial	167	42.8
Cranial + brachial	56	14.4
Cranial + axial	14	3.6
Segmental brachial	83	21.3
Segmental axial	31	7.9
Segmental crural	13	3.3
Multifocal	26	6.7
	390	100

The symptomatic group is subdivided into those conditions associated with various hereditary neurological disorders, those due to environmental causes, dystonia associated with parkinsonism, and psychogenic dystonia (Fahn et al., 1987; Calne and Lang, 1988; Fahn and Williams, 1988) (Table 7). A major portion of the clinical investigation of dystonia (Fahn et al., 1987) concerns the tests required to uncover the etiology of symptomatic dystonia. Yearly, new etiologies of symptomatic dystonia are reported, such as toxoplasmosis (in AIDS) (Tolge and Factor, 1991), disulfiram intoxication (Krauss et al., 1991), and Creutzfeldt-Jakob disease (Sethi and Hess, 1991). In persons infected with the human immunodeficiency virus, dystonia can occur as a result of striatal necrosis (Abbruzzese et al., 1990) or of secondary infections such as toxoplasmosis (Tolge and Factor, 1991).

In a number of cases symptomatic dystonias appear months to years after the cerebral insult, so-called delayed onset dystonia. Often such a delayed onset is seen with perinatal or early childhood asphyxia (Saint-Hilaire et al., 1991). This can be seen also with central pontine myelinolysis (Tison et al., 1991; Maraganore et al., 1992) and cyanide intoxication (Valenzuela et al., 1992).

In idiopathic dystonia, the only neurological abnormality is the presence of dystonic postures and movements. There is no associated loss of postural reflexes, amyotrophy, weakness, spasticity, ataxia, reflex change, abnormality of eye movements, disorder of the retina, dementia, or seizures except where they may be the result of a concomitant problem such as a complication from a neurosurgical procedure undertaken to correct the dystonia, or the presence of some other incidental neurologic disease. Since many of the symptomatic dystonias are associated with these neurological findings, the presence of any of these abnormalities in a patient with dystonia immediately suggests that one is dealing with symptomatic dystonia (Table 8). However, the absence of such neurological findings does not necessarily exclude the possibility of a symptomatic dystonia, which may present as a pure dystonia.

Tardive dystonia is the most common form of symptomatic dystonia seen at the Dystonia Clinical Research Center at Columbia-Presbyterian Medical Center (Table 9). It can appear exactly like idiopathic torsion dystonia, but often there is accompanying classical tardive dyskinesia or tardive akathisia that establishes the diagnosis. Many patients with tardive dystonia have retrocollis and extension of the elbows with adduction of the shoulders and flexion of the wrists. Recently, the benzamide flecainide was reported to induce a persistent dystonia that would fit with the tardive dystonia syndrome (Miller and Jankovic, 1992).

Table 7 Etiologic Classification of Torsion Dystonia

I. Idiopathic (primary)
    A. With hereditary pattern
        1. Autosomal dominant
        2. X-linked recessive
    B. Without hereditary pattern
II. Symptomatic
    A. Associated with hereditary neurological syndromes and with known enzyme defect
        1. Wilson's disease
        2. GM_1 gangliosidosis
        3. GM_2 gangliosidosis
        4. Hexosaminidase A and B deficiency
        5. Metachromatic leukodystrophy
        6. Lesch-Nyhan syndrome
        7. Homocystinuria
        8. Glutaric acidemia
        9. Triosephosphate isomerase deficiency
       10. Methylmalonic aciduria
    B. Associated with probable hereditary neurological syndromes, without known enzyme defect, but with a chemical marker
        1. Leigh's disease
        2. Familial basal ganglia calcifications
        3. Hallervorden-Spatz disease
        4. Dystonic lipidosis (sea-blue histiocytosis)
        5. Juvenile neuronal ceroid-lipofuscinosis
        6. Ataxia-telangiectasia
        7. Neuroacanthocytosis
        8. Hartnup's disease
        9. Intraneuronal inclusion disease
    C. Associated with hereditary neurological syndromes, without known enzyme defect or chemical marker
        1. Huntington's disease
        2. Hereditary juvenile dystonia-parkinsonism
        3. Pelizaeus-Merzbacher disease
        4. Progressive pallidal degeneration
        5. Joseph's disease
        6. Rett's syndrome
        7. Spinocerebellar degenerations
        8. Olivopontocerebellar atrophies
        9. Hereditary spastic paraplegia with dystonia
    D. Due to known environmental cause
        1. Perinatal cerebral injury
            Athetoid cerebral palsy
            Delayed-onset dystonia
        2. Encephalitic and postinfectious
            Reye's syndrome
            Subacute sclerosing leucoencephalopathy
            Wasp sting
            Creutzfeldt-Jakob disease
        3. Head trauma
        4. Thalamotomy
        5. Brain stem lesion, including pontine myelinolysis

Table 7 Continued

      6. Focal cerebral vascular injury
      7. Arteriovenous malformation
      8. Brain tumor
      9. Multiple sclerosis
    10. Cervical cord injury
    11. Peripheral injury
    12. Drugs
        D_2 receptor antagonists
        Levodopa
        Ergotism
        Anticonvulsants
    13. Toxins
        Mn, CO, carbon disulfide, cyanide, methanol, disulfiram
    14. Metabolic
        Hypoparathyroidism
  E. Dystonia associated with parkinsonism
  F. Psychogenic dystonia
  G. Pseudodystonia
      1. Sandifer syndrome
      2. Stiff-man syndrome
      3. Rotational atlanto-axial subluxation
      4. Soft tissue nuchal mass
      5. Bone disease
      6. Ligamentous absence, laxity or damage
      7. Congenital muscular torticollis
      8. Congenital postural torticollis
      9. Congenital Klippel-Feil syndrome
    10. Posterior fossa tumor
    11. Syringomyelia
    12. Arnold-Chiari malformation
    13. Trochlear nerve palsy
    14. Vestibular torticollis

Source: Modified from Fahn, et al., (1987) and Calne and Lang (1988). Those reviews should be consulted for references regarding the literature citations for these etiologies.

Table 8 Clues That Dystonia Is Symptomatic

1. History of possible etiologic factor: e.g., head trauma, peripheral trauma, encephalitis, toxin exposure, drug exposure, perinatal anoxia.
2. Presence of neurologic abnormality: e.g., dementia, seizures, ocular, ataxia, weakness, spasticity, amyotrophy.
3. Presence of false weakness or sensory exam, or other clues of psychogenic etiology (see Table 10)
4. Onset of rest instead of action dystonia.
5. Early onset of speech involvement.
6. Hemidystonia.
7. Abnormal brain imaging.
8. Abnormal laboratory work-up.

Table 9   Common Causes of Torsion Dystonia
at Columbia-Presbyterian Medical Center

Idiopathic	1762
Tardive dystonia	184
Birth injury	83
Psychogenic	64
Peripheral trauma	51
Head injury	39
Stroke	27
Encephalitis	24
Miscellaneous	164
	234

Acute dystonic reactions from drugs that block dopamine receptors are widely recognized and easily treated with antihistaminics and anticholinergics. Acute dystonia has recently been reported with exposure to domperidone (Bonuccelli et al., 1991) and to amitriptyline (Ornadel et al., 1992). Since the former drug is a peripherally acting dopamine receptor blocker, the acute dystonic reaction suggests that some of the drug entered the central nervous system of the affected patient, who had polycystic ovary syndrome. Amitriptyline would ordinarily not be expected to produce such a reaction; the clinical description was typical of acute dystonia after use of a neuroleptic, but no such drug was known to have been taken by the patient.

Head trauma and peripheral trauma can induce generalized and segmental dystonia and focal dystonia, respectively, Trauma may provoke the onset of idiopathic torsion dystonia in a person who carries the gene for this disorder (Fletcher et al., 1991c). Recently, segmental axial dystonia was described with a closed head injury with small areas of encephalomalacia, including the caudate nucleus (Jabbari et al., 1992).

Perhaps the most difficult form of dystonia to diagnose is psychogenic dystonia, which can occur in up to 5% of children presenting with what otherwise appears to be idiopathic dystonia. Clues suggesting a psychogenic etiology are false (give-way) weakness, false sensory findings, inconsistent movements with changing patterns of involvement, incongruent movements not fitting with typical organic dystonia, self-inflicted injuries, deliberate slowness of movement, and multiple types of abnormal dyskinesia that do not fit into a single organic etiology (Fahn and Williams, 1988). Table 10 lists the clinical situations that provide clues one may be encountering a psychogenic movement disorder.

PATHOPHYSIOLOGY AND PATHOANATOMY

A major characteristic of dystonic movements is the presence of sustained simultaneous contractions of agonist and antagonist muscles (Yanagisawa and Goto, 1971; Rothwell et al., 1983; Rothwell and Obeso, 1987). There are also contractions of adjoining and distant muscles, so-called overflow, particularly during a voluntary movement. Also, rhythmical contractions frequently occur on voluntary movement. None of these physiologic features is specific for dystonia.

Although idiopathic dystonia is not associated with any known pathological lesion,

Table 10 Clues Suggesting Psychogenic Dystonia

Clues relating to the movements
1. Abrupt onset
2. Inconsistent movements (changing characteristics over time)
3. Incongruous movements and postures (movements do not fit with recognized patterns or with normal physiological patterns
4. Presence of additional types of abnormal movements that are not consistent with the basic abnormal movement pattern or are not congruous with a known movement disorder, particularly:
    rhythmical shaking
    bizarre gait
    deliberate slowness carrying out requested voluntary movement
    bursts of verbal gibberish
    excessive startle (bizarre movements in response to sudden, unexpected noise or threatening movement
5. Spontaneous remissions
6. Movements that disappear with distraction
7. Response to placebo, suggestion, or psychotherapy
8. Presence as a paroxysmal disorder
9. Dystonia beginning as a fixed posture

Clues relating to the other medical observations
1. False weakness
2. False sensory complaints
3. Multiple somatizations or undiagnosed conditions
4. Self-inflicted injuries
5. Obvious psychiatric disturbances
6. Employment in the health profession or in insurance claims
7. Presence of secondary gain, including continuing care by a "devoted" spouse
8. Litigation or compensation pending

symptomatic dystonia often involves the basal ganglia, particularly the putamen (Burton et al., 1984). Actually, lesions can involve not only the basal ganglia, but also connections to and from these nuclei, such as the thalamus and the cortex (Marsden et al., 1985). However, one should not assume that the basal ganglia are always the site of physiological pathology in idiopathic dystonia. It has been shown, for example, that the rostral brain stem can be pathologically damaged in some cases of secondary blepharospasm (Jankovic and Patel, 1983). Lesions from stroke, multiple sclerosis, and encephalitis have all been seen. Moreover, this is the region found to be associated with abnormal blink reflexes in idiopathic cranial and cervical dystonias (Berardelli et al., 1985; Tolosa et al., 1988). There is increased amplitude and duration of the R1 and R2 blink responses. This finding implies either excess physiological excitatory drive to or deficient inhibition in this midbrain region. In limb dystonia, there is an abnormality of the normal reciprocal inhibition between agonist and antagonist muscles. The second phase of reciprocal inhibition is much reduced or even absent in affected limbs in dystonia (Nakashima et al., 1989). This has been interpreted as evidence for reduced presynaptic inhibition of muscle afferent input to the inhibitory interneurons as a result of defective descending motor control.

BIOCHEMISTRY

There are no consistent morphological abnormalities in idiopathic torsion dystonia as seen on brain imaging (Rutledge et al., 1987) or histological examination (Zeman, 1976). Hornykiewicz et al. (1986) examined the biochemistry of the brain in two patients with childhood-onset generalized idiopathic dystonia, and Jankovic et al. (1987) studied a single case of adult-onset idiopathic cranial segmental dystonia. There were changes in norepinephrine, serotonin, and dopamine levels in various regions of brain. It is not clear which, if any, of these alterations is related to the pathophysiology of dystonia. In a patient with symptomatic dystonia due to neuroacanthocytosis, de Yebenes et al. (1988) found large increases in norepinephrine in the caudate nucleus, putamen, globus pallidus, and dentate nucleus. Again, it is not clear whether changes in norepinephrine levels are related to dystonia. Many more biochemical studies need to be carried out. In the meantime, fluorodeoxyglucose PET studies have revealed some regional hypometabolism in the frontal cortex and lenticular nucleus (Karbe et al., 1992; Eidelberg et al., 1992).

TREATMENT

Only some symptomatic dystonias, such as Wilson's disease, have a specific therapy directed against the pathophysiological mechanisms; treatment of the idiopathic dystonias is based on the experience of many empirical trials (Fahn and Marsden, 1987). Perhaps the most comprehensive study to date is that by Greene et al. (1988), who reported on drug trials in 358 patients. For the practicing clinician, choosing a treatment strategy is important. I will review the strategy used by the Dystonia Clinical Research Center at Columbia-Presbyterian Medical Center.

Since no single drug is uniformly effective in treating dystonia, and surgical approaches are not uniformly beneficial or without risk, it is important in selecting the first choice that the risk be minimum. In order to avoid potential harm when searching for effective therapy, surgical procedures and drugs that can cause irreversible complications, such as tardive dyskinesia and tardive dystonia, should be used late in empirical trials of treatments for dystonic patients.

The focal dystonias have the therapeutic advantage that local injections of botulinum toxin (BTX) and peripheral surgical denervation, which have a low risk of serious adverse effects, are effective in many patients. Trials of BTX in patients with various focal dystonias have shown that more than 70% of patients with blepharospasm, adductor laryngeal dystonia, torticollis, and oromandibular dystonia improve for up to 3 months and can have continued improvement with subsequent injections (Brin et al., 1987; Jankovic and Orman, 1987; Brin et al., 1989; Blitzer et al., 1989; Jankovic and Schwartz, 1990; American Academy of Neurology, 1990; Jankovic and Brin, 1991). Botulinum toxin is fast becoming the first line of treatment for these focal dystonias. There has been no major morbidity reported from these injections.

Peripheral surgical denervation and BTX injections cannot be used to treat the segmental and generalized dystonias because of the greater number of muscles involved. Systemic pharmacological agents and stereotactic thalamotomy are the only alternatives. Pharmacological trials are always recommended before considering stereotactic thalamotomies.

Since about 5–10% of children with dystonia respond to levodopa—so-called dopa-responsive dystonia (Nygaard, 1989; Nygaard et al., 1990)—and since there are virtually no adverse effects with the small doses necessary, it is best to begin therapy with a short course of levodopa to see if the patient is in that small subset who respond to this agent. A dose of carbidopa/levodopa 5/50 mg t.i.d. can be used. If this fails, it is reasonable to increase the dose to a maximum of 25/250 mg q.i.d.

The next drug to be tried is an anticholinergic agent. Since their introduction for dystonia, high-dosage anticholinergic drugs have become one of the mainstays of non-specific therapy in dystonia. Although the use of these drugs given in high dosages was based originally on the results of open-label trials (Fahn, 1983), their efficacy has been substantiated by double-blind investigations (Burke et al., 1986b) and by other open-label trials including large numbers of patients (Marsden et al., 1984; Lang, 1986). In general, all these studies show that approximately 50% of children and 40% of adults with idiopathic dystonia obtain moderate to dramatic benefit from this class of drugs.

Dose-limiting problems with anticholinergics are their peripheral and central adverse effects. Peripheral adverse effects such as dry mouth and blurred vision are fairly common, but can often be ameliorated by coadministration of peripherally acting anticholinesterase drugs (such as pyridostigmine) and eyedrops of pilocarpine, a muscarinic agonist. Central adverse effects such as forgetfulness, confusion, hallucinations, or behavioral changes can be overcome only by reducing the dose, and thus lessening the usefulness of the drug. Sometimes, a slow-release preparation (e.g., Artane Sequels) can overcome this problem.

In order to minimize adverse effects, I start with a low dose of an anticholinergic agent and increase the dosage gradually. For children I start with trihexyphenidyl 2.5 mg b.i.d. and increase the daily dosage by 2.5 mg every week. At daily dosages of, for example, 20, 30, 40, or 50 mg/day, I hold the dose constant for 4 weeks before increasing it further, since some patients have a delay before they respond. I maintain the minimum dose that provides adequate benefit. If no benefit is seen, I increase the dose until intolerable adverse effects are encountered. Antidotes for some of the adverse peripheral effects are discussed above. The dosage of ethopropazine is approximately 10 times greater than that of trihexyphenidyl; otherwise the dosing strategy is identical. If anticholinergics provide any benefit, but higher doses cannot be used because of intolerable side effects, then the optimum dose achieved is maintained and a second drug is added.

If further drug trials are needed, I select from among baclofen, the benzodiazepines, and carbamazepine in that order, since these agents do not cause any persistent adverse effects. Baclofen can sometimes produce dramatic results (Greene et al., 1988; Greene and Fahn, 1992). Although dopamine receptor blockers are more effective than these three, the antipsychotics can cause persistent tardive dyskinesia and tardive dystonia. Thus, I use dopamine receptor blockers as a last resort, and when I do use one of these drugs, I combine it with a dopamine-depleting agent such as reserpine in an attempt to avoid tardive dyskinetic syndromes.

As new centrally acting drugs are developed for other neurological conditions, they should be tested in dystonia as well. Through empirical trials, a new effective therapeutic agent may be discovered.

REFERENCES

Abbruzzese G, Rizzo F, Dall'Agata D, Morandi N, Favale E. Generalized dystonia with bilateral striatal computer-tomographic lucencies in a patient with human immunodeficiency virus infection. Eur Neurol 1990;30:271–273.

American Academy of Neurology, Therapeutics and Technology Assessment Subcommittee. Assessment: the clinical usefulness of botulinum toxin-A in treating neurologic disorders. Neurology 1990;40:1332–1336.

Berardelli A, Rothwell JC, Day BL, Marsden CD. Pathophysiology of blepharospasm and oromandibular dystonia. Brain 1985;108:593–609.

Blitzer A, Brin MF, Greene PE, Fahn S. Botulinum toxin injection for the treatment of oromandibular dystonia. Ann Otol Rhinol Laryngol 1989;98:93–97.

Bonuccelli U, Nocchiero A, Napolitano A, Paoletti AM, Melis GB, Corsini GU, Muratorio A. Domperidone-induced acute dystonia and polycystic ovary syndrome. Mov Disord 1991;6:79–81.

Bressman SB, de Leon D, Brin MF, Risch N, Burke RE, Greene PE, Shale H, Fahn S. Idiopathic torsion dystonia among Ashkenazi Jews: evidence for autosomal dominant inheritance. Ann Neurol 1989;26:612–620.

Brin MF, Fahn S, Moskowitz C, Friedman A, Shale HM, Greene PE, Blitzer A, List T, Lange D, Lovelace RE, McMahon D. Localized injections of botulinum toxin for the treatment of focal dystonia and hemifacial spasm. Mov Disord 1987;2:237–254.

Brin MF, Blitzer A, Fahn S, Gould W, Lovelace RE. Adductor laryngeal dystonia (spastic dysphonia): treatment with local injections of botulinum toxin (Botox). Mov Disord 1989;4:287–296.

Burke RE, Brin MF, Fahn S, Bressman SB, Moskowitz C. Analysis of the clinical course of non-Jewish, autosomal dominant torsion dystonia. Mov Disord 1986a;1:163–178.

Burke RE, Fahn S, Marsden CD. Torsion dystonia: a double-blind, prospective trial of high-dosage trihexyphenidyl. Neurology 1986b;36:160–164.

Burton K, Farrell K, Li D, Calne DB. Lesions of the putamen and dystonia: CT and magnetic resonance imaging. Neurology 1984;34:962–965.

Calne DB, Lang AE. Secondary dystonia. Adv Neurol 1988;50:9–33.

Chan J, Brin MF, Fahn S. Idiopathic cervical dystonia: clinical characteristics. Mov Disord 1991;6:119–126.

Cohen LG, Hallett M, Sudarsky L. A single family with writer's cramp, essential tremor, and primary writing tremor. Mov Disord 1987;2:109–116.

De Leon D, Brin MF, Murphy P, Bressman SB, Ozelius L, Cardon N, Reich S, Breakefield XO, Fahn S. Genetic counseling for idiopathic torsion dystonia: first use of DNA based carrier detection in Ashkenazic Jews. Mov Disord 1991;6:273–274.

Eidelberg D, Dhawan V, Takikawa S, Redington K, Chaly T, Greene P, Fahn S. Regional metabolic covariation in idiopathic torsion dystonia: [^{18}F]fluorodeoxyglucose PET studies. Mov Disord 1992;7:297.

Elble RJ, Moody C, Higgins C. Primary writing tremor: a form of focal dystonia. Mov Disord 1990;5:118–126.

Eldridge R. The torsion dystonias: literature review and genetic and clinical studies. Neurology 1970;20(no. 11, part 2):1–78.

Fahn S: High dosage anticholinergic therapy in dystonia. Neurology 1983;33:1255–1261.

Fahn S. Generalized dystonia: concept and treatment. Clin Neuropharmacol 1986;9(suppl 2):S37–S48.

Fahn S. Concept and classification of dystonia. Adv Neurol 1988;50:1–8.

Fahn S. Dystonia: Where next? In: Quinn NP, Jenner PG, eds. Disorders of movement: clinical, pharmacological and physiological aspects. London: Academic Press, 1989a:349–359.

Fahn S. Assessment of the primary dystonias. In: Munsat TL, ed. Quantification of neurologic deficit. Boston: Butterworth; 1989b:241–270.

Fahn S. Clinical variants of idiopathic torsion dystonia. J Neurol Neurosurg Psychiatry Special Supplement 1989c;96–100.

Fahn S. Recent concepts in the diagnosis and treatment of dystonias. In: Chokroverty S, ed. Movement disorders. Costa Mesa, California: PMA Publishing Corp., 1990:237–258.

Fahn S, Marsden CD. The treatment of dystonia. In: Marsden CD, Fahn S, eds. Movement Disorders 2. London: Butterworths, 1987:359–382.

Fahn S, Marsden CD, Calne DB. Classification and investigation of dystonia. In: Marsden CD, Fahn S, eds. Movement disorders 2. London: Butterworths, 1987:332–358.

Fahn S, Marsden CD, Calne DB, eds: Dystonia 2. Advances in Neurology, vol. 50. New York: Raven Press, 1988.

Fahn S, Moskowitz C. X-Linked recessive dystonia and parkinsonism in Filipino males. Ann Neurol 1988;24:179.

Fahn S, Williams DT. Psychogenic dystonia. Adv Neurol 1988;50:431–455.

Fish DR, Sawyers D, Allen PJ, Blackie JD, Lees AJ, Marsden CD. The effect of sleep on the dyskinetic movements of Parkinson's disease, Gilles de la Tourette syndrome, Huntington's disease, and torsion dystonia. Arch Neurol 1991;48:210–214.

Flatau E, Sterling W. Progressiver Torsionspasms bei Kindern. Z Gesamte Neurol Psychiat 1911;7:586–612.

Fletcher NA, Harding AE, Marsden CD. A case-control study of idiopathic torsion dystonia. Mov Disord 1991a;6:304–309.

Fletcher NA, Harding AE, Marsden CD. Intrafamilial correlation in idiopathic torsion dystonia. Mov Disord 1991b;6:310–314.

Fletcher NA, Harding AE, Marsden CD. The relationship between trauma and idiopathic torsion dystonia. J Neurol Neurosurg Psychiatry 1991c;54:713–717.

Greene PE, Fahn S. Baclofen in the treatment of idiopathic dystonia in children. Mov Disord 1992;7:48–52.

Greene P, Kang U, Fahn S, Brin MF, Moskowitz C, Flaster E. Double-blind, placebo controlled trial of botulinum toxin injection for the treatment of spasmodic torticollis. Neurology 1990;40:1213–1218.

Greene P, Shale H, Fahn S. Analysis of open-label trials in torsion dystonia using high dosages of anticholinergics and other drugs. Mov Disord 1988;3:46–60.

Hornykiewicz O, Kish SJ, Becker LE, Farley I, Shannak K. Brain neurotransmitters in dystonia musculorum deformans. N Engl J Med 1986;315:347–353.

Jabbari B, Paul J, Scherokman B, Vandam B. Posttraumatic segmental axial dystonia. Mov Disord 1992;7:78–81.

Jankovic J, Brin MF. Therapeutic uses of botulinum toxin. N Engl J Med 1991;324:1186–1194.

Jankovic J, Fahn S. Physiologic and pathologic tremors. Diagnosis, mechanism, and management. Ann Intern Med 1980;93:460–465.

Jankovic J, Fahn S. Dystonic syndromes. In: Jankovic J, Tolosa E, eds. Parkinson's disease and movement disorders. Baltimore: Urban and Schwarzenberg; 1988:283–314.

Jankovic J, Orman J. Botulinum A toxin for cranial-cervical dystonia: a double-blind, placebo-controlled study. Neurology 1987;37:616–623.

Jankovic J, Patel SC. Blepharospasm associated with brainstem lesions. Neurology 1983;33:1237–1240.

Jankovic J, Schwartz K. Botulinum toxin injections for cervical dystonia. Neurology 1990;40:277–280.

Jankovic J, Svendsen CN, Bird ED. Brain neurotransmitters in dystonia. N Engl J Med 1987;316:278–279.

Jedynak CP, Bonnet AM, Agid Y. Tremor and idiopathic dystonia. Mov Disord 1991;6:230–236.

Karbe H, Holthoff VA, Rudolf J, Herholz K, Heiss WD. Positron emission tomography demonstrates frontal cortex and basal ganglia hypometabolism in dystonia. Neurology 1992;42:1540–1544.

Kramer PL, Ozelius L, de Leon D, Risch N, Brin MF, Bressman SB, Burke RE, Kwiatkowski DJ, Schuback DE, Shale H, Gusella JF, Breakefield XO, Fahn S. Dystonia gene in Ashkenazi Jewish population located on chromosome 9q32–34. Ann Neurol 1990;27:114–120.

Krauss JK, Mohadjer M, Wakhloo AK, Mundinger F. Dystonia and akinesia due to pallidoputaminal lesions after disulfiram intoxication. Mov Disord 1991;6:166–170.

Kupke KG, Graeber MB, Muller U. Dystonia-parkinsonism syndrome (XDP) locus–flanking markers in Xq12–q21.1. Am J Hum Genet 1992;50:808–815.

Kupke KG, Lee LV, Muller U. Assignment of the X-linked torsion dystonia gene to Xq21 by linkage analysis. Neurology 1990;40:1438–1442.

Kurlan R, Behr J, Medved L. Shoulson I. Myoclonus and dystonia: a family study. Adv Neurol 1988;50:385–389.

Kwiatkowski DJ, Nygaard TG, Schuback DE, Perman S, Trugman J, Bressman SB, Burke RE, Brin MF, Ozelius L, Breakefield XO, Fahn S, Kramer PL. Identification of a highly polymorphic microsatellite VNTR within the argininosuccinate synthetase locus: exclusion of the dystonia gene on 9q32–34 as a cause of dopa-responsive dystonia in a large kindred. Am J Hum Genet 1991;48:121–128.

Lang AE. High dose anticholinergic therapy in adult dystonia. Can J Neurol Sci 1986;13:42–46.

Lee LV, Kupke KG, Caballar-Gonzaga F, Hebron-Ortiz M, Muller U. The phenotype of the X-linked dystonia-parkinsonism syndrome—an assessment of 42 cases in the Philippines. Medicine 1991;70:179–187.

Lee LV, Pascasio FM, Fuentes FD, Viterbo GH. Torsion dystonia in Panay, Philippines. Adv Neurol 1976;14:137–152.

Lou JS, Jankovic J. Essential tremor: clinical correlates in 350 patients. Neurology 1991;41:234–238.

Maraganore DM, Folger WN, Swanson JW, Ahlskog JE. Movement disorders as sequelae of central pontine myelinolysis: report of three cases. Mov Disord 1992;7:142–148.

Marsden CD. The focal dystonias. Clin Neuropharmacol 1986;9 (suppl 2):S49–S60.

Marsden CD, Harrison MJG, Bundey S. Natural history of idiopathic torsion dystonia. Adv Neurol 1976;14:177–187.

Marsden CD, Marion M-H, Quinn N. The treatment of severe dystonia in children and adults. J Neurol Neurosurg Psychiatry 1984;47:1166–1173.

Marsden CD, Obeso JA, Zarranz JJ, Lang AE. The anatomical basis of symptomatic hemidystonia. Brain 1985;108:463–483.

Miller LG, Jankovic J. Persistent dystonia possibly induced by flecainide. Mov Disord 1992;7:62–63.

Nakashima K, Rothwell JC, Day BL, Thompson PD, Shannon K, Marsden CD. Reciprocal inhibition between forearm muscles in patients with writer's cramp and other occupational cramps, symptomatic hemidystonia and hemiparesis due to stroke. Brain 1989;112:681–697.

Narbona J, Obeso JA, Tunon T, Martinez-Lage JM, Marsden CD. Hemi-dystonia secondary to localized basal ganglia tumour. J Neurol Neurosurg Psychiatry 1984;47:704–709.

Nutt JG, Muenter MD, Aronson A, Kurland LT, Melton LJ, Epidemiology of focal and generalized dystonia in Rochester, Minnesota. Mov Disord 1988;3:188–194.

Nygaard TG. Dopa-responsive dystonia: 20 years into the L-dopa era. In: Quinn NP, Jenner PG, eds. Disorders of movement: clinical, pharmacological and physiological aspects. London:Academic Press, 1989:323–337.

Nygaard TG, Marsden CD, Fahn S. Dopa-responsive dystonia: long-term treatment response and prognosis. Neurology 1991;41:174–181.

Nygaard TG, Trugman JM, de Yebenes JG, Fahn S. Dopa-responsive dystonia: the spectrum of clinical manifestations in a large North American family. Neurology 1990;40:66–69.

Obeso JA, Rothwell JC, Lang AE, Marsden CD. Myoclonic dystonia. Neurology 1983;33:825–830.

Ornadel D, Barnes EA, Dick DJ. Acute dystonia due to amitriptyline. J Neurol Neurosurg Psychiatry 1992;55:414.

Oppenheim H. Uber eine eigenartige Krampfkrankheit des kindlichen und jugendlichen Alters (Dysbasia lordotica progressiva, Dystonia musculorum deformans). Neurol Centralbl 1911;30:1090–1107.

Ozelius L, Kramer PL, Moskowitz CB, Kwiatkowski DJ, Brin MF, Schuback DE, Falk CT, Haines J, Bressman SB, DeLeon D, Burke RE, Gusella JF, Fahn S, Breakefield XO. Human gene for torsion dystonia located on chromosome 9q32–34. Neuron 1989;2:1427–1434.

Pauls DL, Korczyn AD. complex segregation analysis of dystonia pedigrees suggests autosomal dominant inheritance. Neurology 1990;40:1107–1110.

Pettigrew LC, Jankovic J. Hemidystonia: a report of 22 patients and a review of the literature. J Neurol Neurosurg Psychiatry 1985;48:650–657.

Quinn NP, Rothwell JC, Thompson PD, Marsden CD. Hereditary myoclonic dystonia, hereditary torsion dystonia and hereditary essential myoclonus: an area of confusion. Adv Neurol 1988;50:391–401.

Risch N, Bressman SB, deLeon D, Brin MF, Bruke RE, Greene PE, Shale H, Claus EB, Cupples LA, and Fahn S. Segregation analysis of idiopathic torsion dystonia in Ashkenazi Jews suggests autosomal dominant inheritance. Am J Hum Genet 1990;46:533–438.

Rosenbaum F, Jankovic J. Focal task-specific tremor and dystonia: categorization of occupational movement disorders.Neurology 1988;38:522–527.

Rothwell JC, Obeso JA. The anatomical and physiological basis of torsion dystonia. In: Marsden CD, Fahn S, eds. Movement disorders 2. London: Butterworths, 1987:313–331.

Rothwell JC, Obeso JA, Day BL, Marsden CD. The pathophysiology of dystonias. Adv Neurol 1983;39:851–863.

Rutledge JN, Hilal SK, Silver AJ, Defendini R, Fahn S. Study of movement disorders and brain iron by MR. Am J Neuroradiol 1987;8:397–411.

Saint-Hilaire M-H, Burke RE, Bressman SB, Brin MF, Fahn S. Delayed-onset dystonia due to perinatal or early childhood asphyxia. Neurology 1991;41:216–222.

Sawle GV, Leenders KL, Brooks DJ, Harwood G, Lees AJ, Frackowiak RSJ, Marsden CD. Dopa-responsive dystonia: [F-18]dopa positron emission tomography. Ann Neurol 1991;30:24–30.

Segawa M, Hosaka A, Miyagawa F, Nomura Y, Imai H. Hereditary progressive dystonia with marked diurnal fluctuation. Adv Neurol 1976;14:215–233.

Sethi KD, Hess DC. Creutzfeldt-Jakob's disease presenting with ataxia and a movement disorder. Mov Disord 1991;6:157–162.

Shale HM, Truong DD, Fahn S. Tics in patients with other movement disorders. Neurology 1986;36(suppl 1):118.

Stone LA, Jankovic J. The coexistence of tics and dystonia. Arch Neurol 1991;48:862–865.

Tison FX, Ferrer X, Julien J. Delayed onset movement disorders as a complication of central pontine myelinolysis. Mov Disord 1991;6:171–173.

Tolge CF, Factor SA. Focal dystonia secondary to cerebral toxoplasmosis in a patient with acquired immune deficiency syndrome. Mov Disord 1991;6:69–72.

Tolosa E, Montserrat L, Bayes A. Blink reflex studies in focal dystonias: enhanced excitability of brainstem interneurons in cranial dystonia and spasmodic torticollis. Mov Disord 1988;3:61–69.

Valenzuela R, Court J, Godoy J. Delayed cyanide induced dystonia. J Neurol Neurosurg Psychiat 1992;55:198–199.

Waddy HM, Fletcher NA, Harding AE, Marsden CD. A genetic study of idiopathic focal dystonias. Ann Neurol 1991;29:320–324.

Wilhelmsen KC, Weeks DE, Nygaard TG, Moskowitz CB, Rosales RL, dela Paz DC, Sobrevega EE, Fahn S. Genetic mapping of ''lubag'' (X-linked dystonia-parkinsonism) in a Filipino kindred to the pericentromeric region of the X chromosome. Ann Neurol 1991;29:124–131.

Yanagisawa N, Goto A. Dysotnia musculorum deformans: analysis with electromyography. J Neurol Sci 1971;13:39–65.

Yanagisawa N, Goto A, Narabayashi H. Familial dystonia musculorum deformans and tremor. J Neurol Sci 1972;16:125–136.

de Yebenes JG, Vazquez A, Martinez A, Mena MA, del Rio RM, et al. Biochemical findings in symptomatic dystonias. Adv Neurol 1988;50:167–175.

Zeman W. Dystonia: an overview. Adv Neurol 1976;14:91–103.

Zeman W, Dyken P. Dystonia musculorum deformans; clinical, genetic and pathoanatomical studies. Psychiat Neurol Neurochir 1967;70:77–121.

Zilber N, Korczyn AD, Kahana E, Fried K, Alter M. Inheritance of idiopathic torsion dystonia among Jews. J Med Genet 1984;21:13–20.

13

Botulinum Toxin for Blepharospasm

John S. Elston
Oxford Eye Hospital, Radcliffe Infirmary, National Health Service Trust, Oxford, England

INTRODUCTION

The development over the past decade of a simple, safe, and effective treatment for idiopathic blepharospasm has brought relief to thousands of people suffering from this formerly intractable condition. It has also raised awareness of the disease among both the public and the medical profession. Patients who may have been misdiagnosed or told that there was no treatment are revisiting doctors, and new cases are now more likely to be correctly diagnosed and sympathetically treated. Increased interest among ophthalmologists and neurologists has led to better documentation of cases and more careful study of the disorder. The spectrum of the disorder, its associations, and its natural history are becoming clearer. Nevertheless, its epidemiology is not established and, as with other forms of focal dystonia, its cause is not known.

In this chapter, the symptomatology of idiopathic blepharospasm and the assessment of the patient will be outlined, and a management plan with particular emphasis on botulinum toxin (BTX) treatment will be proposed. The problem of treatment failures and the possibility of future therapeutic developments will also be considered.

SYMPTOMATOLOGY

Idiopathic blepharospasm invariably begins in adult life, most commonly in the sixth or seventh decade. The sex ratio is two to three women to one man. The earliest symptoms are often sensory. The eyes or eyelids are sore, gritty, or itching and may feel dry or sometimes water excessively (1). Photophobia is prominent and may predate other symptoms by many years. The initial symptoms may date from a specific episode of eyelid inflammation, infection, or other interference with ocular surface dynamics (2). Slit-lamp examination of the eyelids shows that blepharitis and disorders of meibomian gland function are very common. Such abnormalities persist after successful treatment of blepharospasm with BTX and therefore do not appear to be secondary to the excessive lid movements. They may trigger the onset of the disease in susceptible persons. Other possible triggers are hormonal factors (onset of menopause) or drugs such as phenothiazines.

An increased periodic blink rate may be observed in the early stages. There is then usually a progression from an awareness of excessive blinking or fluttering of the eyelids to intermittent spasms of eye closure that interfere with visual function. Typically, the spasms become more frequent and severe and involve the preseptal, pretarsal, and orbital orbicularis oculi muscle. They often result in functional blindness within 2 to 3 years of the onset of symptoms. The speed of onset and severity of the disorder may vary considerably. Occasionally patients have a spontaneous remission.

The spasms may extend into the midfacial and lower facial muscles and occasionally to the jaw and neck. Rarely the spread is reversed from the lower facial muscles to the orbicularis oculi (3). Diagnostic confusion as to the presence of lower facial dystonia may arise, since patients often use stereotyped voluntary movements of the lower face, such as mouth opening, to facilitate eye opening.

In a variant of idiopathic blepharospasm, abnormal muscle contraction is confined to the pretarsal and preseptal orbicularis oculi without brow spasm. The brows are therefore often elevated, especially on attempted eye opening, due to frontalis muscle overactivity. The lids may appear to be passively shut but resist opening by the examiner's fingers. This clinical picture (formerly known erroneously as apraxia of eye opening or levator inhibition) may also be seen in Parkinson's disease and progressive supranuclear palsy (4).

Variability of symptoms and signs is characteristic and is influenced particularly by environmental conditions. Worsening in bright or reflected lighting conditions is usual. There is often a predictable diurnal variation, such as worsening as the day goes on. Spasms may improve on down gaze or when the patient is engrossed. Eating or talking may lessen symptoms, and walking often worsens them. Social stress usually exacerbates the condition but paradoxically may lead to improvement—for example, on consultation with the doctor. In these circumstances, there are no abnormal signs and the diagnosis may have to rest on the history and the reports of relatives. A "geste antagonistique"—such as pressing firmly with a finger on the temple—may be seen or described.

There is some evidence for a genetic susceptibility to the development of idiopathic blepharospasm; in a series of 194 patients, there was a family history among first-degree relatives of focal dystonia for 6%, essential tremor for 12%, and tics for 4.5% (5). Patients in whom the disease appears to be triggered by ocular surface disorders, are on average younger than others and more likely to have a family history of a movement disorder (2). Some patients with eye winking tics in childhood and a family history of tics develop blepharospasm in early adult life (6).

The cause remains elusive; the condition may occur in patients with symptomatic dystonia, generalized idiopathic dystonia, and Parkinson's disease. Pretarsal blepharospasm (see above) may also be seen in progressive supranuclear palsy. The facial tics of Tourette's syndrome may occasionally include sustained spasms of eye closure. There is therefore a suspicion that the underlying abnormality in idiopathic blepharospasm is in the extrapyramidal system. Blink reflex studies suggest that the facial nucleus is hyperexcitable and fails to habituate to repeated stimuli, possibly because of disinhibition (7). Saccadic eye movement abnormalities compatible with extrapyramidal dysfunction have been described (8). Results of neuro-imaging and postmortem studies are normal, and a defect of neurotransmission appears likely. However, positron emission tomography (PET) scanning is inconclusive, and there is no consistent response to pharmacological treatment.

The differential diagnosis includes ocular myasthenia gravis and myotonia of the lids. Blepharoclonus may occur in multiple sclerosis, when it is often gaze-evoked. Hemifacial spasm may very rarely be bilateral.

ASSESSMENT

Clinical assessment must include a full ophthalmological examination to exclude secondary blepharospasm caused by ocular disorders such as trichiasis. Relatively minor ocular surface disorders are frequently found, but appropriate treatment has no effect on the blepharospasm. From the neurological point of view, the extent of craniocervical or generalized involvement should be assessed.

There is no way of objectively measuring the impact of idiopathic blepharospasm on the patient. This includes the visual problems, the sensory symptoms, and the psychological and social sequelae of the disorder. Unfortunately, partly because of the sensitivity of the condition to social and environmental factors, the doctor's assessment of its effect on the patient may be wrong, and this effect is in any case difficult to quantitate. Self-scoring by the patient using analogue scores and questionnaires has been attempted, along with videotaping. However, the problem remains and has hampered the investigation of the effects of treatment and retarded product licence applications for BTX.

INVESTIGATION

In general there is no indication for investigation, including neuro-imaging, in typical adult-onset idiopathic blepharospasm. In cases of doubt, blink reflex studies may be diagnostic. As with other chronic illnesses for which there is no adequate explanation, some patients may become secondarily depressed and require psychiatric referral.

There is a subgroup of patients in whom it appears that minor ocular surface disorders are accompanied by an exaggerated motor response. Other patients with blepharospasm have personality traits suggesting that the condition may be psychogenic. In my experience, neither of these groups benefits from psychiatric interventions, and all patients with the symptom-sign complex of idiopathic blepharospasm should be managed in the same way, regardless of speculation as to the origin of the problem.

MANAGEMENT

Patients with blepharospasm are often distressed by the disorder and confused about its origins. Family, friends, and work colleagues as well as medical practitioners have frequently offered diagnoses that may be dismissive or insulting. If a patient has been in touch with one of the patient help groups (e.g., The Dystonia Society in the United Kingdom), his or her expectations of the effects of BTX treatment may be inappropriately optimistic.

The patient should be given an explanation of the problem as an organic disorder of an isolated part of the movement control centers of the brain.

There are no extensive controlled studies of any form of treatment—surgery, pharmacological therapy, or BTX injection—in idiopathic blepharospasm. In the past, this was partly due to the small numbers of patients studied. The difficulty of objectively quantifying the disease, and consequent reliance on patients' impressions of the effects of treatment, have made such studies difficult to design. Moreover, to the physicians (and patients) who dealt with the condition before the advent of BTX treatment, the beneficial effects of the injections are so self-evident as not to need further research. Jankovic and Orman, in a well-designed placebo-controlled, double-blind study, have demonstrated a significant benefit for BTX treatment of blepharospasm as judged by self-assessment, physical examination, and before-and-after videotapes (9). There is now a substantial body of published literature that strongly supports the contention that BTX injection is the treatment of choice (10); with repeated injections the beneficial effects are sustained for 10 or more years.

It is important to appreciate that childhood-onset dopa-sensitive dystonia may be clinically indistinguishable from idiopathic torsion dystonia. Because of the overlap between generalized and focal dystonia, a trial of dopa treatment may be worthwhile in cases where there is doubt about the diagnostic category of the patient. The low frequency and poor quality of the response to other drugs—including anticholinergics—means they should not be used as first-line treatment.

METHODS OF TREATMENT

While recognizing the inherent difficulties involved, it is important to try to establish some form of pre- and post-treatment assessment of the patient's sensory symptoms and visual difficulties. This can be correlated with data on the site and dose of injections, side effects, and duration of benefit to establish a long-term treatment schedule for the individual patient.

Two different preparations of BTX-A are available—Oculinum (also registered as Botox, Allergan Inc., Irvine, CA) and Dysport (Porton Products, Maidenhead, UK.). The doses used for treatment are measured in units, defined by acute toxicity tests in mice. These have established an LD_{50} of 50 pg for Dysport and of 400 pg for Oculinum. The reason for this difference is not fully understood but is probably related to differences in specific toxicity (mouse LD_{50}/mg of protein) of the two products and possibly to differences in assay procedures. In practice, experience has shown that 1 U of Oculinum is equivalent to 4 U of Dysport. The manufacturer's instructions should therefore be carefully followed, but both products have an identical therapeutic effect.

Dysport is supplied in vials containing 500 U as a freeze-dried powder. It is dissolved in 2.5 ml of sterile, preservative-free saline and then injected subcutaneously using a 1-ml syringe and a 27- or 29-gauge needle. Injections of 40 U at the junction of the orbital and preseptal orbicularis oculi (at the orbital rim) on the upper lids medially and laterally, and on the lower lids laterally only, are recommended. Injections on the upper lids are angled laterally away from the center of the lid to minimize intraorbital spread. For Oculinum, vials contain 100 U, and the amount of preservative-free sterile saline that is used to dilute the contents determines the dose per injection using a standard 0.1-ml injection. In practice, most operators dilute with 4 ml, giving 2.5 U per 0.1 ml. Injections of 1.25–2.5 U are given into the pretarsal orbicularis oculi of the upper lid laterally and medially and the lower lid laterally, together with 2.5-U injections lateral to the lateral canthus and into the brow medially (total 6.25–12.5 U per eye). Both Dysport and Oculinum should be used within 4 hours of reconstitution. Subsequent injections of Oculinum can be increased up to twofold, whereas for Dysport the same or a reduced unit dose is recommended.

Experienced physicians will modify the dose and site of injection for individual patients to deal with specific muscle spasms. The injection sites for Dysport are chosen to weaken primarily the orbital orbicularis oculi, with spread to the pretarsal and preseptal portions of the muscle by diffusion. The Oculinum method directly weakens the pretarsal portion of the muscle with separate brow and lateral orbital treatments. An overall weakening of the orbicularis oculi, without spread to other muscles, is the aim of both methods, and despite the considerable variations in dose and technique described above, results reported with the two products are similar (1,9). Ptosis is documented slightly less frequently as a side effect with the Dysport method, and there is no doubt that the exact injection placement is important with respect to this complication. Jankovic has shown, in a single-blind study, that pretarsal injections of Oculinum produce a mild ptosis in fewer than 10% of patients, whereas over 80% of those injected in the preseptal area developed ptosis (J. Jankovic, personal communication).

Because of practical difficulties, most physicians re-treat patients after a fixed period (usually 8–10 weeks), but an ''open door'' policy that allows re-treatment when symptoms recur is ideal.

RESULTS

Most published reports rely on the patient's perception of change of symptoms as a result of treatment to judge the efficacy. On this basis, numerous open clinical trials have confirmed the initial favorable clinical impressions (10). In general, approximately 70% of patients benefit, and of these roughly half regain normal or near-normal visual function. The benefit lasts about 8 weeks and appears to be repeatable indefinitely. There is some evidence for a slight increase in the duration of benefit with repeated treatments (11), but there may be a reduction in the perception of beneficial effect.

Although side effects are relatively common, occurring in 15–50% of patients, they are usually mild and well tolerated. The large variation is determined by the method of assessment rather than the treatment technique. A 1- to 2-mm ptosis due to accumulation of tissue fluid in the first few days after treatment is common, while ptosis due to spread to the levator generally develops after a week to 10 days. Midfacial weakness, particularly affecting the upper lip muscles, may be troublesome. Entropion usually responds to taping of the lid. Double vision can be managed with Fresnel prisms. There are no systemic side effects.

Successful treatment may unmask a levator disinsertion ptosis caused by the prolonged forceful blinking. This can be successfully treated surgically.

Many patients report improvement in sensory symptoms such as irritation and photophobia after treatment. Also, successful treatment of blepharospasm may be accompanied by a reduction in midfacial and lower facial spasm that is not due to spread of weakness to the muscles concerned. The mechanisms involved in these aspects of the response are unclear. Hyperexcitability of the facial nucleus and failure of habituation of the blink reflex are characteristic of blepharospasm. In these circumstances, the normal sensory stimulation that accompanies a periodic blink could result in an abnormal excessive motor response. The clinical progression of the disease, with spread of spasms from around the eyes to the middle and lower face, suggests that there may be a somatotopic spread of hyperexcitability within the facial nucleus. Botulinum toxin treatment, by weakening the orbicularis oculi and reducing both normal and abnormal motor activity, will reduce sensory input from the eyelids, conjunctiva, ocular surface, and upper facial musculature.

It is possible that this reduction in sensory input has a beneficial damping effect on facial nucleus hypersensitivity, so that abnormal movements in the face as a whole are to some extent suppressed.

TREATMENT FAILURES

If a patient fails to respond at all to BTX therapy when adequate orbicularis oculi weakness has been achieved, the diagnosis should be reviewed. If the problem is pretarsal blepharospasm, the pretarsal orbicularis oculi needs to be weakened. However, the majority of primary treatment failures cannot be predicted on clinical or other grounds. These patients may have a different underlying disorder that produces hyperexcitability of the facial nucleus coupled with an abnormality of reciprocal innervation of the levator muscle. In some patients, persistence of Bell's phenomenon of tonic (usually) upward deviation of the eyes with passive lid closure due to levator inhibition is responsible for the failure to respond. Other measures such as anticholinergic drugs or surgery (such as facial nerve avulsion) may be indicated for these patients, although there is no guarantee that there will be a response.

Secondary treatment failure, a perception by the patient that the treatment that originally worked no longer does so, is more difficult to interpret. Second and subsequent treatments are almost always given before the symptoms have recovered fully and when the orbicularis oculi is still weakened, so the effect is necessarily less dramatic. The patient's expectations of subsequent treatments may therefore not be fulfilled. In others, the underlying disease process may have progressed to disrupt facial muscle control more severely. Antibodies to BTX do not develop when normal blepharospasm treatment doses are used but many do so if concurrent torticollis is being treated. Some secondary treatment failures will respond to some extent to the addition of systemic drugs, such as anticholinergics, while surgical treatment will help others.

THE FUTURE

Improvements in the understanding of the underlying pathophysiology of idiopathic blepharospasm may eventually allow the development of more rational systemic treatment.

Muscles that have been denervated by BTX recover function as a result of nodal and terminal axonal sprouting and the establishment of new neuromuscular junctions. If this process could be prevented, the effects of a single injection could be prolonged indefinitely. Theoretical antisprouting factors exist, but none has so far been isolated for potential use. Until then, empirical treatment with BTX is the best available.

REFERENCES

1. Grandas F, Elston JS, Quinn N, Marsden CD. Blepharospasm: a review of 264 patients. J Neurol Neurosurg Psychiatry 1988;51:767–772.
2. Elston JS, Marsden CD. The significance of ophthalmological symptoms in idiopathic blepharospasm. Eye 1988;2:435–439.
3. Marsden CD. Blepharospasm—oromandibular dystonia (Brueghel's syndrome). A variant of adult onset torsion dystonia. J Neurol Neurosurg Psychiatry 1976;39:1204–1209.
4. Elston JS. A new variant of blepharospasm. J Neurol Neurosurg Psychiatry 1992;55:369–371.

5. Elston JS. Idiopathic blepharospasm, MD thesis, University of London, 1990.

6. Elston JS, Cranje F, Lees AJ. The relationship between eye winking tics, frequent eye blinking and blepharospasm. J Neurol Neurosurg Psychiatry 1989;52:477–480.

7. Berardelli A, Rothwell J, Day BL, Marsden CD. The pathophysiology of blepharospasm and oromandibular dystonia. Brain 1985;108:593–608.

8. Lueck CJ, Tanyeri S, Crawford TJ, Elston JS, Kennard C. Saccadic eye movements in essential blepharospasm. J Neurol 1990;237:226–229.

9. Jankovic J, Orman J. Botulinum A toxin for cranial-cervical dystonia: a double blind placebo controlled study. Neurology 1987;37:616–623.

10. Jankovic J, Brin MF. Drug therapy; therapeutic uses of botulinum toxin. N Engl J Med 1991;324:1186–1194.

11. Elston JS. Management of blepharospasm and hemifacial spasm. J Neurol 1992;239:5–8.

14

Acute and Chronic Effects of Botulinum Toxin in the Management of Blepharospasm

Jonathan J. Dutton
Duke University Eye Center, Durham, North Carolina

INTRODUCTION

Botulinum toxin type A has been used in the treatment of blepharospasm since 1983. Results have been reported for more than 5000 patients worldwide. This substance has proved to be effective in controlling involuntary spasms of the eyelids in a number of neuromuscular disorders, most notably essential blepharospasm, hemifacial spasm, and myokymia (1–8). Around the eyes botulinum toxin (BTX) has also been used for the temporary control of lower eyelid entropion (9,10) and for the induction of upper eyelid ptosis in patients with corneal ulcers (11).

Although the long-term consequences of chronic BTX use are still not clearly understood, many short- and long-term effects have been documented, and others have been suggested by clinical observation (5,10,12–17). These effects can be grouped as either acute (immediate), in which the result becomes manifest within days, or chronic (delayed), where the effect may develop over some time and only after repeated exposure. Although most of these effects are seen locally near the sites of injection, some may occur distant from the area of treatment and are therefore truly systemic in nature.

ACUTE LOCAL EFFECTS OF BOTULINUM TOXIN

Certainly the most important effect of BTX is its ability to chemodenervate cholinergic striated muscles (18–21). Botulinum toxin is now known to work through presynaptic block of the neuromuscular junction. The drug is taken up at special receptors on the presynaptic terminal, internalized, and results in intracellular blockade of neurotransmitter release. This effect appears to be permanent, and recovery of neuromuscular function occurs through nerve sprouting and new terminal formation (22–25). This neuromuscular blockade is the clinically desired effect in the management of facial dyskinesias and the reason for treatment. During the relatively denervated stage, the target muscle is weakened, resulting in reduced contractility and relief of dystonic movement.

The overall results of BTX therapy for blepharospasm have been gratifying, with 93.3% of treated patients reporting a clinically noticeable decrease in spasm intensity (Table 1). All patients recover orbicularis oculi neuromuscular function over time, with a mean duration of beneficial effect of 12.9 weeks. Of the 6.7% of patients who do not experience improvement, the majority show only sporadic poor response. It is not uncommon for a patient to show little or no benefit from one treatment session, only to experience adequate response with subsequent injections. Some patients do not achieve control of spasms with the usual dose of 12.5 to 25 U per eye but respond to higher doses in the range of 30 to 75 U. A small percentage of patients in whom treatment fails will show an initial beneficial response to toxin therapy over five or more sets of injections, but then gradually experience decreasing effect with further treatments. We have observed

Table 1 Response Rate and Duration of Orbicularis Oculi Neuromuscular Inhibition with Botulinum Toxin in the Treatment of Blepharospasm

Author and reference	No. of patients	No. of treatments	Response rate (%)	Duration of effect (weeks)	Toxin dose (U)
Lingua (10)	13	29	100	12	15.5
Scott (12)	39	124	—	9.9	20
Shorr (35)	22	57	—	6.1–12.3	12.5
Elston (26)	34	89	97	11	12.5
Frueh (13)	48	116	94	12	6.25–25
Savino (37)	15	20	100	12.2	12.5
Burns (36)	44	—	—	—	—
Cohen (2)	75	224	86	12.4	12.5
Perman (28)	28	56	96	12	25
Shore (29)	26	41	96	8.5	12.5–25
Gonnering (30)	15	41	100	15.6	12.5
Kristan (38)	12	20	100	14.8	20–45
Engstrom (3)	76	220	95	16.7	20
Mauriello (8)	100	372	97	12.6–17.3	12.5
Dutton (5)	232	1044	97	13.3	12.5–25
Kalra (16)	106	381	99	—	5–25
Elston (6)	101	404	77	9	10
Saraux (44)	32	32	—	24	—
Carruthers (9)	58	114	100	12–16	12.5
Ruusuvaara (31)	62	138	89	5.9	25–30
Biglan (40)	105	350	—	18–26	25–30
Kraft (1)	76	248	87	14.1	20–25
Taylor (7)	365	1418	98–100	14.4	15–30
Grandas (4)	151	151	75	10	—
Elston (32)	307	—	75	12–15	4
Thill (33)	18	36	100	6	10
Arthurs (42)	27	50	90	8–11	—
Roggenkämper (34)	55	55	98	7.5	—
Totals	2242	5830	93.3	12.9	

this phenomenon in about 1.5–2.0% of our patients. The etiology of this response pattern remains uncertain. Another small group of patients (about 2%) may be considered true nonresponders and will not experience any relief of spasms with BTX at any reasonable dose. For all of these treatment failures, surgical myectomy, either radical or limited, may be necessary.

Despite the desired effect of BTX in the control of involuntary spasms, restriction of denervation to the target muscles of clinical interest cannot always be specifically obtained. Adjacent muscles may occasionally be affected. Although weakness of the target muscle into which the toxin is directly injected persists for 3 to 4 months before recovery of function, the peripheral effect on nearby muscles is usually of much shorter duration, typically 1 to 4 weeks.

The chemodenervating mechanism of BTX on adjacent muscle groups is responsible for many of the acute local side effects reported in nearly every large study (Table 2). These are usually considered "complications," although more properly some are expected and acceptable consequences of treatment. The exact incidence of these side effects is difficult to ascertain, since many reports mention only the most common ones. It is not clear in most cases whether other effects did not occur at all or were not specifically noted, since in many cases patients are not examined again until after the recovery of

Table 2 Side Effects of Botulinum Toxin in the Treatment of Blepharospasm

Side effect	References	Number reported (total N = 5830)	Overall incidence (% of 5830)	Observed range (%)
Ptosis	1,2,4–10,12,13,16,27, 29,30,31,32,34–36,38, 40,42,43	715	12.3	0–52.3
Keratitis	7,13,16,35,40,41,43	243	4.3	0–46.2
Epiphora	1,2,5,7,8,16,37,43	205	3.5	0–20.0
Dry eyes	1,5,8,12	145	2.5	0–18.2
Diplopia	1,2,5–9,12,13,16,31, 34,40,44	122	2.1	0–17.2
Lid edema	5,6,43	96	1.6	0–30.4
Facial weakness	4,5,7,16,31,43,50	53	0.9	0–4.6
Lagophthalmos	2,35,37,40	3	0.5	0–63.6
Ecchymosis	4,5,34,35,40,42	18	0.3	0–9.0
Entropion/ectropion	2,4,5,8,13,37,40	16	0.3	0–6.7
Local pain	4,5,38	14	0.2	0–100
Blurred vision	16,37	10	0.2	0–2.1
Facial numbness	5,43	6	0.1	0–4.0
Hematoma	5	3	0.05	0–0.05
Pruritus	5	3	0.05	0–0.3
Weakness	5,50	3	0.05	0–5.9
Dysphagia	37,44	3	0.05	0–3.4
Nausea	5,50	2	0.03	0–5.9
Brow droop	16,37	2	0.03	0–0.7
Headache	44	1	0.02	0–0.3
Dysphonia	4	1	0.02	0.–0.7
Totals		1665	28.6	0–100

orbicularis oculi function. Our experience includes data on more than 400 patients who received over 4300 treatment sessions over a 9-year interval. A review of the published literature has provided data on 2242 patients, and 5830 treatments. The percentages given below indicate the minimum incidence based on all reported patients taken together, as well as the maximum incidence seen in selected reports.

Ptosis

Clinically, the most important side effects of BTX are related to the anatomy of the eyelids and face. The orbicularis oculi muscle is part of a thin sheet of striated muscle fibers that lies just beneath the skin of the face and neck. Around the eyelids, the orbicularis oculi is less than 1 mm in thickness, and it runs circumferentially within the mobile portion of the lid and around the bony orbital rim as far as the brow and temple hair line. Immediately below the muscle is a loose areolar connective tissue layer, the post-orbicular fascial plane, that allows easy diffusion of fluid. Within the mobile portion of the eyelid, just posterior to this fascial plane, is the orbital septum. This is a thin membrane that anatomically and physiologically separates the eyelid proper from the orbital compartment. The orbital septum is a critical layer that normally resists the posterior diffusion of blood and edema. In elderly persons the septum may be attenuated and therefore provide less of a barrier. Also, inadvertent penetration of the septum during toxin injection can result in posterior deposition of drug and weakness or paralysis of the levator muscle. This is a common cause of ptosis as a complication of BTX used for blepharospasm.

Ptosis is seen in 12.3% (range 0–52.3%) of treatments with BTX for blepharospasm (1,4,6,27,30,35,37). It is now well established that the degree of ptosis, as well as the incidence, is related to the toxin dose. Dutton and Buckley (5) reported an incidence of 6.4% with doses of 12.5 to 25 U per eyelid. This rose to 13.3% for doses of 30 to 70 U. A similar finding was reported by Carruthers and Stubbs (9). In the hands of inexperienced resident physicians, the incidence of ptosis was 40% (5). Also, the levator muscle seems to be more sensitive to the effects of BTX, since the superior rectus muscle is rarely, if ever, affected simultaneously with the levator, despite the fact that these two muscles lie in apposition to each other. Placement of toxin into the central upper eyelid is also associated with a higher occurrence of ptosis (9).

Some patients experience ptosis as a frequent side effect, on nearly every injection, despite careful selection of the site. Others never have this complication, even after 25 to 30 injections. It seems probable that the sensitivity of the levator to peripheral effects of toxin varies considerably among patients. In those who experience ptosis more frequently, the dose should be minimal in the upper lid, and the injection sites should be as far medial and lateral as possible. It may be necessary to avoid injections in the upper lid altogether. Limiting toxin to the brow may provide adequate orbicularis denervation. However,this usually requires higher doses, which may be associated with a significant incidence of ptosis (35). The role of antitoxin in limiting the undesirable local side effects of BTX shows some promise and is currently under further investigation (39).

Diplopia

Orbital contamination by BTX can also cause ocular motility disturbance, most commonly affecting the inferior oblique muscle. The latter lies immediately inside the inferior orbital rim, just behind the orbital septum, and is therefore vulnerable to local effects of toxin injected deep into the midportion of the lower eyelid. Symptomatic diplopia occurs in 2.1% of treatments (range 0–17.2%) (4,5,7,9,40). Frueh and Musch (13) showed a significantly higher incidence of diplopia with increasing dose of toxin, from 6.3% at 6.2 U per eyelid up to 50% at 25 U per lid. As with ptosis, the occurrence of diplopia may be higher (20%) when toxin is injected by inexperienced workers, presumably because of deep placement of toxin behind the orbital septum (5). Recovery of extraocular motility usually occurs after 1 to 6 weeks.

Lower Facial Weakness

Below the eyelids, striated fibers are divided into a number of functional groups and form a series of distinct muscles for facial expression. They lie above the fibrofatty layer known as the temporoparietal fascia (SMAS). Between the SMAS and the facial muscles is a relatively loose connective tissue layer that allows easy dissection of edema and blood from the eyelids to the lower face. This situation is seen frequently following eyelid surgery. The injection of BTX into this layer allows the drug to diffuse downward under the influence of gravity, resulting in weakness of the lower face and mouth. Although this is usually only of minor consequence, marked mouth droop and drooling may rarely be seen. The overall incidence of this complication is about 0.9% (range 0–4.6%) when the toxin is administered around the orbicularis oculi muscle alone. When injections are given into the middle and lower face for hemifacial spasm or oromandibular dystonia, the incidence climbs to about 12% (5). This complication can be minimized by restricting injections to the brow and eyelids. When control is needed in the middle and lower face, no more than 1 U should be injected at each site, and this should be directly into the muscle to avoid unnecessary diffusion.

Dry Eyes and Epiphora

Dry eyes and epiphora are common side effects of BTX treatment for blepharospasm, undoubtedly underreported in the literature. Most treated patients will show an impaired blink due to orbicularis oculi muscle weakness. This results in some degree of lagophthalmos, with a reported incidence as high as 63.6% (35). Increased surface evaporation causes inferior corneal exposure and symptoms of dry eyes. Frank superficial punctate keratopathy may be seen in 4.3% (range 0–46.2%) of cases (7,40,41). Symptoms include burning, scratchiness, and photophobia. Most patients do not complain of these symptoms when they are minimal, unless specifically questioned. The reported incidence of symptomatic dry eyes is 2.5% (range 0–18.2%). In our experience, dry eyes were the most common side effect mentioned by patients (7.5%) (5). All patients should be placed on artificial tears routinely during toxin treatment. Reflex lacrimation, combined with an impaired lacrimal pump mechanism from loss of lower eyelid tone, may cause epiphora, even in the presence of a normal lacrimal drainage system. Epiphora has been noted in 3.5% (range 0–20.0%) of treatments (2,5,7,8,16,35). Again, the true incidence is probably higher.

Entropion and Ectropion

Malpositions of the lower eyelid generally result from laxity of lower eyelid support structures, most notably the lateral canthal tendon. Such malpositions are an unusual complication of toxin therapy and probably relate to preexisting involutional horizontal eyelid laxity and redundancy of the lower eyelid retractors. Botulinum toxin wakening of the orbicularis oculi muscle may potentiate these anatomical abnormalities in predisposed patients by reducing or eliminating anterior lamellar tone (15). The overall incidence of these malpositions is 0.3% (range 0–6.7%) (4,5,8,37). In such patients the mechanical corneal irritation may be more bothersome than the spasms, and it is best here to avoid toxin injections into the lower eyelid.

Pain and Local Bruising

Local discomfort is not reported in most studies, but was noted in 100% of injections by Kristan and Stasior (38). It is likely that all but the most stoic patients experience some minimal discomfort, but since this is expected from any percutaneous injection by both the patient and the physician, it is rarely reported as a side effect. However, significant local pain was seen in about 0.2% of treatments (4,5) and is probably related more to technique and individual patient pain threshold.

Ecchymosis and hematoma formation relate to injection technique and are more common in patients with telangiectasia or friable blood vessels, or those taking medications that predispose to easy bruising, such as steroids or aspirin. The overall incidence is less than 0.3% (range 0–9.0%) (4,5,35,40,42). The true incidence is probably higher, since most workers do not consider small ecchymoses a complication. These usually resolve without sequelae within 1 to 2 weeks.

Eyelid edema lasting for several days to a week after toxin injection has been reported by some patients. Although the overall incidence is about 1.6%, Elston (6) reported this in nearly a third of his patients. As with ecchymoses, a minimal occurrence of eyelid edema is likely to go unmentioned by the patient and unnoticed by the physician unless the patient is carefully examined.

Rare Local Effects of Botulinum Toxin for Blepharospasm

In addition to the above side effects, a number of unusual local complications have been reported. The relationship to toxin injection is not always established. Facial numbness in the distribution of the infraorbital nerve (maxillary division of the trigeminal) has been reported in two separate series (5,43). Dutton and Buckley (5) suggested mechanical injury or compression due to local injection near the infraorbital foramen to explain this phenomenon.

Brow ptosis is common among elderly patients as a result of involutional loss of forehead fascial attachments. In predisposed persons, further weakening of the frontalis muscle with BTX may result in a manifest brow droop (16,37). As with some other complications, this is probably not often recognized by the examiner, so that its true incidence remains uncertain. In most cases, however, it is of little clinical consequence unless associated with significant eyelid ptosis and loss of superior visual field.

Blurred vision associated with toxin injection has been mentioned in several reports (16,44), and I have had patients with similar complaints. In most cases this results from corneal exposure and an irregular tear film. In patients who experience significant epiphora, the increased lacrimal tear lake may cause blurring in downgaze during reading. Kalra and Magoon (16) listed 8 patients (2.6%) who experienced "focusing problems," but the nature of this complication was not further discussed. Biglan et al. (40) reported two patients with unexplained accommodative insufficiency following toxin injection to the orbicularis oculi muscle. Pupillary dilation and poor reaction to both light and accommodation are frequent sequelae of botulism in humans (45), and toxic effects on the ciliary ganglion have been seen following retrobulbar injection of BTX in rabbits (46). However, Elston (47) found no evidence of pupillary involvement after orbital injection of BTX toxin for strabismus, nor did Helveston and Pogrebniak (48) in the treatment of nystagmus. Levy et al. (49) have shown immediate mydriasis and supersensitivity denervation of the ciliary ganglion at doses of 0.5 ng in the rat. It is possible that posterior injection of BTX behind the orbital septum may result in subtle accommodative dysfunction in some patients.

ACUTE DISTANT EFFECTS OF BOTULINUM TOXIN FOR BLEPHAROSPASM

Acute effects occurring some distance from the site of BTX injection within 1 to 5 days of treatment have been reported in an increasing number of patients. The exact relationship to this drug remains open to speculation in many cases, but repeated episodes of these phenomena in the same patients make some causal relationship likely. Nausea has been seen in 0.1% to 5.9% of cases in several series following local injection of toxin (4,5,50). Overall, however, this is exceedingly rare, occurring in fewer than 0.03% of all treatments. Generalized pruritus was reported by Dutton and Buckley (5) in 0.3% of their large series ($\frac{3}{1044}$ treatments) and has also been noted in patients receiving toxin for spastic dysphonia (51) and torticollis (52). In none of these cases was pruritus associated with a rash.

A flu-like syndrome occasionally is reported by patients within several days of toxin administration. Although it is difficult to establish a firm relationship with treatment, in several cases this complaint has been associated with repeated injections. Drowsiness, fatigue, and malaise have been reported following toxin therapy for blepharospasm, and in several series for torticollis these were seen in 10% to 20% of treatments (53–55). Many elderly patients with blepharospasm may also be taking other drugs that interfere with neuromuscular transmission, such as antibiotics, cardiovascular drugs, and psychotropics (56), and these drugs can themselves produce a myasthenia-like syndrome. The potentiating effect of BTX on these drugs remains unknown.

Grandas et al. (4) reported one case of dysphonia and two occurrences of dysphagia following toxin therapy for blepharospasm. Several other authors have reported dysphagia following the usual small eyelid doses (37,44). Saraux (44) also reported another patient who experienced respiratory difficulties and cyanosis requiring hospitalization, which was attributed to BTX injection for blepharospasm. Stell et al. (53) reported two patients with vocal cord paralysis following injection of toxin into the sternocleidomastoid muscle. They felt that this could not be explained by local diffusion.

CHRONIC LOCAL EFFECTS OF BOTULINUM TOXIN FOR BLEPHAROSPASM

The long-term local effects of BTX remain unknown. It was originally hoped that repeated injections would result in some degree of muscle atrophy so that more permanent control could be obtained. Experimental studies have shown muscular atrophy following loss of the normal neurotrophic influence of nerve on muscle in botulism (57), and the changes seen are the same as those associated with surgical denervation of muscle. However, in the clinical use of BTX all reports have shown recovery of neuromuscular function over several months, and the symptom-free interval between repeat injections does not increase with multiple injections (5).

Wojno et al. (58) histologically examined orbicularis oculi muscle in one patient after six repeated injections of BTX over a 1-year interval. They demonstrated fatty and fibrotic degeneration of individual muscle fibers and areas of muscle atrophy. These changes were attributed to the toxin and not to aging phenomena in this patient. However, the majority of the muscle sample was histologically normal. Similar alterations in response to BTX were reported in experimental studies (59). In a more recent report, Adams and Dilly (60) examined the levator muscle in a patient treated with toxin to induce a protective ptosis. They found abnormal and thrombosed blood vessels, perivascular lymphocytic cuffing, evidence of regenerating necrotic muscle, and injury to both axons and myelin sheaths. However, it seems more likely that most, if not all, of these changes were the result of ischemia from a complicating carotid-cavernous fistula.

Although significant toxin-induced changes in the orbicularis oculi muscle have not been documented, it is unclear what effect may be seen with very long-term use of this treatment modality over many years.

CHRONIC DISTANT EFFECTS OF BOTULINUM TOXIN FOR BLEPHAROSPASM

The chronic effects of BTX distant from the site of injection are more difficult to establish, and reports have been isolated and largely unsubstantiated. Certainly the most potentially significant effect is generalized weakness reported in 0.06% of all treatments for blepharospasm. In the two series noting this complication, the incidence was 0.2% and 2.0% (4,5). Generalized weakness or severe tiredness has also been reported following toxin administration for torticollis, with an incidence as high as 5–20% (53,54). Sanders et al. (61) reported abnormal neuromuscular transmission in arm muscles of four patients following periocular injection of 12.5 U around each eye for blepharospasm. The pattern of decreasing jitter with increasing firing rate supported BTX as the causative agent. Although none of these patients demonstrated clinical weakness of muscles remote from the eyelids, the authors raised the concern of a possible additive effect with repeated toxin administration. Similar findings were reported by Olney et al. (52) with higher doses of toxin (280 U) for torticollis. Lange et al. (63) reported abnormal jitter measurements in arm muscles persisting at least 4 months in patients receiving over 245 U of toxin for torticollis and oromandibular dystonia, but no abnormalities in patients receiving 100 U or less.

We have observed one patient who received 15 toxin injections at a dose of 25 U per eye over a 4-year period and who reported generalized weakness following the last four sets of injections. Single-fiber electromyographic studies demonstrated increased jitter and blocking, with a slight increase in fiber density in all tested muscle groups including the frontalis, extensor digitorum communis, and anterior tibialis muscles, consistent with repeated exposure to BTX. Over a period of 2 years without further treatment, mild abnormalities persisted in all muscle groups despite some interval improvement with further increase in fiber densities, suggesting reinnervation. Using ^{125}I-labeled BTX, Wiegand et al. (64) suggested that, in addition to hematogenous spread of toxin to other nerve endings, intraspinal transfer of BTX toxin may occur by movement with axonal flow in the cat's peripheral nervous system. Although such distant manifestations in humans are only rarely seen clinically, the potential long-term effects of chronic toxin use in susceptible patients remain to be determined.

Botulinum toxin is a potent neurotoxin that is capable of inducing humoral antibodies in humans. The formation of such antibodies in blepharospasm patients undergoing toxin therapy has been a matter of some concern. Frueh et al. (41) reported that response to toxin treatment decreased with increasing number of injections. They speculated that antibodies could account for this observation. I have observed a small subset of our patients (about 2.0%) who initially show excellent response to toxin, but after 10 to 15 injections obtain decreasing effectiveness, in some cases falling to no response. Biglan et al. (65) tested 28 patients who had received multiple doses of toxin as high as 50 U per injection and could find no detectable antibody. Such antibodies have been detected in patients receiving multiple injections in excess of 300 U per session for torticollis. It is generally believed that the usual doses employed for the treatment of blepharospasm are below the threshold for inducing antibodies. However, there are now several anecdotal reports of antibody formation at doses below 50 to 75 U. Whether this will become more of a problem with prolonged administration of the drug remains to be determined.

REFERENCES

1. Kraft SP, Lang AE. Botulinum toxin injections in the treatment of blepharospasm, hemifacial spasm, and eyelid fasciculations. Can J Neurol Sci 1988;15:276–280.
2. Cohen DA, Savino PJ, Stern MB, Hurtig HI. Botulinum injection therapy for blepharospasm: a review and report of 75 patients. Clin Neuropharmacol 1986;9:415–429.
3. Engstrom PF, Arnoult JB, Mazlow ML, et al. Effectiveness of botulinum toxin therapy for essential blepharospasm. Ophthalmology 1987;94:971–975.
4. Grandas F, Elston J, Quinn N, Marsden CD. Blepharospasm: a review of 264 patients. J Neurol Neurosurg Psychiatry 1988;51:767–772.
5. Dutton JJ, Buckley EG. Long-term results and complications of botulinum A toxin in the treatment of blepharospasm. Ophthalmology 1988;95:1529–1534.
6. Elston JS. Long-term results of treatment of idiopathic blepharospasm with botulinum toxin injections. Br J Ophthalmol 1987;71:664–668.
7. Taylor JDN, Kraft SP, Kazdan MS, et al. Treatment of blepharospasm and hemifacial spasm with botulinum A toxin: a Canadian multicentre study. Can J Ophthalmol 1991;26:133–138.
8. Mauriello JA Jr, Coniaris H, Haupt EJ. Use of botulinum toxin in the treatment of one hundred patients with facial dyskinesias. Ophthalmology 1987;94:976–979.
9. Carruthers J, Stubbs HA. Botulinum toxin for benign essential blepharospasm, hemifacial spasm and age-related lower eyelid entropion. Can J Neurol Sci 1987;14:42–45.
10. Lingua RW. Sequelae of botulinum toxin injection. Am J Ophthalmol 1985;100:305–307.
11. Adams GG, Kirkness CM, Lee JP. Botulinum toxin A induced protective ptosis. Eye 1987;1:603–608.
12. Scott AB, Kennedy RA, Stubbs HA. Botulinum toxin injection as a treatment for blepharospasm. Arch Ophthalmol 1985;103:347–350.
13. Frueh BR, Musch DC. Treatment of facial spasm with botulinum toxin: an interim report. Ophthalmology 1986;93:917–923.
14. Dutton JJ, Buckley EG. Botulinum toxin in the management of blepharospasm. Arch Neurol 1986;43:380–382.
15. Patrinely JR, Whiting AS, Anderson RL. Local side effects of botulinum toxin injections. In: Jankovic J, Tolosa E, eds. Advances in neurology. Vol. 49. New York: Raven Press, 1988:493–500.

16. Kalra HK, Magoon EH. Side effects of the use of botulinum toxin for treatment of benign essential blepharospasm and hemifacial spasm. Ophthalm Surg 1990;21:335–338.

17. American Academy of Ophthalmology: Botulinum toxin therapy of eye muscle disorders. Safety and effectiveness. Ophthalmology (Instrument and Book Issue), 1989:37–41.

18. Gundersen CB. The effects of E toxin on the synthesis, storage and release of acetylcholine. Prog Neurobiol 1980;14:99–119.

19. Simpson LL. Molecular pharmacology of botulinum toxin and tetanus toxin. Annu Rev Pharmacol Toxicol 1986;26:427–453.

20. Black JD, Dolly JO. Interaction of ^{125}I-labeled botulinum neurotoxins with nerve terminals. I. Ultrastructural autoradiographic localization and quantitation of distinct membrane acceptors for types A and B on motor nerves. J Cell Biol 1986;103:521–534.

21. Black JD, Dolly JO. Interaction of ^{125}I-labeled botulinum neurotoxins with nerve terminals. II. Autoradiographic evidence for its uptake into motor nerves by acceptor-mediated endocytosis. J Cell Biol 1986;103:535–544.

22. Duchen LW, Strich SJ. The effects of botulinum toxin on the pattern of innervation of skeletal muscle in the mouse. Q J Exp Physiol 1968;53:84–89.

23. Angaut PD, Molgo J, Comella JX, et al. Terminal sprouting in mouse neuromuscular junctions poisoned with botulinum type A toxin: morphological and electrophysiological features. Neuroscience 1990;37:799–808.

24. Diaz J, Molgo J, Pecot-Dechavassine M. Sprouting of frog motor nerve terminals after long-term paralysis by botulinum type A toxin. Neurosci Lett 1989;96:127–132.

25. Holds JB, Alderson K, Fogg, SG, Anderson RL. Motor nerve sprouting in human orbicularis muscle following botulinum A injection. Invest Ophthalmol Vis Res 1990;31:964–967.

26. Elston JS, Russell RWR. Effect of treatment with botulinum toxin on neurogenic blepharospasm. Br Med J (Clin Res) 1985;290:1857–1859.

27. Dutton JJ. Treatment of hemifacial spasm and essential blepharospasm with botulinum toxin. In: Wilkins RH, Rengachary SS, eds. Neurosurgery update I. Diagnosis, operative technique, and neuro-oncology. New York: McGraw-Hill, 1990:138–141.

28. Perman KI, Bayliss HI, Rosenbaum AL, et al. The use of botulinum toxin in the medical management of benign essential blepharospasm. Ophthalmology 1986;93:1–3.

29. Shore JW, Leone CR Jr, O'Connor PS, et al. Botulinum toxin for the treatment of essential blepharospasm. Ophthalm Surg 1986;17:747–753.

30. Gonnering RS. Treatment of hemifacial spasm with botulinum A toxin: results and rationale. Ophthalm Plast Reconstr Surg 1986;2:143–146.

31. Ruusuvaara P, Setälä K. Long-term treatment of involuntary facial spasms using botulinum toxin. Acta Ophthalmol 1990;68:331–338.

32. Elston JS. Botulinum toxin A in clinical medicine. J Physiol (Paris) 1990;84:285–289.

33. Thill R, Költringer P, Reisecker F, et al. Botulinum Toxin A in der Therapie von kraniozervikalen Dystonien und Hemispasmus facialis. Acta Medica Austriaca 1991;18:125–129.

34. Roggenkämper P.Blepharospasmus-Behandlung mit Botulinus-Toxin (Verlaufsbeobachtungen). Klin Mbl Augenheilk 1986;189:283–285.

35. Shorr N, Seiff SR, Kopelman J. The use of botulinum toxin in blepharospasm. Am J Ophthalmol 1985;99:542–546.

36. Burns CL, Gammon JA, Gemmill MC. Ptosis associated with botulinum toxin treatment of strabismus and blepharospasm. Ophthalmology 1986;93:1621–1627.

37. Savino PJ, Sergott RC, Bosley TM, et al. Hemifacial spasm treated with botulinum toxin injection. Arch Ophthalmol 1985;103:1305–1306.

38. Kristan RW, Stasior OG. Treatment of blepharospasm with high dose brow injection of botulinum toxin. Ophthalm Plast Reconstr Surg 1987;3:25–27.

39. Scott AB. Antitoxin reduces botulinum side effects. Eye 1988;2:29–32.

40. Biglan AW, May M, Bowers RA. Management of facial spasms with Clostridium botulinum toxin, type A (Oculinum). Arch Otolaryngol Head Neck Surg 1988;114:1407–1412.

41. Frueh BR, Felt DP, Wojno TH, Musch DC. Treatment of blepharospasm with botulinum toxin. A preliminary report. Arch Ophthalmol 1984;102:1464–1468.

42. Arthurs B, Flanders M, Codère F, et al. Treatment of blepharospasm with medication, surgery and type A botulinum toxin. Can J Ophthalmol 1987;22:24–28.

43. Ruusuvaara P, Setälä K. Use of botulinum toxin in blepharospasm and other facial spasms. Acta Ophthalmol 1987;65:313–319.

44. Saraux H: Traitement des blépharospasmes et des hémispasmes faciaux par injection de toxine botulique. J Fr Ophthalmol 1988;11:237–240.

45. Tyler HR. Physiological observations in human botulism. Arch Neurol 1963;9:661.

46. Kupfer C. Selective block of synaptic transmission in ciliary ganglion by type A botulinum toxin in rabbits. Proc Soc Exp Biol Med 1979;99:474–483.

47. Elston JS. The use of botulinum toxin A in the treatment of strabismus. Trans Ophthalmol Soc UK 1985;104:208–210.

48. Helveston EM, Pogrebniak AE. Treatment of acquired nystagmus with botulinum A toxin. Am J Ophthalmol 1988;106:584–586.

49. Levy Y, Kremer I, Shavit S, Korczyn AD. The pupillary effects of retrobulbar injection of botulinum toxin A (Oculinum) in albino rats. Invest Ophthalmol 1991;32:122–125.

50. Yoshimura DM, Aminoff MJ, Olney RK. Botulinum toxin therapy for limb dystonias. Neurology 1992,42:627–630.

51. Brin MF, Blitzer A, Fahn S, et al. Adductor laryngeal dystonia (spastic dysphonia): treatment with local injections of botulinum toxin (Botox). Mov Disord 1989;4:287–296.

52. Lorenz IT, Subramanaian SS, Yiannikas C. Treatment of idiopathic spasmodic torticollis with botulinum toxin A: a double-blind study on twenty-three patients. Mov Disord 1991;6:145–150.

53. Stell R, Thompson PD, Marsden CD. Botulinum toxin in spasmodic torticollis. J Neurol Neurosurg Psychiatry 1988;51:920–923.

54. Gelb DJ, Lowenstein DH, Aminoff MJ. Controlled trial of botulinum toxin injections in the treatment of spasmodic torticollis. Neurology 1989;39:80–84.

55. Greene P, Fahn S, Brin M, et al. Double-blind, placebo-controlled trial of botulinum toxin injections for the treatment of spasmodic torticollis. Neurology 1990;40:1213–1218.

56. Argov Z. Disorders of neuromuscular transmission caused by drugs. N Engl J Med 1979;301:409–413.

57. Lewis GE. Biomedical aspects of botulism. New York: Academic Press, 1981:81–91.

58. Wojno T, Campbell P, Wright J. Orbicularis muscle pathology after botulinum toxin injection. Ophthalm Plast Recontr Surg 1986;2:71–74.

59. Drachman AB. Atrophy of skeletal muscle in chick embryos treated with botulinum toxin. Science 1964;145:719–721.

60. Adams GGW, Dilly PN. Pathological changes in levator palpebrae superioris muscle treated with botulinum toxin in a case of carotid-cavernous fistula. Br J Ophthalmol 191;75:181–184.

61. Sanders DB, Massey EW, Buckley EG. Botulinum toxin for blepharospasm: single-fiber EMG studies. Neurology 1986;36:545–547.

62. Olney RK, Aminoff MJ, Gelb DJ, Lowenstein DH. Neuromuscular effects distant from the site of botulinum neurotoxin injection.Neurology 1988;38:1780–1783.

63. Lange DJ, Brin MF, Warner CL, et al. Distant effects of local injection of botulinum toxin. Muscle Nerve 1987;10:552–555.

64. Wiegand H, Erdmann G, Wellhöner HH. ^{125}I-labeled botulinum A neurotoxin: pharmacokinetics in cats after intramuscular injection. Naunyn-Schmiedebergs Arch Pharmacol 1976;292:161–165.

65. Biglan AW, Gonnering R, Lockhart LB, et al. Absence of antibody production in patients treated with botulinum A toxin. Am J Ophthalmol 1986;101:232–235.

15

Clinical Assessments of Patients with Cervical Dystonia

Earl S. Consky
Toronto, Ontario, Canada

Anthony E. Lang
The Toronto Hospital and University of Toronto, Toronto, Ontario, Canada

INTRODUCTION

Cervical dystonia (CD) is the commonest focal dystonia (1). It is also one of the most underrecognized movement disorders (2). Botulinum toxin (BTX) injection therapy is now the most reliably effective symptomatic treatment of cervical dystonia (3–5). Accurate characterization of the dystonic movements, including the determination of which neck muscles most actively contribute to the abnormal head position, is critical in assessing the response to therapy, guiding the ongoing management of patients, and helping to clarify remaining methodological treatment issues. In this chapter a number of clinical features that are important to recognize in evaluating a patient with CD are first reviewed, and the various methods that have been used to assess and quantitate the severity of CD are then examined.

CLINICAL FEATURES OF CERVICAL DYSTONIA

The Spectrum of Dystonic Head Movements

The clinical spectrum of involuntary movements or abnormal postures of the head and neck produced by cervical dystonia is remarkably varied in terms of the rhythmicity, speed, amplitude, duration, and direction of the dystonic movements. Patients with cervical dystonia may exhibit irregular, arrhythmic, "spasmodic" rapid clonic jerks with less rapid recovery phases toward the neutral position, slow rhythmic deviations, sustained (tonic) movements with maintenance of the terminal posture for seconds to minutes, or permanent fixed postural deformities. Superimposed on the large-amplitude movements may be smaller-amplitude, higher-frequency horizontal, vertical, or mixed tremulous oscillations (tremor). Deviations may occur in any single plane or combination of directions in which the head may voluntarily move. Rotational torticollis (turning) rotates the nose and chin around the longitudinal axis toward the shoulder. Laterocollis (tilting) bends the head laterally in the coronal plane, moving the ear toward the ipsilateral shoulder. Anterocollis (forward flexion) deviates the chin downward in the sagittal plane toward the chest, while retrocollis (extension) produces upward excursion of the chin. Sagittal or lateral deviation of the base of the neck from the midline (shift) may be evident, usually with associated axial deformity (kyphoscoliosis). Anterior sagittal shift deviates the chin forward rather than downward, and posterior sagittal shift is a backward displacement of the head in the horizontal plane without upward deviation of the chin. Sagittal shift and anterocollis (or retrocollis) are not mutually exclusive, but differentiation may be difficult when they are concurrently present. Lateral shift involves horizontal displacement of the head in the absence of downward tilting of the ear toward the ipsilateral shoulder unless accompanied by laterocollis which, when present, is usually in the opposite direction. Intermittent or sustained elevation or anterior displacement of the shoulder, most commonly ipsilateral to the direction of the turn or tilt, is commonly seen.

The relative frequency of occurrence of each of these subtypes of cervical dystonia has been evaluated recently in five separate Movement Disorder Clinic studies describing cohorts of CD totaling 966 patients (6–10). The commonest type of deviation in each study was torticollis, with some degree of rotation noted in 82% (7) to 97% (6) of patients. Rotation was characterized as the dominant deviation in 72% (9). Isolated "pure" rotational torticollis was present, however, in only 19% (6) to 37% (8) of patients. In the series of 199 patients reported by Rondot et al. (8), approximately 37% of CD patients exhibited "simple" torticollis, while 22% had torticollis combined with laterocollis, 17.5% torticollis with retrocollis, and 16% torticollis in combination with both laterocollis and retrocollis. While earlier reports (11–13) have suggested a preponderant laterality of turn to the left, three of the above cited series (6–8) noted no definite predilection for either side, and the leftward/rightward rotation ratios of the two others—1.5:1 (9) and 1.3:1 (10)—were not statistically significant.

Laterocollis was the second most common deviation type observed, occurring in 42% (7) to 74% (10) and as the predominant deviation in 18% (9). Pure laterocollis was rare, noted in only 2% (6) to 3.8% (8) of CD patients. In nearly 85% (8) of patients exhibiting some degree of laterocollis, it occurred in combination with rotational torticollis plus or minus retrocollis. Combined laterocollis and rotational torticollis occurs in either an "ipsilateral pattern," in which the turn of the chin and the tilt of the ear are directed toward the same shoulder, or in a "contralateral pattern," in which turn and tilt are in opposite directions.

Retrocollis occurred in 24% (10) to 38% (8) of patients and was predominant in 10% (9), but it rarely occurred in isolation: 1% (6,8). Anterocollis was documented in 11% (10) to 25% (7). Pure anterocollis was never observed in these studies. Lateral shifting of the head was noted in 10% (10) to 21% (6) and sagittal shift in 9% (10) to 21% (6) (19% with anterior displacement, 2% with posterior). Jankovic et al. (7) noted scoliosis in 39% of cervical dystonia patients. Elevation or anterior displacement of the shoulder was noted in 54% (7) to 76% (6). Concomitant head tremor was present in 28% (6) to 60% (7). "Spasmodic" features (head jerks and spasms) were noted in 62% of patients in one series (6). As noted by Jankovic et al. (7) and Chan et al. (6), the traditional designation "spasmodic torticollis" is an inaccurate descriptor, since many patients may have neither simple rotation nor spasmodic movements. They have advocated the generic term "cervical dystonia" as a more accurate designation that recognizes this condition as a form of dystonia with several subtypes.

Diagnostic Features

Diagnostic evaluation of patients with abnormal head movements or postures requires a determination of (1) whether the observed deviations represent dystonia, nondystonic torticollis, or another type of hyperkinetic dyskinesia; (2) whether the dystonia is localized to the neck region or is a component of a segmental or generalized pattern of distribution; (3) whether the etiology of the cervical dystonia is idiopathic or symptomatic; and (4) whether other associated movement disorders (e.g., postural tremor), other neurological deficits (e.g., dysphagia), or secondary complications of cervical dystonia (e.g., cervical spondylosis) are present.

In addition to the typical head deviations,the presence of several other characteristic clinical features, such as sensory tricks, morning benefit, common exacerbating factors, neck pain or extranuchal dystonia and muscle hypertrophy and tenderness on palpitation, is often diagnostically helpful.

Sensory Tricks

The transient correction of head position with the use of sensory tricks (gestes antagonistiques) (11) is a unique pathognomonic feature of CD. Patients with CD almost universally develop a repertoire of maneuvers such as touching various locations on the face, neck, or head (either ipsilateral or contralateral to the direction of deviation) with the hand or an object such as a pencil or eyeglasses. In our cohort of 80 CD patients participating in a factorial clinical trial (14), touching the face and holding the back of the head were the most common sensory tricks, each occurring in approximately 85% of patients, while holding the chin occurred in 65%, leaning against a high-back chair in 65%, holding or pulling the hair in 15%, placing something in the mouth in 8%, and a variety of other tricks in 20% of patients (10). Complete or partial suppression of neck muscle electromyographic (EMG) activity, including both phasic or tonic patterns and tremor bursts, during the application of a sensory trick has been documented (9). Suppression was noted more commonly in rotational torticollis and less frequently in cases of retrocollis, laterocollis, or complex patterns of deviation regardless of the severity or duration of the dystonia. The mechanism by which these tactile or altered proprioceptive inputs (15,16) temporarily alleviates the dystonic movements is unknown, but the reported concurrent reductions in EMG activity are not supportive of the suggestion that correction is due to simple counterpressure (17). While the efficacy of sensory tricks varies considerably among patients and may wane over time, the frequency of their use by patients who find them effective usually reflects severity and may decrease significantly following successful BTX treatments (10).

Exacerbating Factors

As occurs in other forms of dystonia and other movement disorders, the severity of CD may be affected by a number of aggravating factors including fatigue, emotional stress, observation, and specific motor tasks such as driving, writing, or walking and by ameliorating factors such as relaxation and recumbency. Jankovic et al. (7) noted worsening of symptoms with stress in 68% of their CD patients, with activity in 35%, and with fatigue in 23%. Clinical assessment of CD patients should therefore include a number of exacerbating maneuvers such as repetitive arm movement and walking as well as observation while the patient is supine.

Morning Benefit

Early in their course, particularly, patients may experience ''morning benefit,'' an absence or reduction of symptoms after awakening, lasting minutes to hours. At entry,

33% of the 80 patients we studied were currently experiencing morning benefit, 13% had previous but not current morning benefit, and 54% had never experienced morning benefit (10). Morning benefit may occasionally return or occur for longer periods following BTX injections.

Pain

In CD, unlike other movement disorders, including most other forms of dystonia, pain is a frequent and prominent feature that often contributes significantly to disability. Duane (18) noted that pain was not a frequent early feature in his CD patients but that it may become more prominent after the first year of symptoms. In contrast, approximately 40% of our 80 patients recalled some degree of discomfort at the onset of their symptoms, and 15% considered it a major early feature of their condition (10). Nearly 85% had pain at some point over the course of their illness, and approximately two-thirds considered pain a major but not the sole source of their disability. Patients with constant as opposed to intermittent head turning, greater severity of head turning, and forceful, sustained contractions (spasm) more frequently experience marked pain (6). Pain may be localized to the posterior triangle region, the trapezius and posterior-cervical muscles ipsilateral to the turn or tilt, or the mastoid insertion of the sternocleidomastoid, but occasionally it may be diffuse. "Radicular" pain has been reported in 5% (18) to 31% (7) of CD patients. Premature cervical degenerative joint disease secondary to recurrent abnormal neck movements and asymmetric postures may contribute to deep cervical pain and the restriction of range of motion (18). While some patients may develop a radiculopathy or exhibit mechanical features to suggest a nonmuscular source of pain, the cause of neck pain in many patients is multifactorial, and distinctions may be difficult.

Extranuchal Dystonia

At least one-third of patients with CD have evidence of extranuchal dystonia (7,11,18–23), particularly segmental cranial (blepharospasm and oromandibular dystonia), brachial (writer's cramp) and axial (trunk dystonia). Jankovic (7) noted dystonic involvement of the oral region in 16%, involvement of facial muscles in 12%, mandibular involvement in 12%, blepharospasm in 10%, involvement of the arm or hand in 10%, and laryngeal involvement in 7% of his 300 patients. Fourteen percent of his patients reported onset of dystonia initially elsewhere before the neck was affected. Jahanshahi et al. (23) reported progression of dystonia to extranuchal sites in 32% of 72 patients with adult-onset idiopathic CD, most commonly to the arm (17%), hand (writer's cramp) (7%), and oral mandibular region (11%).

Other Neurological Deficits

Riski et al. (24) found swallowing abnormalities in 22 of 43 patients not treated with BTX. Delayed initiation of the swallowing reflex and the presence of vallecular residue were the commonest abnormalities. Swallowing disturbances were present in patients who did not have subjective complaints. A neurogenic etiology for dysphagia appeared to be more frequent than postural or mechanical dysphagia in these patients. Comella et al. (25) noted radiological evidence of peristaltic abnormalities in 22% and clinical symptoms of dysphagia in 11% of 18 CD patients before BTX injections. Preexisting dysphagia did not appear to constitute an increased risk factor for an exacerbation of dysphagia following BTX injections in this cohort. The results of these two studies, however, indicate the need for careful inquiry regarding swallowing function in CD patients.

Secondary complications of CD include cervical spondylosis with radiculopathy and rarely myelopathy. Occasionally patients develop a compressive ulnar neuropathy secondary to repeated use of the limb in performing sensory tricks. Reactive depression may occur, but numerous studies have failed to document a higher incidence of preexisting psychiatric disorders in CD (20,26).

Disability

The term "impairment" denotes an anatomical, physiological, or psychological abnormality that can be objectively determined (e.g., a restricted range of cervical movement) (27). A "functional limitation" is the restriction or lack, as a result of the impairment, of ability to perform a task or activity in a manner considered normal for the person (e.g., difficulty looking over a shoulder while driving) (27). "Disability" is task-specified and can be defined as a behavioral response to functional limitations resulting in prevention of the performance of usual activities, assumption of usual obligations, and fulfillment of the normal role of the affected person (e.g., inability to drive a car (27). Disability in CD patients is common and may vary from minimal incapacity to "exceeding adverse effects on the life and happiness" of many patients (20). Rondot et al. (8) noted at least some degree of "social consequences" in 99% of CD patients, ranging from mild ("subjective feeling of discomfort in social conditions without objective consequences on social life") in 40% and moderate ("subjective feeling of discomfort leading to modification of the qualitative aspects of social life but without lessening of the occupational level") in 42% to severe ("both qualitative and quantitative modification of the occupational level with resulting impairment of social life") in 17%. A wide variation in the perception of the social consequences of CD among patients with approximately equivalent severity was noted.

Variation in disability secondary to CD relates in part to its task-specific nature. Specific actions or tasks such as walking, writing, or use of the hands commonly aggravate the torsional movements limiting the patient in tasks at work, in recreation, and in activities of daily living. Patients commonly employ compensatory strategies including sensory tricks as well as sitting or lying in specific positions while carrying out certain functions to limit interference by the head movements.

The degree of disability experienced by an individual patient may vary not only with the severity of the dystonic movements and associated pain, which is often a significant contributing factor, but also with the psychosocial response of the patient to the impairment (embarrassment, coping strategies) and the response by others such as family members, friends, and employers to the functional limitations (28).

DIFFERENTIAL DIAGNOSIS OF CERVICAL DYSTONIA

Symptomatic Cervical Dystonia

With the exception of neuroleptic-induced tardive dystonia and psychogenic and possible trauma-related cases, a symptomatic cause for adult-onset CD is rare (29,30). Wilson's disease was not present in any of Duane's (18) more than 1000 CD cases, and intracranial neoplasms were found in only two of his patients. Other rarely reported symptomatic cases include head trauma with basal ganglia damage (30–33), arteriovenous malformations (31), central nervous system lupus (34), perinatal asphyxia (35), and possible microvascular compression of the spinal accessory nerve (36,37). Podivinsky (38) suggested that most cases of CD were postencephalitic, but this contention has never been confirmed.

Tardive dystonia secondary to antecedent neuroleptic use most frequently affects cranial and cervical muscles (39,40). Neuroleptic exposure within 3 months of the onset of CD was reported in 6% of cases in Jankovic's survey (7). Our experience as well as that of others (40) indicates an unexpectedly high incidence of retrocollis in patients with tardive cervical dystonia.Severe isolated anterocollis has been reported to occur disproportionately in patients with pathologically proven multiple system atrophy (41–42).

Patients with CD are frequently advised that their symptoms are secondary to stress or an emotional disorder. Psychogenic dystonia, however, is uncommon (43,44). It may be suggested by findings of false weakness, false sensory complaints, multiple somatizations, obvious psychiatric disturbances, inconsistency of dystonic movements and postures, and relief or exacerbation with suggestion, psychotherapy, or placebo (45). The absence of muscle hypertrophy and the lack of use of sensory tricks may be additional features consistent with a psychogenic etiology.

Preceding peripheral injury as a cause of dystonia is controversial, but the association of neck or head trauma with CD has been noted in 9% (6,46) to 11% (7) of patients. Whether trauma represents a specific cause or a nonspecific trigger in an otherwise predisposed person remains undetermined (46–51).

Nondystonic Torticollis

A variety of orthopedic, neurological, neuro-ophthalmologic, infectious, and congenital abnormalities may cause abnormal head postures (52,53), simulating torticollis (Table 1) (54). Mechanical causes may be distinguishable by their persistence during sleep, their unresponsiveness to sensory tricks and typical exacerbating factors, and the lack of appropriate muscle hypertrophy. Lesions of the spine, craniovertebral junction, spinal cord, or posterior fossa may have additional findings on neurological examination. In children without evidence of dystonia elsewhere, a congenital muscular abnormality or infectious cause of acute ''wry neck'' should be sought.

Other Hyperkinetic Movement Disorders

Motor tics may include simple random head jerks or complex head shaking but are rarely continual, can be temporarily suppressed, and are often associated with the subjective urge to perform the movements. Sensory tricks and muscle hypertrophy are rarely present, and neck pain is not as common or as prominent as in CD. Tics and dystonia may coexist (55–57), but it is not clear whether this concurrence is more common than expected by chance. Myoclonic jerks may be repetitive or rhythmic but are usually not twisting. The designation ''myoclonic dystonia'' has been advocated to characterize the shock-like jerks seen in some patients (58), but this feature is not uncommon in typical CD, and the term may lead to confusion with the inherited syndrome of alcohol-sensitive myoclonus and dystonia in which myoclonus is present in extranuchal areas (59,60). Choreic movements can be distinguished from dystonic head movements by the lack of repetitive twisting, pain, and response to sensory tricks.

Tremor frequently occurs in patients with CD. Distinguishing coexistent ''postural head tremor'' (similar to that of essential tremor) from ''dystonic head tremor'' at times is difficult, particularly in cases in which head tremor is the presenting symptom without prominent head deviation (61). Jankovic et al. (7) noted head tremor in 60% of patients

Table 1   Disorders Simulating Cervical Dystonia

1. ''Orthopedic''
    A.   Rotational atlantoaxial subluxation
    B.   Ligamentous absence, laxity, or injury
    C.   Herniated cervical disk
    D.   Klippel-Feil syndrome
    E.   Acquired bony abnormalities (degenerative, infectious, neoplastic)
2. ''Neurological''
    A.   Posterior fossa tumor
    B.   Syringomyelia with spinal cord tumor
    C.   Arnold-Chiari malformation
    D.   Focal seizures
    E.   Bobble-head doll syndrome (with third ventricle cyst)
    F.   Extraocular muscle palsies, strabismus
    G.   Head thrusts with oculomotor apraxia
    H.   Hemianopia
    I.   Congenital nystagmus
    J.   Spasmus nutans
3. Miscellaneous
    A.   Hiatus hernia in childhood (Sandifer's syndrome)
    B.   Congenital muscular lesions (trauma, hemorrhage, tumor)
    C.   Abnormal posture in utero
    D.   Local factors (e.g., adenitis) producing ''acute wry neck''
    E.   Paroxysmal torticollis in infancy
    F.   Acute infectious torticollis
    G.   Labyrinthine disease

Source: Ref. 54.

with CD dystonia and classified the tremor as ''dystonic'' in 37%, ''essential'' in 30%, and combined ''dystonic/essential'' in 8%. Dystonic tremor is often less rhythmic and may show a directional preponderance, with increased amplitude when the head is voluntarily deviated opposite to the direction in which the head is being pulled involuntarily, and may show a dampening when the head is allowed to deviate fully. Coexistent postural head tremor is usually continuous and independent of the head position relative to the direction of deviation, with similar amplitude in both the neutral and the deviated posture. The presence of associated postural tremor of the extremities may not assist in this differentiation, since between 23% (6) and 87% (62) of patients with CD have evidence of at least mild coexisting essential-like tremor of the upper extremities. Rivest and Marsden (61) have suggested that head tremor may represent an isolated presenting feature of CD. In such cases the tremor tends to occur more often in the horizontal plane, as opposed to the more common involvement of the vertical plane in typical essential head tremor. Other characteristics of isolated dystonic head tremor are its greater irregularity, responsiveness to sensory tricks, and potential benefit from anticholinergic medications (61).

EXAMINATION OF THE PATIENT WITH CERVICAL DYSTONIA

A diagnosis of CD is often apparent before formal physical examination. Clinical methods, however, may clarify the components of the dystonic movements, especially in patients with complex patterns, provide evidence of secondary complications, and help exclude a symptomatic cause.

In complex deviations one component is often dominant. Exacerbating maneuvers such as walking, alternating repetitive movements of the upper extremities, or observation while the patient is writing may help clarify the dominant subtype and the minor components. On occasion patients with chaotic or bidirectional movements may require prolonged observation. Darkening the room or asking the patient to close his or her eyes, relax, and allow the head to deviate maximally at times may promote the emergence of the dominant direction of movement. Assessing the speed of side-to-side excursions may also be instructive, as the fast component tends to be dystonic and the slower recovery phase in the opposite direction compensatory (63).

Occasionally patients will utilize compensatory movements in overcoming the forceful dystonic posturing, and these must be distinguished from involuntary deviations. Tilting the head in the direction opposite to that of a dystonic rotation or depressing the head downward to initiate a return to the primary position are in this case compensatory rather than primary components of the CD. Patients with lateral shift may exhibit a contralateral compensatory tilt to maintain a midline position. Patients with anterior sagittal shift may similarly compensate by extension, and patients with retrocollis by an anterior shift or flexion of the thorax to maintain the head in a horizontal position.

Examination of the range of active movement may supplement the clinical impression of direction of deviation. Limitations are usually in the direction opposite to the involuntary pull. Difficulty in passively reducing the deviation may be indicative of a mechanical component such as contractures or cervical spondylosis, which may develop in long-standing cases.

Distinction between dystonic and postural head tremors, as previously discussed, may be made by observation of the amplitude and regularity of the tremor with the head held in the primary, fully deviated, and extreme contralateral positions.

The characterization of the deviation provides a basis for the identification of specific muscles contributing to the abnormal movement. While there are 27 pairs of muscles in the neck, only six pairs are easily identifiable on clinical examination (64). Rotation is usually produced primarily by the contralateral sternocleidomastoid, ipsilateral splenius capitis, and ipsilateral trapezius muscles. Any or all of the ipsilateral splenius, trapezius, levator scapulae, scalenus medius, and sternocleidomastoid may contribute to laterocollis. Anterocollis may be produced by bilateral activation of the sternocleidomastoid, scalene, and submental muscles as well as inaccessible prevertebral flexors. Bilateral splenius, trapezius, and paraspinal muscle activation results in retrocollis. (See chapter 16 for a review of the anatomy and physiology of the neck.) While the involvement of a particular muscle may be suggested by the nature of the deviation, confirmation of this impression requires the presence of muscle hypertrophy, evidence of contraction or spasm on palpation or EMG recording, or muscle tenderness. Asymmetry in muscle size is more accurately assessed by comparing pairs of muscles with the head held in the midposition and at full excursion in the plane in which the particular muscles are usually most active.

The character of deviation may occasionally change following BTX injection, possibly as a result of recruitment of additional neck muscles (65) or the unmasking of components of deviation originally present but compensated for by involuntarily opposing dystonic antagonist muscles. Consequently reduction in these forces following BTX toxin may release a new deviation vector.

Investigations

There is no laboratory test for dystonia. Diagnosis is based on clinical assessment. In patients with a compatible history and without atypical features on examination, the likelihood of finding a symptomatic etiology for cervical dystonia is remote. Even routine investigations in this situation are usually unrevealing. Therefore, in an adult with typical CD we do not recommend a standard battery of blood tests, and adequate imaging is often limited by the extent of the abnormal head movements. More extensive investigations are indicated in patients with childhood or juvenile-onset, atypical presentations or unusual clinical features (29).

CERVICAL DYSTONIA RATING SCALES

Evaluating the efficacy of therapy, especially BTX injections, in reducing the symptoms of CD requires accurate quantitative assessment of the severity of dystonic movements, associated pain, and functional disability. While treatment with BTX has been recognized as a safe and effective therapy for CD, currently there is no consensus regarding several methodological issues. Treatment protocols differ considerably in several respects including the dose per muscle and total dose per treatment session, the distribution of the dose within a given muscle (location and number of injection sites), and the utilization of EMG control of injections. Progress in clarifying these issues and in defining other effective therapies will require reliable and valid CD rating instruments that accurately document changes in severity following treatment. In addition to their value in clinical trials, practical subjective and objective rating scales may be useful as a supplement to global clinical impressions and video recording in the ongoing management of individual patients, in which injection parameters may require adjustment from treatment to treatment to optimize benefit and minimize side effects.

The utility of a rating scale depends on its ease of use; its *reliability*, the extent to which it yields reproducible results; and its *validity*, the extent to which it accurately measures what it is designed to measure. Validity is in part dependent on the extent to which a scale includes all relevant dimensions of the condition being assessed and the degree to which it represents them in reasonably weighted proportions (content validity) and the extent to which the scale is responsive in identifying actual change in clinical status (convergent validity) (66,67). Ideally, torticollis rating scales should encompass the heterogeneity and variability of the clinical features of CD described previously and include an assessment not only of the magnitude of dystonic movements but also of functional limitations and pain. In addition, a quality of life assessment (e.g., the Sickness Impact Profile) should also be considered for patients with CD. To date, none of the rating scales to be reviewed below has included this assessment approach.

Early attempts to evaluate objectively the severity of cervical dystonia include Swash et al.'s (68) use of randomized film segments taken before, during, and after treatment with tetrabenazine showing patients at rest, during walking, and during performance of a simple manual task. Blinded observers ranked the sequences as "least severe" and "most severe." Bernhardt et al. (69) assessed the duration of dystonic movements by using a horizontal grid placed over a videotape monitor to determine the percentage of time during a 10-minute session for which a subject's nose (presumably with retrocollis) deviated above a horizontal line. Couch (62) described a simple clinical rating scale in which he designated severity as absent (0), mild (1), moderate (2), severe (3), and very severe and incapacitating (4) and frequency as absent (0); occasional (1); intermittent, occurring less than 50% of the time (2); intermittent, occurring 50–80% of the time (3); and continuous (4). In this and other similar scales, criterion definitions of the ordinal designations "mild", "moderate," and "severe" are not specified and are therefore highly subjective. Tolosa (70), in addition to designating severity as "absent", "mild," "moderate," or "severe" while lying and sitting, asked patients with CD to hold their heads in a midline position and recorded the time to the initial deviation and to reach the original maximum deviation. The time maintained in a midline position as a singular index of severity is of limited utility because of variability and difficulty with timing accuracy, especially in patients with superimposed tremor and jerky head movements. These early attempts at objectively estimating severity appear somewhat crude, but components of these scales may be found in currently used objective and subjective rating scales.

The Fahn and Marsden Rating Scale for Torsion Dystonia

Fahn and Marsden (71) developed a quantitative rating instrument for the primary torsion dystonias composed of movement and disability subscales. The movement scale score is the sum of the weighted products of a severity factor (0–4) for each of nine body regions multiplied by a provoking factor score (0–4) that rates the circumstances in which the dystonia is evident (specific use of the specified area, regional action, overflow secondary to action of some other area of the body, and at rest). The disability scale includes the patient's subjective impairment in a variety of activities of daily living including speech, handwriting, feeding, eating, hygiene, dressing, and walking. Reliability and validity testing of the Fahn and Marsden scale demonstrated a high degree of both intra-rater and inter-rater reliability and validity (72). While extremely useful for the assessment of generalized torsion dystonia, this scale is significantly less sensitive to changes in focal dystonia and, therefore, far less useful for assessing the severity of CD in clinical trials.

Torticollis Rating Scale of Lang et al.

Lang, Sheehy, and Marsden (73) developed a separate CD scale for a trial of parenteral anticholinergics in adult-onset dystonia. This scale was subsequently refined by Lang (74). The degrees of turn and tilt (0 = 0, 1 = 1–15°, 2 = 16–30°, 3 = 31–45°, 4 = 46–60°, 5 = 61–75°, and 6 = 76–90°) are added to the sagittal deviation (0 = absent, 1 = mild, 2 = moderate, and 3 = severe). A total score is obtained by multiplying this deviation scale by a severity factor score in which 0 = none; 1 = occasional deviation only; 2 = mild, deviation present 45% of the time; 3 = moderate, excursion to maximal deviation present 50% of the time *or* deviation present most of the time but excursions largely submaximal; and 4 = severe, excursions to maximal deviation present 75–100% of the time. In addition to this product, the time (mean of two trials) to a maximum of 60 seconds that the patient is able to hold the head fixed (to the first twitch) in the central position is also measured. No validity testing has been performed on this scale, and it was subsequently altered and expanded to form the TWSTRS Severity Scale described below.

The Columbia Torticollis Rating Scale

Fahn (75) later developed a specific scale for the assessment of torticollis. This composite scale consists of torticollis rating and disability scales. The torticollis scale documents the direction of movement, the circumstances when the head deviation is present, the duration of deviation while sitting, the range of active movement, the excursion amplitude, the duration and severity of pain while sitting, the degree of reduction in deviation with the use of sensory tricks, the average frequency, duration and severity of forceful spasms, the presence of tremor and gross jerking movements of the head, and the presence of "essential tremor" of the hands. Dystonia elsewhere in the body is rated, but does not contribute to the total score. The disability scale (functional capacities or CAP scale) assesses limitation of functional activities such as driving, reading, watching television, going out to movies, shopping, walking about, feeding, falling asleep, and performance of housework or outside work.

Formal reliability and validity testing of the Columbia Torticollis Scale has not been undertaken. The value of this complex, detailed scale for descriptive clinical assessment was demonstrated in Chan, Brin, and Fahn's recent study defining the clinical characteristics of a large cohort of CD patients (6). Its utility, however, in clinical trials is less clear. The scale was employed by the Columbia investigators in a double-blind, controlled trial of BTX for CD (76). Blinded observers, however, rated videotapes made using a standardized protocol only with respect to head turning at rest, the number of degrees of head turning while walking, the maximum degree of volitional range of movement opposite to the direction of dystonic deviation, and the number of seconds that the patient's head could be maintained straight ahead. There was good inter-rater reliability for the degree of head turning at rest and while walking and for the maximum amplitude of rotation opposite to the direction of torticollis. The duration of time in the midline was poorly reproducible and was excluded from the analysis. Additional subjective scales were employed, including the patient's global assessment of improvement (RES scale: $+3$ = markedly improved, very happy with results; $+2$ = moderately improved, happy with results; $+1$ = slightly improved but not significantly; 0 = no change; -1 = slightly worse, but not significantly; -2 = definitely worse) and a PAIN scale (0–100, 0 representing no difference in pain following the injections and 100 representing complete relief). The functional capacity scale of the Columbia Rating Scale (CAP scale) was rated by an unblinded physician at each visit. A significant change in the RES, PAIN, and CAP scales was documented after treatment. The reduction in the CAP scale scores, however, was not statistically significant when the Bonferoni correction for multiple tests was applied. Component and total Columbia Torticollis Rating Scale scores are not included in the report of this study. Some scale items require specific patient inquiry and therefore could not be ascertained by blinded videotape raters. "Live" rater scores were not included because of the double-blind study design. The overall complexity of this scale was probably an additional factor limiting its use in this study. The responsiveness of the scale to change in severity following treatment is undetermined. To date, the scale has not been employed in other published therapeutic trials in cervical dystonia.

The Tsui Rating Scale

The objective Torticollis Rating Scale developed by Tsui and colleagues (77) for the first double-blind trial of BTX published has been widely used by other investigators in subsequent clinical trials. This scale evaluates the amplitude and duration of both sustained and spasmodic (tremulous) movements and the presence of shoulder elevation (Table 2).

The inter-rater reliability testing of two blinded videotape raters using the clinical scoring protocol for 88 observations showed a correlation coefficient of $r = 0.86$. A

Table 2 Tsui Torticollis Rating Scale

A. Amplitude of sustained movements (0–9):
    Rotation (0 = absent, 1 = < 15°, 2 = 15–30°, 3 = > 30°)
    Tilt (0 = absent, 1 = < 15°, 2 = 15–30°, 3 = > 30°)
    Ante/retro (0 = absent, 1 = mild, 2 = moderate, 3 = severe)
    Combined = score A
B. Duration of sustained movements (0–2):
    1 = intermittent, 2 = constant
C. Shoulder elevation (0–3):
    0 = absent, 1 = mild and intermittent, 2 = mild and constant,
    or severe and intermittent, 3 = severe and constant
D. Head tremor (0–4):
    Severity (1 = mild, 2 = severe)
    Duration (1 = occasional, 2 = continuous)
    Severity × duration = score D
Total torticollis score = [A × B] + C + D (0–25)

---

formal assessment of validity was not performed. While changes in post injection clinical scores from their preinjection baseline in patients receiving BTX were statistically significant by Wilcoxon's signed rank test and were not significant after placebo, Gelb's (78) reanalysis of the original Tsui data found no statistically significant difference comparing each individual patient's postplacebo and post-BTX scores in this crossover-design study. In their clinical trial, Gelb et al. (78) were unable to demonstrate objective benefit using the Tsui scale, despite significant improvement on composite subjective scales for severity of head movements (0–10) and pain (0–10) following treatment. While these investigators noted a strong inter-rater correlation ($r = 0.87$) for two independent blinded video raters, there was a large degree of scatter between scores of the video raters for any individual patient, typically ranging from three to four points, as well as considerable scatter between direct examination scores and video scores in magnitudes equivalent to or greater than the typical overall reduction of the total scale scores following treatment considered indicative criteria for "substantial" improvement.

Several other investigators have found applying the Tsui scale problematic. Stell et al. (79) used the Tsui scale for clinical examination but did not use this scale for their blinded videotape assessments. Blackie and Lees (80) noted poor correlation between videotape scorers ($r = 0.64$) and with patients' subjective symptoms, and they did not use the scale in the final analysis of their double-blind study. Moore and Blumhardt (81) reported better correlation between video observers ($r = 0.87$) but noted a scattering of scores as high as six points. They also noted poorer intra-observer reliability ($r = 0.64$) comparing the live clinical ratings and videotape ratings performed at different times by the same individual rater. Lorentz et al. (82) were able to document improvement of two points or greater on the Tsui scale in 20 of 23 patients by "live" examination but in only 14 of these 23 patients on video assessment. Poewe et al. (83) were, however, able to document a 50% reduction in Tsui scale score in 32 of 37 patients following their first BTX treatment, but this was with unblinded assessment.

Some of the difficulties illustrated by these studies using the Tsui scale are related in part to the inherent difficulty of measuring the severity of CD because of its variability secondary to emotional stress, fatigue, and activity and in part to particular difficulties encountered in the assessment of videotape recordings. As noted by Marsden and Schacter

(71), video provides only a brief two-dimensional visual image of the patient in which ambiguities may be difficult to resolve without prolonged observation and the performance of a variety of exacerbating tasks that may be used during an individualized live clinical assessment. In addition, however, there are inherent limitations in the Tsui Rating Scale related to generic problems of all rating scales and to the coarseness and lack of criterion definition of the ordinal scores using the "mild", "moderate," and "severe" designations. Measurement of sustained movement amplitudes are extremely difficult because of variation from moment to moment. Maximal excursions may be sustained for only a short duration, and submaximal deviations may be otherwise constantly evident. In addition, the duration of different components of complex deviations may vary considerably. Specification of the maximum observed amplitude and duration of the dominant deviation may reduce variation in scores. The multiplicative transformation of amplitude times duration amplifies the imprecision of these indices. The coarseness of the amplitude scores for rotation may additionally result in underestimation of change following treatment, since patients may improve from 90° of turn to 31° without a reduction in overall score. The inclusion of a tremor component that is unclearly defined and may include unsustained spasmodic jerky deviations, tremulous movements, dystonic head tremor, or coexisting postural head tremor is problematic. Finally, the scale lacks an assessment of associated disability. Despite these limitations, the Tsui scale has substantially contributed to many of the assessments of the efficacy of BTX that are detailed elsewhere in this volume.

Jankovic's Rating Scales

Jankovic has developed a number of practical scales derived from an original Hyperkinesia Rating Scale (84) for assessing severity of CD and response to BTX injections (85). These scales include a severity scale that is determined by the clinical observer and can also be self-rated by the patient on a regular basis following treatment. This ordinal severity scale (0–4) consists of the following designations: 0 = no spasm or movement; 1 = mild, barely noticeable spasms; 2 = moderate, but without functional impairment; 3 = moderate spasm or movement with moderate functional impairment; 4 = severe, incapacitating spasm or movement. The maximum benefit following treatment ("peak effect") is also rated on a 0 to 4 scale, where 0 = no effect; 1 = mild improvement, but no improvement in function; 2 = moderate improvement, but no change in function; 3 = moderate improvement in severity and function; 4 = marked improvement in severity and function. A "global rating" score as a measure of overall response is calculated from the "peak effect" score by subtracting one point for a mild complication associated with the injections and two points for severe or disabling complications. Benefit was defined as a "global rating" score greater than or equal to 2. Initial use of these scales in a double-blind study (86) did not show significant change following BTX injections, but this may have been the result of dose and design limitations. Subsequent open-label trials demonstrated significant change in "peak effect" and "global rating" scores following treatment (85).

These ordinal scales provide an overall subjective impression of severity and functional improvement. They do not specifically include an assessment of pain, and no objective assessments of the magnitude or duration of head deviations are included. These scales may be particularly useful in clinical practice for following the progress of individual patients. They also supplement objective clinical assessment, which, by its nature, may represent only a brief period of observation in an artificial environment and may therefore not always provide an accurate appraisal of the actual response to treatment.

The Toronto Western Spasmodic Torticollis Rating Scale (TWSTRS)

The Toronto Western Spasmodic Torticollis Rating Scale (TWSTRS, pronounced "twisters") (87) was developed for use in a factorial clinical trial comparing differing BTX treatment regimens (14). This is a composite scale with subscales for clinical severity, disability, and pain (see Appendix A).

The Severity Scale is scored on the basis of standardized clinical examination and videotape protocols. The maximum amplitude of excursion (A) (sustained or unsustained) is determined for all subtypes of head deviation: rotational (0–4), lateral (0–3), anterocollis or retrocollis (0–3), and lateral and sagittal shift (0–1). The maximal excursion is determined after activating and distracting manoeuvers, walking and sitting, with the patient asked to allow the head to deviate fully without resistance. Criteria for demarcation of scale grades were defined as clearly as possible.

The duration factor (B) (0–5) for the dominant deviation is estimated through the course of the standardized examination, excluding the period when the patient is specifically asked to allow the head to deviate maximally. To account for variability, the duration factor assesses first the proportion of time there is any deviation from a neutral position and second, the proportion of time that the head deviation is most often maximal or submaximal in amplitude. We chose to use an additive duration factor which was arbitrarily weighted $\times$ 2 rather than a product of amplitude and duration to avoid amplification of imprecise indices as noted previously.

The effect of sensory tricks (C) (0–2), shoulder displacement (D) (0–3), the range of motion (E) (0–4) without the aid of sensory tricks, and the average time (F) (0–4) the patient is able to maintain the head within 10° of a neutral position on two attempts with active resistance but without the use of sensory tricks are also quantitated. The total Severity Scale score is obtained from the sum of all component scores.

The Disability Scale of the TWSTRS comprises a broadly based assessment of performance of daily activities that may be affected by CD, developed in part from the functional capacities component of the Columbia scale. General as well as specific categories are assayed, including work performance (job or domestic), activities of daily living (feeding, dressing, hygiene), driving, reading, television viewing, and leisure activities outside the home. The extent to which social embarrassment rather than head deviation or pain specifically contributes to limitation of activities was initially included as an inverse item but was deleted in later versions of the scale.

The TWSTRS Pain Scale consists of a dimensional severity score (0–10) for the patient's usual, best, and worst pain as well as a duration component and an assessment of the contribution of pain to disability. The pain severity score was added to a later version of TWSTRS after the initial reliability and validity testing was completed.

We examined the reliability of the TWSTRS scales by analyzing the interobserver agreement using the intraclass correlation coefficient (ICC) based on a mixed-effects linear model with a random rater effect. This provides a measure of agreement sensitive to both random and systematic error. The Severity Scale was initially elevated on 12 untreated CD patients. A standardized videotape (see Appendix B) for each patient was scored by four independent raters. The ICCs for each component and for the whole scale were determined. The ICC for the Disability/Pain Scale score was determined from the

Table 3 TWSTRS Inter-rater Reliability

	ICC[a]
1. Severity Scale (3 video raters—26 of 40 patients)	0.79
2. Severity Scale change in score post Botox (3 video raters—26 of 40 pts)	0.85
3. Disability/Pain Scales—Pre Botox (4 raters—11 pts)	0.74
4. Severity Scale (3 video raters vs. direct observer scores—20 pts)	0.71

[a] < 0 = poor; 0–0.2 = slight; 0.2–0.4 = fair; 0.4–0.6 = moderate; 0.6–0.8 = substantial; 0.8–1.0 = almost perfect.
TWSTRS = Toronto Western Spasmodic Torticollis Rating Scale; ICC = intraclass correlation coefficient.

scores of 11 patients obtained by three independent interviewers and, in addition, patient self-rating. The reliability and validity of the scales for detecting change in severity was assessed by determining the ICCs for the change in the score of three independent "blinded" observers scoring standardized, random-order videotapes of 20 patients made before and 6 weeks after BTX injections, as well as the score changes of a direct ("live") examiner. The ICC for the scores from videotape raters versus the direct observer was also determined. The validity of the scales was determined by calculation of Pearson correlation coefficients comparing changes in severity scores from videotape raters and the direct observers with the patients' self-reported overall "percent improvement" and changes in disability and pain scores following treatment. The results of the inter-rater reliability and validity assessments are shown in Tables 3 and 4.

The intraclass correlation coefficients for both videotape analysis of severity and interview scores for disability and pain showed substantial agreement between raters. Reliability of most but not all subcomponents as well as the scale as a whole was demonstrated for both single determinations and for changes in scores after treatment. The degree of reliability reflects the extent to which scale grades are clearly defined as well as the familiarity of the individual raters with the scoring system. Our initial validity testing did not assess intra-observer reliability because of the potential for significant recall bias (from repeated rating of the same videotape after a short interval) resulting in an overestimation of reliability.

The responsiveness of TWSTRS to changes in torticollis severity (convergent validity) is demonstrated by the magnitude of the correlation coefficient between objectively

Table 4 TWSTRS Validity Assessment

			Pearson correlation coefficients
1. Change in total severity score of 3 videotape raters	and	Patient perception of overall improvement	0.68
2. Change in total severity score of direct observer	and	Patient perception of overall improvement	0.61
3. Change in total severity score of 3 videotape raters	and	Change in disability and pain scores	0.65

TWSTRS = Toronto Western Spasmodic Torticollis Rating Scale.

documented changes in videotape-rater severity scores and direct-observer scores, and patients' perception of "percent improvement" as well as changes in disability and pain scores following BTX injections. The changes in severity scores were therefore more reflective of actual changes in clinical status than of observer differences. In addition, the substantial correlation between scores of the three "blinded" videotape raters and the direct observer indicates the utility of the TWSTRS videotape protocol.

The TWSTRS obviates several of the problems described in the discussion of previous rating scales, specifically the absence of disability assessment, the lack of validity in inter-rater reliability testing, and questionable correlation with change in disease severity. Further data-driven refinement and testing of the TWSTRS is ongoing, but initial experience with this scale by our group and others (88,89) suggests its potential usefulness for assessing clinical severity and associated pain and functional disability of CD in clinical trials. As a supplement to TWSTRS, we have also developed a subjective observer-rated response scale, which is provided in Appendix C.

SUPPLEMENTARY ASSESSMENT METHODS

Instrumental Methods

A number of instrumental methods for measuring the severity of head deviation have been developed but at present are not widely used. Ansari and Webster (90) devised a method for quantitative measurements of head rotation and head tremor in patients with CD using a pointer affixed to a headband that pointed to a rotary scale attached to a stand placed behind the patient's head. The frequency and amplitude of head tremor were measured with a piezoelectric transducer. A major limitation of this and other methods of "objectively" measuring head position is the requirement that the patient remain seated in a chair, although many patients find that the deviation is maximal only with activity such as walking. In addition, it is also possible that the elaborate headband device could alter the severity of deviations in a fashion similar to sensory tricks. Schatz and Urist (91), using a protractor attached to a curved plate that rested on the head, were able to quantitate separately rotation of the head in any of the three axes, vertical, anterior-posterior, or transverse, in patients with ocular torticollis. More recently, van Hoof et al. (92) measured the deflection of the head in the horizontal, sagittal, and coronal planes by means of a protractor that did not touch the patient's head but required maintenance of a seated position. Lye, Roots, and Rogers (93,94) developed a computer graphics method in which videotape recordings of patients with CD were digitized and the movement of a reference marker placed on the patient's nose was tracked along the horizontal and vertical axes. Shann et al. (95) used an overhead television camera to track a light-emitting diode attached to a hat as a reference marker. The video signal was converted through a computer to calculate displacement, velocity, and acceleration of head movements. Most recently, Dykstra et al (96) tested a three-dimensional cervical range of motion system (EMROM) that employs an electromagnetic tracking system with a headpiece sensor and a chest harness source unit. This device provides information on range of motion but is confounded by the effects of cervical jerks or tremor and must be used in a seated position.

None of the currently available instrumental methods are entirely satisfactory because of constraints that do not allow measurement during ambulation, when a patient's head movements may be most active, but future technological developments may provide useful adjunctive measurements to complement clinical ratings scales.

Pain Scales

A variety of instruments designed to measure clinical pain have been developed and tested, and several may be potentially adaptable to therapeutic trials for CD or for clinical practice.

Simple verbal descriptor scales consist of ranked ordinal descriptions such as 1 = none, 2 = slight, 3 = mild, 4 = moderate, and 5 = severe (97). While relatively easy to complete, this type of scale assesses only the intensity dimension of pain and is highly subjective.

Visual analogue scales (VAS) are one of the most frequently used methods for measuring pain (98). The "absolute" VAS consists of a straight line, usually 10 cm in length, representing a continuum of pain intensity,with verbal descriptions defining each end in terms of the extreme limits of pain ("no pain" and "pain as bad as you have ever experienced"). The distance from the zero-pain end to a mark placed along the line is measured as an index of severity. Change in pain intensity is calculated as the difference between the pre- and posttreatment measures. The "comparative" VAS directly assesses change in pain intensity by measuring the distance marked by the patient along a line from a midpoint designated "unchanged" toward either end defined in terms of degree of pain relief ("less severe" and "more severe"). Reliability testing of the various visual analogue scales has yielded contradictory data (98). Some patients find the measure too abstract and confusing, and CD patients with high-amplitude or chaotic head deviations may experience physical difficulty marking the line. In addition, the scale is unidimensional, estimating pain intensity only.

The McGill pain questionnaire (MPQ) (99) is a multidimensional instrument for the measurement of clinical pain consisting of a determination of the location of pain, an evaluation of sensory, affective, and evaluative qualities of the pain, an assessment of the change in pain over time, and an evaluation of intensity using a 1–5 scale corresponding to "mild," "discomforting," "distressing," "horrible," and "excruciating." Reliability and validity testing of the MPQ has indicated its usefulness in assessing both the physical and the emotional response to therapeutic interventions for pain. Its limitations include its relative complexity and the time (15–30 min) required for completion. The Dartmouth pain questionnaire (100) has been developed as an adjunct to the MPQ and includes measures of impaired functioning, remaining positive aspects of function, and changes in self-esteem.

While components of several complementary indices may be potentially useful, further assessment of the suitability of these established scales for assessing pain in CD is required.

Quality-of-Life Assessment

There is increasing interest in evaluating the impact of various movement disorders on quality of life. A review of the scales designed to measure this feature is beyond the scope of this chapter; however, brief mention will be made of possibly the best-known tool utilized in assessing quality of life, the Sickness Impact Profile (SIP). This is a broadly applicable behaviorally based measure of perceived health status designed to detect changes in health status over time (101). It consists of 136 statements concerning health-related dysfunction in 12 areas of daily activities, including sleep and rest, eating, work, home management, recreation and pastimes, ambulation, mobility, body care and movement, social interaction, alertness behavior, emotional behavior, and communication.

Reliability and various components of validity have been demonstrated through extensive testing (101).

To date, correlative testing of existing CD disability scales (TWSTRS Disability Scale and the Columbia CAP scale) with the SIP has not been undertaken. The SIP may potentially provide a sensitive index of the impact of CD on "quality of life."

CONCLUSIONS

The clinical assessment of CD requires an understanding of the varied nature of the disorder. Diagnosis is usually straightforward, but despite this, misdiagnosis remains relatively common. Accurate assessment methodologies that facilitate the collection of meaningful outcome data are necessary for the validation of the effectiveness of new therapies and to allow optimization of benefit and minimization of side effects with available treatment approaches. To be valid a rating scale must evaluate the relevant clinical dimensions of CD and be responsive to change in clinical status. A variety of approaches have been used to assess CD. Which of the currently available subjective and objective rating instruments is most appropriate strongly depends on the clinical circumstances and the needs of the "operator." To encourage consistency in clinical evaluation in the future, it may be appropriate to consider the formulation of a "Unified Cervical Dystonia Rating Scale," with input from a number of investigators with interest and experience in the care and management of this common focal dystonia.

ACKNOWLEDGMENT

This work was supported in part by a grant from Physicians' Services Incorporated (PSI) of Ontario.

APPENDIX A: THE TORONTO WESTERN SPASMODIC TORTICOLLIS RATING SCALE (TWSTRS)

    I. TORTICOLLIS SEVERITY SCALE
        A. MAXIMAL EXCURSION
            Rate maximum amplitude of excursion asking patient not to oppose the abnormal movement; examiner may use distracting or aggravating maneuvers. When degree of deviation is between two scores, chose the higher of the two.
            1. Rotation (turn: right or left)
                0 None
                1 Slight ($<$ 1/4 range) (1–22°)
                2 Mild (1/4–1/2 range) (23–45°)
                3 Moderate (1/2–3/4 range) (46–67°)
                4 Severe ($>$ 3/4 range) (68–90°)
             2. Laterocollis (tilt: right or left) (exclude shoulder elevation)
                0 None
                1 Mild (1–15 degrees)
                2 Moderate (16–35 degrees)
                3 Severe ($>$ 35 degrees)

   3. Anterocollis/retrocollis (a *or* b)
      a) Anterocollis
      0 None
      1 Mild downward deviation of chin
      2 Moderate downward deviation (approximates 1/2 possible range)
      3 Severe (chin approximates chest)
      b) Retrocollis
      0 None
      1 Mild backward deviation of vertex with upward deviation of chin
      2 Moderate backward deviation (approximates ½ possible range)
      3 Severe (approximates full range)
   4. Lateral shift (right or left)
      0 Absent
      1 Present
   5. Sagittal shift (forward or backward)
      0 Absent
      1 Present
B. DURATION FACTOR
   Provide an overall score estimated through the course of the standardized examination after estimating maximal excursion (exclusive of asking patient to allow
   head to deviate maximally). Weighted × 2 (see schematic representation of
   scoring duration)
      0 None
      1 Occasional deviation (< 25% of the time), most often submaximal
      2 Occasional deviation (< 25% of the time), often maximal
         or
         Intermittent deviation (25–50% of the time), most often submaximal
      3 Intermittent deviation (25–50% of the time) often maximal
         or
         Frequent deviation (50–75% of the time), most often submaximal
      4 Frequent deviation (50–75% of the time), often maximal
         or
         Constant deviation (> 75% of the time), most often submaximal
      5 Constant deviation (> 75% of the time), often maximal
C. EFFECT OF SENSORY TRICKS
      0 Complete relief by one or more tricks
      1 Partial or only limited relief by tricks
      2 Little or no benefit from tricks
D. SHOULDER ELEVATION/ANTERIOR DISPLACEMENT
      0 Absent
      1 Mild (< 1/3 possible range), intermittent or constant
      2 Moderate (1/3–2/3 possible range) and constant (> 75% of the time) or
         severe (> 2/3 possible range) and intermittent
      3 Severe and constant
E. RANGE OF MOTION (without aid of sensory tricks). If limitation occurs in
   more than one plane of motion use individual score that is highest.
      0 Able to move to extreme opposite position
      1 Able to move head well past midline but not to extreme opposite position

    2   Able to move head barely past midline
    3   Able to move head toward but not past midline
    4   Barely able to move head beyond abnormal posture
  F. TIME (up to 60 sec) for which patient is able to maintain head within 10° of
      neutral position without the use of sensory "tricks" (mean of two attempts)
        0   > 60 sec
        1   46–60 sec
        2   31–45 sec
        3   16–30 sec
        4   < 15 sec
      TOTAL SEVERITY SCORE = sum of A–F. Maximum score = 35.

  B. DURATION FACTOR (Schematic representation)*

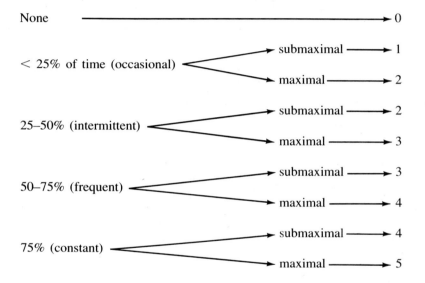

II. DISABILITY SCALE
    1. WORK (occupation or housework/home management)
        0   No difficulty
        1   Normal work expectations with satisfactory performance at usual level of
            occupation but some interference by torticollis
        2   Most activities unlimited, selected activities very difficult and hampered
            but still possible with satisfactory performance
        3   Working at lower than usual occupational level; most activities ham-
            pered, all possible but with less than satisfactory performance in some
            activities
        4   Unable to engage in voluntary or gainful employment; still able to
            perform some domestic responsibilities satisfactorily
        5   Marginal or no ability to perform domestic responsibilities

*The rater simply determines the proportion of time that the dystonic head posturing is present (left column) and
then decides whether the deviations are most often maximal or submaximal, having previously determined the
maximal excursion score (A).

2. ACTIVITIES OF DAILY LIVING (e.g., feeding, dressing, hygiene, including washing, shaving, makeup, etc.)

   0 No difficulty with any activity
   1 Activities unlimited but some interference by torticollis
   2 Most activities unlimited, selected activities very difficult and hampered but still possible using simple tricks
   3 Most activities hampered or laborious but still possible; may use extreme "tricks"
   4 All activities impaired; some impossible or require assistance
   5 Dependent on others in most self-care tasks

3. DRIVING

   0 No difficulty (or has never driven a car)
   1 Unlimited ability to drive but bothered by torticollis
   2 Unlimited ability to drive but requires "tricks" (including touching or holding face, holding head against head rest) to control torticollis
   3 Can drive only short distances
   4 Usually cannot drive because of torticollis
   5 Unable to drive and cannot ride in a car for long stretches as a passenger because of torticollis

4. READING

   0 No difficulty
   1 Unlimited ability to read in normal seated position but bothered by torticollis
   2 Unlimited ability to read in normal seated position but requires use of "tricks" to control torticollis
   3 Unlimited ability to read but requires extensive measures to control torticollis or is able to read only in nonseated position (e.g., lying down)
   4 Limited ability to read because of torticollis despite tricks
   5 Unable to read more than a few sentences because of torticollis

5. TELEVISION

   0 No difficulty
   1 Unlimited ability to watch television in normal seated position but bothered by torticollis
   2 Unlimited ability to watch television in normal seated position but requires the use of tricks to control torticollis
   3 Unlimited ability to watch television but requires extensive measures to control torticollis or is able to view only in nonseated position (e.g., lying down)
   4 Limited ability to watch television because of torticollis
   5 Unable to watch television for more than a few minutes because of torticollis

6. ACTIVITIES OUTSIDE THE HOME (e.g., shopping, walking about, movies, dining, and other recreational activities)

   0 No difficulty
   1 Unlimited activities but bothered by torticollis
   2 Unlimited activities but requires simple "tricks" to accomplish
   3 Accomplishes activities only when accompanied by others because of torticollis

    4 Limited activities outside home; certain activities impossible or given up because of torticollis

    5 Rarely if ever engages in activities outside the home

TOTAL DISABILITY SCORE = sum of 1–6. Maximum score = 30.

III. PAIN SCALE (Preliminary Version)

    1. Rate the severity of neck pain during the last week on a scale of 0–10 where a score of 0 represents no pain and 10 represents the most excruciating pain imaginable

Best	0–10	Severity = [(2 × usual) + best + worst]/4
Worst	0–10	
Usual	0–10	Maximum Score = 10

    2. Rate the duration of neck pain

        1 None

        1 Present < 10% of the time

        2 Present 10%–< 25% of the time

        3 Present 25%–< 50% of the time

        4 Present 50%–< 75% of the time

        5 Present > 75% of the time

    3. Rate the degree to which pain contributes to disability

        0 No limitation or interference from pain

        1 Pain is quite bothersome but not a source of disability

        2 Pain definitely interferes with some tasks but is not a major contributor to disability

        3 Pain accounts for some (less than half) but not all disability

        4 Pain is a major source of difficulty with activities; separate from this, head pulling is also a source of some (less than half) disability

        5 Pain is the major source of disability; without it most impaired activities could be performed quite satisfactorily despite the head pulling

TOTAL PAIN SCALE SCORE = sum of 1–3. Maximum score = 20.

APPENDIX B: TWSTRS—VIDEOTAPE PROTOCOL

1. Standing—viewed from front, side, and back × 10 sec each
2. Walking—20 feet back and forth
    a) without instructions × 2
    b) with instructions not to resist deviation (i.e., allow head to deviate to maximum) × 2
3. Sitting—in preferred or most comfortable position
    a) without instructions × 30 sec and
    b) with instructions not to resist deviation × 30 sec
4. Distracting or activating maneuvers: (sitting) (R and L separately) each × 10 seconds
    a) finger tapping
    b) opening and closing fist
    c) pronation and supination forearm
    d) arms outstretched, held under nose, finger to nose × 3
    e) foot tapping
5. Time in midline

With active resistance to deviation but without aid of sensory tricks or support. Patient asked to maintain head in midline for as long as possible—maximum 60 seconds × 2 attempts. Patient instructed not to talk.

6. Effect of ''tricks''
Including touching side of face, holding chin, holding back of neck or head, pressing against wall behind head, and other preferred tricks used by patient

7. Active range of movement (× 2 each time)
Rotation, lateral flexion, forward flexion, extension

8. Writing name, sentence, repetitive words or phrase × 10 seconds

9. Lying supine × 20 seconds

APPENDIX C: TWSTRS RESPONSE SCALE

-1 = Worse

0 = No benefit

1 = Minimal or questionable reduction in dystonia and pain with no functional improvement

2 = Mild response with some reduction in dystonia and/or pain, little functional improvement

3 = Moderate response with definite reduction in dystonia and/or pain and some functional improvement

4 = Marked response of dystonia and/or pain dystonia still evident, excellent functional improvement

5 = Striking improvement with little or no dystonia or pain remaining

REFERENCES

1. Nutt JG, Muenter MD, Aronson A, Kurland LT, Melton LJ. Epidemiology of focal and generalized dystonia in Rochester, Minnesota. Mov Disord 1988;3:188–194.
2. Fahn S. The varied clinical expressions of dystonia. Neurol Clin 1984;2:541–554.
3. Report of the Therapeutics and Technology Assessment Subcommittee of the American Academy of Neurology. Assessment: the clinical usefulness of botulinum toxin-A in treating neurologic disorders. Neurology 1990;40:1332–1336.
4. Consensus Statement: Clinical use of botulinum toxin. NIH Consensus Development Conference, November 12–14, 1990;8:1–20.
5. Jankovic, J, Brin MF. Therapeutic uses of botulinum toxin. N Engl J Med 1991;324:1186–1193.
6. Chan J, Brin MF, Fahn S. Idiopathic cervical dystonia—clinical characteristics. Mov Disord 1991;6:119–126.
7. Jankovic J, Leder S, Warner D, Schwartz K. Cervical dystonia—clinical findings and associated movement disorders. Neurology 1991;41:1088–1091.
8. Rondot P, Marchand MP, Dellatolas G. Spasmodic torticollis—review of 220 patients. Can J Neurol Sci 1991;18:143–151.
9. Deuschl G, Heinen F, Kleedorfer B, Wagner M, Lucking CH, Poewe W. Clinical and polymyographic investigation of spasmodic torticollis. J Neurol 1992;239:9–15.
10. Consky ES, Lang AE. Unpublished data.
11. Patterson RM, Little SC. Spasmodic torticollis. J Nerv Ment Dis 1943;98:571–559.
12. Stejskal L, Tomanek Z. Postural laterality in torticollis and torsion dystonia. J Neurol Neurosurg Psychiatry 1981;44:1029–1034.
13. Gauthier S. Idiopathic spasmodic torticollis. Pathophysiology and treatment. Can J Neurol Sci 1986;13:88–90.

14. Consky ES, Basinki A, Belle-Scantlebury L, Lang AE. Comparison of botulinum toxin treatment variables for spasmodic torticollis. Neurology 1991;41(suppl l):273.

15. Fahn S. Torsion dystonia: clinical spectrum and treatment. Semin Neurol 1982;2:316–323.

16. Weiner WJ, Nora LM. "Trick" movements in facial dystonia. J Clin Psychiatry 1984;45:519–521.

17. Stejskal L. Counterpressure in torticollis. J Neurol Sci 1980;48:9–19.

18. Duane DD. Spasmodic torticollis. In: Jankovic J, Tolosa E, eds. Facial dyskinesias. Advances in neurology, vol. 50. New York: Raven Press, 1988:135–150.

19. Herz E, Glaser GH. Spasmodic torticollis, II: clinical evaluation. Arch Neurol Psychiatry. 1949;61:227–239.

20. Matthews WB, Beasley P, Parry-Jones W, Garland G. Spasmodic torticollis: a combined clinical study. J Neurol Neurosurg Psychiatry 1978;41:485–492.

21. Lowenstein D, Aminoff MJ. The clinical course of spasmodic torticollis. Neurology 1988;38:530–532.

22. Marsden CD. The problem of adult-onset idiopathic torsion dystonia and other isolated dyskinesias in adult life (including blepharospasm, oromandibular dystonia, dystonic writer's cramp and torticollis, or axial dystonia). Adv Neurol 1976;14:259–276.

23. Jahanshahi M, Marion MH, Marsden CD. Natural history of adult-onset idiopathic torticollis. Arch Neurol 1990;47:548–552.

24. Riski JE, Horner J, Nashod BS. Swallowing function in patients with spasmodic torticollis. Neurology 1990;40:1443–1445.

25. Comella CL, Tanner CM, DeFoor-Hill L, Smith C. Dysphagia after botulinum toxin injections for spasmodic torticollis: clinical and radiologic findings. Neurology 1992;42:1307–1310.

26. Jahanshahi M, Marsden CD. Personality in torticollis: a controlled study. Psychol Med 1988;18:375–387.

27. Vasudevam SV. Clinical perspectives on the relationship between pain and disability. In: Portenoy RK, ed. Pain: mechanism and syndromes. Neurology clinics, vol. 7. Philadelphia: W.B. Saunders, 1989:429–440.

28. Melvin JL, Nagi SZ. Factors in behavioural responses to impairments. Arch Phys Med Rehabil 1970;51:552–557.

29. Marsden CD. Investigation of dystonia. In: Fahn S, Marsden CD, Calne DB, eds. Dystonia 2. Advances in neurology, vol. 50. New York: Raven Press, 1988:35–44.

30. Calne DB, Lang AE. Secondary dystonia. In: Fahn S, Marsden CD, Calne DB, eds. Dystonia 2. Advances in neurology, vol. 50. New York: Raven press, 1988:9–33.

31. Marsden CD, Obeso JA, Zarrantz JJ, Lang AE. The anatomical basis of symptomatic hemidystonia. Brain 1985;108:463–483.

32. Isaac K, Cohen JA. Post-traumatic torticollis.Neurology 1989;39:1642–1643.

33. Krauss JK, Mohadjer M, Braus DF, Wakhloo AK, Nobbe F, Mundinger F. Dystonia following head trauma: a report of nine patients and review of the literature. Mov Disord 1992;3:263–272.

34. Rajagopalan N, Humphrey PRD, Buchnall RC. Torticollis and blepharospasm in systemic lupus erythematosus. Mov Disord 1989;4:345–348.

35. Sainte Hilaire M-H, Burke RE, Bressman SB, Brin MF, Fahn S. Delayed-onset dystonia due to perinatal or early childhood asphyxia. Neurology 1991;41:216–222.

36. Pagni CA, Naddeo M, Faccani G. Spasmodic torticollis due to neurovascular compression of the 11th nerve. J Neurosurg 1985;63:789–791.

37. Shima F, Fukui M, Kitamura K, Kuromatsu C, Okamura T. Diagnosis and surgical treatment of spasmodic torticollis of 11th nerve origin. Neurosurgery 1988;22:358–363.

38. Podivinsky F. Torticollis. In: Vinken PJ, Bruyn GW, eds. Handbook of clinical neurology. Vol. 6. Amsterdam: North Holland, 1968:567–603.

39. Burke RE, Fahn S, Jankovic J, Marsden CD, Lang AE, Gollomp S, Ilson J. Tardive dystonia: late-onset and persistent dystonia caused by antipsychotic drugs. Neurology 1982;32:1335–1346.
40. Kang UJ, Burke RE, Fahn S. Natural history and treatment of tardive dystonia. Mov Disord 1986;1:193–208.
41. Quinn N. Disproportionate antecollis in multiple system atrophy. Lancet 1989;1:844.
42. Rivest J, Quinn N, Marsden CD. Dystonia in Parkinson's disease, multiple system atrophy and progressive supranuclear palsy. Neurology 1990;40:1571–1578.
43. Lesser RP, Fahn S. Dystonia: a disorder often misdiagnosed as a conversion reaction. Am J Psychiatry 1978:135:349–352.
44. Fahn S, Williams D, Reches A, Lesser RP, Jankovic J, Silberstein SD. Hysterical dystonia, a rare disorder: report of five documented cases. Neurology 1983;33(suppl 2):161.
45. Fahn S, Williams D. Psychogenic dystonia. In: Fahn S, Marsden CD, Calne DB, eds. Dystonia 2. Advances in neurology, vol. 50. New York: Raven Press, 1988:431–456.
46. Sheehy MP, Marsden CD. Trauma and pain in spasmodic torticollis. Lancet 1981;1:777–778.
47. Jankovic J, Van der Linden C. Dystonia and tremor induced by peripheral trauma: predisposing factors. J Neurol Neurosurg Psychiatry 1988;51:1512–1519.
48. Schott GD. The relationship of peripheral trauma and pain to dystonia. J Neurol Neurosurg Psychiatry 1985;48:698–701.
49. Koller WC, Wong GF, Lang AE. Posttraumatic movement disorders: a review. Mov Disord 1989;4:20–36.
50. Truong DD, Dubinsky RM, Hermanowicz N, Olson WL, Silverman B, Koller WC. Posttraumatic torticollis. Arch Neurol 1991;48:221–223.
51. Fletcher NA, Harding AE, Marsden CD. The relationship between trauma and idiopathic torsion dystonia. J Neurol Neurosurg Psychiatry 1991;54:713–717.
52. Suchowersky O, Calne DB. Non-dystonic causes of torticollis. In: Fahn S, Marsden CD, Calne DB, eds. Dystonia 2. Advances in neurology, vol. 50. New York: Raven Press, 1988;501–508.
53. Kiwak KJ. Establishing an etiology for torticollis. Postgrad Med 1984;75:126–134.
54. Weiner WJ, Lang AE. Movement disorders, a comprehensive survey. Mount Kisco, New York: Futura, 1989;394.
55. Lees AJ, Robertson M, Trimble MR, Murray NMF. A clinical study of Gilles de la Tourette syndrome in the United Kingdom. J Neurol Neurosurg Psychiatry 1984;47:1–8.
56. Shale HM, Truong DD, Fahn S. Tics in patients with other movement disorders. Neurology 1986;36(suppl l):118.
57. Stone LA, Jankovic J. The coexistence of tics and dystonia. Arch Neurol 1991;48:862–865.
58. Obeso JA, Rothwell JC, Lang AE, Marsden CD. Myoclonic dystonia. Neurology 1983;33:825–830.
59. Quinn NP, Rothwell JC, Thompson PD. Hereditary myoclonic dystonia, hereditary torsion dystonia and hereditary essential myoclonus: an area of confusion. In: Fahn S, Marsden CD, Calne DB, eds. Dystonia 2. Advances in neurology, vol. 50. New York:Raven Press, 1988;391–401.
60. Kurlan R, Behr J, Medved L, Shoulson I. Myoclonus and dystonia: a family study. In: Fahn S, Marsden CD, Calne DB, eds. Dystonia 2. Advances in neurology, vol. 50. New York: Raven Press, 1988:385–390.
61. Rivest J, Marsden CD. Trunk and head tremor as isolated manifestation of dystonia. Mov Disord 1990;5:60–65.
62. Couch JR. Dystonia and tremor in spasmodic torticollis. Adv Neurol 1976;14:245–258.
63. Truong DD, Hermanowicz NS. Clinical evaluation of bidirectional torticollis. Mov Disord 1990;5:181.

64. Tsui JKC, Calne DB. Botulinum toxin in cervical dystonia. In: Jankovic J, Tolosa ES, eds. Facial Dyskinesias. Advances in neurology, vol. 49. New York: Raven Press, 1988;473–478.

65. Gelb DJ, Yoshimura DM, Olney RK, Lowenstein DH, Aminoff MJ. Change in pattern of muscle activity following botulinum toxin injections for torticollis. Ann Neurol 1991;29:370–376.

66. LaRoca NG. Statistical and methodologic considerations in scale construction. In: Munsat TL, ed. Quantification of neurologic deficit. London: Butterworths, 1989:49–67.

67. Feinstein AR. Clinimetrics. New Haven, Connecticut: Yale University Press, 1987:190–211.

68. Swash M, Roberts AH, Zakko H, Heathfield KW. Treatment of involuntary disorders with tetrabenazine. J Neurol Neurosurg Psychiatry 1972;35:186–191.

69. Bernhardt AJ, Hersen M, Barlow DH. Measurement and modification of spasmodic torticollis: an experimental analysis. Behav Therap 1972;3:294–297.

70. Tolosa ES. Modification of tardive dyskinesia and spasmodic torticollis by apomorphine. Arch Neurol 1978;35:459–462.

71. Marsden CD, Schachter M. Assessment of extrapyramidal disorders. Br J Clin Pharmacol 1981;11:129–151.

72. Burke RE, Fahn S, Marsden CD, Bressman SB, Moskowitz C, Friedman J. Validity and reliability of a rating scale for the primary torsion dystonias. Neurology 1985;35:73–77.

73. Lang AE, Sheehy MP, Marsden CD. Anticholinergics in adult-onset dystonia. Can J Neurol Sci 1982;9:313–319.

74. Weiner WJ, Lang AE. Movement disorders, a comprehensive survey. Mount Kisco, New York: Futura, 1989:712–713.

75. Fahn S. Assessment of the primary dystonias. In: Munsat TL, ed. Quantification of neurologic deficit. London: Butterworths, 1989:241–270.

76. Greene P, Kang U, Fahn S, Brin M, Moskowitz C, Flaster MS. Double-blind, placebo-controlled trial of botulinum toxin injections for the treatment of spasmodic torticollis. Neurology 1990;40:1213–1218.

77. Tsui JKC, Eisen A, Stoessl AJ, Calne DB. Double-blind study of botulinum toxin in spasmodic torticollis. Lancet 1986;2:245–247.

78. Gelb DJ, Lowenstein DH, Aminoff MJ. Controlled trial of botulinum toxin injections in the treatment of spasmodic torticollis. Neurology 1989;39:80–84.

79. Stell R, Thompson PD, Marsden CD. Botulinum toxin in spasmodic torticollis. J Neurol Neurosurg Psychiatry 1988;51:920–923.

80. Blackie JD, Lees AJ. Botulinum toxin treatment in spasmodic torticollis. J Neurol Neurosurg Psychiatry 1990;53:640–643.

81. Moore AP, Blumhardt LD. A double-blind trial of botulinum toxin "A" in torticollis, with one year follow-up. J Neurol Neurosurg Psychiatry 1991;54:813–816.

82. Lorentz IT, Shanthi Subramaniam S, Yiannikas C. Treatment of idiopathic spasmodic torticollis with botulinum toxin A: a double-blind study on twenty-three patients. Mov Disord 1991;6:145–150.

83. Poewe W, Schelosky L, Kleedorfer B, Heinen F, Wagner M, Deuschl G. Treatment of spasmodic torticollis with local injections of botulinum toxin. One-year follow-up in thirty seven patients. J Neurol 1992;239:21–25.

84. Jankovic J. Treatment of hyperkinetic movement disorders with tetrabenazine: a double-blind crossover study. Ann Neurol 1982;11:41–47.

85. Jankovic J, Schwartz K. Botulinum toxin injections for cervical dystonia. Neurology 1990;40:277–280.

86. Jankovic J, Orman J. Botulinum A toxin for cranial-cervical dystonia. Neurology 1987;37:616–623.

87. Consky ES, Basinki A, Belle L, Ranawaya R, Lang AE. The Toronto Western Spasmodic Torticollis Rating Scale (TWSTRS): assessment of validity and inter-rater reliability. Neurology 1990;40(suppl l):445.

88. Comella CL, Buchman AS, Tanner CM, Brown-Toms NC, Goetz CG. Botulinum toxin injection for spasmodic torticollis: increased magnitude of benefit with electromyographic assistance. Neurology 1992;42:878–882.

89. Dubinsky RM. Electromyographic guidance of botulinum toxin treatment in torticollis. Abstracts NIH Consensus Development Conference on the clinical use of botulinum toxin Nov 12–14 1990;8:73–77.

90. Ansari KA, Webster DD. Quantitative measurements in spasmodic torticollis. Dis Nerv Syst 1974;35:44–47.

91. Schatz H, Urist M. An instrument for measuring ocular torticollis (head turn, tilt, and bend). Trans Am Acad Ophthalmol Otolaryngol 1971;75:650–653.

92. Van Hoof JJ, Horstink MI, Berger HJ, van Spaendonck KP, Cools AR. Spasmodic torticollis: the problem of pathophysiology and assessment. J Neurol 1987;234:322–327.

93. Rogers GW, Rootes M, Lye RH. Computer/video analysis of movement disorders. J Audiov Media Med 1985;8:101–107.

94. Lye RH, Rootes M, Rogers GW. Computer graphics in the assessment of severity of spasmodic torticollis: potential role in the evaluation of surgical treatment. Surg Neurol 1987;27:357–360.

95. Shann RT, Lye RH, Rogers GW. Severity in movement disorders: a quantitative approach. Acta Neurochirurg 1987;suppl 39:77–79.

96. Dykstra D, Ellingham C, Belfie A, Baxter T, Lee M, Voelker A. Quantitative measurement of cervical range of motion in patients with torticollis treated with botulinum A toxin. Mov Disord 1993;8:38–42.

97. Keele KD. The pain chart. Lancet 1948;2:6–8.

98. Carlsson AM. Assessment of chronic pain. I: Aspects of the reliability and validity of the visual analogue scale. Pain 1983;16:87–101.

99. Melzack R. The McGill pain questionnaire. Major properties and scoring methods. Pain 1975;1:277–299.

100. Corsan JA, Schneider M. The Dartmouth pain questionnaire: an adjunct to McGill pain questionnaire. Pain 1984;19:59–69.

101. Bergner M, Bobbitt RA, Carter WB, Gilson BS. The Sickness Impact Profile: development and final revision of a health status measure. Med Care 1981;19:787–805.

16

Anatomy and Neurophysiology of Neck Muscles

Richard M. Dubinsky
University of Kansas Medical Center, Kansas City, Kansas

INTRODUCTION

Knowledge of the major muscles of the neck that are involved in head and neck movement is a prerequisite to the successful treatment of cervical dystonia with botulinum toxin (BTX). It is only by knowing which muscles can produce the observed movement that rational selection of muscles can be made. When the abnormal neck posture returns after BTX injections, and the previously injected muscles are still atrophic (e.g., the sternocleidomastoid and splenius capitis muscles), it is obvious that other muscles are producing the movement. It is these "newly" involved muscles that must be sought out and injected (1).

ANATOMY OF THE MAJOR NECK MUSCLES

The major neck muscles and their innervations can be divided anatomically into the anterolateral and posterior groups (Tables 1 and 2). They can also be divided by their actions (Table 3). The muscles will be presented with a brief description of their course, major and minor actions, and where appropriate, suggestions for needle placement (2).

Platysma. This subcutaneous muscle consists of a broad sheet that extends from the fascia overlying the pectoralis muscles to the mandible and the subcutaneous structures of the face. Although not involved in head movement, the platysma is involved in cervical and craniocervical dystonia. Contraction of the platysma gives the appearance of widening the neck while making the vertical folds of skin overlying the laryngeal strap muscles more prominent. Insertion of the needle may be made almost anywhere in the anterior skin of the neck at a depth of 0.5 cm.

Sternocleidomastoid. The sternal and clavicular heads join together into a strong band of muscle below the middle of the neck that inserts into the lateral aspect of the mastoid

Table 1 Anterolateral Muscles of the Neck Involved in Head and Neck Movement

Muscle	Innervation
Superficial	
Platysma	CN VII
Lateral cervical	
Sternocleidomastoid	CN XI
Trapezius	CN XI
Anterior vertebral	
Longus colli	C 1,2,3
Longus capitis	C 1,2,3
Rectus capitis anterior	C 1, anterior rami
Rectus capitis lateralis	C 1, anterior rami
Lateral vertebral	
Scalenus anterior	C 5,6, anterior rami
Scalenus medius	C 3–8, anterior rami
Scalenus posterior	C 6–8, ventral primary divisions

process. This muscle is frequently hypertrophied in cervical dystonia. The sternocleidomastoid acts to rotate the head to the opposite side and to tilt the head to the same side. Acting together, the two sternocleidomastoids flex the neck. Needle insertion is suggested in the upper half, where the two heads have fused.

Trapezius (upper portion). The trapezius arises from the occipital protuberance, the ligamentum nuchae, and the spinous processes of C7 and the upper thoracic vertebrae. It inserts into the posterior border of the lateral third of the clavicle. This muscle primarily functions to rotate the scapula and to elevate the shoulder. In cervical dystonia the trapezius works to rotate the head and neck toward the opposite side. The needle may be inserted into either the lateral fibers of the upper portion at the upper border of the shoulder or into the posterior neck portion, two finger breadths lateral to the spinous process of C7, at a depth of 1.0 cm.

Longus colli. The longus colli arises from the bodies of the thoracic vertebrae and inserts into the bodies of the upper cervical vertebrae (Fig. 1). This muscle functions to flex the neck and can also be involved in neck rotation and lateral flexion. If the needle is advanced to the vertebral column, posterior to the clavicular head of the sternocleidomastoid muscle and halfway between the mandible and the clavicle, it will be in the longus colli and longus capitis. These muscles are extremely close to the posterior pharyngeal muscles.

Longus capitis. The longus capitis arises from the transverse processes of C3–6 and inserts into the base of the occipital bone (Fig. 1). This muscle flexes the head and the upper cervical spine.

Rectus capitis anterior. This muscle originates from the transverse process of the atlas and inserts into the base of the occipital bone, just anterior to the foramen magnum. It passes deep to the longus capitis (Fig. 1). The rectus capitis anterior stabilizes the atlantooccipital joint and flexes the head.

Rectus capitis lateralis. The rectus capitis lateralis originates from the transverse process of the atlas and inserts into the occipital bone at the jugular process (Fig. 1). This muscle, like the rectus capitis anterior, stabilizes the atlantooccipital joint. It also bends the head laterally.

Table 2   Major Muscles of the Posterior Neck and Thorax

Muscle	Innervation
Splenius muscles	
Splenius capitis	C 3–6, dorsal rami
Splenius cervicis	C 5–8, dorsal rami
Levator scapulae	C 5, dorsal rami
Erector spinae	
Iliocostalis cervicis	Dorsal primary rami of the spinal nerves
Longissimus cervicis	Dorsal primary rami of the spinal nerves
Longissimus capitis	C 3–8, dorsal rami
Spinalis thoracis, cervicis, and capitis	Dorsal primary rami of the spinal nerves
Semispinalis thoracis	Dorsal primary rami of the thoracic spinal nerves
Semispinalis cervicis	Dorsal primary rami of the cervical spinal nerves
Semispinalis capitis	Dorsal primary rami of the cervical spinal nerves
Multifidus	Dorsal primary rami of the cervical spinal nerves
Rotatores cervicis	Dorsal primary rami of the cervical spinal nerves
Interspinales cervicis	Dorsal primary rami of the cervical spinal nerves
Intertransversarii cervicis	Ventral rami of the cervical spinal nerves
Suboccipital	
Rectus capitis posterior major	Suboccipital nerve
Rectus capitis posterior minor	Suboccipital nerve
Obliquus capitis inferior	Suboccipital nerve
Obliquus capitis superior	Suboccipital nerve

Source: Ref. 2.

Scalenus anterior. This muscle arises from the transverse processes of C3–6, passes vertically downward, behind the sternocleidomastoid, inserting into the first rib at the scalene tubercle (Fig. 1). The scalenus anterior functions to elevate the first rib during respiration. The brachial plexus passes between the scalenus anterior and scalenus medius. Attempted injection into the scalenus anterior or medius muscles has been reported to result in inadvertent injection into the brachial plexus (3).

Scalenus medius. The scalenus medius, the largest muscle of the scalenus group, arises from the transverse processes of the cervical vertebrae and inserts into the superior portion of the first rib (Fig. 1). This muscle can elevate the first rib or bend and rotate the neck. A needle can be placed into the scalenus medius muscle by palpating the belly of the muscle, in the floor of the posterior triangle, two finger breadths anterior to the anterior border of the trapezius muscle. At this point the muscle is just beneath the skin. The upper portion can be inserted by placing the needle just anterior to the lateral edge of the splenius capitis muscle to a depth of 1.5 to 3.0 cm.

Table 3 Actions of Major Neck Muscles Accessible to Electromyography[a]

Contralateral rotators	Ipsilateral rotators
Sternocleidomastoid	Splenius capitis and cervicis
Trapezius	Levator scapulae
Scalenus medius	Longissimus cervicis and capitis
Semispinalis thoracis, cervicis, and capitis	Multifidus
	Rotatores cervicis
Neck extensors	Neck flexors
Levator scapulae (B)	Longus colli and capitis
Splenius capitis and cervicis (B)	Sternocleidomastoids (B)
Iliocostalis cervicis	
Longissimus cervicis and capitis (B)	Lateral flexors
Spinalis capitis, cervicis, and thoracis (B)	Sternocleidomastoid
Semispinalis capitis, cervicis, and thoracis (B)	Trapezius
Rotatores cervicis (B)	Scalenus medius and posterior
Interspinales cervicis	Splenius capitis and cervicis
Intertransversarii cervicis (B)	Longissimus cervicis and capitis
	Multifidus
	Intertransversarii cervicis

[a](B) indicates that the action results from the combined contraction of the muscle on each side of the neck.

Scalenus posterior. This muscle arises from the posterior portion of the transverse processes of C5–6, passing medially and posteriorly to the scalenus medius, and inserts into the outer surface of the second rib, deep to the attachment of the serratus anterior (Fig. 1). The scalenus posterior elevates the second rib or bends and slightly rotates the neck.

The scalenus group serves to elevate the rib cage or to bend the neck to the side. Both scalene groups, contracting together, slightly flex the neck.

Splenius capitis. The splenius capitis arises from the nuchal line and the spinous process of C7 and T1–3. It courses beneath the upper portion of the trapezius and inserts deep to the sternocleidomastoid muscle into the mastoid process (Fig. 2). This muscle serves to rotate the head toward the same side and to bend the head laterally. Together the splenius capitis muscles extend the neck. A needle may be inserted in the middle portion, where the muscle lies just beneath the skin lateral to the border of the trapezius muscle, or two finger breadths lateral to the spinous process of C7 at a depth of 2.0 cm.

Splenius cervicis. This muscle arises from the spinous processes of T3–6. It courses inferiorly to the splenius capitis and inserts into the transverse processes of C2 and C3 (Fig. 2).

The splenius cervicis, like the splenius capitis, rotates the head toward the same side. Together, the two splenius cervicis muscles extend the neck. Electromyographically, the splenius cervicis cannot be readily differentiated from the splenius capitis muscle.

Levator scapulae. This muscle originates on the anterior aspect of the scapula and inserts into the mastoid process. It travels beneath the upper fibers of the trapezius. The levator scapulae acts to elevate the scapula or to extend the neck and rotate the head toward the same side.

Iliocostalis cervicis. The iliocostalis cervicis arises from the angles of the third through sixth ribs and inserts into the transverse processes of C4–6. (Fig. 3). This muscle bends the neck to the same side. Acting together, these muscles extend the vertebral column.

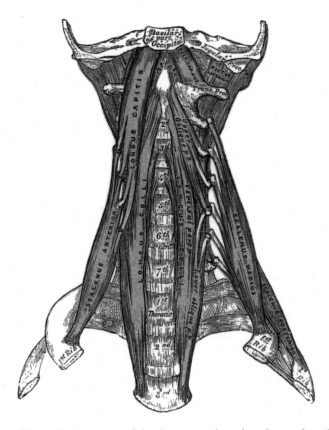

Figure 1 Anatomy of the deep anterolateral neck muscles. (From Ref. 2.)

Longissimus cervicis. This muscle arises from the transverse process of T1–4 and inserts into the transverse processes of C2–6. It courses between the iliocostalis cervicis and the longissimus capitis on top of the rib cage (Fig. 3). The longissimus cervicis bends the neck to the same side. When the longissimus cervicis muscles are active bilaterally they extend the neck.

Longissimus capitis. This muscle arises from the transverse processes of T1–4 and C5–8. It travels between the longissimus cervicis and semispinalis capitis, inserting into the mastoid process (Fig. 3). Acting alone, the longissimus capitis turns the head toward the same side and tilts the face toward the same shoulder. Together, the two longissimus capitis muscles extend the neck.

Spinalis thoracis, cervicis, and capitis. These three muscles are an extension of the erector spinae muscles. They originate along the spinous processes of the thoracic and cervical vertebrae and insert into spinous processes of the upper thoracic vertebrae (spinalis thoracis), cervical vertebrae (spinalis cervicis), and axis (spinalis capitis) (Fig. 3). Together they extend the neck.

Semispinalis thoracis. This muscle originates from the transverse processes of T6–10 and courses along the lateral and posterior aspects of the vertebral bodies to insert into the spinous processes of C6–7 and T1–4 (Fig. 3).

Semispinalis cervicis. The semispinalis cervicis originates from the transverse processes of T1–5 and inserts into the spinous processes of the axis to C5. It courses deep to the

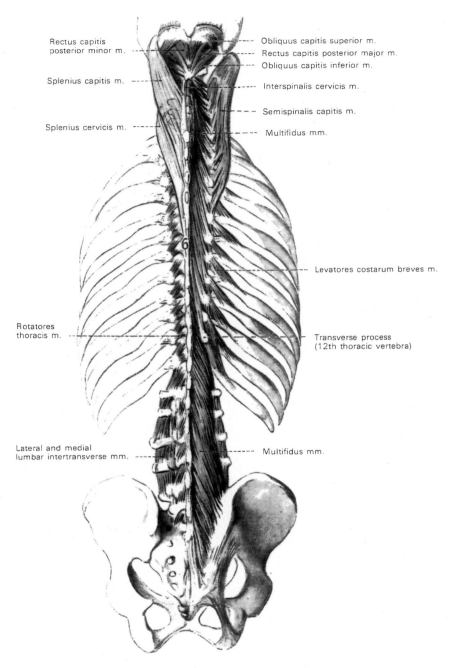

Rectus capitis
posterior minor m.

Splenius capitis m.

Splenius cervicis m.

Rotatores
thoracis m.

Lateral and medial
lumbar intertransverse mm.

Obliquus capitis superior m.
Rectus capitis posterior major m.
Obliquus capitis inferior m.

Interspinalis cervicis m.

Semispinalis capitis m.

Multifidus mm.

Levatores costarum breves m.

Transverse process
(12th thoracic vertebra)

Multifidus mm.

Figure 2 Anatomy of the superficial and deep neck and back muscles. (Courtesy of Urban and Schwarzenberg, Munich, Germany.)

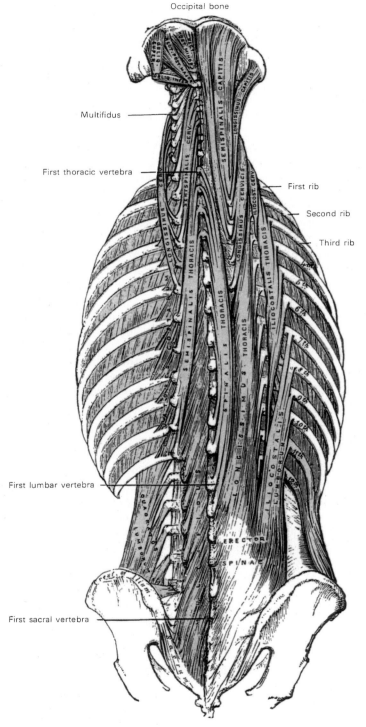

Figure 3 Anatomy of the intermediate and deep muscles of the neck and suboccipital regions. (From Ref. 2.)

semispinalis capitis (Fig. 3). The semispinalis thoracis and cervicis extend the vertebral column and rotate it toward the opposite side.

Semispinalis capitis. This muscle originates from the tips of the transverse processes of T1–6, C7, and the articular processes of C4–6. It inserts into the occipital bone, between the superior and inferior nuchal lines. This large muscle courses beneath the splenius capitis (Fig. 3). The semispinalis capitis extends the neck and rotates the head and neck so that the face is rotated toward the opposite side. Needle placement is the same as for the splenius capitus, but at a depth of 3.0 to 5.0 cm. Because of its opposite rotatory action, when compared to the splenius capitus, electromyography (EMG) is the only way to separate these two muscles for the purpose of BTX injections.

Multifidus. The multifidus muscles course in the groove between the spinous and transverse vertebral processes, deep to the semispinalis muscles. The cervical multifidus muscles arise from the articular processes of C4–7 and course diagonally and superiorly for two to three vertebral bodies, inserting into the spinous processes of the upper cervical vertebrae (Figs. 3 and 4). These muscles act to bend the neck to the same side and to rotate the neck toward the opposite side.

Rotatores cervicis. These small muscles originate from transverse spinous processes, course diagonally and superiorly, and insert into the base of the spinous process of the next cervical vertebrae (Fig. 2). They act to extend the neck and to rotate it toward the opposite side.

A needle may be placed into the multifidus or rotatores cervicis muscles by inserting the needle two finger breadths lateral to the spinous process and advancing the needle until the vertebral body is reached.

Interspinales cervicis. The interspinales muscles are six distinct pairs of muscles coursing between the spinous processes of the cervical vertebrae, the first pair from the axis to the spinous process of C3 and the last pair from the spinous process of C7 to T1 (Fig. 4). These muscles extend the neck.

Intertransversarii cervicis. These muscles are paired, with the anterior and posterior intertransversarii cervicis muscles coursing between the transverse processes of the cervical vertebrae, with the first set between the atlas and the axis and the last set between C7 and T1. Acting along they bend the neck toward the same side, and acting together they extend the neck.

Rectus capitis posterior major. The rectus capitis posterior major muscle arises from the spinous process of the axis. It courses superiorly and laterally to insert into the occipital bone, at the lateral part of the inferior nuchal line (Fig. 4). Acting alone this muscle rotates the head toward the same side. Acting together, the two rectus capitis posterior major muscles extend the neck. Needle insertion into this and the following three muscles is not advised because of the close proximity of the vertebral artery, occipital artery, and greater occipital nerve.

Rectus capitis posterior minor. This muscle arises from the tubercle on the posterior arch of the atlas, and coursing superiorly it inserts into the inferior nuchal line of the occipital bone (Fig. 4).

Obliquus capitis inferior. The obliquus capitis inferior arises from the spinous process of the axis. It courses laterally to the transverse process of the atlas (Fig. 4). This muscle rotates the head toward the same side.

Obliquus capitis superior. This muscle originates from the transverse process of the atlas, courses superiorly, and inserts into the occipital bone, between the inferior and superior nuchal lines (Fig. 4). The obliquus capitis superior extends the head and bends it laterally.

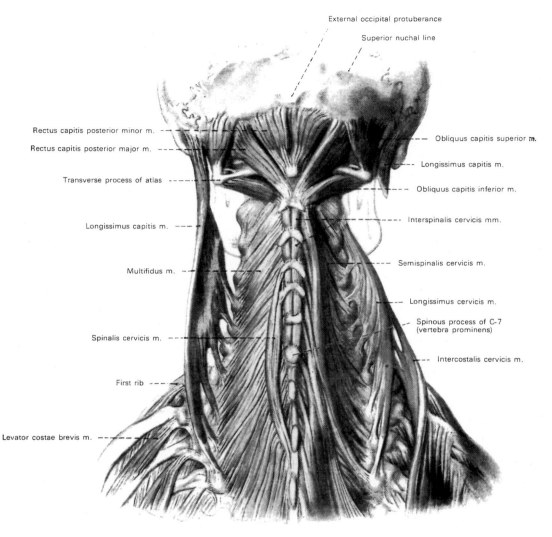

Figure 4 Anatomy of the suboccipital muscles. (Courtesy of Urban and Schwarzenberg, Munich, Germany.)

NEUROPHYSIOLOGY OF HEAD CONTROL

Central Control

The position of the head and neck is influenced by several reflex mechanisms (4). The vestibulocollic reflex is a closed-loop reflex that serves to right the head in response to angular momentum and perturbations in body posture. The vestibulo-ocular reflex is an open-loop reflex that serves to compensate for changes in head position in order to maintain a fixed or constant direction of gaze. The cervico-ocular reflex serves to maintain a constant direction of gaze in response to changes in the position of the head and neck. In normal primates this reflex is suppressed and supplanted by the vestibulo-ocular reflex (5). In addition, there are static postural reflexes such as the tonic neck reflex that are incorporated into the maintenance of posture, including head position. (For a review of these reflexes see Ref. 4.)

Bronstein and Rudge investigated the vestibulocollic response in cervical dystonia patients and in normal subjects (6). They found significant asymmetry in the response from cervical dystonia subjects. However, the directional preponderance of the abnormal response was not associated with the direction of abnormal movement caused by the dystonia. Stell et al. studied the vestibulo-ocular reflex in patients with cervical dystonia (7). They found a highly asymmetric vestibulo-ocular response in four of eight patients, with the slow phase of the response more active ipsilaterally to the direction of chin movements caused by torticollis. This asymmetry persisted after injections of BTX effectively improved head and neck position. Stell et al. (8) found that the cervico-ocular reflex is suppressed or absent in subjects with cervical dystonia, as it is in normal subjects. They concluded that the cervico-ocular reflex was not responsible for the abnormal head position in cervical dystonia. In part, these studies rely on the saccadic eye movements elicited by vestibular or proprioceptive stimulation. Saccadic function in response to visual targets is normal in cervical dystonia (9). These studies indicate that there are abnormalities in the reflex control of head, neck, and ocular movement in patients with cervical dystonia. These abnormalities appear to be due to inhibition or alteration of descending control from centers above the brain stem and not to vestibular abnormalities.

Many studies have demonstrated abnormalities in brain stem and spinal cord level reflexes in patients with dystonia. Panizza et al. (10) and Nakashima et al. (11) showed diminished reciprocal inhibition of H-reflexes in patients with different types of dystonia, including cervical dystonia. Nakashima et al. found diminished inhibition of the H-reflex specific for control of the sternocleidomastoid, but not for the masseter. They concluded that the descending control of these reflexes must be abnormal in cervical dystonia. Tolosa et al. (12) demonstrated that the R2 component of the blink reflex recovery curve, elicited by paired electrical stimuli, was abnormal in patients with cervical dystonia, blepharospasm, and cranial dystonia, in that there was diminished inhibition. Nakashima et al. (13) demonstrated similar abnormalities.

Basal ganglia control of the neck muscles is through the thalamocortical projections to the primary and supplementary motor areas or through the descending pallidal and nigral pathways to the midbrain and brainstem nuclei. Kavaklis et al. (14) have studied the basal ganglia control of the sternocleidomastoid muscle in the cat. They studied the firing rate of sternocleidomastoid motor neurons after stimulation of the globus pallidus–entopeduncular nucleus complex or cortical ablation. Repetitive stimulation of the ipsilateral globus pallidus–entopeduncular nucleus complex increased the rate of discharge, while contralateral stimulation decreased the rate of discharge. This persisted even after ablation of the motor and premotor cortices, indicating that the output from globus pallidus to the sternocleidomastoid must be through the pallidothalamic or another similar pathway. This pathway influences the pontine and medullary reticular formation, which are involved in the innervation of neck muscles (see below). Other potential pathways are the pallidonigral and nigrotectal (15), which influence saccadic eye movements (16).

Motoneurons of the Cervical Musculature

The precise locations of the cervical motor neurons for the neck muscles have not been fully established in humans. They have been studied thoroughly in the cat. Trapezius motoneurons arise from the spinal accessory nucleus, which forms a column from C1 to C5 in the lateral portion of the ventral horn in the upper segments and in the central portion in the cervical enlargement. The motoneurons for the sternocleidomastoid muscle are believed to arise from medial portion of lamina VIII near the trapezius motoneurons. The splenius motoneurons are located near the dorsal border of the ventromedial nucleus, corresponding to the ventral portion of lamina VIII and XI. The motoneurons of the suboccipital muscles have been localized to the ventromedial nuclei of C1 and C2, where they are intermingled with the motoneurons of the dorsal neck muscles (17).

The spinal accessory nerve originates from the ventral gray substance of the first five cervical segments. The fibers exit the spinal cord and ascend to join with the cranial portion of cranial nerve (CN) XI as the nerve passes through the jugular foramen. The spinal accessory nerve has two major branches to the sternocleidomastoid and trapezius muscles (2).

Innervation of Neck Muscles

The major neck muscles are innervated by a combination of cranial nerves and spinal nerves. The sternocleidomastoid and trapezius muscles are innervated by CN XI. The rest of the neck muscles are innervated by the cervical spinal nerves (2).

The ventral divisions of the first four cervical nerves join in the cervical plexus, which consists of three loops with numerous branches. The rectus capitis branches supply the rectus capitis anterior and rectus capitis lateralis. The longus capitis and longus colli branches innervate their respective muscles with branches from the first four cervical nerves. Proprioceptive fibers from the trapezius and sternocleidomastoid muscles are carried in the second and third cervical nerves. Deep branches from the third and fourth cervical nerves innervate the levator scapulae and scalenus medius muscles (2).

The dorsal divisions of the first three cervical nerves innervate the suboccipital muscles. There is considerable overlap in the innervation of the suboccipital, cervical, and thoracic muscles that are involved in neck movement. The first cervical nerve, known as the suboccipital, innervates the rectus capitis major and minor and obliquus capitis superior muscles. The second cervical nerve innervates the obliquus capitis inferior and splenius capitis muscles. The third cervical nerve innervates the splenius capitis, semi-spinalis cervicis, and obliquus capitis inferior muscles. The dorsal primary division of the fourth and fifth cervical nerves innervate the semispinalis cervicis and semispinalis capitis muscles. The sixth, seventh, and eighth divisions innervate the semispinalis cervicis, semispinalis capitis, multifidus, interspinales, splenius cervicis, iliocostalis cervicis, longissimus capitis, and longissimus cervicis muscles. The dorsal divisions of the thoracis spinal nerves innervate the spinalis thoracis and semispinalis thoracis (2).

NECK MUSCLE INVOLVEMENT IN CERVICAL DYSTONIA

Background

Cervical dystonia is the most common form of focal dystonia, yet the treatment of this disorder has been largely unrewarding until the recent application of BTX. Several prior studies have looked at muscle involvement in cervical dystonia through the use of surface electrodes, with recordings made on an electroencephalograph (18–22). One of the major drawbacks of these studies is the difficulty of differentiating the recordings obtained from overlapping neck muscles.

In order to understand better the involvement of neck muscles in cervical dystonia, we undertook a study of four pairs of major neck muscles in patients with cervical dystonia in comparison with normal controls, utilizing intramuscular recording techniques that have been previously applied to other forms of focal dystonia (23,24).

Methods

We studied 12 patients (six men and six women) who had idiopathic cervical dystonia, without evidence of other focal dystonias. Their mean age was 47 years (range 32–85), and the mean duration of their disease was 7.8 years. Patients with prior neck surgery, neck trauma, or injection of BTX were excluded from this study. For controls, four normal subjects (three men and one woman) were used, with a mean age of 53 years (range 44–77). Informed consent was obtained, and this study was approved by the Human Subjects Committee of the University of Kansas Medical Center.

Electromyographic activity was recorded from bilateral sternocleidomastoid, scalenus medius, trapezius, and splenius capitis muscles with the subjects seated on a chair that provided back, but not head, support. Recordings were made from pairs of stainless steel Teflon-coated wires (diameter 0.008 cm) introduced into the muscle belly of the selected muscles with a 22-gauge needle (23). The correct position of the needle was verified by EMG monitoring of active voluntary contraction of the selected muscles. Once the placement of the wires was verified the needle was withdrawn, leaving the wires in place, allowing the subjects to move their head and neck freely without moving the recording electrodes.

Electromyographic activity was amplified and recorded using a five-channel TECA Mystro (Pleasantville, New York) with a band pass of 100 to 10,000 Hz. The relatively high low-frequency filter was used in order to diminish the movement artifact in the recordings. Because of the recording limitation to five simultaneous channels, combinations of antagonist muscles were analyzed to provide the best recordings. The recordings were stored on-line in 1- to 10-second epochs for later analysis.

All 12 subjects with cervical dystonia were studied with their heads held in their usual positions. Four of them were able to bring the head to a midline position for a brief period and were studied under that condition as well. These four did not use a geste antagonistique to bring their heads to a midline position. The four normal subjects were studied with the head held in midline position and rotated 45° to the side.

Results

In the four normal subjects with their heads held in midline, very little muscle activity was noted (Fig. 5). With deviation of the head to the side at 45°, mild to moderate low-amplitude activity was noted from the contralateral sternocleidomastoid and trapezius muscles (Fig. 6).

In all 12 subjects with cervical dystonia, cocontraction of the contralateral sternocleidomastoid and ipsilateral splenius capitis muscles was noted. In addition, cocontraction was found in the ipsilateral scalenus medius (nine), contralateral splenius capitis (eight), contralateral scalenus medius (four), ipsilateral sternocleidomastoid (four), ipsilateral trapezius (five), and contralateral trapezius (five). Primarily a bursting pattern of contraction was noted in eight subjects, and a steady contraction pattern in four (Fig. 7A and B).

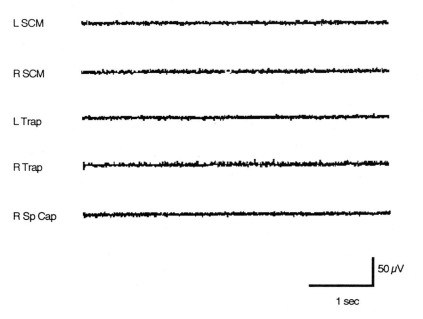

Figure 5 Multichannel fine-wire electromyographic recording of a 43 year old man, holding his head in the midline. L = left; R = right; SCM = sternocleidomastoid; Trap = trapezius; Sp Cap = splenius capitis.

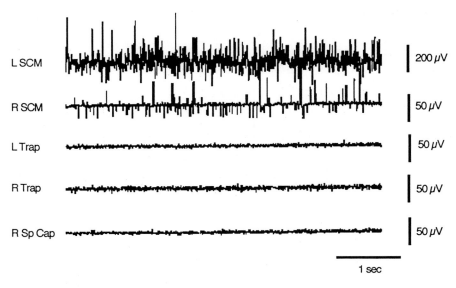

Figure 6 Multichannel fine-wire electromyographic recording of a 43 year old man, turning his head toward the right. L = left; R = right; SCM = sternocleidomastoid; Trap = trapezius; Sp Cap = splenius capitis.

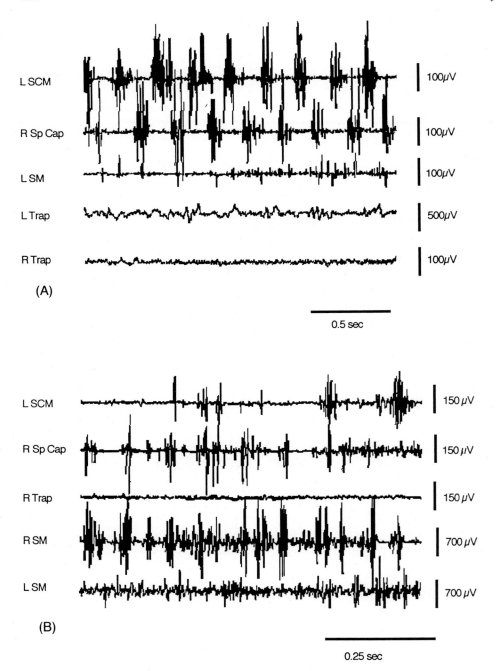

Figure 7 (A) Multichannel fine-wire electromyographic (EMG) recording of a 37-year-old woman with torticollis who has involuntary turning of her head toward the right. (B) Multichannel fine-wire EMG recording of a 57-year-old woman with torticollis who has involuntary turning of her head toward the right and tilting toward the left. L = left; R = right; SCM = sternocleidomastoid; Sp Cap = splenius capitis; SM = scalenus medius; Trap = trapezius.

Four patients with cervical dystonia were able to hold their heads in a midline position. Under this condition all four had cocontraction of the sternocleidomastoid, scalenus medius, and splenius capitis muscles (Fig. 8), and in two cases the trapezius muscles were active as well.

Discussion

As in all forms of dystonia, cervical dystonia is characterized by unusually sustained postures or muscle contractions. Prior studies have been performed with either bipolar surface electrodes or monopolar electrodes referenced to the forehead. Recordings have been performed from the sternocleidomastoid, trapezus, and splenius capitis muscles (18–22,25).

In normal subjects Podivinsky (20) found that the ipsilateral splenius capitis and contralateral sternocleidomastoid muscles provide most of the muscle activity with simple torsion, while the sternocleidomastoid muscles alone are involved with torsion combined with sagittal movement. In subjects with cervical dystonia, various patterns have been recognized including single agonist muscle involvement of either the trapezius or the sternocleidomastoid muscles (20), multiple agonist involvement (22), and various combinations of antagonist muscles (18–22,25).

Clinically, several distinct clinical patterns are seen in subjects with cervical dystonia. Pure torticollis or laterocollis is rare. Many subjects have various combinations of rotation, bending of the neck, and neck extension or flexion. The two most frequent combinations seen at our institution are turning and tilting toward the same side and crossed turning and tilting, which is often combined with mild retrocollis.

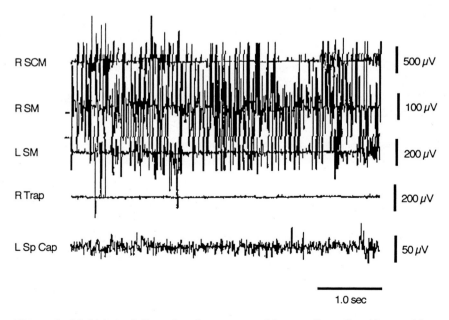

Figure 8 Multichannel fine-wire electromyographic recording of a 44-year-old woman with torticollis with involuntary turning of her head toward the left. She was instructed to try to bring her head to the midline. L = left; R = right; SCM = sternocleidomastoid; SM = scalenus medius; Trap = trapezius; Sp Cap = splenius capitis.

In our four dystonic subjects who were able to bring the head to a midline position, an increase in muscle activity was noted. These subjects did not make use of a geste antagonistique to bring their heads to midline. Buchman et al. (26) have recently presented an EMG study of cervical dystonia patients utilizing turns analysis as a measure of EMG activity. The subjects were studied with the head in the "usual" position as well as while holding the head in the midline, with or without the use of a geste antagonistique. They found a significant decrease in the number of turns for both midline conditions compared with the "usual" neck position. There was a further decrease in turns for the geste antagoniste condition, but this was not significantly different from the non–geste antagoniste position. Leis et al. (27), in a study of sensory modification of cervical dystonia, also found a decrease in muscle activity when the subject used a geste antagonistique.

Major drawbacks of former studies of muscle involvement in cervical dystonia include the imprecise localization provided by surface electrodes, attenuation of the EMG signal through the skin, the paucity of muscles that could be recorded simultaneously, and the lack of investigation of the scalenus medius muscle, which is a major muscle involved in tilting and torsion of the neck. Since this study was undertaken, additional studies performed by Thompson et al. (28) and Deuschl et al. (29) have demonstrated similar findings when recording from the superficial neck muscles. The study by Deuschl et al. (29) is of interest in that eight of their subjects with rotational torticollis had involvement of only the contralateral sternocleidomastoid muscle. Single-muscle involvement in torticollis has not been previously reported (20,26,28). One explanation is that deeper cervical muscles were involved but not recorded. Clinical experience in the treatment of cervical dystonia with the use of EMG guidance has documented that numerous muscles are active (29,30).

The present study has shown that while the primarily involved muscles in cervical dystonia are the sternocleidomastoid and splenius capitis, other muscles contribute to the abnormal torsion of the neck. This distinct pattern of cocontraction of an antagonist pair of muscles (which is the physiological hallmark of dystonia) in combination with the excessive activity required to hold the head in a midline position demonstrates the complexity of this disorder.

The complexity of the muscle involvement, reported here and by others, could explain the relatively poor results of selective peripheral nerve sectioning as well as of myotomy and myectomy (32,33). In addition, since we have demonstrated that several muscles with separate innervations are involved, microvascular decompression of the spinal accessory nerve (34) could be predicted not to be efficacious in the long-term treatment of cervical dystonia.

The application of multichannel electromyography with wire or needle recordings, demonstrating cocontraction of antagonist muscle pairs, can be of benefit in the diagnosis of cervical dystonia. In addition, accurate localization of the involved muscles would be of paramount importance in the treatment of cervical dystonia with focal injections of BTX (22).

ACKNOWLEDGMENTS

The author wishes to thank Carolyn Gray, RN and Helga Wycoff, RN, for invaluable technical support and also Steve Moon, MD, and Craig Packard, PhD, for providing the necessary translations.

REFERENCES

1. Gelb DJ, Yoshimura DM, Olney RK, Lowenstein DH, Aminoff MJ. Change in pattern of muscle activity following botulinum toxin injections for torticollis. Ann Neurol 1991;29: 370–376.
2. Clemente CD, ed. Gray's anatomy. 30th American Edition. Philadelphia: Lea & Febiger, 1985;452–475.
3. Glanzman RL, Gelb DJ, Drury I, Bromberg MB, Truong DD. Brachial plexopathy after botulinum toxin injections. Neurology 1990;40:1143.
4. Brooks VB. The neural basis for motor control. New York: Oxford University Press, 1986: 160–180.
5. Bronstein AM, Hood DJ. The cervico-ocular reflex in normal subjects and patients with absent vestibular function. Brain Res 1986;373:399–408.
6. Bronstein AM, Rudge P, The vestibular system in abnormal head postures and in spasmodic torticollis. In: Fahn S, Marsden CD, Calne DB, eds. Dystonia 2. Advances in neurology, vol. 50. New York: Raven Press, 1988: 493–500.
7. Stell R, Bronstein AM, Marsden CD. Vestibulo-ocular abnormalities in spasmodic torticollis before and after botulinum toxin injections. J Neurol Neurosurg Psychiatry 1989;52:57–62.
8. Stell R, Gresty M, Metcalfe T, Bronstein AM. Cervico-ocular function in patients with spasmodic torticollis. J Neurol Neurosurg Psychiatry 1991;54:39–41.
9. Stell R, Bronstein AM, Gresty M, Buckwell D, Marsden CD. Saccadic function in spasmodic torticollis. J Neurol Neurosurg Psychiatry 1990;53:496–501.
10. Panizza M, Lelli S, Nilsson J, Hallett M. H-reflex recovery curve and reciprocal inhibition of H-reflex in different kinds of dystonia. Neurology 1990;40:824–828.
11. Nakashima K, Thompson PD, Rothwell JC, et al. An exteroceptive reflex in the sterno-cleidomastoid muscle produced by electrical stimulation of the supraorbital nerve in normal subjects and patients with spasmodic torticollis. Neurology 1989;39:1354–1358.
12. Tolosa E, Montserrat L, Bayes A. Blink reflex studies in focal dystonias: enhanced excitability of brainstem interneurons in cranial dystonia and spasmodic torticollis. Mov Disord 1988;3:61–69.
13. Nakashima K, Rothwell JC, Thompson PD, et al. The blink reflex in patients with idiopathic torsion dystonia. Arch Neurol 1990;47:413–416.
14. Kavaklis O, Shima F, Kato M, Fukui M. Ipsilateral pallidal control on the sterno-cleidomastoid muscle in cats: relationship to the side of thalamotomy for torticollis. Neuro-surgery 1992;30:724–730.
15. Hattori T, Fibiger HC, McGeer PL. Demonstration of pallidonigral projection to dopami-nergic neurons. J Comp Neurol 1975;162:487–504.
16. Hikosaka O, Wurtz RH. Visual and oculomotor function of monkey substantia nigra pars reticulata. IV. Relations of substantia nigra to superior colliculus. J. Neurophysiol 1983; 49:1285–1301.
17. Rose PK, Keeirstead SA. Cervical motoneurons. In: Peterson BW, Richmond FJ, eds. Control of head movement. New York: Oxford University Press, 1988;37–49.
18. Hertz E, Hoeffer PFA. Spasmodic torticollis. I. Physiologic analysis of involuntary motor activity. Arch Neurol Psychiatry 1949;61:129–136.
19. Tournay A, Paillard J. Torticollis spasmodique et électromyographie. Rev Neurol 1955; 93:347–355.
20. Podivinsky F. Torticollis. In: Vinken PJ, Bruyn GW, eds. Handbook of clinical neurology. Vol. 6. Amsterdam: North Holland, 1968:567–603.
21. Raeva SN, Vasin NY, Vainberg VA, Shabalov VA, Medzhidov MR. Electromyography in patients with spasmodic torticollis. Zhurnal Voprosy Neirokhirurgii Imeni N. N. Burdenko. 1987;5:46–53.

22. Tsui JKC, Eisen A, Caine DB. Botulinum toxin in spasmodic torticollis. In: Fahn S, Marsden CD, Calne DB eds. Dystonia 2. Advances in neurology, vol. 50. New York: Raven Press. 1988:593–597.

23. Basmajian JV. Electrodes and electrode connectors. In: Desmedt JE, ed. New developments in EMG and clinical neurophysiology. Vol. 1. Basel: Karger, 1973:502–510.

24. Cohen LG, Hallett M. Hand cramps: clinical features and electromyographic patterns in a focal dystonia. Neurology 1988;38:1005–1012.

25. Vasin NI, Safronov VA, Medzhidov MR, Shabalov VA. Voluntary activity of the neck muscles in patients with spastic torticollis. Nevropatol Psikhiatr 1988;87:7–10.

26. Buchman AS, Comella CL, Stebbins GT, Goetz CG. Quantitative electromyographic assessment of geste antagoniste in cervical dystonia. Muscle Nerve 1992;15:1173.

27. Leis AA, Dimitrijevic MR, Delapasse JS. Sharkey PC. Modification of cervical dystonia by selective sensory stimulation. J Neurol Sci 1992;110:79–89.

28. Thompson PD, Stell R, Maccabe JJ, Day BL, Rothwell JC, Marsden CD. Electromyography of neck muscles and treatment in spasmodic torticollis. In: Berrardelli A, Benecke R, Manfredi M, Marsden CD, eds. Motor disturbances II. London: Harcourt Brace Jovanovich, 1990;289–304.

29. Deuschl G, Heinen F, Kleedorfer B, et al. Clinical and polymyographic investigation of spasmodic torticollis. J Neurol 1992;239:9–15.

30. Dubinsky RM, Gray C, Vetere-Overfield B, Koller WC. Electromyographic guidance of botulinum toxin injections in cervical dystonia. Clin Neuropharmacol 1991;12:262–267.

31. Comella CL, Buchman AS, Tanner CM, Brown-Toms, Goetz CG. Botulinum toxin injections for spasmodic torticollis: Increased magnitude of benefit with electromyographic assistance. Neurology 1992;42:878–882.

32. Xinkang C. Selective resection and denervation of cervical muscles in the treatment of spasmodic torticollis: results in 60 cases. Neuropsychology 1981;8:680–688.

33. Hernesniemi J, Keranen T. Long-term outcome after surgery for spasmodic torticollis. Acta Neurochirurg (Wien) 1990;103:128–130.

34. Sima F, Fukui M, Kitamura K, Kuromatsu C, Okamura T. Diagnosis and surgical treatment of spasmodic torticollis of 11th nerve origin. Neurosurgery 1988;22:358–363.

17

Clinical Neurophysiology of Cervical Dystonia

Michael J. Aminoff and Richard K. Olney
University of California at San Francisco, San Francisco, California

INTRODUCTION

Abnormal cervical postures may result from local musculoskeletal changes (such as fibrotic changes in the neck muscles or fracture-dislocations of the cervical spine), but the term "cervical dystonia" implies an abnormal cervical posture produced by muscular overactivity resulting from dysfunction of the central nervous system, and in particular the basal ganglia. Dystonic movements are distinguished from normal voluntary movements by the high degree of coactivation of agonist and antagonist muscles. Dystonic movements may occur spontaneously or may be precipitated by voluntary activity. In cervical dystonia the abnormal contraction of muscles in the neck leads to abnormal movements or postures involving the head.

ELECTROMYOGRAPHIC STUDIES

Herz and Hoefer (1) provided a physiological analysis of cervical dystonia and distinguished between several types of involuntary motor activity. First, there was a predominantly tonic pattern, with sustained clinical and electromyographic (EMG) activity. Second, quick jerking movements occurred at irregular intervals and with varying duration. Third, rhythmic activity was seen to occur either alone or superimposed on more continuous dystonic activity. Muscles on both sides of the neck were found to be involved far more frequently than had previously been appreciated, and in most cases the pattern of activity was more complex than was suggested by the clinical appearance.

When relaxed patients are studied in the EMG laboratory as they are lying quietly on the examination couch, little—if any—involuntary muscle activity may be recorded. However, involuntary movements or postures may persist to some extent and lead either to periods of continuous EMG activity interrupted by short periods of electrical silence or to repetitive bursts of EMG activity that occur regularly or irregularly and last for a variable period (usually 1–2 sec). Rapid, irregular, brief (100 msec) jerks reminiscent of myoclonus may also be found (2). During voluntary contraction of the cervical muscles or with postural maintenance, there is coactivation of agonist and antagonist muscles. In addition, patients with torticollis may have an associated postural tremor in the outstretched arms, with a frequency of between 6 and 10 Hz.

Many patients with cervical dystonia find that light touch or pressure on parts of the face or neck reduces the severity of abnormal posturing. The physiological basis for this so-called *geste antagonistique* of counterpressure is uncertain. Sherrington (3) found that pressure on the skin around the muzzle of a decerebrate cat brought about a relaxation of previously contracted muscles in the neck. Other authors have described or speculated about the phenomenon without really advancing matters, attributing it to proprioceptive reflexes without further elaboration.

Stejskal (4) studied a group of 65 patients with cervical dystonia to determine the characteristics of the geste antagonistique and found that both the location and the direction of any counterpressure were important. Electromyographic analysis suggested that counterpressure could either inhibit the muscles (and their synergists) primarily responsible for the dystonic movements or postures, activate antagonistic neck muscles in order to enable voluntary correction of the abnormal head position, or produce a general inhibition of the activity of neck muscles. The most common EMG change induced by the counterpressure was decrease or extinction of activity in the muscles primarily responsible for the abnormal head posture, and in any synergistic muscles in the neck, together with activation of the contralateral antagonist muscles. Stejskal (4) suggested that counterpressure was neither a proprioceptive reflex nor the result of nociceptive stimulation in the trigeminal area, and that it did not depend on tonic neck reflexes. Instead, it was held to be a voluntary device serving to counteract (by some ill-defined mechanism) the abnormal postures or movements of cervical dystonia because their plane and direction were predictable.

The control system for neck movement has been referred to as overcomplete because there are more muscles available than are required to accomplish specific movements (5,6). As a consequence, any specific neck movement may be produced by several different patterns of muscle activity (7). For any particular task, electrophysiological studies have shown that individual neck muscles participate in a consistent manner (5,8). With different tasks, different patterns of activity in the neck muscles may produce the same head position. Accordingly, in different patients with cervical dystonia an abnormal head posture of identical appearance may be produced by the abnormal or excessive activity of different combinations of neck muscles. This is of major clinical relevance with regard to the treatment of cervical dystonia. In most patients who are to be treated by injection of botulinum toxin (BTX), the muscles to be injected are selected on clinical grounds based primarily on the observed head posture. Clearly, however, this is not completely reliable in itself, and a poor response to treatment may reflect the injection of muscles that were not primarily responsible for the abnormal head posture.

Gelb et al. (9) studied 20 patients with cervical dystonia by EMG examination of their neck muscles, performed before and after a series of therapeutic injections with BTX. The pattern of muscle activity was found to have changed after the injections, even when head position had returned to baseline, and there was an increase in EMG activity in noninjected muscles. Such a change in the pattern of muscle activity did not depend on whether clinical benefit followed the injections. Such results suggest that the underlying abnormality in patients with cervical dystonia involves a general motor program for head position, rather than the selective overactivity of individual muscles.

From the study of Gelb et al. (9), it is apparent that EMG studies may be helpful in identifying the most actively involved muscles in patients with cervical dystonia who are to be treated by injections of BTX. This may be of particular relevance when a patient who initially responded well to BTX subsequently becomes less responsive, because the EMG findings will then be useful in guiding any adjustment of the injection sites.

Neurophysiological techniques have also been used as a means of providing sensory feedback therapy (biofeedback) to patients with cervical dystonia. An attempt is made to improve volitional control of the overactive muscle groups by means of audiovisual displays of the activity monitored from affected muscles. In one study, for example, each of 13 patients with cervical dystonia was able to maintain the head in the neutral position for much longer after an 8- to 12-week course of therapy by this means than before such treatment (10). The mechanisms of improvement after EMG feedback therapy are poorly understood (11).

Another therapeutic approach to cervical dystonia is selective peripheral denervation, with sparing of muscles having normal function. Accordingly, it is of paramount importance to distinguish between normally and abnormally active muscles as completely as possible by EMG examination, with simultaneous recording from both agonist and antagonist muscles. Usually more muscles are involved than is clinically suspected. In one study, the most striking feature electrophysiologically was the degree to which antagonists of the active muscles were sometimes inhibited (12). The patient may therefore need biofeedback to learn to use the inhibited muscles following surgical treatment. In some instances, as when there is pronounced laterocollis, any retraining may be complicated by the fact that the muscles have been stretched for a long time.

EXTEROCEPTIVE REFLEXES

The overactivity of muscles in cervical dystonia differs from voluntary activation in the reduced depth of inhibition produced by exteroceptive stimuli. Nakashima and co-workers (13) examined the activity level of the sternocleidomastoid muscles and the time course of its inhibition (or silent period) following supraorbital nerve stimulation in 10 normal subjects and in nine patients with cervical dystonia. In normal subjects, a suppression of the surface-recorded, rectified, integrated EMG activity began around 35 msec after stimulation and persisted for about 35 msec. The depth of this suppression had a mean of 37% ipsilaterally and 41% contralaterally in comparison with the prestimulus (background) level of sternocleidomastoid muscle activity. In patients with cervical dystonia, the time course for this suppressive phase was similar, but the mean depth of suppression was significantly less, being 23% ($p < 0.05$) ipsilateral to supraorbital stimulation and 17% contralaterally ($p < 0.001$). These investigators also examined suppression of masseter muscle activity following supraorbital nerve stimulation (the masseter silent period). The depth of the masseter silent period was similar for normal subjects and patients. Thus, the reduction in depth of the silent period was seen in muscles affected by dystonia, but not in a clinically unaffected muscle. These data suggest that cervical dystonia is associated with a reduced function of inhibitory interneural networks that act on the lower motor neuron pool of affected muscles.

VESTIBULAR REFLEXES

Whereas the preceding EMG and exteroceptive reflex studies reflect abnormalities that may be the result or expression of cervical dystonia, other types of neurophysiological investigation have identified abnormalities in patients with cervical and other dystonias that may reflect the underlying central dysfunction. Perhaps the most long-standing suggestion in this regard is that the vestibular system may be involved in patients with cervical dystonia. In 1926, Lord Brain (14) reviewed the extensive literature that described unilateral lesions of the internal ear and eighth nerve as a cause for abnormal head postures in experimental animals and in humans. More contemporary, systematic investigation of vestibular function in patients with cervical dystonia but no other neurological or otological symptoms was begun by Bronstein and Rudge in 1986 (15). In more than 70% of 35 cases, they found a directional preponderance of vestibular nystagmus in the dark, in a direction contralateral to the side to which the chin pointed. They concluded that there was primary involvement of the vestibular system in cervical dystonia, perhaps as part of a dysfunction of central mechanisms conveying sensory information responsible for orientation of the head and eyes. However, this initial study left unanswered whether the vestibular abnormalities were primary or secondary to the cervical dystonia. Others have reported abnormalities of otolith function in patients with cervical dystonia, as indicated by measurement of ocular counter-rolling evoked at low-frequency rotation, as well as evidence of central vestibular dysfunction (16).

In a more recent study of patients with cervical dystonia, the vestibulo-ocular reflex was studied before and after correction of head posture with BTX (17). Stell et al. found that four of their eight patients showed a significantly asymmetric response, with the slow phase of the vestibulo-ocular reflex being more active on the same side as the chin. The asymmetry of vestibular function persisted despite marked improvement in head posture after injection with BTX, suggesting that the reflex abnormalities were not caused by the head posture itself but reflected primary vestibular involvement. Support for this concept is derived from the observations of Denny-Brown (18), who described patients in whom the severity of torticollis was markedly affected by turning. Stell and associates (17) pointed out that there are at least two ways in which cervical dystonia and the vestibular system may be related. First, cervical dystonia may be due, at least in part, to hyperactive, disinhibited, or otherwise abnormal vestibulocollic reflexes that serve in animals to maintain the head in a stable position in space. The importance of such reflexes in humans is unclear, however, and Stell et al. therefore favored a second possibility, in which there is a more widespread, central derangement of various sensorimotor mechanisms controlling head posture in cervical dystonia. This latter possibility is favored by their more recent investigation, in which they studied the cervico-ocular reflex and interactions between the cervico-ocular and vestibulo-ocular reflexes in seven patients with cervical dystonia and in six normal controls (19). They further concluded that the frequent asymmetry in vestibulo-ocular reflexes is primary in cervical dystonia because (1) the cervico-ocular reflex was weak or absent in both groups; (2) the vestibulo-ocular reflex gain was similar in the two groups but asymmetric only in five patients; and (3) there was no evidence of abnormal cervicovestibular interaction during active head rotation.

The primary nature of vestibular hyperactivity has been challenged by others. Huygen and co-workers (20) found significantly elevated gain to the vestibulo-ocular reflex in seven of eight patients with cervical dystonia. Because this type of abnormality usually produces vertigo in humans, rather than abnormal head posture, they concluded that the vestibular hyperactivity is secondary to, rather than causative of, cervical dystonia.

Although asymmetries in the vestibulo-ocular reflex are frequent in cervical dystonia, this type of abnormality is neither necessary (30% of patients with cervical dystonia did not have such an abnormality in the study of Bronstein and Rudge [15]) nor sufficient to explain fully the physiological basis for the dystonia.

BLINK REFLEX RECOVERY CURVES

Increased excitability of brain stem interneurons based on enhanced blink reflex recovery curves was first demonstrated in patients with blepharospasm (21,22) and oromandibular dystonia (21) in 1985, and later in patients with cervical dystonia. To obtain a blink reflex recovery curve, paired stimuli of equal intensity are delivered to the supraorbital nerve at varying interstimulus intervals. The intensity is set at a level to produce an R1 reflex of maximal amplitude in response to the first (''conditioning'') stimulus. The second (or ''test'') stimulus is delivered at varying intervals after the normal reflex response. The reflex is held to have recovered completely at interstimulus intervals in which its amplitude or area in response to the test stimulus equals that to the conditioning stimulus. The *blink reflex recovery curve* is a plot of the amplitude or area of the response from the test stimulus (usually expressed as a percentage of the conditioned response) over time (expressed as the interstimulus interval between conditioning and test stimuli).

Tolosa and co-workers (23) included eight patients with cervical dystonia in their 1988 study of 31 patients with various focal dystonias. Blink reflexes were recorded with surface electrodes from the ipsilateral orbicularis oculi muscle. For statistical analysis, area of the R2 response was estimated by the product of amplitude and duration. Recovery curves were constructed by expressing estimated area of the test response as a percentage of the estimated area of the conditioned response. Patients with blepharospasm, cervical dystonia, or spasmodic dysphonia had an abnormally rapid recovery of the R2 component of the blink reflex, which started around 300 msec. Furthermore, half of the patients with blepharospasm (but not those with cervical dystonia) had an initial facilitation of the R2 response between 30 and 250 msec, whereas there was virtually complete suppression of the R2 response over this time in control subjects. Patients with brachial dystonia had normal recovery curves for the R2 response. All groups of these dystonias had normal recovery curves for the R1 response.

Nakashima and colleagues (24) examined the blink reflex recovery to paired stimuli in 25 normal controls and 57 patients with various forms of idiopathic dystonia, including 19 with cervical dystonia. None of the patients had blepharospasm. Area was measured by the rectified, integrated, surface-recorded EMG activity. The amplitude and latency of the R1 and R2 components of the blink reflex were similar in patients and controls, except for an increase in ipsilateral R2 amplitude in patients with generalized dystonia. Recovery curves with multiple interstimulus intervals from 100 msec to 2000 msec were constructed for 31 patients and 10 controls, and they suggested that the 500-msec interval produced the greatest difference between control subjects and dystonic patients. Accordingly, all 57 patients and 25 controls were studied with an interstimulus interval of 500 msec. A significant enhancement of R2 reflex recovery was found in patients with cervical dystonia, segmental dystonia (cervical and arm involvement), or generalized dystonia, but not in patients with arm dystonia (without associated cervical involvement). At this interval, the R2 had recovered 35% of its conditioned value in normal subjects but about 60% in patients with cervical dystonia. Blink reflex recovery of the R1 response was normal for all groups.

Because the R1 response of the blink reflex and the R1 recovery curves are normal, oligosynaptic pontine interneuronal interactions appear to be normal in dystonias. However, the early and enhanced recovery of the R2 response demonstrates abnormal inhibitory, polysynaptic interneuronal networks in patients with cervical dystonia, blepharospasm, oromandibular dystonia, and generalized dystonia, but not in patients with brachial dystonia.

H-REFLEX RECOVERY CURVE AND RECIPROCAL INHIBITION OF THE H-REFLEX

Among the idiopathic dystonias, reciprocal inhibition of the H-reflex of the flexor carpi radialis muscle was studied first in patients with writer's cramp and other dystonias that affected forearm muscles (2,25,26). To determine reciprocal inhibition, single and paired stimuli are applied alternately. One stimulus (the test stimulus) is always delivered and is selected to elicit an H-reflex of standard amplitude or area; when delivered alone, it produces an unconditioned H-reflex. The other stimulus (the conditioning stimulus) is delivered at varying intervals relative to the test stimulus. For these studies of reciprocal inhibition, the conditioning stimulus was an electrical stimulus delivered to the radial nerve near the elbow, with an intensity at or near motor threshold.

Three phases of reciprocal inhibition were found in control subjects. The first occurred when the conditioning and test stimuli were applied simultaneously. In patients with writer's cramp, this phase of inhibition was found to be reduced by some authors (26) but not by others (25). The second phase of inhibition occurred in controls when the conditioning stimulus was delivered 10 to 20 msec before the test stimulus, and this phase was reduced in patients with writer's cramp (25,26). Panizza and colleagues (26) analyzed the third phase of inhibition, which was maximal at a 75-msec interstimulus interval in controls, and this also was reduced in patients with writer's cramp.

Panizza and colleagues (27) later extended their observations to include patients with other forms of dystonia, including 10 with cervical dystonia, and they also studied the H-reflex recovery curve. The *recovery curve for the H-reflex* of the flexor carpi radialis is analogous to the recovery curve for the blink reflex, as discussed earlier in this chapter, except that the conditioning and test stimuli are delivered to the median nerve just above the elbow, and the intensity of the conditioning stimulus is set at a level to produce an H-reflex of standard amplitude or area. In healthy control subjects, the recovery curve had a phase of partial recovery or facilitation at an interstimulus interval of 200 msec, between two phases of inhibition. The mean level of recovery in normal subjects was 66% at 200 msec, whereas patients with cervical dystonia had a more complete recovery (mean 90%) at this interval. Patients with generalized dystonia had not only a modest ''potentiation'' (mean 104%) at 200 msec but also less inhibition before and after this potentiation. H-reflex recovery in the groups with blepharospasm and writer's cramp was the same as in control subjects.

With measurement of reciprocal inhibition of the forearm H-reflex, the depth of inhibition in control subjects had a mean amplitude that was 47% of unconditioned amplitude with the 0-msec interstimulus interval (simultaneous stimuli), a mean of 61% at the 10-msec interval, and a mean of 69% at the 75-msec interval. Groups of patients with cervical dystonia, blepharospasm, or generalized dystonia had less inhibition at 0 msec and 10 msec. Furthermore, patients with cervical or generalized dystonia had potentiation rather than inhibition at intervals of 75 msec (means of 105% and 122%, respectively) and 200 msec (means of 119% for each group).

Thus, patients with cervical dystonia have abnormal potentiation of H-reflex recovery at the 200-msec interval between paired stimuli, reduced reciprocal inhibition of the forearm H-reflex when 0 or 10 msec separate the conditioning and test stimuli, and modest "potentiation" rather than reciprocal inhibition at interstimulus intervals of 75 msec and 200 msec.

H-reflex recovery curves and studies of reciprocal inhibition of the H-reflex identify reduced inhibition or enhanced facilitation of interneuronal networks that influence muscles not affected clinically by cervical dystonia. H-reflex recovery at the 200-msec interval may be mediated by cutaneous afferents through segmental or long-loop reflex mechanisms (27). Abnormal potentiation of recovery at this interval is not specific for cervical or generalized dystonia, because it may also be seen in Parkinson's disease, spasticity, and cerebellar disorders (25,28–30). The first phase of reciprocal inhibition of the H-reflex is mediated by Ia interneurons and the second phase by presynaptic inhibition (31,32). Both of these types of inhibition are reduced in dystonias, including blepharospasm and limb, cervical, or generalized dystonia. The physiological basis for the third period of reciprocal inhibition is uncertain but probably is polysynaptic (27). The net potentiation observed in cervical and generalized dystonia may result from functional loss of inhibitory interneurons or an enhanced influence of facilitatory ones.

EVOKED POTENTIALS

Multimodality evoked potentials have been recorded in small groups of patients with idiopathic cervical dystonia. In one such study, 10 patients with cervical dystonia were studied by visual, auditory, and short-latency median and peroneal somatosensory evoked potentials in order to detect any evidence of physiological dysfunction along these major afferent pathways, but normal results were obtained in every case (33). More recently, Reilly and co-workers (34) recorded the short-latency median-derived somatosensory evoked potential in 10 patients with focal, segmental, or generalized dystonia. They recorded from multiple sites on the scalp with linked earlobes as reference and directed their attention at the P15, N20, P45, and N30 components of the response. The only abnormality detected was that the amplitude of the frontal N30 was greater than in controls, but this finding is of particular interest because this same component is diminished in amplitude in patients with Parkinson's disease (35). The N30 is thought to arise from the region of the supplementary motor area, which is a major cortical target for efferent pathways from the basal ganglia, and changes in amplitude of N30 may therefore reflect basal ganglia dysfunction.

REFERENCES

1. Herz E, Hoefer PFA. Spasmodic torticollis. 1. Physiologic analysis of involuntary motor activity. Arch Neurol Psychiatry 1949;61:129–136.
2. Rothwell JC, Obeso JA, Day BL, Marsden CD. Pathophysiology of dystonias. In: Desmedt JE, ed. Motor control mechanisms in health and disease. New York: Raven Press, 1983: 851–863.
3. Sherrington CS. Cited by Stejskal L. Counterpressure in torticollis. J Neurol Sci 1980;48: 9–19.

4. Stejskal L. Counterpressure in torticollis. J Neurol Sci 1980;48:9–19.
5. Keshner EA, Peterson BW. Motor control strategies underlying head stabilization and voluntary head movements in humans and cats. Prog Brain Res 1988;76:329–339.
6. Pellionisz AJ, Peterson BW. A tensorial model of neck motor activation. In: Peterson BW, Richmond FJ, eds. Control of head movement. New York: Oxford University Press, 1988: 178–186.
7. Abbs JH, Cole KJ. Neural mechanisms of motor equivalence and goal achievement. In: Wise SP, ed. Higher brain functions: recent explorations of the brain's emergent properties. New York: John Wiley & Sons 1987:15–43.
8. Keshner EA, Campbell D, Katz RT, Peterson BW. Neck muscle activation patterns in humans during isometric head stabilization. Exp Brain Res 1989;75:335–344.
9. Gelb DJ, Yoshimura DM, Olney RK, Lowenstein DH, Aminoff MJ. Change in pattern of muscle activity following botulinum toxin injections for torticollis. Ann Neurol 1991;29: 370–376.
10. Brudny J, Korein J, Levidow L, Grynbaum BB, Lieberman A, Friedmann LW. Sensory feedback therapy as a modality of treatment in central nervous system disorders of voluntary movement. Neurology 1974;24:925–932.
11. Korein J, Brudny J. Integrated EMG feedback in the management of spasmodic torticollis and focal dystonia: A prospective study of 80 patients. In: Yahr MD, ed. The basal ganglia. New York: Raven Press, 1976:385–424.
12. Bertrand C, Negro PM, Martinez SN. Technical aspects of selective peripheral denervation for spasmodic torticollis. Appl Neurophysiol 1982;45:326–330.
13. Nakashima K, Thompson PD, Rothwell JC, Day BL, Stell R, Marsden CD. An exteroceptive reflex in the sternocleidomastoid muscle produced by electrical stimulation of the supraorbital nerve in normal subjects and patients with spasmodic torticollis. Neurology 1989;39: 1354–1358.
14. Brain WR. On the rotated or "cerebellar" posture of the head. Brain 1926;49:61–76.
15. Bronstein AM, Rudge P. Vestibular involvement in spasmodic torticollis. J Neurol Neurosurg Psychiatry 1986;49:290–295.
16. Diamond SG, Markham CH, Baloh RW. Ocular counterrolling abnormalities in spasmodic torticollis. Arch Neurol 1988;45:164–169.
17. Stell R, Bronstein AM, Marsden CD. Vestibulo-ocular abnormalities in spasmodic torticollis before and after botulinum toxin injections. J Neurol Neurosurg Psychiatry 1989;52:57–62.
18. Denny-Brown D. Clinical symptomatology of diseases of the basal ganglia. In: Vinken PJ, Bruyn GW, eds. Handbook of clinical neurology. Vol 6. Amsterdam: Elsevier, 1968; 133–172.
19. Stell R, Gresty M, Metcalfe T, Bronstein AM. Cervico-ocular function in patients with spasmodic torticollis. J Neurol Neurosurg Psychiatry 1991;54:39–41.
20. Huygen PLM, Verhagen WIM, Van Hoof JJM, Horstink MWIM. Vestibular hyperreactivity in patients with idiopathic spasmodic torticollis. J Neurol Neurosurg Psychiatry 1989;52: 782–785.
21. Berardelli A, Rothwell JC, Day BL, Marsden CD. Pathophysiology of blepharospasm and oromandibular dystonia. Brain 1985;108:593–608.
22. Tolosa ES, Montserrat L. Depressed blink reflex habituation in dystonic blepharospasm. Neurology 1985;35(Suppl 1):271.
23. Tolosa E, Montserrat L, Bayes A. Blink reflex studies in patients with focal dystonias. In: Fahn S et al, eds. Dystonia 2. Advances in neurology, vol. 50. New York: Raven Press, 1988:517–524.
24. Nakashima K, Rothwell JC, Thompson PD, et al. The blink reflex in patients with idiopathic torsion dystonia. Arch Neurol 1990;47:413–416.
25. Nakashima K, Rothwell JC, Day BL, Thompson PD, Shannon K, Marsden CD. Reciprocal inhibition between forearm muscles in patients with writer's cramp and other occupational cramps, symptomatic hemidystonia and hemiparesis due to stroke. Brain 1989;112:681–697.

26. Panizza ME, Hallett M, Nilsson J. Reciprocal inhibition in patients with hand cramps. Neurology 1989;39:85–89.
27. Panizza M, Lelli S, Nilsson J, Hallett M. H-reflex recovery curve and reciprocal inhibition of H-reflex in different kinds of dystonia. Neurology 1990;40:824–828.
28. Olsen PZ, Diamantopoulos E. Excitability of spinal motor neurones in normal subjects and patients with spasticity, Parkinsonian rigidity, and cerebellar hypotonia. J Neurol Neurosurg Psychiatry 1967;30:325–331.
29. Yap C-B. Spinal segmental and long-loop reflexes on spinal motoneurone excitability in spasticity and rigidity. Brain 1967;90:887–896.
30. McLeod JG. H reflex studies in patients with cerebellar disorders. J Neurol Neurosurg Psychiatry 1969;32:21–27.
31. Day BL, Marsden CD, Obeso JA, Rothwell JC. Reciprocal inhibition between the muscles of the human forearm. J Physiol 1984;349:519–534.
32. Berardelli A, Day BL, Marsden CD, Rothwell JC. Evidence favouring presynaptic inhibition between antagonist muscle afferents in the human forearm. J Physiol 1987;391:71–83.
33. Narayan TM, Ludwig C, Sato S. A study of multimodality evoked responses in idiopathic spasmodic torticollis. Electroencephalogr Clin Neurophysiol 1986;63:239–241.
34. Reilly JA, Hallett M, Cohen LG, Tarkka IM, Dang N. The N30 component of somatosensory evoked potentials in patients with dystonia. Electroencephalogr Clin Neurophysiol 1992; 84:243–247.
35. Rossini PM, Babiloni F, Bernardi G, et al. Abnormalities of short-latency somatosensory evoked potentials in parkinsonian patients. Electroencephalogr Clin Neurophysiol 1989; 74:277–289.

18

Experience with Botulinum Toxin in Cervical Dystonia

W. Poewe and Jörg Wissel
Free University of Berlin, Berlin, Germany

INTRODUCTION

Botulinum toxin (BTX) type A was first used therapeutically to correct strabismus by temporarily paralyzing extraocular muscles (1). Subsequently it was used successfully for essential blepharospasm and Meige syndrome, and the American Academy of Neurology has recommended local BTX injections as a first-line treatment of these types of cranial dystonia (2).

Following an initial double-blind study by Tsui and colleagues (3), cervical dystonia has developed into the second major neurological indication for local BTX injections. Published reports now cover several thousands sets of injections in hundreds of patients, and this chapter will review the experience with BTX treatment of cervical dystonia that has accumulated in the literature over the past 6 years.

INJECTION TECHNIQUE AND DOSES

Selection of Muscles

Correct identification of the muscles responsible for abnormal postures and movements is an essential prerequisite for successful local BTX injections in cervical dystonia. Muscle selection for injections can be based on four sets of criteria:

Analysis of apparent head deviation
Dystonic muscle activation as indicated by hypertrophy and/or stiffening of muscles
Localization of neck pain
Electromyographic (EMG)-polygraphic features

To derive useful conclusions from observable head deviations it is essential to be aware of the major biomechanical forces exerted on the head and cervical spine by various neck

Table 1 Biomechanical Action of Major Neck Muscles

Muscle	Action on head position
Splenius capitis and cervicis	Ipsilateral rotation and lateroflexion; retroflexion (synergistic with contralateral splenius)
Sternocleidomastoid	Contralateral rotation; ipsilateral lateroflexion; anteflexion (synergistic with contralateral splenius)
Trapezius	Contralateral rotation; ipsilateral lateroflexion; retroflexion (synergistic with contralateral trapezius); ipsilateral shoulder elevation
Levator scapulae	Ipsilateral lateroflexion and rotation; ipsilateral shoulder elevation
Deep neck extensors (semispinalis capitis and cervicis; longissimus capitis and cervicis)	Retroflexion with bilateral activation; ipsilateral lateroflexion and rotation
Suboccipital muscles (rectus capitis posterior major and minor; obliquus capitis inferior and superior)	Ipsilateral rotation; retroflexion with bilateral activation

muscles. Table 1 lists the main actions of the most important neck muscles on head position. Not all of these muscle are accessible for local BTX injections.

The prevailing patterns of head deviation in cervical dystonia are shown in Fig. 1 and include rotational torticollis, laterocollis, retrocollis, and complex patterns (Fig. 1a–c). In studying 100 patients with cervical dystonia clinically and by means of polymyography, Deuschl and colleagues (4) were able to identify characteristic patterns of dystonic muscle activation in three of these four clinical types (Fig. 2).

In routine practice, localization of neck pain is another useful criterion for muscle selection, since pain frequently corresponds to areas of maximal muscle stiffening. A clinical approach using visible hypertrophy, palpable muscle stiffening, analysis of head deviation, and localization of pain will thus lead to correct identification of dystonically active muscles in many patients. In cases of complex multidimensional head deviation or for patients failing to respond adequately to an injection, polymyography may be useful in identifying further muscles involved (4,5).

Injection Techniques

Injections can be made from tuberculin syringes using 27-gauge hypodermic needles for superficial neck muscles such as the sternocleidomastoid, trapezius, and splenius capitis muscles. For deeper layers of muscles EMG guidance using Teflon-coated 24-gauge needles may be appropriate. Figure 3 illustrates the anatomical localization of the most frequently used injections into the sternocleidomastoid, splenius capitis, and trapezius muscles. It is sufficient to place injections into the middle portion of a muscle belly without further EMG-guided localization of the motor point (see Fig. 4).

In several studies Botulinum toxin type A (BTX-A) was injected at multiple sites along the muscle belly in order to achieve evenly distributed chemical denervation (6–8), while

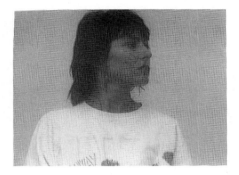

(a)

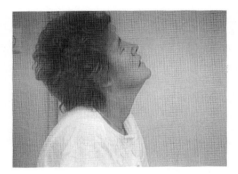

(b)

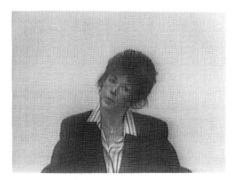

(c)

Figure 1 Prevailing patterns of head deviation in cervical dystonia: (a) rotational torticollis; (b) retrocollis; (c) laterocollis.

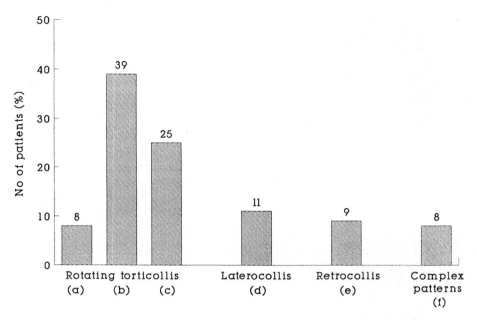

Figure 2 Distribution of dystonic electromyographic activity in 100 patients with cervical dystonia. (a) One muscle (ipsilateral splenius capitis or contralateral sternocleidomastoid). (b) Two muscles (ipsilateral splenius capitis and contralateral sternocleidomastoid). (c) Three muscles (contralateral sternocleidomastoid and bilateral splenius capitis). (d) Two or three ipsilateral muscles (splenius capitis and/or sternocleidomastoid and/or trapezoid). (e) Two to four muscles (splenius capitis and/or trapezoid bilaterally). (f) Variable multiple muscles. (From Ref. 4.)

others have restricted injections to one or two sites per muscle (5,9,10). Both types of approach appear to produce similar degrees of clinical improvement or muscle hypotrophy. There is, however, one study directly comparing efficacy of single versus multiple-point injections in 49 patients with cervical dystonia, and these authors found greater improvement on several measures with multiple-point injections (11).

There is no general agreement about the optimal volume to be injected. Since there is a possibility that small injection volumes might minimize local or systemic toxin spread (9,10), many centers now tend to use concentrated BTX solutions of 800 or more mouse units (Dysport) per milliliter of saline.

Only a few authors have advocated the use of EMG-guided injections for BTX treatment of cervical dystonia (5,12), and the major relevant neck muscles can be confidently localized without such guidance (see above). Electromyographically guided injections through Teflon-coated needles can be useful, however, in patients with numerous previous injections, since fibrous muscle changes make it more difficult to localize injections into an active part of the muscles. Injections into posterior neck muscles in obese patients will also be more precise if performed under EMG guidance, and the same is true for injections into the scalenus or levator scapulae muscles.

Polygraphic multichannel EMG recordings can be helpful for dystonic muscle identification in patients with complex clinical patterns of cervical dystonia or in those with an insufficient response to a preceding injection.

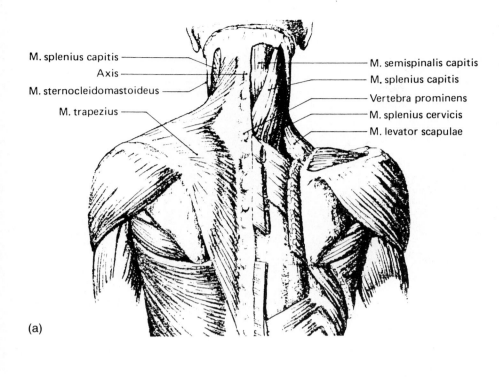

M. splenius capitis —————————

Axis —————

M. sternocleidomastoideus —————

M. trapezius —————

————— M. semispinalis capitis

————— M. splenius capitis

————— Vertebra prominens

————— M. splenius cervicis

————— M. levator scapulae

(a)

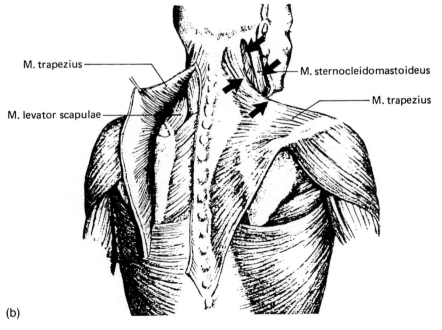

M. trapezius —————

M. levator scapulae —————

————— M. sternocleidomastoideus

————— M. trapezius

(b)

Figure 3 (a) Anatomical location of relevant muscles for botulinum toxin treatment of cervical dystonia. (b) Sites of most frequently used injections of botulinum toxin in cervical dystonia: splenius capitis (uppermost arrow), sternocleidomastoid, and trapezoid muscles. (Modified from The Ciba Collection of Medical Illustrations, Vol. 8, Musculoskeletal System Part I: Anatomy, Physiology and Metabolic Disorders; Frank H. Netter, M.D.; with permission).

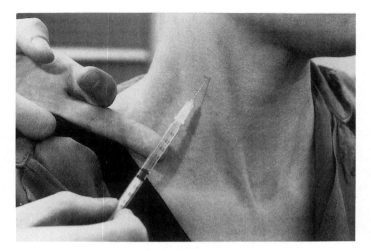

Figure 4 Placement of botulinum toxin injections into midpart of sternocleidomastoid muscle.

Types of Toxin and Doses to Be Injected

So far only BTX-A has been used for the treatment of cervical dystonia, although very preliminary experience with the use of BTX-F does exist (13). There is a considerable variation in the doses of BTX-A that have been employed in the different series of patients reported in the literature, with respect both to doses injected per muscle and to total doses per treatment session. Doses per muscle range from 50 to more than 600 mouse units and totals per session from 100 to 1200 mouse units (Table 2). Part of this discrepancy appears to arise from differences in potency between the two preparations of BTX used (14). The majority of European studies have used the preparation distributed by Porton Products, England (Dysport), while North American studies have employed the product supplied by Allergan Inc. (Botox). Unfortunately there are no published guidelines for calculating equipotent doses of these two preparations. Theoretically there should be equipotency when strength is expressed as mouse units. The standard dose for the treatment of blepharospasm is 20–40 mouse units per site with Dysport. In studies of cervical dystonia, Dysport doses have on average been three to four times above those of Botox in otherwise comparable series (Table 2). From the information available it would thus appear that 1 Botox unit is equivalent to 3–5 Dysport units (Table 2).

Another source of variation in dose ranges among studies lies in a trend toward lower doses in European studies over the last few years, as experience has accumulated showing that efficacy can be maintained with lesser amounts of toxin than had been employed in early studies (15,16).

Although there is still no consensus about "standard" or "optimal" doses for the treatment of cervical dystonia, many authors now consider 200 to 300 mouse units of Dysport per muscle as sufficient for initial injections in de novo patients (9). For Botox, the majority of studies have used 100 units per muscle. There is also emerging agreement that doses for the sternocleidomastoid muscles should be lower than those for the splenius capitis to avoid dysphagia (see below). Most authors user lower doses for repeat injections than for the initial treatment session. There is less variation and uncertainty about the

Table 2 Botulinum Toxin Type A in Cervical Dystonia: Treatment Results

Study	Number of patients	Mean dose (mouse units)		Response rate (%)		Rating scale	Degree of response (%)
		Per muscle	Per session	Posture	Pain		
Tsui et al., 1986[a]	19	50[c]	100[c]	63	87	Tsui	30
Gelb et al., 1989[a]	20	90[c]	280[c]	15	50	Tsui	20
Gelb et al., 1991[a]	28	90[c]	280[c]	32	64	Tsui	20
Perlmutter et al., 1989[a]	21	50[c]	100[c]	Significant improvement	Significant improvement	?	?
Blackie and Lees, 1990[a]	19	480	960	84	75	Tsui	22
Blackie and Lees, 1990[b]	50	396	875	83	77	Tsui	22
Greene et al., 1990[b]	34	118[c]	240[c]	74	?	GIR(0–3)	33
Lorentz et al., 1991[a]	21	50[c]	150[c]	87	63	Tsui	?
Ceballos-Baumann et al., 1990[b]	45	?	692	73	78	Tsui	25
Stell et al., 1988[b]	10	600[d]	1200[d]	90	100	Tsui	47
Jankovic and Schwarz 1990[b]	205	105[c]	209[c]	71	76	GIR)–4)	?
Tsui et al., 1988[b]	19	50[c]	100[c]	53	?	Tsui	?
Jankovic et al., 1990[b]	195	100[c]	209[c]	90	93	GIR(0–4)	>50
Lees et al., 1992[b]	89	200[d]	666[d]	62	68	Tsui	?
Brin et al., 1987[b]	28	?	276[c]	64	74	?	?
D'Costa and Abbott, 1991[b]	12	?	520[d]	91	91	GIR(0–5)	>40
Comella et al., 1992[b]	52	40-120[c]	374[c]	71	86	TWSTRS	>10
Poewe et al., 1992[b]	37	312[d]	632[d]	86	84	Tsui	>50
Wissel and Poewe, 1992[b]	108	254[d]	594[d]	85	85	Tsui	>50

[a]Double-blind.
[b]Open trial.
[c]Botox.
[d]Dysport.
TWSTRS = Toronto Western Spasmodic Torticollis Rating Scale; GIR = Global Improvement Rating.

number of neck muscles to be injected per treatment session, the majority of patients showing dystonic involvement of two or three muscles (Fig. 2).

THERAPEUTIC EFFICACY

Published series of local BTX therapy for cervical dystonia now cover more than 1000 patients, and the number of those treated by this approach worldwide probably reaches several thousand. Despite the degree of variation in doses indicated above, the results obtained in 19 studies published between 1986 and 1992—13 open (5,7–10,12,15–21) and six double-blind (3,6,9,22–24)—are remarkably similar (Table 2). The percentage of responders as judged on clinical grounds and by score improvement on rating scales ranged from 53% to 90%. Only two small double-blind studies by the same group have found low responder rates of 15% and 32%, respectively. The magnitude of response as assessed by various rating scales (most often the one proposed by Tsui and colleagues [3]) is less well documented. Only 13 of 19 studies give information on score changes during treatment, and this was 30% or greater in seven. It has to be borne in mind, however, that rating scores will not always adequately reflect clinical improvement in patients with cervical dystonia. For example, the Tsui scale does not assess pain as a major determinant of disability in this disorder. Furthermore, improvement of postural deviation by 15–30° in one plane or disappearance of dystonic head tremor may be highly meaningful for a patient but will not improve the subject's Tsui score by more than one or two points.

Latency between injections and onset of clinical benefit has been around 7 days in most studies, but it may not be before 3 weeks that a plateau of clinical improvement is reached (18). Duration of effect has averaged 3 months in the great majority of published series.

RISKS AND SIDE EFFECTS

The most common side effects and their frequencies are listed in Table 3. Local pain at or near injection sites, neck weakness, and swallowing problems are the most prevalent complications. According the majority of studies 20–30% of injections will be complicated by the subsequent development of some degree of dysphagia, and up to 50% of all patients treated chronically will develop dysphagia on one or several occasions (9,10). Such swallowing problems are usually of mild to moderate severity and rarely require nasogastric tube feeding. Their onset is usually close to the onset of clinical benefit, and their duration has been around 3 weeks in most published series. The occurrence of dysphagia seems to be related to dose, and incidences have been lower in series using less than 300 U per session (Table 3). Incidences of swallowing problems of 7% or less have been noted in series where only 50 mouse units of Botox per muscle were given (3,6,7,23,24). In all studies using higher doses, with one exception (12), more than 20% of patients developed dysphagia, and this figure was 90% in one series using doses of 600 mouse units of Dysport per muscle (15). Such dose-response relationships are not apparent for the incidences of neck weakness in the various reports, and the reasons for this discrepancy are not clear.

Dysphagia may also be more common in female than in male patients, and injections into the sternocleidomastoid muscle are more likely to produce this side effect than administration of the toxin into posterior neck muscles (8,9,21). The occurrence of both dysphagia and neck weakness may be related to smaller neck muscle mass (25). The

Table 3 Frequency of Side Effects in 17 Studies

Study	Number of patients	Mean dose per session	Side effects						
			Dysphagia	Weak neck	Local pain	Lethargy	Dysphonia	Vertigo	Dry Mouth
Tsui et al., 1986	19	100[a]	—	10%	5%	—	—	—	—
Gelb et al., 1989	20	280[a]	7%	20%	28%	—	—	—	—
Perlmutter et al., 1989	21	100[a]	—	10%	—	—	—	—	—
Blackie and Lees, 1990	19	960[b]	16%	10%	36%	20%	—	20%	—
Blackie and Lees, 1990	50	875[b]	28%	5%	?	9%	2%	3%	1%
Greene et al., 1990	28	145[a]	11%	7%	18%	—	—	—	—
Lorenz et al., 1991	21	150[a]	—	—	38%	—	—	—	—
Ceballos-Baumann et al., 1990	45	692[b]	6%	31%	9%	—	—	—	—
Stell et al., 1988	10	1200[b]	90%	—	10%	20%	50%	—	20%
Jancovic et al., 1990	195	209[a]	23%	12%	2%	—	2%	—	—
Jancovic and Schwarz, 1990	205	209[a]	17%	8%	—	—	—	—	3%
Lees et al., 1992	89	666[b]	22%	2%	2%	5%	—	—	—
Brin et al., 1987	28	276[a]	—	7%	—	—	—	—	—
D'Costa and Abbott, 1991	12	520[b]	25%	—	—	—	—	—	—
Comella et al., 1992	52	374[a]	31%	44%	—	—	—	—	—
Poewe et al., 1992	37	632[b]	22%	10%	—	—	—	—	—
Wissel and Poewe, 1992	108	594[b]	32%	17%	6%	—	—	—	—

[a]Botox.
[b]Dysport.

mechanisms leading to dysphagia are not entirely clear, but hematogenous spread is the most likely explanation, since esophageal end plates are known to be particularly sensitive to the blocking effects of BTX (26).

While pain at or near injection sites is another commonly observed complaint following local BTX treatment, a number of other side effects have been noted only in a minority of studies (Table 3). It seems quite possible that this reflects underreporting whenever these latter complications are not specifically mentioned.

Severe immunological reactions to repeated BTX injections have not been reported, but some patients will produce neutralizing antibodies during the course of multiple treatment sessions. The latter is the prime reason for secondary refractoriness to injections (see below).

The risks of injecting BTX during pregnancy and lactation are not clearly defined, and most clinicians would at present exclude such patients from treatment. This also applies to patients with bleeding disorders and those receiving anticoagulant medication. Special consideration should be given to those with preexisting dysphagia or any concomitant neuromuscular disorder. In general, however, there are very few patients with cervical dystonia who cannot be safely treated with BTX.

PRIMARY AND SECONDARY NONRESPONDERS

Some 15% of patients with cervical dystonia will not adequately respond to the first injection of BTX (8–10). In the authors' experience about half of them will subsequently profit from dose adjustments and/or modifications of the original injection pattern (10). Occasionally, detailed polygraphic simultaneous EMG recordings from many neck muscles will be needed before the relevant dystonic muscles can be properly identified. There remains, however, a group of patients in whom BTX injections fail to produce clinical benefit even after such measures have been exploited. The reasons for such primary unresponsiveness are unclear, but they may include dystonic activity of deep neck muscles that cannot be reached by conventional injection techniques. Some authors believe that this is so in cases of pure antecollis in which bilateral sternocleidomastoid injections remain ineffective. Whether there are differences in responsiveness between idiopathic cervical dystonia and symptomatic forms such as tardive dystonia has not been sufficiently investigated.

Secondary nonresponsiveness, on the other hand, is generally related to the development of neutralizing antibodies to BTX. One study identified 10 secondary nonresponders among several hundred patients receiving regular injections of BTX for cervical dystonia and found neutralizing antibodies in six of them, while only one patient of 10 matched patients with a continuing clinical response had low antibody concentrations (27).

Another study found neutralizing antibodies in five of 14 nonresponders as opposed to none of 23 responders (25). There are no consistent data yet on how frequently neutralizing antibodies develop during treatment or how their production might be related to treatment factors such as volume of injection, dose, and intervals between injections. Most authors now believe that fewer than 5% of patients are likely to produce antibodies with prolonged treatment (28). Such patients currently have no prospect of gaining further benefit from BTX-A injections, but preliminary experience with BTX-F suggests that other serotypes of toxin remain effective in patients with type A antibodies (13).

CONCLUSIONS

Idiopathic cervical dystonia, like other adult-onset focal dystonias, has been notoriously difficult to treat. Multiple approaches, including systemic drug treatment with anticholinergics, antidopaminergics, anticonvulsants, muscle relaxants, and many other drugs as well as physiotherapy and psychotherapy, usually lead only to temporary amelioration in a minority of patients. Selective surgical EMG-controlled denervation of dystonic neck muscles produces better and, in the hands of some, lasting improvement, but is invasive and as such less well accepted by patients.

Local injections of BTX are strikingly successful in improving postural deviation and pain in about 80% of patients. They can be made on an outpatient basis and appear to be safe even over many repeat sessions. Dysphagia is the potentially most serious side effect but can be decreased in incidence and severity by injection lower doses, particularly into the sternocleidomastoid. Major drawbacks at present are a lack of prospective data to establish guidelines for optimal dose and volume of injection and the need to continue indefinitely with repeat injections approximately every 3 months.

REFERENCES

1. Scott AB. Botulinum toxin injection into extraocular muscles as an alternative to strabismus surgery. Ophthalmology 1980;87:1044–1049.
2. American Academy of Neurology Assessment: The clinical usefulness of botulinum toxin-A in treating neurologic disorders. Neurology 1990;40:1332–1336.
3. Tsui JK, Eisen A, Stoessel AJ, Calne S, Calne DB. Double-blind study of botulinum toxin in spasmodic torticollis. Lancet 1986:245–246.
4. Deuschl G, Heinen F, Kleedorfer B, Wagner M, Lücking CH, Poewe W. Clinical and polymyographic investigation of spasmodic torticollis. J Neurol 1992;239:9–15.
5. Comella CL, Buchman AS, Tanner CM, Brown-Toms NC, Goetz CG. Botulinum toxin injections for spasmodic torticollis: increased magnitude of benefit with electromyographic assistance. Neurology 1992;42:878–882.
6. Greene P, Kang U, Fahn S, Brin M, Moskowitz C, Flaster E. Double-blind, placebo-controlled trial of botulinum toxin injections for the treatment of spasmodic torticollis. Neurology 1990;40:1213–1218.
7. Gelb DJ, Lowenstein DH, Aminoff MJ. Controlled trial of botulinum toxin injections in the treatment of spasmodic torticollis. Neurology 1989;39:80–84.
8. Jankovic J, Schwartz K. Botulinum toxin injections for cervical dystonia. Neurology 1990;40:277–280.
9. Blackie JD, Lees AJ. Botulinum toxin treatment in spasmodic torticollis. J. Neurol Neurosurg Psychiatry 1990;53:640–643.
10. Poewe W, Schelosky L, Kleedorfer B, Heinen F, Wagner M, Deuschl G. Treatment of spasmodic torticollis with local injections of botulinum toxin: one-year follow-up in 37 patients. J Neurol 1992;239:21–25.
11. Borodic GE, Pearce LB, Smith K, Joseph M. Botulinum A toxin for spasmodic torticollis: multiple vs single injection points per muscle. Head Neck 1992;1:33–37.
12. Ceballos-Baumann AO, Konstanzer A, Dengler R, Conrad B. Lokale Injektionen von Botulinum-Toxin A bei zervikaler Dystonie: Verlaufsbeobachtungen an 45 Patienten. Akt Neurol 1990;17:139–145.
13. Ludlow CL, Hallett M, Rhew K, Cole R, Shimizu T, Sakaguchi G, Bagley JA, Schulz GM, Yin SU, Koda J. Therapeutic use of type F botulinum toxin. N Engl J Med 1992;326:349–350.

14. Jankovic J, Brin MF. Therapeutic uses of botulinum toxin. N Engl J Med 1991;324:1186–1194.

15. Stell R, Thompson PD, Marsden CD. Botulinum toxin in spasmodic torticollis. J Neurol Neurosurg Psychiatry 1988;51:920–923.

16. D'Costa DF, Abbott RJ. Low dose botulinum toxin in spasmodic torticollis. J Royal Soc Med 1991;84:650–651.

17. Tsui JK, Eisen A, Calne DB. Botulinum toxin in spasmodic torticollis. Adv Neurol 1988; 50:593–597.

18. Jankovic J, Schwartz K, Donovan DT. Botulinum toxin treatment of cranial-cervical dystonia, spasmodic dysphonia, other focal dystonias and hemifacial spasm. J Neurol Neurosurg Psychiatry 1990;53:633–639.

19. Lees AJ, Turjanski N, Rivest J, Whurr R, Lorch M, Brookes G. Treatment of cervical dystonia, hand spasms and laryngeal dystonia with botulinum toxin. J Neurol 1992;239:1–4.

20. Brin MF, Fahn S, Moskowitz C, Friedman A, Shale HM, Greene P, Blitzer A. Localized injections of botulinum toxin for the treatment of focal dystonia and hemifacial spasm. Mov Disord 1987;2:237–254.

21. Wissel J, Poewe W. Dystonia—a clinical, neuropathological and therapeutic review. J Neural Transm 1992;38:91–104.

22. Gelb DJ, Yoshimura DM, Olney RK, Lowenstein DH, Aminoff MJ. Change in pattern of muscle activity following botulinum toxin injections for torticollis. Ann Neurol 1991;29:370–376.

23. Perlmutter JS, Tempel LW, Burde R. Double-blind, placebo-controlled, crossover trial of botulinum-A toxin for torticollis. Neurology 1989;39:352.

24. Lorentz IT, Subramaniam SS, Yiannikas C. Treatment of idiopathic spasmodic torticollis with botulinum toxin A: a double-blind study on twenty-three patients. Mov Disord 1991;6:145–150.

25. Jankovic J, Schwartz KS. Clinical correlates of response to botulinum toxin injections. Arch Neurol 1991;48:1253–1256.

26. Nix AW, Eckart VF, Kramer G. Reversible esophageal motor dysfunction in botulism. Muscle Nerve 1985;8:791–795.

27. Hambleton P, Cohen HE, Palmer BJ, Melling J. Antitoxin and botulinum toxin treatment. Br Med J 1992;304:959–960.

28. Jankovic J, Schwartz KS. Longitudinal experience with botulinum toxin injections for treatment of blepharospasm and cervical dystonia. Neurology 1993 (in press).

19

Controlled Trials of Botulinum Toxin for Cervical Dystonia: A Critical Review

Paul Greene
Columbia-Presbyterian Medical Center, New York, New York

INTRODUCTION

Cervical dystonia (also called spasmodic torticollis or torticollis) is a form of torsion dystonia affecting the muscles controlling head position. Adult-onset torticollis is difficult to treat with medication, although as many as 40% of patients may achieve some degree of benefit from medication trials (1). Torticollis may occur in children or adolescents, as part of more widespread dystonic involvement, or occasionally as the only dystonic manifestation, and high-dose anticholinergic therapy may produce dramatic benefit in these patients (2). A variety of surgical techniques involving muscle, root, and nerve lesions have been developed, but despite some reports of dramatic success (3), there have been no controlled trials of surgical therapy, and most patients and their neurologists consider surgery a last resort. Similarly, the success rate of bilateral thalamotomy in torticollis has not been documented by prospective study, and the procedure entails significant risk of speech impairment (4).

Since 1984, neurologists have been treating torticollis with injections of botulinum toxin (BTX) into excessively contracting muscles (5). Uncontrolled trials (5) indicate that these injections are more successful than medication. Despite the success in open trials, prospective studies are necessary to confirm the usefulness of BTX. The symptoms of torticollis may vary from day to day, and even from hour to hour, depending on such factors as the type and extent of physical activity and the emotional state of the patient. This makes it difficult to assess the outcome of treatment and raises concern about the contribution of the placebo effect. In addition, spontaneous remissions occur (6). To document the efficacy of BTX, there have been eight prospective, placebo-controlled studies of the use of BTX in treating torticollis (7–14). All of these were double-blind, except for one study (9) in which the investigators were aware of the contents of injection but the patients were not and videotapes were assessed in random order, to provide blinded objective assessments. There was statistically significant improvement in objective measures of torticollis compared with placebo in five of the eight studies (7,10,11, 13,14). There was statistically significant improvement in subjective measures in four of six studies (7,10,13,14), and in the remaining two studies (9,11) there was substantial subject improvement that was not statistically analyzed.

Most of the studies used toxin distributed in the United States, but two studies (11,13) used toxin distributed in the United Kingdom. This makes comparison of doses difficult: there is an unexplained disparity between the U.S. and U.K. toxins as measured either by weight of toxin or in units (a unit of BTX is the mouse LD_{50} by intraperitoneal injection) (15). A patient with torticollis in the United States will receive approximately 100–300 U per treatment, which is 40–120 ng of toxin-hemagglutinin complex. Patients in the United Kingdom receive about 1000 U of U.K. toxin, which is about 25 ng of toxin-hemagglutinin complex of U.K. toxin. I will express all amounts of BTX in units: ''U'' for U.S. units and ''U-U.K.'' for U.K. units. Until the disparity in toxin measurement is explained, the experience in treating blepharospasm affords the best comparison between U.S. and U.K. toxins, since the dose for blepharospasm tends to vary much less from center to center than the dose for torticollis. In the United States, a dose of about 25 U per eye is adequate for many (but not all) patients (16); a comparable dose in the United Kingdom appears to be about 120 U-U.K. per eye (17), a ratio of U.S./U.K. units of about 1/5.

METHODS

Dystonia of the neck may produce any combination of movements available to the neck: rotation, tilt, anterocollis, retrocollis, and shift of the neck laterally, forward, or backward. The shoulder ipsilateral to the direction of head turning is often elevated or displaced forward. Jerky movements or regular tremor are sometimes superimposed on tonic deviation. Constant pain in contracting muscles, or brief, painful spasms may be present in addition to head deviation. Patients also may have dystonic contraction and pain in neck muscles that do not contribute to the abnormal movements (cocontraction of agonist and antagonist muscles). Because torticollis varies considerably from patient to patient, most studies had some flexibility in the injection schedule. The exception was the study of Koller et al. (12), in which the same muscles were injected in all patients, with a fixed dose per muscle: sternocleidomastoid (SCM) contralateral to direction of rotation and trapezius (TRP) on both sides to a total dose per patient of 150 U. The injection strategy of the other studies is described in order of increasing flexibility. In the series of Jankovic and Orman (8), two patients with anterocollis were injected in both SCMs, one patient was injected in a single SCM, and four patients with rotational torticollis were injected in the SCM and TRP contralateral to the direction of head turning, to a total dose of 100 U in each of the six patients. All other studies included injection of the SCM contralateral to the direction of rotation and the TRP ipsilateral to the direction of rotation. In two studies, two of the most actively contracting muscles (selected from the SCM, TRP, and splenius capitis) were injected to a fixed total dose per patient of 100 U (7) or 960 U-U.K. (11). In two studies, separate injection protocols were used for lateral tilt, retrocollis, and pure rotation, with a fixed dose per muscle to a total per patient of 150 U (14) or 140–165 U (10). In the series of Moore and Blumhardt (13), a total dose of 1000 U-U.K. was used for all patients, but the muscles and dose per muscle were determined by clinically estimating the contribution of the muscle to the dystonia. The actual muscles, dose per muscle, and number of sites per muscle were not specified. Finally, Gelb et al. (9) not only determined the muscles and dose per muscle by clinical assessment, but had three dose schedules: medium (90–140 U), low (one-half medium), and high (twice medium). The total dose per patient ranged between 45 and 280 U, but the mean low, medium, and high doses were not specified.

Aside from the choice of muscle and dose per muscle, other aspects of injection strategy may have affected outcome or adverse effects but were not studied. The concentration of toxin varied from 25 to 100 U/ml in the U.S. studies, and from 200 to 800 U-U.K./ml in the United Kingdom; the volume of toxin per injection site varied from 0.1 to 0.5 ml; the number of sites per muscle varied from two to 11. One study (12) did not specify the toxin concentration, and two studies did not specify volume per site or number of sites per muscle (12,13). Three studies (7,8,11) used electromyographic (EMG) recordings in at least some patients to help choose target muscles, but none of these state that injections were performed via hollow-core needles using EMG control.

RATING SCALES

Five of the eight studies used the composite score of Tsui et al. (7) to measure objective change (7,9,11,13,14). This score combines:

A = amplitude of head deviation
Rotation, tilt: 0: absent; 1: $< 15°$; 2: 15–30°; 3: $>30°$
Antero/retrocollis: 0 = absent; 1 = mild; 2 = moderate; 3 = severe
A = sum of rotation, tilt, and antero/retrocollis
B = duration of head deviation
1 = intermittent; 2 = constant
C = shoulder elevation
0 = absent; 1 = mild, intermittent; 2 = mild, constant or severe, intermittent; 3 = severe, constant
D = tremor in the following formula:
Severity: 1 = mild; 2 = severe
Duration: 1 = occasional; 2 = continuous
D = severity × duration

to yield a score, as follows: $[(A) \times (B)] + (C) + (D)$

The maximum (worst) potential score is thus $[9 \times 2] + 3 + [2 \times 2] = 25$. In fact, it is difficult to distinguish tilt and retrocollis in the presence of severe rotation, so a more reasonable maximum potential score is $[6 \times 2] + 3 + 4 = 19$. This score has the advantage of representing severity with a single number. However, the scale for amplitude of rotation and tilt assigns 3 to any degree of rotation between 30° and 90°. Thus, a 60° change of rotation from 75° to 15° in a severely affected patient, a dramatic improvement, would produce the same change in score (1 or 2 points) as a 15° change from 30° to 15° in a mildly to moderately affected patient. Objective measures were not described in detail in the study of Koller et al (12), but they included magnitude of head deviation, time the patient could hold the head straight and at the extremes of deviation, number of forceful spasms per day, and a global assessment. Jankovic and Orman (8) used a rating scale for the objective examination and had blinded neurologists who rated videotapes for global severity of torticollis. Greene et al. (10) estimated the angle of head deviation at rest, walking, and turned maximally against the direction of torticollis. Tremor was not rated.

There was more variation in subjective rating scales, which were not described in detail in four studies (7,8,12,13). In all studies patients were asked to estimate the results of injections or absolute severity of torticollis. All studies but that of Koller et al. (12) considered pain independently from other subjective factors. Four studies (8,10,12,14) included some measure of the impact of torticollis on functional capacity.

OUTCOME

The percentage of patients improving in objective measures varied from 20% (8) to 87% (14) (Table 1). The magnitude of objective change could be estimated in some studies. The mean improvement in Tsui scale was 1.8 points above placebo in the study of Tsui et al. (7), 2.3 points in that of Blackie and Lees (11), and 4.2 points in that of Moore and Blumhardt (13), and the median improvement was 4.5 points with BTX versus a median worsening of 0.2 with placebo in the study of Lorentz et al. (14). Because of the composite nature of the Tsui score, the magnitude of these changes is hard to interpret. Three studies (9,10,12) specifically addressed the magnitude of objective change after BTX treatment. In two of these, objective improvement was not statistically significant: no patient had marked improvement with BTX in the study of Koller et al. (12), and three of 18 BTX-treated patients (17%) had substantial objective improvement in the study of Gelb et al. (9), but so did two of 18 placebo-treated patients (11%). Greene et al. (10) looked at the 17 of 28 BTX-treated patients (50%) who reported subjective improvement: in these patients, blinded observers estimated a mean improvement of 17° in head position while sitting (from a mean initial head rotation of about 60°) and mean improvement of 22° in head position while walking (from a mean initial head rotation of about 50°).

Most studies reported subjective improvement after BTX treatment (Table 1). In four studies, subjective improvement was analyzed and was statistically significant: about 80% of patients improved in two studies (13,14), and about 50% improved in two studies (7,10). In two studies, subjective improvement rates were substantially higher than with placebo—74% (versus 5% with placebo) in the series of Blackie and Lees (11) and 80% (versus 25% with placebo) in the series of Gelb et al. (9)—but were not statistically analyzed. Only 11–15% of patients reported marked improvement in the studies analyzing magnitude of improvement (9–11). Pain also improved in most studies (Table 1). In two studies, 63% (14) and 88% (7) of patients had pain improvement that was statistically significant compared with placebo. In the study of Blackie and Lees (11), 12 of 16 patients (75%) had pain improvement, but this was not statistically analyzed. Similarly, 16 patients with pain improved in the study of Gelb et al. (9), but the total number of patients with pain and the number with pain improvement after placebo were not given. In the study of Greene et al. (10), the mean magnitude of pain improvement for BTX-treated patients was 63% (percentage improvement compared with baseline pain, as estimated by the patients), which was statistically significant in comparison with the placebo group. In the remaining three studies, pain was not mentioned (12); was decreased, but the decrease was not statistically significant (13); or was decreased, but the decrease was not analyzed statistically (8). The magnitude of pain improvement was addressed in two studies in addition to the series of Green et al. (10): pain improvement was substantial in 10 of 20 (50%) of the patients of Gelb et al. (9), and pain severity score improved from a mean 6.1 to 3.3 (score of 0–10) in the patients of Blackie and Lees (11).

Table 1 Outcome

Study	Group	Number with objective improvement (%)	Number with subjective improvement (%)	Number with pain improvement (%)	Number with objective worsening (%)	Number with subjective worsening (%)
Tsui et al. (7)	BTX	12/19 (63%)[a]	10/19 (53%)[a]	14/16 (88%)[a]	2/19 (11%)	
	Placebo	7/20 (35%)	3/20 (15%)	4/17 (24%)	11/20 (55%)	
Jankovic and Orman (8)	BTX	3/5 (60%)	2/5 (40%)		1/5 (20%)	1/5 (20%)
	Placebo	2/3 (67%)	2/3 (67%)		1/3 (33%)	2/3 (67%)
Gelb et al. (9)	BTX	12/18 (67%)	16/20 (80%)	16/?[b]	9/18 (50%)	3/20 (15%)
	Placebo		5/20 (25%)			4/20 (25%)
Blackie and Lees (11)	BTX	16/19 (84%)[a]	14/19 (74%)	12/16 (75%)		
	Placebo	1/19 (5%)		2/16 (13%)		
Koller et al. (12)	BTX	15/29 (52%)	11/29 (38%)		0/29	1/29 (3%)
	Placebo	5/29 (17%)	8/29 (28%)		1/29 (3%)	8/29 (28%)
Lorentz et al. (14)	BTX	14/23 (61%)[a]	18/23 (78%)[a]	12/19 (63%)[a]	0/23	0/23
	Placebo	1/23 (4%)	4/23 (17%)	1/19 (5%)	4/23 (17%)	0/23
Moore and Blumhardt (13)	BTX	12/19 (63%)[a]	16/19 (84%)[a]		0/19	
	Placebo	4/19 (21%)	3/19 (16%)		2/19 (11%)	

[a]Results analyzed and statistically significant.
[b]Total number of patients with pain not reported.
Data from the study of Greene et al. (10) are not included in this table, since only group means were analyzed.

Three studies attempted to correlate clinical features of torticollis with outcome. Greene et al. (19) found no significant difference in response between the entire group of 28 BTX-treated patients and the subgroups with retrocollis, tilt, tremor, or jerks; there was also no correlation between outcome and initial severity of torticollis, sex, age, or duration of symptoms. Moore and Blumhardt (13) found significant improvement in tremor as compared with placebo. Blackie and Lees (11) found no correlation between outcome and sex, age, duration or severity of torticollis, or pattern of muscle activation.

ADVERSE EFFECTS

Two studies reported the number of patients without any adverse effect. In the study of Tsui et al. (7), with a total dose of 100 U per patient, 14 of 19 patients (74%) had no adverse effect, whereas in that of Lorentz et al. (14), with a total dose of 150 U per patient, only 8 of 23 patients (35%) had no adverse effect. This difference may have been attributable to the difference in dose or the difference in technique. Adverse effects were generally minor. The most common adverse effect described as severe was pain related to the injections. The exact number of patients with adverse effects could not be calculated in the study of Gelb et al. (9), but local pain was common in placebo- and BTX-treated patients. Dysphagia did not occur in placebo-treated patients and occurred in 15–17 of 162 (9–10%) of BTX-treated patients. It was speculated that dysphagia resulted from direct local spread of the toxin to pharyngeal muscles (10), hematogenous spread (11), mechanical factors (9), or autonomic effects of toxin (13), but the mechanism of dysphagia could not be deduced from the data in these studies. Blackie and Lees (11) found that significantly more women than men got adverse effects, including dysphagia, at a somewhat lower total dose. Local neck weakness (16–22 of 162 BTX-treated patients versus 1 of 160 placebo-treated patients) and generalized weakness (6–7 of 162 BTX-treated patients versus 1 of 160 placebo-treated patients) were reported more frequently with BTX than with placebo. Tiredness and malaise (23–31 of 162 BTX-treated patients) were reported more commonly with BTX, except in the study of Lorentz et al. (14), in which 11 BTX-treated and 11 placebo-treated patients complained of tiredness. In our experience at Columbia-Presbyterian Medical Center subsequent to our double-blind trial, complaints of generalized weakness, malaise, muscle aches, headache, nausea, and low-grade fever tend to cluster together as a ''flu-like'' syndrome after BTX treatment.

STATISTICS

One study used parallel design (10), and the other seven used a randomized crossover design in which 50% of patients received BTX followed by placebo, and 50% received injections in the opposite order. In four of the crossover studies (7,11,13,14), injections were given at a preset interval (2–3 months apart); in 2 (9,12), the second set of injections was performed when there was no objective or subjective evidence of residual benefit from the first injections. Jankovic and Orman (8) treated seven patients with torticollis but only crossed over patients who did not respond to the first treatment, so that only three patients received placebo, and only one patient received both placebo and BTX.

The parallel-design study was analyzed by analysis of covariance with time adjustment for baseline (10). A variety of statistical tests were used in the crossover studies to analyze objective response (used as the primary response variable in these studies): Wilcoxon signed rank test (7,8,9,12), ANOVA (13), Mann-Whitney U test (11), and McNemar's test (14). In addition, Jankovic and Orman (8) analyzed objective scores by paired T-test, Moore and Blumhardt (13) used chi-square to compare numbers of successes and failures, and Tsui et al. (7) analyzed numbers of patients improved in objective, subjective, and pain scores without specifying the nonparametric test. Chi-square and U test are sometimes used to analyze data from crossover studies, but Wilcoxon and McNemar's tests, taking the crossover into account, are more appropriate. Only Blackie and Lees (11) and Moore and Blumhardt (13) performed statistical analyses for carryover effects. In light of the prolonged action of BTX, carry-over of BTX effect into the placebo phase is a potential problem even for the two studies that performed the second injections after effects of the first were not detected by blinded participants.

Many of the studies performed multiple analyses (7,10,11,13,14), but only Green et al. (10) corrected for multiple analyses. Most studies reported dropouts or missing data (7,9,10,12,13): these were simply omitted in the analyses, since only a small amount of data was missing. Botulinum toxin and placebo groups were analyzed for comparability in the parallel study (10).

In addition to muscle weakness, BTX injections produce marked, but temporary, muscle atrophy, which is particularly evident in the case of SCM injections. The potential difficulty of maintaining effective treatment anonymity in patients and examiners in the face of this change was noted by Blackie and Lees (11), several of whose patients reported this change to the examiners. Blackie and Lees felt that anonymity was maintained for the blinded ratings because atrophy was not apparent on videotapes (11), but no report made an attempt to verify the success of the blinding strategy in patients.

DISCUSSION

The primary function of these double-blind studies was to document convincingly benefit from BTX injections in cervical dystonia. Despite the variations in technique and rating, this was clearly accomplished in five of these studies (7,10,11,13,14), which documented objective and subjective improvement. The study of Gelb et al. (9) showed substantial patient satisfaction with BTX injections compared with placebo. This was not statistically analyzed but was significant at the $p < 0.01$ level using chi-square. In the face of this substantial patient satisfaction, it is difficult to understand why they were unable to document objective change. Although 12 of their 18 patients (67%) showed objective improvement, there were nine patients whose condition objectively deteriorated after some dose of BTX. Nonetheless, three of these patients also improved on some dose of BTX, and four of the six others had subjective improvement. Since they used a crossover design, there may have been carry-over effect from BTX injections to subsequent placebo injections. They note considerable interobserver variability in the videotape ratings, but their correlation of 0.83 to 0.87 is comparable to that reported by Tsui et al. (7). Another possibility is that patient satisfaction was determined by factors not apparent in the objective ratings. This possibility is discussed below.

The study of Jankovic and Orman (8) involved only five patients and was probably too small to detect improvement after BTX. Koller et al. (12) randomized 30 patients but failed to show any benefit. This study had a large placebo effect, but not as large as in some other studies that did detect improvement (7). It is difficult to assess the sensitivity of their rating scheme without details. They injected the TRP contralateral to the direction of head rotation in all patients, which may have weakened a muscle opposing head rotation and been counterproductive in some patients. Probably most significantly, this was the only study that did not tailor the injection protocol to the pattern of torticollis.

It is apparent from these studies that improvement in the pain associated with torticollis is a major advantage of BTX injections. All studies but that of Koller et al. (12), which did not mention pain, reported pain improvement, which was statistically significant in three studies (7,10,14) and unanalyzed but probably statistically significant in two other studies (9,11).

The magnitude of improvement after BTX treatment was not a primary concern of most of these studies. Patient satisfaction was high in most studies, and yet the change in objective measures was often modest. After subtracting placebo effect, improvement in mean Tsui scores ranged from about 16% to 30% in the four studies with adequate data (7,11,13,14). Head position improved only 17° to 22° from a mean starting position of 55° to 65° in Greene et al. (10). Since these are all blinded, placebo-controlled studies, the presumption must be that the substantial patient satisfaction represents a change not well measured in these studies. Certainly, improvement in pain accounts for some of the subjective improvement. Another major source of disability in many patients is the constant effort required to fight head deviation. This was not considered in any study. Future studies of treatments for torticollis, including BTX treatment, probably should attempt to measure some of the other sources of disability, which are summarized in Table 2.

These studies, while documenting the usefulness of BTX for torticollis, have only begun to address the problem of maximizing benefit from BTX while minimizing adverse

Table 2 Factors Influencing Disability in Torticollis

I.   Factors measured objectively
   1. Degree of head deviation.
   2. Direction of head deviation: anterocollis or retrocollis are more disabling than rotation for the same degree of deviation; rotation away from the dominant arm is more disabling than rotation toward the dominant arm.
   3. Tremor or jerky movememts: often produce more disability for the same degree of head deviation.
   4. Presence of "sensory tricks": ability to straighten the head by gently touching the cheek, neck or back of head, raising the arms in the air, etc. may allow relatively normal function even in the presence of extreme head deviation. These tricks are often lost as the disease progresses.
   5. Dystonia at other sites.
II. Subjective factors
   1. Difficulty in overcoming head deviation: small degrees of deviation may be disabling if the head cannot be rotated in the opposite direction.
   2. Pain: even mild pain may be disabling if unremitting.
   3. Muscle tension: patients who do not complain of pain may have a constant sensation of pulling, which is distracting and ennervating.
   4. Presence of painful spasms.
III. Factors indirectly related to torticollis
   1. Depression (may actually be part of the underlying disease, or a reaction to the disease).
   2. Insomnia because of pain, spasms, or depression.
   3. Radiculopathy: may be more likely in the presence of torticollis.
   4. Dysphagia: related to extreme head deviation or dystonia in pharyngeal structures.
   5. Disequilibrium.
   6. Compression neuropathy at the elbow from the use of sensory tricks.
   7. Skin abrasion at the chin from rotation of the head into the shoulder, or occassionally from sensory tricks.

effects. Further studies are required to answer such questions as the following: Are there optimal concentrations of toxin, number of sites per muscle, and volume of toxin solution per injection site? Is there an optimal frequency of injection treatments? What is the role, if any, of EMG in BTX treatments? How can dysphagia be avoided? Can benefit be maximized without the risk of excess neck weakness? What is the cause of the "flu-like" syndrome after BTX, and can it be avoided? In addition, because of the short-term nature of these studies, the possibility of long-term problems, such as the appearance of antibodies to botox (16,18–20), remains to be examined.

REFERENCES

1. Greene P, Shale S, Fahn S. Analysis of open-label trials in torsion dystonia using high dosages of anticholinergics and other drugs. Mov Disord 1988;3:46–60.
2. Burke RE, Fahn S, Marsden CD. Torsion dystonia: a double-blind prospective trial of high-dose trihexyphenidyl. Neurology 1986;36:160–164.
3. Bertrand CM, Molina-Negro P. Selective peripheral denervation in 111 cases of spasmodic torticollis: rationale and results. Adv Neurol 1988;50:637–643.
4. Andrew J, Fowler CL, Harrison MJG. Stereotaxic thalamotomy in 55 cases of dystonia. Brain 1983;106:981–1000.
5. Jankovic J, Brin MF. Therapeutic uses of botulinum toxin. N Engl J Med 1991;324:1186–1194.
6. Friedman A, Fahn S. Spontaneous remissions in spasmodic torticollis. Neurology 1986;36:398–400.
7. Tsui JKC, Eisen A, Stoessl AJ, Calne S, Calne DB. Double-blind study of botulinum toxin in spasmodic torticollis. Lancet 1986;2:245–247.
8. Jankovic J, Orman J. Botulinum A toxin for cranial-cervical dystonia: a double-blind, placebo-controlled study. Neurology 1987;37:616–623.
9. Gelb DJ, Lowenstein DH, Aminoff MJ. Controlled trial of botulinum toxin injections in the treatment of spasmodic torticollis. Neurology 1989;39:80–84.
10. Greene P, Kang U, Fahn S, Brin M, Moskowitz C, Flaster E. Double-blind, placebo-controlled trial of botulinum toxin injections for the treatment of spasmodic torticollis. Neurology 1990;40:1213–1218.
11. Blackie JD, Lees AJ. Botulinum toxin treatment in spasmodic torticollis. J Neurol Neurosurg Psychiatry 1990;53:640–643.
12. Koller W, Vetere-Overfield B, Gray C, Dubinsky R. Failure of fixed-dose, fixed muscle injection of botulinum toxin in torticollis. Clin Neuropharmacol 1990;13:355–358.
13. Moore AP, Blumhardt LD. A double blind trial of botulinum toxin "A" in torticollis, with one year follow up. J Neurol Neurosurg Psychiatry 1991;54:813–816.
14. Lorentz IT, Subramaniam SS, Yiannikas C. Treatment of idiopathic spasmodic torticollis with botulinum toxin A: a double-blind study on twenty-three patients. Mov Disord 1991;6:145–150.
15. Quinn N, Hallett M: Dose standardisation of botulinum toxin. Lancet 1989;1:964.
16. Brin MF, Fahn S, Moskowitz C, Friedman A, Shale HM, Greene PE, Blitzer A, List T, Lange D, Lovelace RE, McMahon D. Localized injections of botulinum toxin for the treatment of focal dystonia and hemifacial spasm. Mov Disord 1987;2:237–254.
17. Elston JS. The management of blepharospasm and hemifacial spasm. J Neurol 1992;239:5–8.
18. Tsui JK, Wong NLM, Wong E, Calne DB. Production of circulating antibodies to botulinum-A toxin in patients receiving repeated injections for dystonia. Ann Neurol 1988;23:181.
19. Hambleton P, Cohen HE, Palmer BJ, Melling J. Antitoxins and botulinum toxin treatment. Br Med J 1992;304:959–960.
20. Jankovic J, Schwartz KS. Clinical correlates of response to botulinum toxin injections. Arch Neurol 1991;48:1253–1256.

20

Electromyography-Assisted Botulinum Toxin Injections for Cervical Dystonia

Cynthia L. Comella
Rush–Presbyterian–St. Luke's Medical Center, Chicago, Illinois

INTRODUCTION

Traditionally, electromyography (EMG) has been applied for the evaluation of neuro-muscular disorders. In dystonia, EMG has been used primarily as an investigative tool to describe the motor phenomenon and try to elucidate underlying pathophysiology (1–5). With the recent introduction of local injections of botulinum toxin (BTX) for the treatment of focal dystonia (6–8), a new role for EMG as a therapeutic tool has emerged. This chapter will (1) discuss the rationale for electromyography (EMG) as an adjunct to the clinical examination for BTX injections in cervical dystonia (CD); (2) review the experience with EMG in focal dystonia and CD; and (3) describe the methods of EMG-assisted injection in CD developed at Rush-Presbyterian-St. Luke's Medical Center (9).

RATIONALE FOR ELECTROMYOGRAPHY-ASSISTED TECHNIQUE

Electromyography is designed to evaluate muscle activity. This would suggest two roles for EMG as an adjunct to the clinical examination for the BTX treatment of CD. First, EMG may be used to identify which muscles contribute to the dystonic posture of the head and neck. Identifying the pattern of muscle involvement may further serve to predict the outcome of treatment. Second, EMG provides a method whereby the BTX may be accurately injected into the involved muscles.

Identifying Patterns of Muscle Involvement with Electromyography

The primary reason cited in favor of EMG-assisted injections is the ability to identify abnormally contracting muscles that contribute to the dystonic posture of the head and neck (10). Although more than 26 muscle pairs control head and neck movements (11), only six of these pairs are routinely accessible to injection with BTX, including the sternocleidomastoid (SCM), scalene complex (SCA), levator scapulae (LEV), splenius (SPL), trapezius (TRAP), and deep postvertebrals (VERT), consisting of the semispinalis and longissimus capitis muscles. Of these six muscle pairs, three (SCM, TRAP, SPL) are easily palpable from the surface. The other three (SCA, LEV, VERT) are in large part concealed under other more superficial muscles (11).

The pattern of activation of cervical muscles has been demonstrated to be variable even with the same general abnormal head position. Studies of abnormal patterns of cervical muscle activity have largely been restricted to more superficial muscles using surface electrodes. Podvinsky (3) evaluated the EMG activity of the sternocleidomastoid, splenius capitis, and trapezius muscles bilaterally. Patterns of activation were categorized into five types: (1) sternocleidomastoid type; (2) splenius type; (3) trapezius type; (4) unilateral muscle involvement; and (5) bilateral muscle involvement. Podvinsky points out that when electromyographic recordings are made, "various types of involuntary motor activity can then be differentiated with a high degrees of precision."

Deuschl et al. (12) evaluated three muscle pairs (sternocleidomastoid, splenius, trapezius) electrophysiologically in 100 CD patients. They categorized their patients according to the predominant head position. Predominant rotational torticollis was the most common (N = 72), followed by laterocollis (N = 11), retrocollis (N = 9), and complex activation patterns (N = 8). These investigators demonstrated that in rotational torticollis, the pattern of electrically active muscles varied, eight patients having single-muscle involvement, 39 involvement of two muscles, and 25 involvement of three muscles. The trapezius muscle was involved in only seven patients, although in some reports this muscle is one of the more frequently injected. The small number of patients having laterocollis, retrocollis, or complex activation patterns had more predictable muscle-activation patterns. This study, based on only three muscle pairs, was limited in that the levator scapulae, scalene complex, and deep paraspinals (longissimus capitis and semispinalis capitis) were not studied.

Following BTX treatment, the pattern of muscle involvement may change. Gelb et al. (13) studied the pattern of muscle activation in CD patients before and after BTX treatment. They found that in the same patient following treatment, other previously inactive cervical muscles may become activated and result in the pretreatment abnormal head posture.

The EMG pattern of activation may also be useful in predicting outcome following BTX treatment. Tsui at al. (14), using surface EMG, reported that the patterns of electrically active muscles in CD may predict responsiveness to BTX injections. In their group of 19 patients, they studied the sternocleidomastoid, splenius, and trapezius and defined two groups of patients: (1) agonist type, in which all involved muscles act together in the same direction, and (2) antagonist type, in which the overactive muscles act in opposite directions. Following BTX treatment, 82% of the agonist type had a good response, whereas only 12% of the antagonist type achieved similar benefit. Studies of larger numbers of patients are needed to confirm this observation.

Targeting Botulinum Toxin Injection into Muscle with Electromyography

A second rationale for EMG-assisted BTX injections is the ability to accurately inject the toxin directly into the muscle by using a hollow recording needle and injecting only when the full recruitment pattern of the targeted muscle is obtained. Borodic and his colleagues (15) found that following injections of BTX into the longissimus dorsi of mice, acetylcholinesterase staining activity reflecting the effect of the toxin extended only 30 mm from the injection site. At 45 mm from the injection site, no BTX effect was apparent. This suggests that the accuracy of the injection into the muscle may be crucial. However, with the larger doses used in humans and injection into actively contracting dystonic muscle, the effect of the toxin may extend further.

PAST EXPERIENCE WITH ELECTROMYOGRAPHY-ASSISTED TECHNIQUE

Electromyography-Assisted Botulinum Toxin Injections for Focal Dystonia

Electromyography has been used routinely in conjunction with the clinical examination for the BTX treatment of certain types of focal dystonia. Botulinum toxin injections for spasmodic dysphonia (16,17), hand and foot dystonia (18–22), jaw opening oromandibular dystonia (7), and lingual dystonia rely on EMG to accurately identify involved muscles and to direct the injection in the muscle. These focal dystonias all have in common muscles not visible or easily palpable from the surface. In contrast, blepharospasm results from the abnormal contraction of superficially located orbicularis oculi muscle, and BTX is injected subcutaneously over the muscle (23–25). Hence BTX treatment of blepharospasm is rarely performed with EMG.

Electromyography-Assisted Botulinum Toxin Injections for Cervical Dystonia

When BTX was first introduced as a treatment for CD, EMG was frequently used in conjunction with the physical examination. Initially, EMG was used to identify sites for injection closest to the motor end plates, but this did not enhance the results and so was abandoned (26). As further experience with BTX injections was gained, many experts began to reserve EMG only for those patients with obese necks (8), those who failed to benefit from clinically directed injections, and those in whom there was uncertainty as to which muscles were involved (17).

In the largest series of BTX-treated CD patients with adequate follow-up, Jankovic and Schwartz (27) did not use EMG. Of their 205 CD patients, 71% were found to improve to a moderate or marked degree by subjective patient report. Similar outcomes have been reported by other investigators who injected BTX solely on the basis of the physical examination without any additional information provided by EMG (28–30) (Table 1).

Alternatively, some experienced investigators have continued to use an EMG-assisted technique to inject BTX in their CD patients. Dubinsky and his associates demonstrated the safety of the EMG technique (36). In their study, EMG served both to select the muscles and to target the BTX injections directly into the involved muscle through a hollow, Teflon-coated electrode. Of their 84 patients undergoing 225 injection sessions, moderate improvement was found in 79%. While dysphagia was reported in 11.1% and neck weakness in 16% of injection series, no unique complications were reported as a result of EMG use.

A comparison of clinical outcome among different investigators, however, has not been possible, as the methods of injection differ not only in the utilization of EMG, but also in other technical issues, including number of injection sites per muscle, dose of BTX administered, and concentration of BTX injected. In addition, the lack of a universal rating scale for the evaluation of cervical dystonia has led to the use of many different

Table 1 Botulinum Toxin Treatment for Cervical Dystonia: Differing Injection Techniques and Outcome

Study	Number of patients	Use of electromyography (EMG)	Patients improving (objective[a])
Tsui et al. 1987 (31)	56	EMG-assisted for (surface) muscle selection	66%
Stell et al., 1988 (32)	10	EMG-assisted (needle) for muscle selection	100%
Shannon et al., 1989 (33)	18	EMG-assisted (needle) muscle selection and injection	83%
Gelb et al., 1989 (34)	20	Clinically based technique without EMG use	No objective benefit, 80% with subjective benefit
Jankovic and Schwartz, 1990 (27)	205	Clinically based technique without EMG use	71%
Blackie and Lees, 1990 (35)	19	EMG-assisted (surface) for muscle selection	74%
Greene et al., 1990 (29)	28	Clinically based technique without EMG use	61%
Moore and Blumhardt 1991 (28)	20	Clinically based technique without EMG use	63%
Dubinsky et al., 1991 (36)	84	EMG-assisted (needle) for muscle selection and injection	79%
Lorentz et al., 1991 (37)	23	Clinically based technique without EMG use	65%
Borodic et al., 1991 (30)	33	Clinically based technique without EMG use	80% combined subjective and objective
Poewe et al., 1992 (38)	37	EMG-assisted for muscle selection	86%

[a]Objective outcome as determined by the application of different rating scales of cervical dystonia. The outcome is therefore not directly comparable among the different studies.

scales to determine outcome of therapy (31,39,40). In the absence of compelling data, many investigators have devised their own injection techniques, some abandoning EMG altogether, others using EMG routinely, and yet others using EMG in a limited fashion (Table 1).

In order to determine whether EMG offered any advantage, Comella and her colleagues conducted a prospective, blinded study directly comparing the outcome of EMG-assisted BTX injections with that of clinically directed injections (9). Fifty-two CD patients were randomized into two groups. One group was treated by means of a Teflon-coated, hollow monopolar electrode and EMG in conjunction with the clinical examination to select and direct injections; the other group was treated with the same type of needle but without connection to the EMG, relying solely on clinical examination. The dilution and total dose of BTX were the same in both groups. Benefit following injection was determined from randomized videotape segments rated by an investigator blinded to the treatment grouping of the patient, using the same rating scale. Their results demonstrated that there was no significant difference in the number of patients improved whether EMG was used or not, but that the number of patients with marked improvement was greater in the EMG-assisted group (Table 2). In particular, there was a greater magnitude of benefit in the EMG-assisted treatment group for retrocollis, head tilt, and shoulder elevation. Adverse effects did not differ between the groups, with no additional complications arising from the use of EMG.

Table 2 A Comparison of Electromyography-Assisted Botulinum
Toxin Injections and Clinically Based Injections for Cervical Dystonia:
Percentage of Patients Improved Following Botulinum Toxin

Measure	EMG-CLIN	CLIN	*p* value
Objective measures			
Any improvement	82%	58%	NS
Marked improvement	50%	8%	0.003
Subjective improvement			
Any improvement	86%	79%	NS
Marked improvement			
Global CD scale	46%	17%	0.049
Head position	61%	25%	0.021
Mobility	54%	18%	0.026
Pain	73%	38%	NS

Cervical dystonia (CD) patients receiving botulinum toxin injections with electromyographic assistance (EMG-CLIN) and those treated solely on the basis of clinical
examination (CLIN) are compared for the percentage of patients with any improvement
and those with marked improvement, defined as the upper 75% percentile of change for
both objective and subjective measures.
Source: Ref. 9.

The value of EMG as applied to BTX injections for the treatment of CD is not
resolved. Some experts feel that clinically guided BTX injections for CD result in
symptomatic benefit in most patients and that routine use of EMG is more expensive and
time-consuming, offering no practical advantage (8,27,28). Others believe that the
increased ability to identify involved cervical muscles and to target injections directly into
the muscle improves the outcome and warrants the extra time and expense of the EMG-
assisted technique (10,33,36).

TECHNIQUE OF ELECTROMYOGRAPHY-ASSISTED INJECTION

Among investigators using EMG, the technique has varied. Surface, needle, and wire
electrodes have all been utilized either separately or in combination (41). Surface electrodes, while not invasive, allow only for recordings of superficial muscles and do not
permit directed injections. Wire electrodes are particularly useful for defining the simultaneous activation patterns of deeper cervical muscles without displacement of the
electrode caused by movement, but do not permit targeted injections into the muscle.
Needle electrodes (monopolar or concentric) allow for conventional EMG analysis of
motor unit activity. Needle electrodes, however, tend to change position if left in the
muscle and are suboptimal in simultaneous recordings. They also cause greater pain than
either surface or wire electrodes (42). Teflon-coated, hollow monopolar needle electrodes (Fig. 1), although sharing the drawbacks of other needle electrodes, allow for targeted injections of BTX directly into the overactive muscle. These hollow needles are
used at Rush-Presbyterian-St. Luke's Medical Center and are used in the technique
reported below.

In addition to the specialized needle electrode, other equipment required includes a
standard EMG machine, an alligator clip or customized clip to fit the electrode hub, and

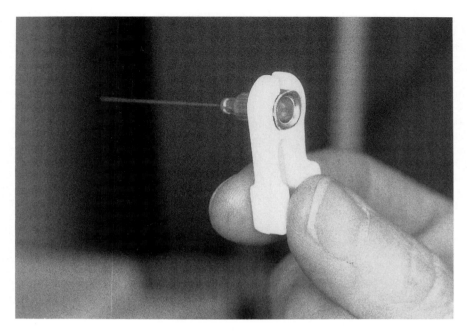

Figure 1 The Teflon-coated, hollow monopolar electrode. The Teflon coating extends along the needle shaft, leaving the hub and the tip exposed. The customized clip (shown here) is attached to the hub. The hollowed electrode may be used both for selecting muscles and for injecting directly into the muscle.

cable for connection of the needle to the EMG machine. The additional time for the EMG technique is approximately 15 minutes (9,36). The EMG band passes are standard. The hollow, Teflon-coated needle is used to evaluate muscle activity and to target the injection of BTX directly into the muscle. The hollow electrode is connected to the EMG apparatus by a specialized cable (Fig. 2). Botulinum toxin is drawn up into a tuberculin syringe, and the syringe is attached to the needle before insertion into the muscle. The patient is seated in front of the EMG machine (Fig. 3). The cervical region is first examined clinically according to the methods outlined in the previous section. The muscles likely to be involved in the abnormal movement as determined by the position of the head at rest and the clinical evaluation are then examined with EMG by inserting the needle electrode. Electrode placement is based on standard anatomical landmarks. Once the electrode is inserted, the needle is positioned so that a full recruitment pattern is demonstrated with voluntary activation of the muscle. The needle is held in position as the patient again resumes the relaxed position with the spontaneous abnormal posture. The syringe is aspirated to ensure that the tip is not within a blood vessel, and the appropriate amount of BTX is then directly injected through the electrode into the muscle. This procedure can be used for either single- or multiple-site injections into the same muscle. After the injection is completed, the needle is withdrawn and may be used to inject other muscles in the same patient during that session. At the completion of the session, the needle is discarded. During the injection, leakage of toxin may occur around the hub of the needle at its attachment to the syringe. Should a droplet form at this attachment, tightening the

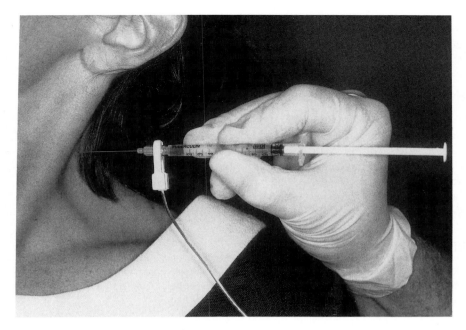

Figure 2 A demonstration of the electromyography (EMG)-assisted technique. In this figure, the sternocleidomastoid muscle is being targeted for injection. The tuberculin syringe containing botulinum toxin is attached directly to the electrode, and will be injected through the electrode when a full recruitment pattern appears on the EMG oscilloscope.

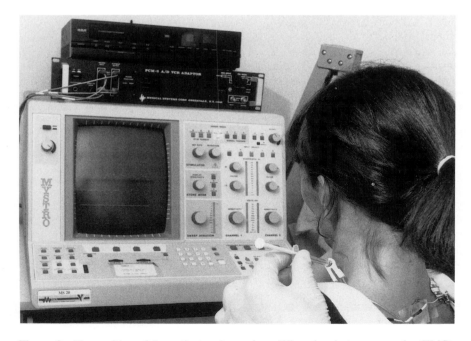

Figure 3 The position of the patient and examiner. When the electromyography (EMG)-assisted technique is used, the patient is seated in front of the EMG machine, and the treating physician is positioned behind the patient, permitting a full view of the EMG oscilloscope tracing.

connection or changing syringes and reattaching the needle will prevent an expensive leak.

CONCLUSION

The EMG-assisted technique for BTX treatment of CD does not replace the physical examination but rather augments it with electrophysiological information. Although injections based solely on clinical evaluation are effective, this simple technique may allow for a greater magnitude of benefit following treatment, particularly for patients with activation of deeper muscles, those who have failed to achieve a satisfactory response to clinically administered BTX injections, those with obscured surface cervical anatomy, and those with complex patterns of muscle activation.

REFERENCES

1. Rothwell JC, Obeso JA, Day BL, Marsden CD. Pathophysiology of dystonia. In: Desmedt JE, ed. Motor control mechanisms in health and disease. New York: Raven Press, 1983:851–868.
2. Nakashima K, Thompson PD, Rothwell JC, Day BL, Stell R, Marsden CD. An exteroceptive reflex in the sternocleidomastoid muscle produced by electrical stimulation of the supraorbital nerve in normal subjects and patients with spasmodic torticollis. Neurology 1989;39:1354–1358.
3. Podivinsky F. Torticollis. In: Vinken PJ, Bruyn GW, eds. Handbook of clinical neurology. Vol. 6. Amsterdam: North Holland, 1968:567–603.
4. Tournay A, Paillard J. Torticollis spasmodique et electromyographie. Rev Neurol 1955; 93:347–355.
5. Stejskal L. Counterpressure in torticollis. J Neurol Sci 1980;48:9–19.
6. National Institutes of Health Consensus Development Conference: Clinical Use of botulinum toxin. Arch Neurol 1991;48:1294–1298.
7. Report of the Therapeutics and Technology Assessment Subcommittee of the American Academy of Neurology. Assessment: the clinical usefulness of botulinum toxin-A in treating neurologic disorders. Neurology 1990;40:1332–1336.
8. Jankovic J, Brin M. Therapeutic applications of botulinum toxin. N Engl J Med 1991; 324:1186–1194.
9. Comella C, Buchman AS, Tanner CM, Brown-Toms NC, Goetz CG. Botulinum toxin injection for spasmodic torticollis: increased magnitude of benefit with electromyographic assistance. Neurology 1992;42:878–882.
10. Stell R, Thompson PD, Marsden CD. Botulinum toxin in torticollis (letter). Neurology 1989;39:1403–1404.
11. Berkovitz BKB, Moxham BJ. A textbook of head and neck anatomy. London: New York Medical Publishers, 1988.
12. Deuschl G, Heinen F, Kleedorfer B, Wagner M, Lucking CH, Poewe W. Clinical and polymyographic investigation of spasmodic torticollis. J Neurol 1992;239:9–15.
13. Gelb DJ, Yoshimura DM, Olney RK, Lowenstein DH, Aminoff MJ. Change in pattern of muscle activity following botulinum toxin injections for torticollis. Ann Neurol 1991;29:370–376.
14. Tsui JK, Eisen A, Calne DB. Botulinum toxin in spasmodic torticollis. Adv Neurol 1988;50:593–597.
15. Borodic GE, Joseph M, Fay L, Cozzolino D, Ferrante RJ. Botulinum A toxin for the treatment of spasmodic torticollis: dysphagia and regional toxin spread. Head Neck 1990; 12:392–399.

16. Ludlow CL, Nauton RF, Sedory SE, Schulz GM, Hallett M. Effects of botulinum toxin injections on speech in adductor spasmodic dysphonia. Neurology 1988;38:1220–1225.

17. Jankovic J, Schwartz K, Donovan DT. Botulinum toxin treatment of cranial-cervical dystonia, spasmodic dysphonia, other focal dystonias and hemifacial spasm. J Neurol Neurosurg Psychiatry 1990;53:633–639.

18. Brin MF, Fahn S, Moskowitz C, Friedman A, Shale HM, Greene PE, Blitzer A, List T, Lange D, Lovelace RE, McMahon D. Localized injection of botulinum toxin or the treatment of focal dystonia and hemifacial spasm. Adv Neurol 1988;50:599–608.

19. Yoshimura Y, Aminoff MJ, Olney RK. Botulinum toxin therapy for limb dystonias. Neurology 1992;42:627–630.

20. Rivest J, Lees AJ, Marsden CD. Writer's cramp: treatment with botulinum toxin injections. Mov Disord 1991;6:55–59.

21. Cohen LG, Hallett M, Geller BD, Hochberg F. Treatment of focal dystonia of the hand with botulinum toxin injections. J Neurol Neurosurg Psychiatry 1989;52:355–363.

22. Lees AJ, Turjanski N, Rivest J, Whurr R, Lorch M, Brookes G. Treatment of cervical dystonia, hand spasms, and laryngeal dystonia with botulinum toxin. J Neurol 1992;239:1–4.

23. Cohen DA, Savino PJ, Stern MB, Hurtig HI. Botulinum injection therapy for blepharospasm: a review and report of 75 patients. Clin Neuropharmacol 1986;9:415–429.

24. Dutton J, Buckley EG. Long-term results and complications of botulinum A toxin in the treatment of blepharospasm. Ophthalmology 1988;95:1529–1534.

25. Kennedy RH, Bartley GB, Flanagan JC, Waller RR. Treatment of blepharospasm with botulinum toxin. Mayo Clin Proc 1989;64:1085–1090.

26. Tsui JK, Eisen A, Mak E, Carruthers J, Scott A, Calne DB. A pilot study on the use of botulinum toxin in spasmodic torticollis. Can J Neurol Sci 1985;12:314–316.

27. Jankovic J, Schwartz K. Botulinum toxin injections for cervical dystonia. Neurology 1990;40:277–280.

28. Moore AP, Blumhardt LD. A double blind trial of botulinum toxin "A" in torticollis, with one year follow up. J Neurol Neurosurg Psychiatry 1991;54:813–816.

29. Greene P, Kang U, Fahn S, Brin M, Moskowitz C, Flaster E. Double-blind, placebo-controlled trial of botulinum toxin injections for the treatment of spasmodic torticollis. Neurology 1990;40:1213–1218.

30. Borodic GE, Mills L, Joseph M. Botulinum A toxin for the treatment of adult-onset spasmodic torticollis. Plast Reconstr Surg 1991;87:285–289.

31. Tsui JKC, Fross RD, Calne S, Calne DB. Local treatment of spasmodic torticollis with botulinum toxin. Can J Neurol Sci 1987;14:533–535.

32. Stell R, Thompson PD, Marsden CD. Botulinum toxin in spasmodic torticollis. J Neurol Neurosurg Psychiatry 1988;51:920–923.

33. Shannon KM, Comella C, Tanner CM. EMG-guided botulinum toxin injections in torticollis: objective clinical improvements (abstr). Neurology 1989;39(suppl 1):352.

34. Gelb DJ, Lowenstein DH, Aminoff MJ. Controlled trial of botulinum toxin injections in the treatment of spasmodic torticollis. Neurology 1989;39:80–84.

35. Blackie JD, Lees AJ. Botulinum toxin treatment in spasmodic torticollis. J Neurol Neurosurg Psychiatry 1990;53:640–643.

36. Dubinsky RM, Grey CS, Vetere-Overfield B, Koller WC. Electromyographic guidance of botulinum toxin treatment in cervical dystonia. Clin Neuropharmacol 1991;14:262–267.

37. Lorentz IT, Subramaniam SS, Yiannikas C. Treatment of idiopathic spasmodic torticollis with botulinum toxin A: a double-blind study on twenty-three patients. Movement Dis 1991;6:145–150.

38. Poewe W, Schelosky L, Kleedorfer B, Heinen F, Wagner M, Deuschl G. Treatment of spasmodic torticollis with local injections of botulinum toxin. J Neurol 1992;239:21–25.

39. Fahn S. Assessment of the primary dystonias. In: Munsat T, ed. Quantification of neurologic deficits. Boston: Butterworths, 1989:241–270.

40. Consky E, Basinski A, Belle L, Ranawaya R, Lang AE. The Toronto Western Spasmodic Torticollis Rating Scale (TWSTRS): assessment of validity and inter-rater reliability. Neurology 1990;40(suppl 1):445.

41. Buchman AS, Comella CL, Garratt MJ, Tanner CM. Quantitative electromyographic analysis of response to botulinum toxin therapy for spasmodic torticollis (abstr). Ann Neurol 1990;28:234.

42. Bouisset S, Maton B. Comparison between surface and intramuscular EMG during voluntary movement. In: Desmedt JE, ed. New developments in electromyography and clinical neurophysiology. Vol. 1. Basel: Karger, 1973:533–539.

21

Botulinum Toxin Treatment of Focal Hand Dystonia

Barbara Illowsky Karp and Mark Hallett
National Institute of Neurological Disorders and Stroke, National Institutes of Health,
Bethesda, Maryland

INTRODUCTION

Descriptions of writer's cramp first appeared in the 18th and 19th centuries. Reports such as those by Solly described "scrivener's palsy or paralysis of writers," a disease that "shows itself outwardly in a palsy of the writing powers. The muscles cease to obey the mandates of the will. It comes on very insidiously, the first indication often being only a painful feeling in the thumb or forefinger of the writing hand, accompanied by some stiffness; these unnatural sensations subside during the hours of rest and sleep, to return with the writer's work on the next day" (1). Although writer's cramp was the most common form of occupational dystonia, similar abnormalities were described in shoemakers, milkers, musicians, seamstresses, cobblers, and others whose work involved frequent repetitive movements (2,3).

Early descriptions of writer's cramp remain valid. The initial symptom is typically a feeling of clumsiness during writing with a loss of speed and fluency of movement. There is a tendency to grip the pen too tightly, and the hand quickly becomes fatigued. Tightness with aching may extend to the forearm or shoulder. Abnormal muscle contraction may lead to distortion of normal posture. The wrist may flex or extend; the fingers may curl into the palm or pull away so that grip on the pen cannot be maintained. The process of writing becomes labored. Although the dystonia is relieved by rest, it quickly reappears as soon as writing resumes and worsens with continued effort. Pain is prominent in some patients. Tremor accompanies dystonia in 25–48% of patients (4–6). Myoclonic jerks, decreased arm swing, or slight increase in tone of the affected arm may also be present (4). In some patients, dystonia remains limited to writing. This has been termed "simple writer's cramp" (7). In "dystonic writer's cramp" the dystonia is present during additional tasks. Patients whose simple writer's cramp evolves into dystonic cramp are said to have "progressive writer's cramp." Writer's cramp can also be classified as "localized" if three or fewer fingers on one hand are affected and as "nonlocalized" if more than three fingers or both hands are involved (8).

Writer's cramp typically begins between ages 20 and 50 (9). Progression usually occurs within the first 6 months of onset but can develop years later. Few patients become totally disabled. Marsden and Sheehy (9) noted that only 17% of patients entirely ceased writing. Spontaneous remission is rare and probably occurs in fewer than 5% of patients. Nutt et al. (10) studied the occurrence of focal dystonias in Rochester, Minnesota. Writer's cramp accounted for 25% of all focal dystonias in their population, with an incidence of $2.7/10^6$ population and a prevalence of $69/10^6$.

The etiology of writer's cramp remains uncertain. Writer's cramp can develop following trauma or in association with peripheral nerve injury (9,11). It is occasionally seen following central nervous system damage. Writer's cramp, along with other focal dystonias, may be a forme fruste of generalized dystonia. A family history of dystonia can be identified in 5–20% of patients with writer's cramp (4,12). The inheritance pattern is most consistent with autosomal dominant transmission with incomplete penetrance.

Electrophysiological studies have identified abnormal muscle activation in writer's cramp (8). There is a loss of the normal alternating pattern of agonist/antagonist contraction. Cocontracting agonist and antagonist muscles have prolonged electromyographic (EMG) bursts and abnormally decreased reciprocal inhibition. Overflow activity is present in muscles not normally involved in the task being performed. Willed voluntary activation may fail to occur.

Many approaches have been taken to treating writer's cramp. Patients often try to switch to writing with their nondominant hand. While this strategy helps many to continue writing, about 25% will develop dystonia in the second hand (9). Physical devices such as splints or braces may occasionally be helpful. Biofeedback, acupuncture, psychotherapy, physical therapy, chiropractic manipulation, relaxation therapy, hypnosis, wax baths, immobilization, transcutaneous nerve stimulation, re-educating the muscles, and avoidance conditioning have not proven useful. Patients have undergone peripheral nerve surgery, such as ulnar nerve transposition, carpal tunnel release, or posterior interosseous nerve release, without benefit. Thalamotomy, tenotomy, and thoracic rib removal are similarly of little use. Percutaneous anti-inflammatory drug or steroid injections have not relieved the dystonia. Medications tried have included dopamine agonists, dopamine antagonists, baclofen, benzodiazepines, alcohol, clonidine, sedatives, muscle relaxants, steroids, propranolol, tricyclic antidepressants, testosterone, dimethyl sulfoxide, phenytoin, primidone, pimozide, amantadine, tryptophan, and nonsteroidal anti-inflammatories. The most effective medications are anticholinergics. Unfortunately, these medications work only rarely and must frequently be used at such high doses that the side effects become intolerable. Botulinum toxin (BTX), which does not have these systemic side effects, has proven useful for writer's cramp. The evaluation and treatment of writer's cramp with BTX is discussed in the sections that follow.

BOTULINUM TOXIN TREATMENT OF WRITER'S CRAMP

Initial evaluation of patients with writer's cramp includes general neurological examination. Sensory loss, weakness, spasticity, or changes in reflexes are not seen with dystonia and may indicate radiculopathy or peripheral nerve entrapment for which specific treatment might be available. Nerve conductions studies may be needed to exclude an ulnar neuropathy or carpal tunnel syndrome. The patient should be examined for abnormal postures in order to determine which muscles are involved in the dystonia. Observations should be made at rest, during the provoking activity, and during a variety of other actions such as using a cup or a comb. Sustained posture of outstretched arms may bring out associated tremor. During examination, the patient should be instructed not to compensate for the dystonia. Abnormal flexion or extension of the wrist or fingers and ease of performance are carefully observed. In some cases, the patient experiences pain or fatigue without a change in posture. Under these circumstances, palpation of the active muscle may detect excessive contraction or tension. Wire electromyography during rest and activity may help identify involved muscles not readily apparent. The selection of muscles for injection therefore depends on clinical evaluation, patient report of local pain or tightness, and/or EMG evidence of excessive activity.

Botulinum toxin is injected into the muscle belly. Although injections that target the motor end plate offer a theoretical advantage in concentrating the toxin at its site of action, clinical experience has shown that the toxin can diffuse 1–2 cm from the site of injection, and precise identification of the motor end plate is not necessary.

Localizing muscles for injection within the forearm may be difficult. The muscle bellies are thin and frequently overlap. At times it is necessary to place the needle in a specific part of a larger muscle, such as the fascicle for movement of a single finger. Verification of needle location is therefore important and can be accomplished in several ways. One can passively stretch the muscle while the needle is in place, looking for needle movement with muscle movement. If a Teflon-coated EMG needle is used, motor unit activity with activation of the muscle can be confirmed. The position of the needle can also be determined by passing a small current through the needle to evoke muscle contraction. Once proper needle location is confirmed, BTX can be injected.

There are few complications associated with BTX injection for writer's cramp. Some patients notice slight pain, similar to that of an EMG or other intramuscular injections. At times, a small hematoma may develop at the injection site.

Common initial doses of BTX for hand cramp are 5 U for small muscles, such as the hand intrinsic muscles, and 10–20 U for the muscles in the forearm. Botulinum toxin should be prepared in concentrations of 2.5–10 U/0.1 ml. Large doses into a single muscle may best be given in multiple sites to aid diffusion of the toxin to a greater number of end plates.

The dose of BTX is initially titrated over several injection sessions, as frequent as every 2 weeks, to the dose that maximizes relief from dystonia while minimizing muscle weakness. Subsequent injections should be given at 2- to 4-month intervals. At each session, the patient should be examined for weakness that might postpone injection or limit the dose. The dystonia should also be reevaluated at each session, since the pattern of muscle contraction can change. Variation in the pattern of muscle contraction may be due to progression of the writer's cramp, alteration as a result of BTX treatment, or unmasking of muscles not previously thought to be involved in the dystonia.

Treatment may lead to improvement in abnormal posture, relief of pain, and/or restoration of normal function. Although benefit may be apparent, it is difficult to describe or quantitate. Correction of abnormal posture can be evaluated visually. Videotapes made before and after injections allow for direct comparison of actions at different times. Evaluation of pain relief relies on patient report. Functional improvement can be assessed by observing the ease and outcome of performance, such as writing samples, before and after injection (Fig. 1).

BEFORE TREATMENT

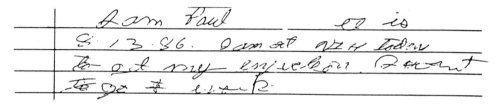

AFTER TREATMENT

Figure 1 Sample of handwriting before and 2 weeks after botulinum toxin treatment in a patient with dystonic writer's cramp. (From Ref. 13.)

The effect of BTX treatment in writer's cramp is usually apparent 5 to 7 days after injection. Curiously, however, some patients report an early change in either strength or writing within a day. Improvement in writing and hand position is usually accompanied by relief from pain. Some patients experience functional improvement while pain persists, whereas others may have an improvement in pain without a change in posture or writing. Benefit peaks about 2 weeks after treatment and generally lasts 3 to 4 months. Occasionally, beneficial effects can persist up to a year.

EFFICACY OF INJECTION

Several studies have addressed the issue of efficacy of BTX for writer's cramp. Cohen et al. studied 19 patients with localized and nonlocalized writer's cramp (13). Finger and forearm flexors and extensors were the muscles most commonly injected. Doses used ranged from 17.5 to 140 U per injection session. Injection intervals ranged from 2 weeks to 6 months. Patients were followed for up to 27 months. Eighty-four percent of patients had significant benefit. All patients who improved also had weakness in the injected muscles. As might be expected, patients with localized dystonia required lower doses than those with nonlocalized dystonia. Unexpectedly, patients with extensor cramp seemed to respond more quickly than those with flexors involved. Two patients (11%) developed antibodies to BTX resulting in loss of response to treatment.

Jankovic et al. (14) included 28 patients with hand dystonia in a larger study of BTX use in a variety of focal dystonias. Of these hand cramp patients, 93% had moderate to marked improvement during at least one injection cycle. However, 48% of all injections, especially early injections, were not effective, and 5% resulted in disabling weakness. The latency to response was 5 days (range 0–28 days), with maximum benefit lasting a mean of 7 weeks (range 0–20 weeks). The total duration of any benefit was 2–4 weeks longer.

Yoshimura et al. (15) conducted a blind, placebo-controlled study of BTX in 17 patients with symptomatic or idiopathic hand dystonia. Patients were injected in four sessions: at an estimated effective dose, at one-half the effective dose, at two times the effective dose, and with placebo. Injections were given in random order and were at least 4 weeks apart. Moderate or major improvement was seen with at least one injection in 82% of patients. The improvement was substantial in 59%. Interestingly, there were no differences in the response to the differing doses. Side effects of treatment included weakness, muscle stiffness, pain, malaise, muscle twitching, paresthesias, and nausea.

Rivest et al. (16) treated 12 hand cramp patients. Finger and wrist flexors and extensors were injected with doses ranging from 40 to 120 U per muscle. Patients were followed for up to 12 months. Eleven of their patients had at least moderate improvement; seven had major development. Eight of the 11 patients who benefited had improvement in writing, and three had correction of abnormal posture. All of 12 patients with painful hand cramp had relief from pain. Patients with localized symptoms had a better outcome than those with nonlocalized dystonias. The patients with nonlocalized dystonias also required more than one injection and higher doses to achieve a beneficial response. The authors also observed that although weakness might be present initially along with improvement in writing, the weakness often resolved within 2 weeks, while benefit continued for 4 to 13 weeks. One of their patients maintained an excellent response for 9 months.

Poungvarin (5) reported results of BTX treatment of 21 writer's cramp patients with doses ranging from 40 to 80 U per session. Sixty-seven percent of their patients had definite improvement in the dystonia lasting 3 to 4 months. All patients with painful dystonia had a decrease in pain. Thirty-three percent of patients experienced weakness that lasted from 2 to 6 weeks.

The five studies mentioned above varied in many ways. Some included patients with both symptomatic and idiopathic writer's cramp, while others treated patients with idiopathic hand cramp only. Electromyography was used to select muscles for injection in some studies, whereas others relied solely on observation. In each study, the dose of toxin injected was individualized on the basis of clinical judgment, resulting in a range of doses from 10 to 120 U per muscle and 10 to 300 U per treatment session. Reinjection intervals ranged from 2 weeks to 9 months. The results of all these studies, however, are remarkably similar. Approximately 80% of patients experience at least moderate improvement in symptoms. Pain relief is more dramatic; almost all patients with painful cramp benefit. Improvement from the injection generally lasts 3 to 4 months, although it can extend much longer. Injections result in weakness in about 50% of injection sessions. The weakness, however, often resolves quickly, resulting in a period of peak benefit beginning approximately 2 weeks after injection.

The cited studies focused on the initial outcome of BTX injections for writer's cramp. It remains to be determined if long-term benefit can be maintained by repeated injections. Preliminary information is available on patients at the National Institutes of Health (NIH) who have been followed for more than 2 years since starting treatment. Forty-five patients who participated in studies from 1986 through October 1992 were contacted. Information on the severity and current treatment of their dystonia was requested. Patients still receiving BTX provided additional information on the current doses and muscles being injected, the interval between injections, and the extent and frequency of weakness accompanying injection. Nine patients did not respond. Information was thus obtained on 36 patients a mean of 4 years after initial BTX treatment.

Twenty-three of the 36 patients are no longer receiving BTX for hand dystonia. Fifteen patients discontinued treatment because of inadequate response. Two patients, who initially responded to treatment but failed to have either benefit or weakness with later injections, were found to have antibodies to botulinum toxin type A. Six patients responded to treatment but were unable to continue because of the expense of the toxin or inability to find a local physician to provide treatment once their participation in NIH protocols ended.

Thirteen patients initially responded to injection and continued treatment. All patients continue to benefit from injections. The dose of toxin injected at each session and the duration of improvement from each injection have remained stable, with benefit lasting approximately 4 months (range 2 weeks to 9 months). No long-term or systemic side effects have been noted.

MUSICIAN'S CRAMP

With the years of practice and repetitive movement required to achieve professional performance, it is not surprising that musicians are prone to overuse syndromes. Pain is common; musculoskeletal disorders and nerve entrapment can occur. They may also develop focal dystonia, which is particularly devastating. Musician's cramp is generally refractory to medical treatment, rest, or physical therapy. Alteration of playing technique may help some patients.

Cole et al. (17) treated 18 musicians with musician's cramp with BTX. These 18 patients partially overlap with the 45 focal hand dystonia patients discussed earlier. Fifteen of these patients were professional musicians; three played only recreationally. The instruments played included piano (five patients), guitar (three patients), trumpet, drum, and flute (two patients each), and violin, clarinet, organ, and bagpipe (one patient each). Patients were screened to exclude those with peripheral nerve damage or a central cause of dystonia. The muscles selected for injection were those that assumed abnormal posture or could not be properly controlled during musical performance. Electromyography recorded through wire electrodes during performance was needed to determine the involved muscles in some cases. The initial BTX dose used was 20 U. Later doses were based on the outcome of prior injections. Patients received up to six injection cycles and were followed a mean of 15 months.

Eighty-three percent of patients had improved instrumental performance in response to at least one injection. The mean dose of BTX used during the best injection cycle was approximately 56 U (range 5–215 U). The duration of benefit was 3 to 4 months.

The extent of improvement and duration of response were unchanged through the initial four injection cycles; slightly less improvement was found with later injections.

Even though most patients did respond to treatment, the magnitude of improvement was only modest compared to their need. Ten patients stopped treatment because they considered the benefit inadequate to maintain the desired level of performance. Three patients had no initial response to injection and withdrew from the study. Three additional patients withdrew when they lost response to treatment. Two of these patients were found to have antibodies to BTX. Thus, by the end of the study, only two patients (11%) considered continued BTX injections worthwhile.

The high withdrawal rate for musicians is disappointing and is largely accounted for by insufficient response to injection. In patients with writer's cramp, even a mild response to treatment may ease or preserve the ability to write. For professional musicians, however, even a marked response to treatment is of no benefit if the ability to play professionally is not maintained. It appears that although BTX injection can decrease spasm and relieve abnormal postures, the loss of coordination that is part of the dystonia may not be restored.

CONCLUSION

The clinical use of BTX for neurological disorders was reviewed in 1990 at an NIH Consensus Development Conference and by the American Academy of Neurology (18,19). At that time little information was available on the efficacy of BTX treatment of focal hand dystonia. Experience over the past several years has shown that many patients with hand cramp unresponsive to other therapies improve with BTX. We therefore suggest that BTX injection be considered for first-line treatment of focal hand dystonia.

REFERENCES

1. Solly S. Scrivener's palsy, or the paralysis of writers. Lancet 1864;2:709–711.
2. Hunter D. The diseases of occupations. 6th ed. London: Hodder & Stoughton, 1978.
3. Gowers WR. A manual of diseases of the nervous system. Philadelphia: P. Blakiston, Son & Co, 1888.
4. Sheehy MP, Marsden CD. Writer's cramp—a focal dystonia. Brain 1982;105:461–480.
5. Poungvarin N. Writer's cramp: the experience with botulinum toxin injections in 25 patients. J Med Assoc Thai 1991;74:239–247.
6. Jedynak CP, Bonnet AM, Agid Y. Tremor and idiopathic dystonia. Mov Disord 1991;6:230–236.
7. Marsden CD. The focal dystonias. Clin Neuropharmacol 1986;9:S49–S60.
8. Cohen LG, Hallett M. Hand cramps: clinical features and electromyographic patterns in a focal dystonia. Neurology 1988;38:1005–1012.
9. Marsden CD, Sheehy MP. Writer's cramp. TINS 1990;13:148–153.
10. Nutt JG, Muenter MD, Aronson A, Kurland LT, Melton LJ. Epidemiology of focal and generalized dystonia in Rochester, Minn. Mov Disord 1988;3:188–194.
11. Scherokman B, Husain F, Cuetter A, Jabbari B, Maniglia E. Peripheral dystonia. Arch Neurol 1986;43:830–832.
12. Waddy HM, Fletcher NA, Harding AE, Marsden CD. A genetic study of idiopathic focal dystonias. Ann Neurol 1991;29:320–324.
13. Cohen LG, Hallett M, Geller BD, Hochberg F. Treatment of focal dystonias of the hand with botulinum toxin injections. J Neurol Neurosurg Psychiatry 1989;52:355–363.
14. Jankovic J, Schwartz K, Donovan D. Botulinum toxin treatment of cranial-cervical dystonia, spasmodic dysphonia, other focal dystonias and hemifacial spasm. J Neurol Neurosurg Psychiatry 1990;53:633–639.
15. Yoshimura D, Aminoff MJ, Olney RK. Botulinum toxin therapy for limb dystonias. Neurology 1992;42:627–630.
16. Rivest J, Lees AJ, Marsden CD. Writer's cramp: treatment with botulinum toxin injections. Mov Disord 1991;6:55–59.

17. Cole RA, Cohen LG, Hallett M. Treatment of musician's cramp with botulinum toxin. Med Prob Perf Art 1991;6:137–143.

18. National Institutes of Health Consensus Development Conference Statement: Clinical use of botulinum toxin. Arch Neurol 1991;48:1294–1298.

19. Report of the Therapeutics and Technology Assessment Subcommittee of the American Academy of Neurology. Assessment: the clinical usefulness of botulinum toxin-A in treating neurologic disorders. Neurology 1990;40:1332–1336.

22

Limb Dystonia: Treatment with Botulinum Toxin

Seth L. Pullman

The Neurological Institute, Columbia-Presbyterian Medical Center, New York, New York

INTRODUCTION

Limb dystonia is characterized by sustained involuntary muscle contractions and abnormal movements in the arm, hand, leg, or foot. As with other types of dystonia, limb dystonia is caused by overactivity in groups of muscles and presents clinically with spasms, abnormal twisting postures, and irregular tremors. Physiological correlates of limb dystonia include cocontraction of antagonist muscles, prolongation of electromyographic (EMG) activity with overflow of activity from prime movers into neighboring muscles, loss of fine motor performance, and dystonic tremors (1). Additionally, there are abnormalities in later phases of reciprocal inhibition and dysfunctional brain stem interneuronal activity (2).

All types of dystonia affect the limbs. Focal limb dystonia typically presents as an "occupational cramp" in which specific learned complex motor tasks (such as writing or playing a musical instrument) trigger muscle spasms and interfere with performance while other actions remain normal. With time, focal limb dystonia may be triggered less specifically and may even occur at rest. Writers' cramp is the most common form of idiopathic limb dystonia (3), and while there are many other known occupational cramps including musicians', typists', stenographers', telegraphers', physicians', and sports players' cramps (and probably several others yet to be reported), writers' cramp has been the most extensively studied (1,3). A clinically useful classification scheme defines simple writers' cramp as muscles spasms only with writing and dystonic writers' cramp as spasms with writing as well as other actions (3). Simple cramp may progress into dystonic cramp over time. Focal limb dystonia usually affects fine control in the hands or feet. Segmental limb dystonia involves several adjacent muscle groups and usually affects the hand or foot as well as more proximal regions such as the upper arm or shoulder. Segmental dystonia may begin more focally and then spread to involve more muscles and actions. Generalized dystonia always involves at least one leg and adjacent body regions and often includes the arms (4). Like segmental dystonia, generalized dystonia characteristically begins more focally and progresses to affect both proximal and distal motor function.

Limb dystonia may be idiopathic (primary) or symptomatic (secondary), and although no cellular or neurotransmitter abnormality has been found for primary dystonia (5), its association with other basal ganglia disorders suggests that striatal or other subcortical regions play a major role in its pathogenesis. Lesions in the striatum account for most of the reported cases of symptomatic dystonia (6). Minor trauma sometimes precedes the onset of limb dystonia, but this relationship is unclear (7,8), and limb dystonia is usually idiopathic. The secondary dystonias typically occur in the setting of a hereditary or acquired condition such as Wilson's disease, Parkinson's disease, or a focal cerebral lesion (9). In these cases, the involved limbs represent only a portion of a more diffuse segmental dystonia, hemidystonia, or generalized dystonia. Any part of the body may be affected, but the foot is often affected in secondary limb dystonias.

Therapy with oral anticholinergics, baclofen, muscle relaxants, clonazepam or other benzodiazepines (3), and acute intravenous anticholinergics (10), and nonmedical approaches such as behavioral therapy (11), have generally been ineffective in treating patients with focal limb dystonias. Botulinum toxin type A injections have become the treatment of choice for most patients with blepharospasm, torticollis, and hemifacial spasm (12), and their use in limb dystonia is limited but growing. Because of its success in cranial/cervical conditions, botulinum toxin (BTX) use in the limbs is becoming a promising alternative to those previously used but less efficacious methods.

Small intramuscular doses of BTX reversibly denervate and locally weaken muscles. Therefore, this method of treatment is empirically well suited to reducing the localized excessive muscle activity characteristic of limb dystonia. A sampling of the early studies from the National Institutes of Health (13), Baylor College of Medicine (14), Columbia-Presbyterian Medical Center (15), The National Hospital at Queen Square (16), Mahidol University, Bangkok (17), and the University of California, San Francisco (18), indicates that injections of BTX have been highly successful in relieving at least some of the symptoms of muscle spasms in 84.2% and pain in 85% of patients with hand cramps (Table 1). The one placebo-controlled blinded study (18) found subjective improvement in 82% of the patients. Preliminary reports are also emerging on the use of BTX in foot dystonias, particularly in Parkinson's disease (19,20).

Any type of dystonia (primary, secondary, focal, segmental, or generalized) affecting the limbs can be treated symptomatically with BTX. The overall improvement in motor disability can be dramatic even if the spasms are only partially treated, as is often the case in segmental and generalized dystonia. Indications for using BTX in limb dystonia are the same for other conditions: prior failure with pharmacological, surgical, or behavioral therapy. In many cases, BTX is becoming the treatment of choice and can be safely used before other types of therapy. We have found at Columbia-Presbyterian Medical Center that BTX can also be safely administered in conjunction with other treatment in more widespread or secondary dystonia.

There are no absolute contraindications to using BTX, although relative contraindications include pregnancy and lactation and significant peripheral nerve or muscle disease, particularly disorders of the neuromuscular junction (12). Consideration should also be given to patients receiving certain antibiotics, anesthetics, or other medications that impair neuromuscular transmission (21). Excess fatigue due to the interaction of such medications with BTX injections, however, has not been reported.

Table 1 Early Hand Dystonia Series

Study	Σ N	Functional improvement after botulinum toxin therapy						Pain relief
		None		Minimal		Major		
Cohen et al., 1989 (13)	19	3	15.8%	3	15.8%	13	68.4%	—
Jankovic et al., 1990 (14)	22	5	22.7%	—	—	17	77.3%	—
Pullman, 1990 (15)	29	4	13.8%	9	31.0%	16	55.2%	80%
Rivest et al., 1991 (16)	12	1	8.3%	4	33.3%	7	58.3%	75%
Poungvarin, 1991 (17)	21	3	14.3%	4	19.0%	14	66.7%	100%
Yoshimura et al., 1992 (18)	17	3	17.6%	—	—	14	82.4%	—
Combined	120	19	15.8%	20	16.7%	81	67.5%	85%
Summary								
No improvement	19	15.8%						
Some improvement	101	84.2%						

GENERAL CONCERNS

Before injecting BTX into limb muscles for dystonia, it is important that the diagnosis is secure and the specific goals and limitations of this treatment are understood. A diagnostic EMG should exclude nerve or muscle disease, although this is not routinely done without a clinical suspicion of such a disorder. It should be recognized that some symptoms of radiculopathy or peripheral neuropathy may be similar to focal or segmental dystonia and that some dystonic conditions predispose the patient to root or peripheral nerve damage. The opposite is also true: dystonia (particularly hand cramps) may present with symptoms resembling peripheral nerve entrapment or joint disease (22). These issues may cause some clinical confusion because nerve entrapments, joint diseases, other limb disorders, and focal dystonia occur in the same population of patients who repeatedly "overuse" their limbs.

The primary muscles involved in the dystonia can be identified by clinical examination and occasionally with the help of EMG. In most situations, the clinical examination alone is sufficient to locate muscles because EMG recordings cannot distinguish dystonic from other contractions better than the examination (16). Furthermore, the pain induced by needle or wire EMG electrodes may alter the spasm patterns and give errant results. Nonetheless, in some cases EMG is very helpful in demonstrating antagonist cocontraction or mirror activity in the opposite limb and thus aids in the diagnosis of dystonia as well as in choice of muscles to be injected. Apart from its use in diagnosis of dystonia, EMG is almost always needed as a tool to guide BTX injections into limb muscles.

Before BTX injection, strength of the involved limb muscles should be documented using a clinical scale (such as Medical Research Council 0–5 scale [23]) to establish baseline measurements and monitor changes after treatment. Some weakness invariably develops, as BTX does not work in limb dystonia unless there is some effect on neuromuscular transmission and at least some initial muscle weakening (13). However, we have found that its effect in ameliorating dystonic symptoms often outlasts the weakness.

Dystonic spasms also must be distinguished from compensatory movements so as not to inject uninvolved muscles. Compensatory movements are voluntary or semivoluntary actions intended to negate the effect of the dystonic spasms. For example, in some forms of writer's cramp, the patient may present with hyperflexion of the thumb and index finger and increased downward pressure on the paper. These are compensatory flexor actions to overcome the extensor dystonic spasms. To treat this, only the extensor muscles need to be injected. This will relax the primary extensor spasms and obviate the compensatory flexion movements. The reverse is also evident: the dystonia would be made worse if the flexor muscles, which provide the opposing actions, were weakened.

Distinguishing between primary, compensatory, and other muscle actions may be difficult, as dystonia characteristically involves cocontracting antagonists and other muscles. To help distinguish between compensatory and dystonic muscle contraction in writer's cramp, the patient can be instructed to write holding the pen or pencil with different finger pairs while the examiner notes the actions of the thumb and index finger. If the same fingers (which previously had been hyperflexing) tend to move into an extended position, it is likely that the underlying dystonia that appeared as flexion is actually one of extension. In addition to understanding compensatory actions, an appreciation of synergist and fixator actions is important to thoroughly examine the clinical patterns of muscular activity and the details of how spasms alter limb movements. Knowing the actions of these other functionally important muscles also avoids injecting them unnecessarily.

Dystonic limb movements should be videotaped with the patient at rest and while performing tasks that induce or relieve spasms. This type of semiobjective documentation can be useful for later clinical comparison, even though no significant changes were found by blinded videotape comparisons before and after BTX injection in the one placebo-controlled study (18). Nonetheless, evidence on videotape of change after BTX treatment can add to the clinical examination and the patient's subjective impressions of improvement on an individual nonblinded patient basis. Other semiquantitative methods of measuring the functional impact of dystonic spasms before and after treatment with BTX include the use of clinical scales and scoring activities of daily living. These can be useful in documenting the effects of motor impairment in such areas as eating, dressing, or hygiene and are most helpful in assessing the effect of BTX in segmental or generalized dystonia.

To partially quantify motor impairment in some of the focal dystonias, handwriting analysis (13,16,18), speed of performance (as in writing or typing), and measurements of agility while playing a musical instrument might be considered. However, it is difficult to measure improvement in motor performance beyond rudimentary skills that are often not affected, and complex learned skills such as playing an instrument are beyond physiological analysis at this time. Complex or highly technical abilities that are disrupted by dystonia can be measured only in subjective terms by the patient, who ultimately decides whether there has been improvement in his or her motor performance after BTX treatment.

Kinesiologic and physiological methods of documenting the type and severity of the dystonia before therapy may be helpful; however, such tests usually are found only at specialized centers and are probably not significantly more beneficial than the clinical examination. These include multichannel EMG analysis of the limb while the patient performs those tasks that induce dystonic spasms, other mechanographic measurements of limb actions such as tremor analysis, and tests of brain stem or segmental spinal activity such as reciprocal inhibition. While of great scientific interest, results from these studies do not usually alter the diagnosis or affect the selection of muscles to be injected (16). Furthermore, many abnormalities such as overflow of muscle activity and the abnormalities in reciprocal inhibition do not improve after administration of BTX (13). If dystonic tremor oscillations are prominent or disabling, objective measurement of limb motion using ultra-light accelerometers can be useful in documenting significant changes in tremor amplitude and irregularity (24).

DETERMINATION OF BOTULINUM TOXIN DOSES

The goal with BTX injections in limb dystonia is to create sufficient localized weakness to ameliorate dystonic spasms while preserving an appropriate amount of strength for the limb to function at an acceptable level of motor performance. Commercial BTX currently is available in 100–mouse unit vials (1 U = 0.4 ng dry toxin) of lyophilized powder that is then dissolved in normal saline for injection. To administer the range of doses needed in limb dystonia, BTX is diluted to concentrations ranging between 1.25 and 20 U/0.1 ml. We have found the most useful dilution to be 5 U/0.1 ml, as this allows the deposition of 5–30 U at one injection site, keeping the volume to 0.6 ml or lower.

Initial BTX doses are either based on previous experience or established empirically. Without prior guidelines, the smallest number of muscles are injected starting with low doses (2.5–25 U) that are incremented weekly until optimal improvement has been achieved. We have injected 88 patients (51 men, 37 women) ranging in age from 12 to 72 years with a variety of primary and secondary limb dystonias (48 focal, 25 segmental, 15 generalized) between 1988 and 1992 (Table 2). During this period, limb muscles were injected a total of 312 times over a range of one to 11 visits, with a median of two visits. Some muscles, such as the extensor carpi radialis in the arm or the tibialis posterior in the leg, were injected substantially more often because of their more typical involvement in

Table 2 Limb Dystonia Patients and botulinum Toxin Injection Data from the Neurological Institute at Columbia-Presbyterian Medical Center, 1988–92

Number of patients	88
Men/women	51/37
Average age ± SD (years) (range)	42.79 ± 15.57 (12–72)
Average age at onset of dystonia (years) (range)	35.32 ± 16.86 (2–56)
Focal/segmental/generalized	48/25/15
Average duration of symptoms (years) (range)	6.75 ± 5.87 (1–24)
Total number of muscles injected over all visits	312
Median number of visits per patient (range)	2 (1–11)
Average botulinum toxin dose per muscle (mouse units) (range)	32.72 ± 31.43 (2.5–200)
Average total botulinum toxin dose per visit (mouse units) (range)	69.79 ± 69.67 (2.5–300)

limb dystonia. Other muscles, such as the biceps or brachialis, have been injected only once. Cumulative data are summarized by type and topography of dystonia (Table 3) and by muscle and function. These injection data have proved useful over time and serve as starting reference values for new patients.

We have found that the effect of BTX injections may vary considerably among patients and even among apparently similar muscles in the same patient. Apart from the type and severity of the underlying dystonia, this disparity of effect is due to many factors, some of which remain elusive. Muscle location, function, and size, muscle interactions, joint actions, and limb biomechanics all probably have a role in determining the ultimate effect of local BTX injections. Because of the varying therapeutic gains achieved with BTX injections, it has been useful to classify limb dystonia functionally according to potential treatment benefit, and not only by severity or topography. This method bases the potential benefit of BTX on several factors: the extent of involvement or ''degree of localization'' of the muscles (13), the complexity of their pattern of interaction, and the severity of underlying dystonia. More severe focal dystonias may be more difficult to treat than mild segmental cases. For example, a violinist's inability to hold the bow properly because of a severe focal misdirected action of the ring finger may be more difficult to correct functionally than a tennis player's segmental excessive arm hyperpronation and hyperextension on serving. In general, musicians as a subgroup of patients with focal dystonia usually do not regain the necessary motor skills to perform as well as they had played before developing dystonia.

It has been useful to categorize patients into three groups according to potential treatment outcome (Table 4). This does not change overall statistics on treatment effect but serves as a guide for understanding the benefits and limitations of BTX. Group I consists of patients with focal or segmental dystonia with localized disability who are injected with the potential of achieving major functional improvement. This group comprises 51 of the 88 patients (58%), and most but not all have focal dystonia. Group I includes 42 of 48 patients with focal dystonia (87.5%) and 9 of 25 patients with segmental dystonia (36%). Typically these patients have mild involvement of the hand, wrist, or arm, with primary involvement of only a few muscles, usually finger or hand extensors. In patients with segmental dystonia, several muscle groups are mildly affected, often including the pronator teres or supinator.

Group II patients have less localized disability and are injected in order to achieve mild to moderate improvement but not necessarily functional return of fine motor tasks. This group is made up of most, but not all, patients with segmental dystonia. Group II patients comprise 22 of our 88 patients (25%) and include 6 of 48 patients with focal dystonia (12.5%) and 16 of 25 patients with segmental dystonia (64%). These are focal dystonia patients with slightly more extensive hand dystonia usually involving flexors (particularly at the metacarpal-phalangeal joint) or with additional involvement of more proximal forearm muscles such as the supinator, or patients with segmental dystonia in the upper arm or in the leg. Success rates are only modest when several proximal arm muscles are involved in addition to the hand dystonia. Treatment of finger flexion movements is further complicated because so many muscles (including wrist flexors and extensors) have synergistic roles in these actions. Lumbrical injection may be necessary in some cases. With dystonic spasms in the leg, the best outcomes result when very few muscles, usually including the tibialis posterior, are predominantly involved. In general, treatment of the leg and foot has proved more difficult and appears to require higher BTX doses, even for smaller muscles.

Table 3 Summary Data of All Botulinum Toxin Injections by Region, Sex, and Type of Dystonia Affecting the Limbs

	Total number of injection visits	Average dose/muscle[a] (range)	Average total dose/visit[a,b] (range)	Median sites/muscle (range)	Median conc./0.1 ml[a] (range)	Average ml/site (range)
Region						
Arms	254	30.23 (2.5–200)	53.87 (2.5–300)	1 (1–4)	5 (1.25–10)	0.33 (0.1–0.7)
Legs	29	48.15 (15–100)	157.43 (50–200)	2 (1–4)	5 (5–10)	0.37 (0.2–0.5)
Hands	19	5.84 (2.5–15)	32.53 (2.5–50)	1 (1–1)	2.5 (1.25–10)	0.18 (0.1–0.3)
Feet	10	46.91 (20–150)	107.49 (50–250)	1 (1–3)	5 (5–20)	0.38 (0.1–0.6)
Region/sex						
Arms/men	156	34.43 (5–200)	65.42 (5–300)	1 (1–4)	5 (1.25–10)	0.34 (0.2–0.7)
Legs/men	14	71.84 (25–150)	90.53 (50–150)	1 (1–4)	10 (5–10)	0.38 (0.2–0.5)
Hands/men	17	5.94 (2.5–15)	32.50 (2.5–50)	1 (1–1)	2.5 (1.25–10)	0.19 (0.1–0.3)
Feet/men	6	47.22 (35–120)	125.00 (50–250)	1 (1–3)	10 (5–20)	0.38 (0.2–0.6)
Arms/women	98	23.54 (5–90)	29.41 (2.5–150)	1 (1–4)	5 (1.25–10)	0.31 (0.2–0.7)
Legs/women	15	63.10 (15–150)	75.50 (50–120)	1 (1–4)	10 (5–10)	0.36 (0.2–0.5)
Hands/women	2	5.00 (2.5–7.5)	8.33 (2.5–10)	1 (1–1)	5 (5–5)	0.13 (0.05–0.2)
Feet/women	4	46.95 (20–150)	98.75 (50–250)	2 (1–3)	10 (10–20)	0.39 (0.1–0.5)
Type of dystonia						
Focal	176	17.98 (2.5–120)	49.14 (2.5–150)	1 (1–3)	5 (1.25–20)	0.28 (0.1–0.7)
Segmental	81	56.70 (5–200)	135.67 (5–300)	2 (1–4)	10 (2.5–20)	0.40 (0.2–0.8)
Generalized	55	55.52 (5–150)	90.63 (10–150)	1 (1–4)	5 (1.25–10)	0.39 (0.2–0.7)
Type of dystonia/sex						
Focal/men	114	18.72 (2.5–120)	57.38 (4.5–90)	2 (1–3)	5 (1.25–20)	0.28 (0.3–0.7)
Segmental/men	50	56.70 (25–200)	142.50 (25–300)	2 (1–4)	10 (2.5–20)	0.40 (0.2–0.8)
Generalized/men	30	57.55 (7.5–150)	137.50 (15–150)	2 (1–4)	5 (1.25–10)	0.41 (0.2–0.7)
Focal/women	62	16.62 (2.5–100)	36.78 (2.5–120)	1 (1–3)	5 (1.25–20)	0.28 (0.1–0.7)
Segmental/women	31	37.30 (15–150)	55.00 (5–180)	2 (1–4)	5 (2.5–20)	0.34 (0.2–0.7)
Generalized/women	25	53.09 (25–90)	43.75 (10–140)	2 (1–4)	5 (1.25–10)	0.37 (0.2–0.5)

[a]Mouse units.
[b]Includes doses for all additional muscles injected.

Table 4 Improvement After Botulinum Toxin Injections for Limb Dystonia at the Columbia-Presbyterian Medical Center Categorized by Topographic and Functional Groups of Dystonia

Topographic categories:

	Σ N		Improvement None		Minimal		Major	
Focal	48	55%	9	18.8%	12	25.0%	27	56.3%
Segmental	25	28%	4	16.0%	8	32.0%	13	52.0%
Generalized	15	17%	3	20.0%	4	26.7%	8	53.3%
Functional categories:								
Group I	51	58%	7	13.7%	11	21.6%	33	64.7%
Group II	22	25%	6	27.3%	9	40.9%	7	31.8%
Group III	15	17%	3	20.0%	4	26.7%	8	53.3%
Total	88	100%	16	18.2%	24	27.3%	48	54.5%

Group composition:

	Focal	Segmental	Generalized	Total
Group I	42	9	0	51
Group II	6	16	0	22
Group III	0	0	15	15
Total	48	25	15	88

Summary

No improvement	16	18.2%
Some improvement	72	81.8%

Patients in group III are all those with generalized dystonia and are injected specifically to relieve pain, prevent skin abrasions, or lessen obtrusive, disabling postures. Fifteen of the 88 patients (17%) belong to this group. These patients are not seeking improvement in motor performance, so there is little concern about causing too much weakness in most cases. In addition to pain relief, primary goals are improvement in hygiene, the prevention of contractures, and the prevention of skin breakdown, as with excessively flexed fingers abrading the palm. Multiple large doses in the forearm, specifically in flexor digitorum profundi to weaken distal interphalangeal joints, and large doses in proximal arm and shoulder muscles sometimes provide significant overall improvement in daily living. The major concern for these patients is the development of antibodies to the toxin, rendering the treatment ineffective, because of the large doses sometimes required.

Using other antigenic strains of BTX, such as type F, can avoid the development of antibodies to type A (25). Although the effect of type F on relieving dystonia is shorter-lived than that of type A, it can be used to determine whether BTX injections would be useful before the administration of type A without worry about antibody formation. Other acute uses of BTX toxin in limb dystonia are perioperative applications. We have found that proximal arm muscles can be injected a few days in advance of tendon-lengthening procedures for flexion contractures at the elbows caused by generalized dystonia. This has allowed for postoperative healing without spasms, which would otherwise tear the tendon stitches. A similar use of BTX has been to create temporary perioperative muscle weakness for repair of a rotator cuff injury in a patient with brachial dystonia and parkinsonism (26).

Despite individual variability, extensor muscles in the forearm generally need approximately half the BTX dose of forearm flexor muscles for all patient groups. Proximal arm and shoulder muscles require larger doses than distal hand muscles, and foot and leg muscles require higher doses than either the hand or the arm. In larger forearm, arm, or leg or foot muscles, multiple injection sites are used. Even certain muscle fascicles, for example those fascicles for digits 3 and 4 in the flexor digitorum superficialis, reveal better susceptibility to BTX than fascicles for digits 2 and 5, for reasons possibly related to their anatomic arrangement. Multiple injection sites allow for better distribution of the toxin in the muscle and minimize pain caused by larger intramuscular volumes. Higher concentrations also reduce injection volume. This is particularly important in the foot, where large doses are needed in small muscles. Women show beneficial results with approximately one-third less toxin for individual forearm muscles than men, although there are no significant sex differences in doses for small foot muscles.

The amount of BTX needed is roughly proportional to muscle size, but this is not the only factor. The relative innervation ratio and end plate density are probably equally or more important in determining BTX doses. This is probably why small muscles with precise movements, such as eye or hand muscles, require proportionally more toxin (for their size) than large limb muscles. Determination of end plate zones for injection has not been found necessary for optimal results (13), although injections are generally placed in or near these regions (usually the muscle belly) when possible. Presumably diffusion of toxin several centimeters from the injection site helps deliver its effect to the end plates; however, other unknown but potentially important factors, such as the effect of BTX on non-alpha motor neurons and the intrafusal muscle fiber system, may contribute to the overall effect.

INJECTION TECHNIQUE

After identification of the involved muscle(s) during active spasms and a decision on the dose(s), BTX is injected with the limb at rest. Under EMG guidance, a hollow-core needle is used to locate the muscle, serving as both a monopolar electrode and a conduit for diluted BTX. The needle is electrically insulated except at the recording tip and hub. Sizes can vary, but the most commonly used is 27-gauge and 1.5 inches long. Longer needles are needed for deeper leg muscles such as the tibialis posterior. An insulated wire with clip connects the needle hub to an EMG machine. To the hub is also attached a removable syringe filled with the diluted BTX. Muscle location is determined with standard EMG technique. Specifically, muscles are identified by recruitment patterns at low and high levels of effort in each of the muscles intended for injection. Muscle location in the forearm may also be achieved through passive joint displacement at the wrist or fingers and noting whether the placed needle moves appropriately. Previously injected muscles will exhibit fibrillations and positive sharp waves within the first 10–20 days after injection; however, these denervation potentials are rarely evident after 3 months.

Among the most commonly injected muscles in limb dystonia are the wrist flexors and extensors and the flexor digitorum superficialis and extensor indicis. Fascicles subserving individual digits in larger muscles (such as the flexor digitorum superficialis or extensor digitorum communis) can be injected to provide more precise control over the effect of BTX on the actions of specific digits. It has been found easier to obtain a good response in some muscles than in others. The hand and finger extensors weaken with an appropriate response relatively easily, while, for unclear reasons, it is more difficult to demonstrate

Table 5 Most Commonly Injected Muscles by Order of Treatment Success Rate

		Improvement (success rate)			
		Min	Major	Total %	N
Arm					
1	Extensor indicis	2 (11%)	16 (89%)	100%	18
2	Extensor digitorum com	2 (13%)	14 (88%)	100%	16
3	Extensor pollicis longus	1 (13%)	6 (75%)	88%	8
4	Extensor carpi radialis	5 (12%)	27 (66%)	78%	41
5	Extensor carpi ulnaris	6 (23%)	14 (54%)	77%	26
6	Flexor pollicis longus	1 (13%)	5 (63%)	75%	8
7	Flexor digitorum profund	3 (43%)	2 (29%)	71%	7
8	Flexor digitorum superficialis, digits 3,4	5 (28%)	7 (39%)	67%	18
9	Pronator teres	1 (9%)	6 (55%)	64%	11
10	Flexor carpi radialis	5 (33%)	4 (27%)	60%	15
11	Flexor carpi ulnaris	6 (18%)	13 (39%)	58%	33
12	Flexor digitorum superficialis, digits 2,5	5 (38%)	2 (15%)	54%	13
Leg					
1	Extensor hallucis longus	3 (60%)	1 (20%)	80%	5
2	Extensor digitorum longus	1 (50%)	0 (0%)	50%	2
3	Tibialis anterior	2 (33%)	1 (17%)	50%	6
4	Tibialis posterior	5 (36%)	1 (7%)	43%	14
Hand					
1	Abductor pollicis brevis	2 (33%)	4 (67%)	100%	6
2	Abductor pollicis	2 (67%)	1 (33%)	100%	3
3	Opponens pollicis	1 (50%)	1 (50%)	100%	2
4	Dorsal interossei	2 (50%)	1 (25%)	75%	4
Foot					
1	Extensor digitorum brevis	2 (67%)	0 (0%)	67%	3
2	Flexor hallucis brevis	1 (50%)	0 (0%)	50%	2
3	Flexor digitorum brevis	2 (40%)	0 (0%)	40%	5

efficacy in small foot muscles. Injecting digit fascicles 2 and 5 in the flexor digitorum superficialis is technically more challenging than injecting digit fascicles 3 and 4. As this is mostly due to the anatomic arrangement of fascicles for digits 2 and 5 and their proximity to deeper tendons in the forearm, injecting laterally from the ulnar aspect of the forearm can help in localization. Those muscles most commonly injected, in order of success rate in reducing dystonic symptoms, are listed in Table 5.

THE QUESTION OF ELECTROMYOGRAPHY

The utility of EMG in administering BTX has been a topic of considerable debate and is of particular importance in limb dystonia. Several issues need to be addressed. The distinction should be made between clinically diagnosing limb dystonia, physiologically investigating dystonia, determining which muscles need to be treated, and actually performing the injections. Expertise and training in EMG is probably of more importance in limb dystonia than other disorders requiring intramuscular injections. Initial work on the use of BTX in hand cramps used multichannel EMG to characterize physiological aspects of the condition and determine the extent and character of the involved muscles (13). This technique enabled the kinesiologic identification of those muscles directly involved in dystonic spasms. However, some muscles found to be active by EMG are not necessarily involved in the dystonia, while others clearly identified by clinical examination are not always found active by EMG (16). Furthermore, multichannel EMG cannot discern compensatory from dystonic activity better than the clinical examination. While important for understanding pathophysiology and pattern development in dystonia, multichannel EMG recordings are most useful as a research tool.

Another issue is the actual injection procedure for BTX in limb dystonia. In other focal dystonias such as blepharospasm, the involved muscles are located subcutaneously; in torticollis the neck muscle are not always subcutaneous but are relatively superficial, few in number, and usually palpable. The involved muscles in limb dystonia are more numerous, often are not superficial, and cannot always be palpated. In several larger forearm muscles such as flexor digitorum superficialis or extensor digitorum communis, individual digital fascicles can be located only by EMG guidance to provide accurate control over specific finger joints involved in the dystonic spasms. Although BTX diffuses a few centimeters when administered (13), and although it remains unclear how close to end plates injections need to be, it is difficult or impossible to inject any limb muscle accurately and reproducibly without EMG guidance. Finally, apart from locating those muscles to inject, the identification of synergists, antagonists, or compensatory muscles may be helpful in determining which muscles not to inject. Without training and competence in EMG, locating and understanding the functional significance of limb muscles for possible injection can be problematic.

TREATMENT OUTCOME

Usually a treatment response occurs within 1–4 days, occasionally as late as 7–10 days after BTX injections. The reduction of dystonic spasms lasts about 3 months once appropriate toxin doses and muscles have been determined. A few patients report lasting benefit for up to 4–6 months. There are cumulative effects in which some patients require less toxin for the same effect in some muscles injected regularly over several years. This long-term ''carry-over'' effect presumably is due to minimal additive residual weakness between injection visits rather than to permanent change in neuromuscular transmission. The effects of prolonged use of chronic BTX injections are not known.

Four possible outcomes result after BTX treatment, each requiring a slightly different approach to follow-up (Table 6). The first is that no weakness and no improvement in dystonia occurs. In this case, the same muscles are usually reinjected 1–2 weeks later with equal or higher doses of BTX on the assumption that at least some weakness is necessary for beneficial effect. Nonresponsiveness can be due to a number of causes, the more common being that the dosage was too low or improperly placed, and the less common that the BTX was ineffective because of a faulty batch, improper handling, or faulty preparation. Antibodies to BTX cause nonresponsiveness only in patients with prior exposure. A second possible outcome is a submaximal or ineffective but otherwise acceptable response. In this case, the same muscles are usually reinjected with 0.5–1 times the original dose. An additional muscle may be injected as well. A third outcome is an incomplete response with overactivity found in noninjected muscles. In this case, too few muscles were originally injected (even with a good response in muscles that were injected). For this, the additionally active muscles are injected within the initial 1–3

Table 6 Treatment Outcomes and Strategy

First visit:	Injection of botulinum toxin with lowest doses per muscle (based on previous experience) in fewest number of muscles.
Next 1 or 2 visits (7–10 days apart):	*No response*—injection of same muscles with same or higher doses. *Submaximal response*—injection of same muscles with same or lower doses, may inject new muscle if necessary. *Incomplete response*—new clinical pattern with overactivity found in non-injected muscles requiring injection of new muscles. *Good response*—no further injections until effect worn off.
Follow-up visit (every 3–4 months):	Same muscles injected with doses equal to total combined amount given during first 2–3 visits for each muscle.

weeks. The final possibility is a good response with the expected improvement in motor performance or relief of pain. When an optimal response is finally obtained, follow-up injections with doses equal to the cumulative amount over the first few weeks are given every 3–4 months. Despite semiobjective methods of measurement, optimal outcome depends on functional improvement and is based mainly on patient judgment.

PAIN

Dystonic spasms can be associated with a significant amount of pain. Several mechanisms probably mediate dystonic pain, including extremes of posture, excessive tendon and joint tension, and direct muscle pain. Botulinum toxin therapy has been shown to be useful in alleviating pain in many of the focal dystonias, particularly in torticollis, where up to 88% of patients were found to have improvement since early in the use of BTX (27). In studies of focal dystonia of the limbs, pain relief was found in from 75–100% of the cases (Table 1) (15–17), and it has been the continued experience at the Neurological Institute that even if there is little improvement in motor function with BTX injections, the pain associated with dystonic spasms is usually abolished. Presumably, pain relief with BTX occurs with even a minimal amount of muscle relaxation, although the mechanisms have not been worked out.

DYSTONIC TREMOR

Tremor is a salient feature of limb dystonia (1) and is characterized by irregular, semirhythmic jerkiness that may be task- or posture-specific (28,29). Dystonic tremor is thought to be partly due to volitional attempts at correcting the twisting posture of the dystonic spasms (28) and is often associated with a "null point" or extreme posture in which the semirhythmic movements disappear. Tremor may be a disabling feature of the limb dystonia, but the involved muscles can be treated with BTX with the same outcome as the underlying dystonia. As in all dystonic spasms, treating the primary muscle(s) responsible for the tremor (which are generally the same as for the dystonia) will significantly reduce the jerky oscillations. Unlike other tremor conditions, such as essential or parkinsonian tremor, where there is a more equal contribution of antagonist muscles causing the oscillations (and which are therefore more difficult to treat with botulinum toxin [30]) the physiological mechanisms are different for dystonic tremor. In dystonic tremor, there is a primary movement in one direction underlying the tremor, and this can be treated.

SIDE EFFECTS

Local side effects consist of ecchymoses, muscle pain, and stiffness at the site of injection, which are infrequent, and excessive weakness, which is relatively common. Weakness is technically not a side effect in injected muscles, as it is the desired effect; however, an argument can be made that excessive weakness is a side effect. Weakness in neighboring muscles not intended for injection also occurs. Excessive weakness can be difficult to avoid, even with extreme care, as doses can be difficult to determine in advance, and the diluted BTX spreads to adjacent muscles and fascicles (13). Fortunately, weakness diminishes over time, and better control can be attempted at the next injection visit.

Systemic side effects are rare. Most studies report no systemic side effects. Malaise, muscle twitching, paresthesias, and nausea have been reported in a small percentage of patients (18). Antibody formation is a systemic side effect with no clinical manifestation other than the development of lack of response to subsequent BTX injections. In limb dystonia, BTX doses are usually small and preclude the development of antibodies; however, when larger proximal muscles (such as the biceps, deltoids or trapezius) are injected for segmental or generalized dystonia, antibody formation is a concern. This might be suspected in a patient who previously did well and becomes a nonresponder. Another subclinical side effect is the development of increased jitter on single-fiber EMG (31). While indicative of systemic spread of BTX, this has been shown not to be of clinical concern, but it should be weighed in patients taking medication that may additionally alter neuromuscular transmission.

CONCLUDING REMARKS

Botulinum toxin type A injections can provide at least some amount of relief for spasms and pain in over 80% of patients with limb dystonia. Overall, major functional improvement in motor performance or activities of daily living may be obtained in over 50% of patients with focal, segmental, or generalized dystonia, and in almost two-thirds of patients with mild focal or segmental dystonia (in group I). Certain motor functions, such as typing, writing, or playing sports are more amenable to treatment than the potentially more complex skills of playing a musical instrument. A large amount of success has been obtained in relieving pain, preventing skin abrasions, and reducing disabling postures in 80% of patients with generalized dystonia. Short-term uses of BTX in limb dystonia include the prevention of postoperative tearing spasms. Although its effect is shorter-lived, BTX type F can be used before the administration of type A to determine whether BTX injections would be efficacious.

There are many issues in need of further research from both a physiological and a functional vantage point. These include clarifying factors behind the clinical variability in patient sensitivity to BTX injections and determining why muscles in the same patient appear to show different susceptibilities to BTX. To what extent BTX diffuses through muscle tissue is still unknown, and therefore the extent to which it is necessary to inject close to the end plate zone needs to be investigated. The time course of weakness in comparison with the lasting effects on spasms, and the cumulative carry-over effect in chronic administration of BTX, remain elusive. The effects of BTX on non-alpha motor neurons and the intrafusal muscle fiber system may play important roles and provide clues to the understanding of many of these issues.

REFERENCES

1. Cohen LG, Hallett M. Hand cramps: clinical features and electromyographic patterns in a focal dystonia. Neurology 1988;38:1005–1012.
2. Rothwell JC, Obeso JA, Day BL, Marsden CD. Pathophysiology of dystonias. In: Desmedt JE, ed. Motor control mechanisms in health and disease. New York: Raven Press, 1983:851–863.
3. Sheehy MP, Marsden CD. Writers' cramp—a focal dystonia. Brain 1982;105:461–480.
4. Fahn S. Concept and classification of dystonia. In: Fahn S, Marsden CD, Caln DB, eds. Dystonia 2. Advances in neurology, vol 50. New York: Raven Press, 1988:1–8.
5. Hedreen JC, Zweig RM, DeLong MR, Whitehouse PJ, Price DL. Primary dystonias: a review of the pathology and suggestion for new directions of study. In: Fahn S, Marsden CD, Calne DB, eds. Dystonia 2. Advances in neurology, vol 50. New York: Raven Press, 1988:123–132.
6. Obeso JA, Gimenez-Roldan S. Clinico-pathological correlation in symptomatic dystonia. In: Fahn S, Marsden CD, Calne DB, eds. Dystonia 2. Advances in neurology, vol 50. New York: Raven Press, 1988:113–122.
7. Schott GD. The relationship of peripheral trauma and pain to dystonia. J Neurol Neurosurg Psychiatry 1985;48:698–701.
8. Jankovic J, van der Linden C. Dystonia and tremor induced by peripheral trauma: predisposing factors. J Neurol Neurosurg Psychiatry 1988;51:1512–1519.
9. Calne DB, Lang AE. Secondary dystonia. In: Fahn S, Marsden CD, Calne DB, eds. Advances in Neurology: Dystonia 2. vol 50. New York: Raven Press, 1988:9–33.
10. Lang AE, Sheehy MP, Marsden CD. Acute anticholinergic action in focal dystonia. Adv Neurol 1983;37:193–200.
11. Bindman E, Tibbetts RW. Writer's cramp—a rational approach to treatment? Br J Psychiatry 1977;131:143–148.
12. National Institutes of Health Consensus Development Conference. Clinical use of botulinum toxin. Arch Neurol 1991;48:1294–1298.
13. Cohen LG, Hallett M, Geller BD, Hochberg F. Treatment of focal dystonias of the hand with botulinum toxin injections. J Neurol Neurosurg Psychiatry 1989;52:355–363.
14. Jankovic J, Schwartz K, Donovan DT. Botulinum toxin treatment of cranial-cervical dystonia, spasmodic dysphonia, other focal dystonias and hemifacial spasms. J Neurol Neurosurg Psychiatry 1990;53:633–639.
15. Pullman S. Limb dystonia: treatment with botulinum toxin. In: The use of botulinum toxin in the treatment of focal dystonia. Columbia University College of Physicians and Surgeons Symposium: Department of Neurology, 1990:97–101.
16. Rivest J, Lees AJ, Marsden CD. Writer's cramp: treatment with botulinum toxin injections. Mov Disord 1991;6:55–59.
17. Poungvarin N. Writer's cramp: the experience with botulinum toxin injections in 25 patients. J Med Assoc Thai 1991;74:239–247.
18. Yoshimura DM, Aminoff MJ, Olney RK. Botulinum toxin therapy for limb dystonias. Neurology 1992;42:627–630.
19. Tsui JKC, Snow B, Bhatt M, Varelas M, Hashimoto S, Calne DB. New applications of botulinum toxin in the lower limbs. Neurology 1990;40(suppl 1):382.
20. Tanner CM, Floss RD, Buchman AS, Comella CL. Botulinum toxin treatment of foot dystonia in Parkinson's disease. Mov Disord 1992;7:301.
21. Argov Z, Mastaglia FL. Disorders of neuromuscular transmission caused by drugs. N Engl J Med 1979;301:409–413.
22. Fry H, Hallett M. Focal dystonia (occupational cramp) masquerading as nerve entrapment or hysteria. Plast Reconstr Surg 1988;82:908–910.
23. Medical Research Council. Aids to the examination of the peripheral nervous system. London: Crown, 1976.

24. Pullman SL, Fahn S, Rueda J. Physiologic characterization of dystonic and essential tremors. Neurology 1992;42(suppl 3):471.
25. Ludlow CL, Hallett M, Rhew K, et al. Therapeutic use of type F botulinum toxin (letter). N Engl J Med 1992;326:349–350.
26. Gasser T, Fritsch K, Arnold G, Oertel W. Botulinum toxin A in orthopaedic surgery (letter). Lancet 1991;338:761.
27. Tsui J, Eisen A, Stoessl AJ, Calne S, Calne DB. Double-blind study of botulinum toxin in spasmodic torticollis. Lancet 1986;2:245–247.
28. Rosenbaum F, Jankovic J. Task-specific focal tremor and dystonia: categorization of occupational movement disorders. Neurology 1988;38:522–527.
29. Jedynak CP, Bonnet AM, Agid Y. Tremor and idiopathic dystonia. Mov Disord 1991;6:230–236.
30. Trosch R, Pullman SL. Botulinum A toxin injections for the treatment of hand tremors. Ann Neurol 1992;32:250.
31. Lange DJ, Brin MF, Fahn S, Lovelace RL. Distant effects of locally injected botulinum toxin: incidence and course. In: Fahn S, Marsden CD, Calne DB, eds. Dystonia 2. Advances in neurology, vol 50. New York: Raven Press, 1988;609–613.

23

Clinical Experience with Botulinum Toxin F

Karen Rhew and Christy L. Ludlow
National Institute on Deafness and Other Communication Disorders, National Institutes of Health, Bethesda, Maryland

Barbara Illowsky Karp and Mark Hallett
National Institute of Neurological Disorders and Stroke, National Institutes of Health, Bethesda, Maryland

INTRODUCTION

As botulinum toxin A (BTX-A) has been used more extensively as a treatment for focal dystonias, several centers have reported patients who have become unresponsive to the injections (1–4). The presence of antibodies to BTX-A in many of this group was confirmed by in vivo mouse assay performed by the Center for Communicable Diseases and later by the Smith-Kettlewell Eye Research Institute, San Francisco, California. Theoretically, it seemed reasonable that one of the six other immunologically different types of botulinum neurotoxin (types B, C, D, E, F, and G) might be used to treat these patients who could no longer benefit from BTX-A. Type F was chosen as the alternative injection material because our first patient to be identified with antibodies to BTX-A had been intentionally inoculated with pentavalent toxoid containing inactivated BTXs of type A, B, C, D, and E (5) to protect him in his work with biological toxins.

Although antibody formation has been found in patients receiving BTX injections for most of the focal dystonias, most reported cases have been found in patients treated for cervical dystonia or torticollis. Development of antibodies in the torticollis patients is assumed to be related in part to the large total dose of toxin (100–500 U or more) required to weaken the overactive cervical muscles (6). Indeed, antibody formation has been less commonly seen in the focal dystonias requiring relatively small total doses (2.5–100 U), such as spasmodic dysphonia, orolingual-mandibular dystonia, blepharospasm, strabismus, and focal hand dystonia.

PATIENT POPULATION

In our clinic, only four of the 350 patients who have received BTX became unresponsive to BTX-A injection because of development of antibodies. The diagnoses of these patients include stuttering (treated with laryngeal injections), orolingual dystonia, and hand cramp in a violinist and a pianist. The occurrence of antibodies in these patients with disorders other than torticollis is a reflection of our patient population, 70% of whom have laryngeal dystonias (spasmodic dysphonia), speech motor disorders (orolingual-mandibular dystonia, stuttering), or vocal tremor. Only 30% had torticollis, blepharospasm, facial spasm, or hand cramp. When BTX-F became available for experimental use in humans in 1991, we recruited seven patients with torticollis from other programs who had positive titers for antibodies to BTX-A. These torticollis patients, in addition to three of our four original patients with antibodies, constituted the initial trial group to receive the first injections of BTX-F used for treatment of movement disorders in humans.

There were five men and five women in this initial treatment group. The time interval between the last BTX-A injection and the first BTX-F injection ranged from 3 to 41 months. Four of the torticollis patients had undergone surgery for selective section of cervical spinal nerves or myectomy for relief of symptoms after they developed antibodies to BTX-A. In all cases there had been an interval of at least 1 year between surgery and their first BTX-F injection. Three of the four patients reported that, although their torticollis symptoms had returned, the spasms were decreased in severity as compared with their presurgical state.

METHODS

The BTX-F used was prepared at the Osaka Prefecture Agricultural College, Osaka, Japan. It was filtered and tested for purity and potency at the Chiba Serum Institute, Chiba, Japan. As is the case with BTX-A, one unit of BTX-F was defined as the LD_{50} for 18- to 20-g female Swiss Weber mice injected intraperitoneally. The preparation used contained 2405 ± 518 U/2 μg of toxin. When the preparation was retested by the FDA after reconstituting the freeze-dried form in 20 ml of normal saline per 2-μg vial, the potency was between 3529 and 4746 U per vial. We therefore took the value of 4000 U/2 μg toxin per vial as the basis for preparing the toxin for injection.

Initially, each patient was treated with BTX-F at a dosage in mouse units equal to one quarter of the dose that was effective when they had responded fully to BTX-A. Muscles selected for injection were clinically involved as evidenced by electromyographic (EMG) studies and physical examination and had been injected with good result with BTX-A when the patient had responded to BTX-A in the past. Two weeks later, after demonstration of no adverse reactions, each patient was given the same treatment, but with the full amount of the previously effective dose. All injections were done using EMG guidance (7,8). The torticollis patients were each injected in two or three neck muscles (trapezius, sternocleidomastoid, or splenius capitis), the patient with hand cramp in one muscle (pronator teres), the patient with orolingual dystonia in the tongue at four different sites, and the stutterer in one thyroarytenoid muscle.

Immediately before and 1 week after the first injection using only one quarter the therapeutic dose, blood samples were drawn for complete blood count, sedimentation rate, immunoglobulin levels, liver and renal functions, and electrolytes. The second injection with the full therapeutic dose was administered if there were no significant changes in these laboratory values and the patient had no signs and symptoms of adverse clinical reaction.

Pre- and postinjection videotaped recordings were used to document changes in speech, head and neck movement, or hand movement. Flexible fiberoptic laryngoscopy was used to examine the vocal folds in the stutterer who received laryngeal injections. Hooked wire electromyography of the clinically involved muscles and at least one uninvolved muscle was done before the first injection and then repeated at the time of peak effect, which was 2 to 3 weeks after the full treatment was completed.

The patients kept daily diaries for three months to document the occurrence and degree of any undesirable side effects as well as the beneficial effects of treatment. Three months after injection, each patient answered a questionnaire in which they compared the effects of BTX-A and BTX-F.

RESULTS

Analysis of the pre- and postinjection results of four of these ten patients were reported in the New England Journal of Medicine in January 1992 (9). A more comprehensive analysis of the test and treatment results of all 10 patients that is currently in preparation for publication will show that our findings were similar for all the patients (10).

In general, there was both objective and subjective evidence that BTX-F produced some degree of symptom reduction and weakness in the injected muscles of all 10 patients. In comparing the effects of BTX-F and BTX-A injections, five patients, all with torticollis, thought that BTX-F was more effective in reducing their symptoms. The other five patients reported that BTX-A produced a better effect.

Patient diaries documented that the onset of muscle weakness and reduction in symptoms after BTX-F was similar to that experienced with BTX-A, occurring within 3 to 8 days after the full therapeutic injection. All of the patients had significant return of symptoms within 6 to 10 weeks, as compared with 10 to 12 weeks with BTX-A.

Electromyographic signals recorded during rest and during gestures that maximally activated the specific muscles being studied were analyzed. Mean activation levels in the injected muscles were found to be markedly decreased when compared with pretreatment levels. This correlated clinically with the decreased muscle mass and strength noted on examination. In addition, video fiberoptic laryngoscopy demonstrated decreased movement of the injected vocal fold in the stutterer, indicating effective weakening of the thyroarytenoid muscle.

Analysis of the videotaped studies was done by trained physician observers blinded as to pre- and posttreatment studies. Using a rating scale in which 0 = severely abnormal, 1 = moderately abnormal, 2 = slightly abnormal, and 3 = normal, the judges gave the posttreatment behaviors in seven of the patients higher scores, indicating reduction of symptoms. No noticeable difference was observed in two patients, one with torticollis and one with orolingual dystonia. Only one torticollis patient was judged as appearing more symptomatic after treatment.

None of the patients demonstrated any significant changes in complete blood count, sedimentation rate, immunoglobulin levels, liver and renal functions, and electrolytes.

SIDE EFFECTS AND ADVERSE REACTIONS

The initial trial injections of BTX-F were successfully completed in the first 10 patients with antibodies to BTX-A, without serious local or systemic adverse reactions. In general, side effects occurred with the same frequency and degree of severity as was experienced with BTX-A treatment. Transient dysphagia occurred in two of the torticollis patients, in the stutterer, and in the patient with orolingual dystonia. Mild flu-like symptoms such as

Table 1 Four Patients' Responses to Type F Botulinum Toxin Injection

Patient age/sex/disorder	Dose of toxin	Activation level (μV)[a]		Mean rating of symptom change		Time to full return of symptoms (days)
		Preinjection	Postinjection	Patients[b]	Examiners[c]	
1. 52/F/torticollis	285 in left trapezius 150 in right sternocleidomastoid	233 ± 288	45 ± 30	0.90	−0.67	82
2. 47/M/torticollis	150 in right splenius capitus 125 in left sternocleidomastoid 125 in right trapezius	363 ± 321	74 ± 99	0.67	0.33	40
3. 61/M/stuttering	40 in left thyroarytenoid	21.3 ± 4.7	6.7 ± 0.6	2.25	0.67	60
4. 65/M/oromandibular dystonia	10 in right genioglossus 10 in right genioglossus 50 in right styloglossus 50 in left styloglossus	Postinjection EMG not done		0.07	0[d]	30

[a]The mean and standard deviation of amplitude of the electromyographic signal of each injected muscle determined for a 20-msec period during a maximum activation gesture.
[b]Mean rating of symptoms by patient diaries in relation to levels before treatment: markedly worse = −3, no change = 0, markedly better = + 3.
[c]Change in mean rating of symptoms according to examiners on a scale relative to normal function: normal = 3, severely impaired = 0.
[d]Patient #4 did not change noticeably to the examiners, although the patient and his speech-language pathologist reported some improvement.

malaise, muscle and joint aching, and headache occurred in two torticollis patients for 2 days and 6 days.

However, we have had a significant adverse reaction in one patient treated with BTX-F in another protocol. The patient was a 54-year-old woman with adductor spasmodic dysphonia who had shown no response to BTX-A injections into laryngeal muscles on seven different visits over a 3-year period. Approximately 36 hours after injection of her left thyroarytenoid with 20 U of BTX-F, she reported development of a puritic rash over her neck, chest, and upper arms. She also experienced nausea with abdominal cramping and mild diarrhea, slight headache, and low-grade fever. These symptoms and the rash resolved after 3 days, although the itching persisted for several more days. At no time did she experience any change in her voice symptoms or show other evidence that the injected BTX-F had caused muscle weakness. Tests on blood samples drawn 10 days after the injection showed no evidence of systemic reaction or other abnormalities.

CONCLUSION

It is apparent from this clinical trial that BTX-F can be used safely and effectively at levels of potency similar to those of BTX-A for treatment of a variety of movement disorders. Patient reports that the length of benefit was shorter are consistent with studies in animals in which BTX-F had a shorter duration of action than BTX-A (11). It is also possible that circulating antibodies to BTX-A may interfere with the action of BTX-F even though antibodies to the other six types of BTX have not been shown to neutralize BTX-F (12). A clinical trial using BTX-F in dystonia patients who respond well to BTX-A could help resolve this question.

REFERENCES

1. Brin MF, Fahn S, Moskowitz C, et al. Localized injections of botulinum toxin for the treatment of focal dystonial and hemifacial spasm. Mov Disord 1987;2:237–254.
2. Holds JB, Fogg SG, Anderson RL. Botulinum A toxin injection: failures in clinical practice and a biomechanical system for the study of toxin-induced paralysis. Opthalm Plast Reconstruct Surg 1990;6:252–259.
3. Jankovic J, Schwartz K, Donovan DT. Botulinum toxin treatment of cranial-cervical dystonia, spasmodic dysphonia, other focal dystonias and hemifacial spasm. J Neurol Neurosurg Psychiatry 1990;53:633–639.
4. Greene P, Fahn S. Development of antibodies to botulinum toxin type A in torticollis patients treated with botulinum toxin injections (abstr). Mov Disord 1992;7:134.
5. Ellis RJ. Immunologic agents and drugs available from the Centers for Disease Control: descriptions, recommendations, adverse reactions, and serologic response. 3rd ed. Atlanta, Georgia: Centers for Disease Control, 1982.
6. Hambleton P, Cohen HE, Palmer BJ, Melling J. Antitoxins and botulinum toxin treatment. Br Med J 1992;304:959–960.
7. Shannon KM, Comella CL, Tanner CM. EMG-guided botulinum toxin (BoTox) injections in torticollis: objective clinical improvement. Neurology 1989;39:352.
8. Comella CL, Buchman AS, Tanner CM, Brown-Toms NC, Goetz CG. Botulinum toxin injection for spasmodic torticollis. Neurology 1992;42:878–882.
9. Ludlow CL, Hallett M, Rhew K, et al. Therapeutic use of type F botulinum toxin. N Engl J Med 1992;326:349–350.

10. Ludlow CL, Hallett M, Rhew K, et al. Botulinum toxin type F treatment of patients with botulinum toxin antibodies. Mov Disord 1992;7;133.

11. Kauffman JA, Way JF, Siegel LS, Sellin LC. Comparisons of the action of types A and F botulinum toxin at the rat neuromuscular junction. Toxicol Appl Pharmacol 1985;79:211–217.

12. Siegel LS. Evaluation of neutralizing antibodies to type A, B, E, F botulinum toxins in sera from human recipients of botulinum pentavalent (ABCDE) toxoid. J Clin Microbiol 1989;27:1906–1908.

HEMIFACIAL SPASM

24

Hemifacial Spasm: Evaluation and Management, with Emphasis on Botulinum Toxin Therapy

Gary E. Borodic
Harvard Medical School, Massachusetts Eye and Ear Infirmary, and Boston University School of Medicine, Boston, Massachusetts

INTRODUCTION

Hemifacial spasm is a disorder of the facial nerve characterized by involuntary synkinetic movement of facial muscles on the afflicted side associated with minimal facial weakness. Management of this disorder has transcended several medical and surgical specialties. The condition has implications for ophthalmological practice because of visual obstruction produced by involuntary eyelid closure, which is most troublesome to patients. Neuro-ophthalmic or neurological evaluation is necessary for accurate diagnosis and exclusion of vascular mass lesions in the posterior fossa, which are very uncommon. Neurosurgical experience has been useful in elucidating the pathogenesis and offering an alternative therapeutic modality. Additionally, since the condition adversely affects a patient's ability to communicate via facial expression and produces substantial disfigurement, a plastic surgeon may occasionally be consulted. This chapter surveys the clinical characteristics of hemifacial spasm and reviews the application of therapy with botulinum toxin type A therapy for this disorder.

CLINICAL CHARACTERISTICS

Hemifacial spasm usually appears between the fourth and fifth decades of life, most often as an involuntary twitch in the orbicularis oculi muscle. The movement begins in the lower eyelid and extends to the upper lid. The involuntary movement progresses to gain sufficient force to cause increased blink rates and forced closure of the eyelids on the involved side. Shortly thereafter, the involuntary muscle twitching becomes more generalized to involve not only the lid protractors but muscles over the upper lip on the affected side. As the condition progresses, the twitching becomes an obvious involuntary movement over all facial muscles on one side as well as the thin superficial muscle of the neck, the platysma (Fig. 1). Involvement of the platysma causes asymmetric bands and twitching of the neck muscles in addition to muscles of facial expression. Occasionally, with involvement of the stapedius muscle of the middle ear, the patients may hear an auditory hallucination characterized as a ''thumping'' associated with the spasm. This auditory hallucination occurs only in a small minority of patients. Occasionally, the patient may complain of hearing loss.

In the most severe forms of involuntary movement, there is a more sustained distortion on muscles on one side of the face (Fig. 1). In more advanced cases, the distortion caused by a mass contraction of all muscles supplied by one facial nerve causes a forced closure of the eyelid, eyebrow elevation, elevation of the nasolabial fold, ectropion of the lower lip with chin deformity, deviation of the tip of the nose toward the left side, and tight band formation within superficial muscles of the neck. The spasms most notably involve the orbicularis oculi, frontalis, zygomaticus major and minor, orbicularis oris, and mentalis muscles on one side of the face. With mass contraction of these muscles, the eyelid is forced closed, the nasolabial fold is prominently pulled up, the vermilion border is displaced toward the involved side, and the lower lip turns outward. Occasionally the eyebrow become elevated during periods of mass contraction.

If the condition exists over a period of many years, the weakness and involuntary movement can cause fixed contractures in which the disfigurement remains constant rather than intermittent (Fig. 2).

Unlike some other movement disorders, hemifacial spasm is clearly an intermittent disease in most situations. This ''on-off'' characteristic can occasionally delay accurate

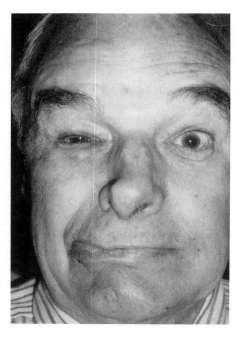

Figure 1   Typical appearance of a patient with advanced hemifacial spasm. Note forced involuntary eyelid closure, elevation of brow, distortion of the lateral angle of the mouth, and ectropion of the lip on the involved side.

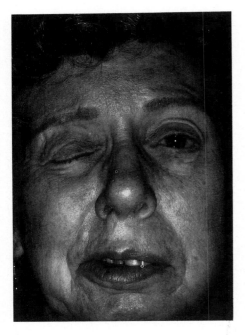

Figure 2 After 35 years of involuntary facial spastic movements associated with facial weakness, this patient with hemifacial spasm developed fixed facial contractures.

diagnosis. When the patient presents to the clinician, often there is no involuntary movement, and the examining physician may be unable to make a clear diagnosis. As the disease progresses, the incidence and duration of the spasms tend to increase. In a 10-hour videotaping review of five patients, the involuntary spasms were present for 5–80% of the observation period.

The involuntary movements may be classified into several types. Increased blinking associated with synchronous lower face twitching is most characteristic. The average blink rate of a normal eyelid is 15–25/min with a normal distribution (Fig. 3). When blink rate is quantified over a substantial period for the lid involved with hemifacial spasm, the blink rate can be seen to be distributed over two superimposed normal statistical curves (Fig. 3). One curve represents the blink rate when the spasms are ''off,'' and the other curve represents the blink rate when the spasms are ''on.'' When pathological blinking is seen, there is almost always synchronous twitch of varying degree in muscles in the lower face, and this provides strong evidence of the diagnosis. In certain situations, another characteristic of the movement disorder is continuous stimulation and tone increase of all the facial muscles that is not sufficient to cause the upper eyelid to close. In this situation, the disfigurement is one of asymmetry of the palpebral fissures and alteration of the skin creases on one side of the face. In this case, the increased blink rate may not be the obvious component of the syndrome. When sudden high-intensity bursts of ectopic impulses stimulate the muscles on one side of the face, the eyelid is forced to close, the brow becomes elevated, and there is distortion of the lower face characterized by an updrawn mouth and turned-out lower lip (Fig. 4). This phenomenon is termed a paroxysm and is always associated with forced lid closure.

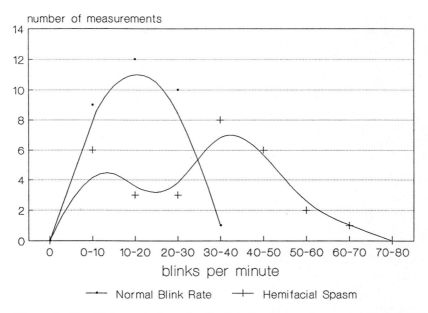

Figure 3 The blink rate is normally distributed, with an average rate of 15–25/min, in patients without facial dyskinesia. Because of the "on-off" phenomenon observed with hemifacial spasm, the blink rate is distributed over two superimposed normal curves, one curve representing the "on" periods and the other curve the "off" periods.

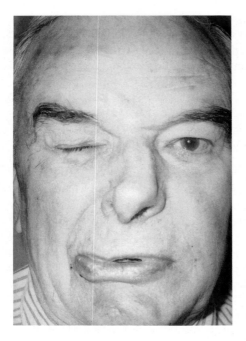

Figure 4 Sudden bursts of ectopic impulses force the lid closed, with maximal facial contraction for periods of 5–60 sec.

Morbidity caused by hemifacial spasm results from visual loss on the affected side due to increased blink rate and involuntary eyelid closure. Impaired facial communication and psychological alterations resulting from the disfigurement inherent in the disease are additional problems for patients. When hemifacial spasm occurs on the side of a patient's only seeing eye, it can have serious visual consequences. More commonly, patients will relate difficulty with interpersonal expression. When casually conversing with such a patient, the average person will not understand the reason for facial movements and will incorrectly interpret the condition as excessive winking due to nervousness or psychological impairment. This disease of facial expression is found most bothersome by patients with occupations requiring frequent interpersonal communication or public speaking.

PATHOPHYSIOLOGY

The exact cause of hemifacial spasm remains uncertain. The best understanding of the disease comes from neurosurgical observation and experience (1) and electromyographic data (2). The working theory is that an aberrantly tortuous blood vessel at the base of the brain results in a displacement of the intracranial portion of the seventh cranial nerve and a pressure phenomenon, with deterioration of the myelin sheath. A focal area of demyelination results in ectopic impulse generation in the facial nerve, with propagation of the impulse through ephaptic transmission, causing the involuntary synchronous motion of half the face. A small degree of facial muscle weakness often accompanies the involuntary movements. Nelson, using electromyographic methods, has described a phenomenon of ectopic impulse generation as well as ephaptic transmission of the impulse down the nerve (2). Ephaptic generation is defined as side-by-side axonal impulse propagation that occurs as a result of damage to the facial nerve. Ephaptic transmission explains the *synchronous movements* of the face observed in physical examination. Although this explanation may account for a number of cases, there are patients with hemifacial spasm who present in their early 20s with no apparent neuroradiological evidence of tortuous blood vessels. Alternative explanations may involve aberrant stimulation of the facial nerve nucleus or fasciculus. In a small percentage of patients ($< 1\%$) (3–5), there may be mass lesions in the posterior fossa. In the Boston experience, the lesions most commonly found were arteriovenous malformations in the region of the cerebral pontine angle (Fig. 5).

It is clear that a pathophysiological explanation of the phenomena of hemifacial spasm must account for a high incidence of negative neuroradiographic findings, a small degree of facial weakness consistently seen in patients, and synchronous contractions on the afflicted side.

DIFFERENTIAL DIAGNOSIS

Hemifacial spasm must be differentiated from many other conditions involving involuntary movement of one side of the face. The most common involuntary movement seen in ophthalmological practice is myokymia of the orbicularis oculi muscle. This movement is characterized by a small twitch in the lower lid interpreted as a nuisance by the person affected. Myokymia, however, never causes contraction within the orbicularis muscle forceful enough to cause complete eyelid closure. Hence, this condition does not really cause involuntary blinking. Orbicularis oculi myokymia has no pathological significance and usually resolves spontaneously. Rarely, localized myokymia may be the first symptom of hemifacial spasm.

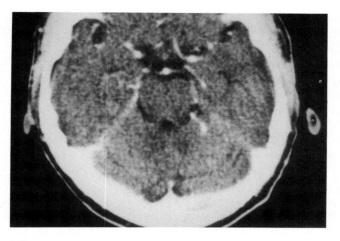

(A)

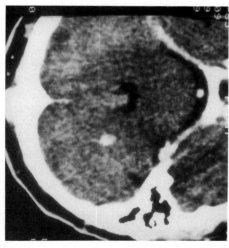

(B)

Figure 5 Arteriovenous malformation in close proximity to the brain stem in the posterior fossa is the cause of hemifacial spasm in this case. However, structural lesions within the neurocranium are very uncommon.

Hemifacial spasm must be differentiated from aberrant regeneration of the facial nerve, as both conditions can produce synchronous contractions on one side of the face. Aberrant regeneration of the facial nerve is distinguished from hemifacial spasm by a preceding bout of facial paralysis, usually from Bell's palsy but occasionally as result of herpes zoster oticus or skull base fracture or following acoustic neuroma resection. Aberrant regeneration of the facial nerve is associated with facial weakness, some degree of hemifacial contracture with constant distortion of facial landmarks, and synkinetic lid closure on the affected side. Synkinetic lid closure is defined as involuntary eyelid closure associated with lower face movements during speech, chewing, or eating (Fig. 6). The

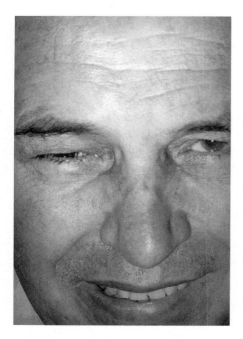

Figure 6 Synkinetic eyelid closure connected with lower facial movement is diagnostic of aberrant regeneration of the facial nerve.

syndrome of aberrant regeneration of the facial nerve also occasionally includes excessive tearing (epiphora) linked with gustatory sensation (crocodile tears). The involuntary movement associated with aberrant regeneration of the facial nerve is distinctly different from hemifacial spasm in that (1) the synkinetic lid closure is constantly present, (2) residual facial weakness usually is more apparent than the mild degree of weakness seen in hemifacial spasm, and (3) epiphora is not seen with hemifacial spasm.

Hemifacial spasm needs to be distinguished from hemifacial myokymia, a distinctly rare condition in which low-amplitude twitches and fibrillations occur in all muscles on one side of the face. Usually, in this condition, not enough force is generated to cause the eyelid to close completely. Hemifacial myokymia is often associated with demonstrable pathology in the posterior fossa (6).

Hemifacial spasm must be distinguished from benign essential blepharospasm and blepharospasm associated with Meige's disease and generalized movement disorders (7–10). The distinction can easily be made, since hemifacial spasm affects muscles only on one side of the face. Essential blepharospasm and blepharospasm associated with Meige's disease and other generalized dystonias are most commonly bilateral, although the presentation rarely may be more unilateral. In patients with unilateral Meige disease, there are asynchronous movements on the involved side.

THERAPY

There are two forms of therapy effective for the treatment of hemifacial spasm, (1) microvascular decompression of the intracranial portion of the seventh cranial nerve via posterior craniotomy and (2) intramuscular injection of botulinum toxin (BTX).

Neurosurgical Decompression of the Intracranial Facial Nerve

Microvascular decompression of the facial nerve was first described by Jannetta et al. (1). In this procedure, a posterior craniotomy is needed to expose the facial nerve in the vicinity of arteries of the ventral brain stem, with use of a neurosurgical operating microscope. Insulating material is placed between the facial nerve and blood vessels of the region. The insulating effect of gelfoam or other neurosurgical material essentially relieves the pressure of the tortuous vessel on the seventh cranial nerve, which is thought to provoke the movement disorder.

There are obvious disadvantages to this approach. The first and most obvious is that patient acceptance of neurosurgical procedures for non-life-threatening conditions is generally low. The efficacy reported for this procedure is approximately 70–89% (1) in the long term. In short-term follow-up, the success rate has been described as approximately 60%. It is clear that the neurosurgeon performing the procedure should be skilled in the technique for the best possible results. Potential complications of this procedure are the second important drawback and have been the major reason for reluctance within the medical community. Complications, although rare, can include quadriplegia from hemorrhage or vasospasm during surgery or in the postoperative period. Hearing loss on the operative side has also been reported. Although complications clearly occur in a very small fraction of cases (fewer than 1%), patients often reject the procedure when advised of the potential risks. Long-term evaluations of this procedure have not been published. It is the opinion of this author that extended videophotographic studies with well-defined efficacy criteria need to be reported for this surgical procedure to fully assess the rates of successful outcomes. Nevertheless, the concept of decompression and its demonstrated efficacy have made a substantial contribution to medical understanding of the cause of hemifacial spasm.

Botulinum Toxin Type A

Botulinum toxin type A (BTX-A) is clearly the first choice for treatment of hemifacial spasm. It is relatively easy to administer and provides relief in the vast majority of patients (over 95%) (11–17). The major disadvantages of the application include (1) the need for repetitive injections indefinitely, (2) potential for lagophthalmos and ophthalmic complications, and (3) facial asymmetry.

Botulinum toxin is quantified with a biological assay assessing the lethality of an injection of a given quantity into a standard white mouse. The international unit is the lethal dose of 50% of a cohort of white mice injected. The total dose used in the treatment of hemifacial spasm should start between 10 and 15 IU. This dose is substantially below the quantity needed to treat other forms of blepharospasm. For instance, Meige's disease and essential blepharospasm should generally be treated with higher doses, 30–40 IU. Table 1 compares dose-response relations for Meige's disease, essential blepharospasm, and hemifacial spasm. The reasons for the differences involve the pathophysiology of hemifacial spasm as compared with Meige's disease and essential blepharospasm. Meige's disease and essential blepharospasm are basically dystonias, that is, movement disorders arising from derangement in information processing within the central nervous system. Central nervous system regulation of facial movement and blink is altered in such a fashion that involuntary impulses arise, with the impulses propagated over normal peripheral nervous structures. Hemifacial spasm is distinctly different as it is associated with facial neuropathy and facial muscle weakness. Partially denervated muscle, such as

Table 1 Dose Response Relations, Comparing the Various Forms of Blepharospasm

	Blepharospasm	Hemifacial spasm	Aberrant regeneration
No. of patients/no. of injections	112/697	71/269	12/40
Mean dose (IU)	35.4790[a]	20.1877[b]	22.4426[b]
Dose: standard deviation	8.4529	1.3919	1.8705
Average no. of injections	6.22	3.79	3.33
Average duration (months)	3.1	5.6	6.28

[a]One-half of the total dose given for blepharospasm is shown, because this condition is bilateral whereas aberrant regeneration is unilateral.
[b]Dose requirements for aberrant regeneration of the facial nerve and hemifacial spasm are significantly lower than requirement for Meige syndrome (blepharospasm), $p < .001$.

occurs with hemifacial spasm, appears to be more sensitive to the weakening effect of BTX (Table 1).

With repeated injections of the toxin, there is some degree of resistance. As the number of BTX treatment sessions received by a patient increases, the dosage needed in subsequent injections generally becomes higher. This is particularly true for Meige's disease and essential blepharospasm, and less so for hemifacial spasm. Comparative dose requirements after multiple injections for various syndromes causing blepharospasm are outlined in Fig. 7.

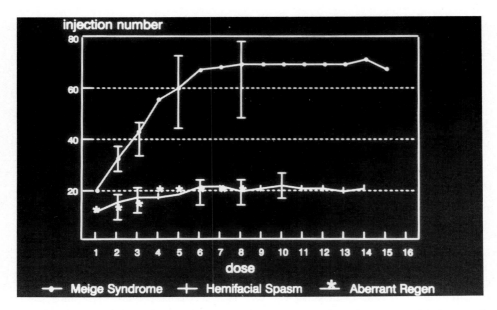

Figure 7 Dose requirement after multiple injection periods over an average of 3–4 years for various syndromes causing blepharospasm (Meige syndrome, aberrant regeneration of the facial nerve, and hemifacial spasm).

Generally, the dose requirements for hemifacial spasm level off between 20 and 25 IU. Injection of higher doses of BTX can result in excessive weakness of the orbicularis oculi muscle, paralytic lagophthalmos, and exposure keratopathy, resulting in pain and blurred vision. Patients with hemifacial spasm are more susceptible to this complication than patients with essential blepharospasm, because of the preexisting weakness associated with the former disease. Occasionally, dose levels of 20–25 IU may be excessive and can cause symptomatic exposure keratitis.

Patients with known dry-eye syndromes should receive especially low starting doses to avoid postinjection keratitis.

As the doses needed to treat facial dyskinesias are very low, there has never been a case report of BTX intoxication in the application of this treatment modality. In contrast, in the treatment of spasmodic torticollis, a form of dystonia, the dose requirements range between 200 and 300 IU. Since the therapeutic index (therapeutic dose/LD_{50}) of BTX-A is low, systemic complications from disseminated weakness are expected to be very rare. The minimal estimated lethal dose of BTX for a human is approximately 2500 IU (18).

The injection sites are important in the treatment of hemifacial spasm as well as other forms of blepharospasm. When BTX is injected for the treatment of hemifacial spasm with involuntary eyelid closure, it is important to target the orbicularis oculi muscle for weakening, as this muscle promotes involuntary eyelid closure and increased blinking. The injection sites for the treatment of hemifacial spasm are shown in Fig. 8A. Although these injection points may be appropriate for most patients, modification of the injection points occasionally is necessary if most of the involuntary movement is in the lower face.

The efficacy of treatment can be measured by assessing blink rate (Fig. 8B) and quantitating palpebral fissure asymmetry (Fig. 8C) during an extended period using video recordings.

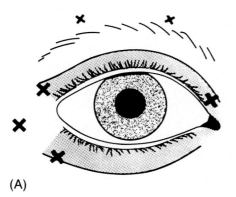

(A)

Figure 8 (A) Injection points used to treat blepharospasm associated with hemifacial spasm. Note that the lateral injections affect the ipsilateral zygomaticus major and minor muscles, which are retractors to the nasolabial fold and the lateral angle of the mouth. Injections points occasionally need to be customized to individual patients, such a those who demonstrate the involuntary movement primarily in the lower face. (B) Efficacy of botulinum toxin injections using blink rate as criterion, before and 2 weeks after injection. Note that there is substantial reduction in the blink rate after treatment. (C) Efficacy of botulinum toxin injections using periods of palpebral fissure asymmetry as criterion, measured over 30–45 min before and after injection. Palpebral fissure closure from orbicularis muscle spasm causes both loss of visual field and disfigurement from hemifacial spasm.

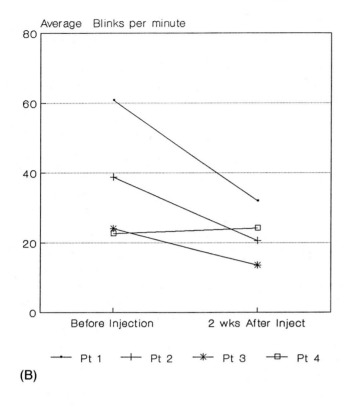

(B)

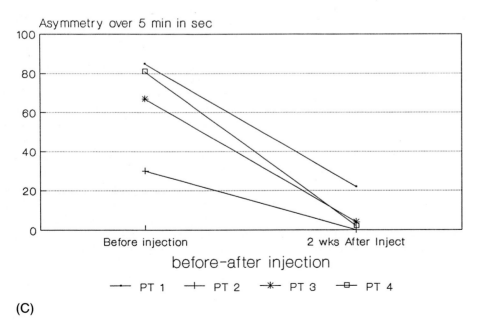

(C)

Over the past 8 years, it has been recognized that the effectiveness and rate of complications of BTX administration can be technique-dependent (19,20). The site of toxin injection is anatomically important and consequential to the effectiveness of the therapy. Botulinum toxin is injected at four points into the orbicularis oculi (Fig. 8A). Two injection points are used in the upper lid, one to the medial extreme of the upper lid and the other on the lateral extreme of the upper lid. A lateral injection point and a lateral inferior lid injection point complete the multiple-point injection strategy. The location of injections over multiple points is important in achieving a diffuse biological effect of the toxin throughout the orbicularis muscle. The lateral orbicularis injections also cover the upper portions of the zygomaticus major and minor muscle, which are responsible for the position of the nasolabial fold and the lip. Another implication of the injection points concerns toxin diffusion to contiguous muscles, which causes complications. For instance, injection in the superior portion of the upper lid into the anatomical lid fold can have deleterious effects caused by diffusion into the levator palpebrae superioris muscle, which keeps the upper lid in the appropriate position (Fig. 9A,B). Toxin diffusion into the levator palpebrae superioris muscle will result in decreased muscle tone, which results in ptosis (drooping of the upper eyelid) (Fig. 10). Ptosis can further obstruct a patient's vision and create further disfigurement in patients with hemifacial spasm. This complication is usually transient, lasting 2–3 weeks. Placing the upper-lid injections close to the lash line and away from the midline of the lid maximizes the distance between the upper-lid points of injection into the orbicularis muscle and the orbicularis muscle's antagonist, the levator palpebrae superioris muscle. In fact, the anatomical remoteness of the pretarsal orbicularis muscle from its antagonist (the levator) is an important reason for the success achieved by regional BTX injections for blepharospasm. Because of this distance, containment of the denervative effect to the orbicularis oculi without weakening the eyelid retractors is possible.

In the lower lid, the injection points should be lateral and, particularly, away from the inner aspect of the lid. Nelson and co-workers (19) have identified another complication, diplopia (double vision), occurring as a result of diffusion of BTX into the inferior oblique muscle from medial lower lid injections. As the inferior oblique muscle is the most anteriorly located extraocular muscle in the orbit, arising posterior to the posterior lacrimal crest along the medial orbit, it is easy to understand that medial lower lid injections can diffuse into this region, causing another complication of therapy. The inferior oblique muscle actually lies very close to medial lower lid skin as it passes through the capsulopalpebral fascia.

Multiple injection points around the orbicularis and other targeted muscles are important for a directed homogeneous effect. In another chapter, it was demonstrated that the diffusion potential of point injection of BTX is clearly dose-dependent. At higher doses, the toxin not only produces a greater degree of weakness of the injected muscle but has the potential to diffuse away from the point of injection and cause complications by affecting nontargeted muscles. Additionally, the multiple-point injection not only allows lower doses in given areas within the muscle, but also, if the muscle's innervation zone is diffuse, it probably saturates the innervation zone more completely. For instance, the innervation zone of the orbicularis oculi muscle is probably very diffuse (21). The facial nerve projects to this muscle from a number of different ramifications from the temporal, zygomatic, and buccal branches. This complex motor nerve network to the orbicularis oculi from multiple branches of the facial nerve affects this muscle's responses to resections and reconstructive surgery of the eyelids. The orbicularis muscle is not easily

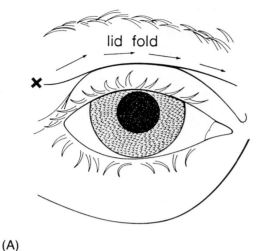

(A)

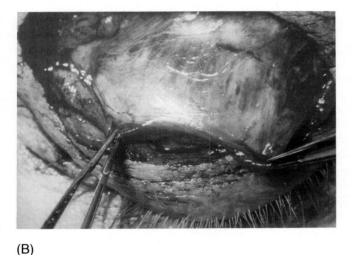

(B)

Figure 9 Injection of botulinum toxin into the lid fold may cause ptosis from diffusion of the biological activity of the toxin into the levator muscle of the eyelid. (A) The thin arrows demonstrate the position of the lid fold. Lid fold injections bring the injection point into close proximity to the muscular portion of the levator palpebrae superioris muscle. Weakening of the levator muscle results in ptosis (see Fig. 10). (B) Part of the surgical field of a ptosis operation (levator advancement), demonstrating the proximity of the muscular portion of the levator to the lid fold.

paralyzed with oculoplastic procedures after large sections of the muscle are resected. This clinical observation suggests that there is a diffuse innervation zone to this muscle. The innervation zone of the orbicularis was studied in strips of muscle taken during ptosis surgery (21,22). Although this was a limited sampling of muscle, it indicated that the distribution of neuromuscular junctions within muscle strips (innervation zone) was diffuse for this muscle. This finding may explain why multiple injections within the

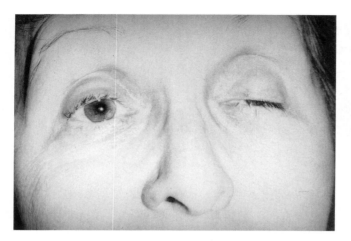

Figure 10 Ptosis as a complication of botulinum toxin injections into the eyelids. Weakening of the muscular portion of the levator palpebrae superioris muscle is the cause.

muscle are probably more effective in producing the most beneficial results. A similar phenomenon may explain why BTX is more effective when used in multiple-point injections in the treatment of adult-onset spasmodic torticollis (23).

Facial dynamic asymmetry is a problem in using BTX for hemifacial spasm. Botulinum toxin weakens injected muscles. Alterations in the injected muscle's resting tone can cause a small degree of resting asymmetry. However, because of depressed contractility of injected facial muscles, there can occasionally be more substantial facial asymmetry during periods of active facial expression, when facial muscle contractility is greatest as compared with periods of neutral facial expression (Fig. 11). It is rewarding to be able to eliminate the amplitude of spasmodic contractions by using BTX injection. However, an unfortunate complication of the injection is that the amplitude of volitional contractions on the side of the face injected is also occasionally noticeably impaired. It is possible to titrate the dose in such a fashion that volitional contractions are much less impaired than the high-velocity contractions associated with the spasm.

The term "facial dynamic asymmetry" is used to advance the concept that facial symmetry needs to be evaluated during periods of active expression, such as smiling and laughing, as well as with facial muscles at rest. Although BTX therapy can rarely cause asymmetry with facial muscles at rest (static asymmetry), the much more common asymmetry occurs during periods of active expression. The static asymmetry is noted by a droop on the lateral angle of the mouth and depression of the nasolabial fold (Fig. 12A,B). This complication would indicate that an excessive dose of BTX was administered. The dynamic asymmetry accentuated during active facial expressions is, again, more common and is demonstrated by symmetry in upper lip excursions and dentition show during smiling, lack of crease accentuation and elevation along the nasolabial fold and other dynamic creases of the lower face, and drooping of the side of the lower lip (Fig. 13A). The major reason for the asymmetry appears to be excessive effect on the zygomaticus major and minor muscles resulting from excessive biological effect diffusing from the more inferolateral injections to the orbicularis oculi muscle. Occasionally, this asymmetry results from injection of excessive amounts of toxin directly into the zygomatic muscles. As BTX tends to reach its peak effect of muscle weakening within 14 to 17 days after the

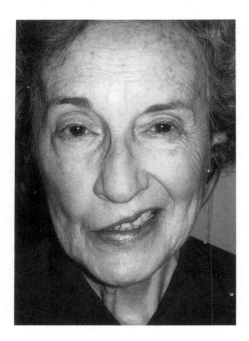

Figure 11 Example of facial dynamic asymmetry. Note asymmetry of upper lip and nasolabial fold excursion and asymmetry of exposure of the teeth.

injection, patients will generally call within 2 weeks with this complaint. The clinician who receives such a complaint has several options. The first is to reassure the patient that the complaint will be temporary and that as the effect of the BTX recedes, the degree of asymmetry will clearly diminish. The patient should be reassured that this complication is always reversible. Another more immediate approach would be to use an injection of BTX contralateral to the side affected (24) (Fig. 13B). This contralateral injection should be placed over the intersection between the zygomaticus major and minor muscles lying over the zygomatic bone. The action of these muscles is primarily to raise the lips, the lateral angle of the mouth, and the nasolabial fold, and injection of BTX to the contralateral side diminishes the contraction amplitude of these facial muscles and yields a more symmetrical dynamic facial appearance with more even dentition show during smiling (Fig. 14). The author has found this approach to be effective in a number of patients (24,25). A dose of 5–15 IU given at three points just over the zygomatic arch on the contralateral side usually suffices to produce this effect (Fig. 13B).

This approach in creating facial symmetry derives from the observation that it is difficult to diagnose patients with simultaneous bilateral facial nerve disease. Because there is symmetry in the paralytic facial movements, the clinician has difficulty perceiving facial weakness. If a patient expresses displeasure with asymmetry of dynamic expression, the asymmetry is reduced by altering contractility of the normal side of her face. A similar approach has been suggested in managing forehead symmetry after frontalis branch damage of the face in patients undergoing cosmetic face-lifts (26). The major side effect encountered with contralateral zygomaticus injections is impaired excursions of the upper lip, which can be noticeable to the patient during speech. Smile characteristics will also change.

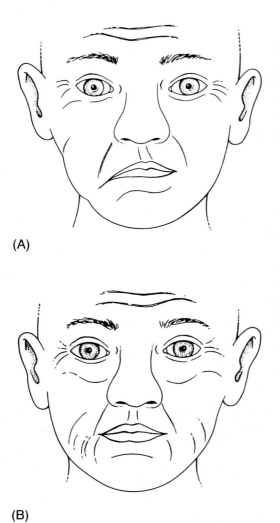

(A)

(B)

Figure 12   Diagram of facial asymmetry (A) with facial muscles at rest, compared with normal appearance (B).

Another problem frequently encountered in patients with hemifacial spasm is a concomitant dry eye syndrome. Dry eye is generally assessed using Schirmer paper wetting over a 5-minute period after topical anesthetic is placed in the conjunctival fornix. Patients with dry eye syndrome may experience more severe exposure faster application of BTX. Decreased blink response seen after administration of the toxin results in excessive evaporation away from the precorneal tear film. Nevertheless, patients with hemifacial spasm and dry eye syndrome can be effectively treated with BTX. The author suggests the use of silicone punctal plugs to halt the egress of tears from the conjunctival fornix into the nasolacrimal sac (Fig. 15). The increased wetting produced by nasolacrimal obstruction allows BTX to be used more effectively in patients with dry eyes. Patients with dry eye syndrome should also be given lower doses (5–10 IU). If this dose is not enough to

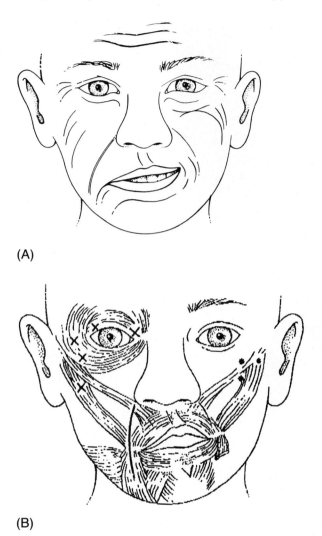

(A)

(B)

Figure 13 Diagram of facial asymmetry with dynamic facial movement. Contralateral injections (asterisks) of smaller doses of botulinum toxin (5–10 IU) help maintain symmetry of important facial landmarks during dynamic expression.

mitigate symptoms, it can be increased in 2 weeks. It is wise to titrate the dose up in these patients, as has been previously mentioned.

In summary, the complications of therapy for hemifacial spasm include

1. Ptosis from toxin diffusion into the muscular portion of the levator palpebrae superioris muscle
2. Double vision, from diffusion of the toxin into the orbit and involvement of the extraocular muscles, particularly the inferior oblique
3. Epiphora from weakening of Horner's muscle, which functions as the lacrimal pump muscle, taking tears from the conjunctiva and delivering into the nose

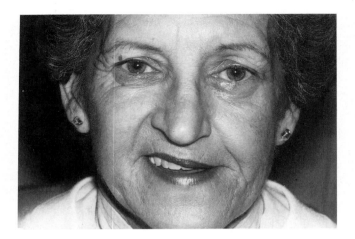

(A)

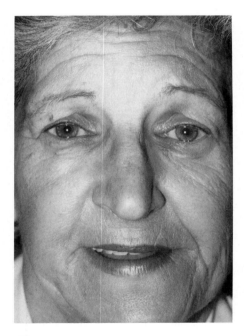

(B)

Figure 14   Before and after contralateral injection of botulinum toxin to increase facial symmetry during active expressions. (A) Asymmetric exposure of teeth and depressed excursions of the nasolabial fold and lateral angle of the mouth during smiling. (B) This asymmetry is corrected by contralateral injections.

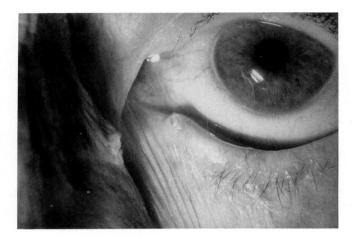

Figure 15 Punctal plugs can be helpful in the treatment of dry eye syndrome, which can be aggravated by the use of botulinum toxin injections to the eyelids. Note the silicone plug placed in the inferior punctum. This plug can be left in place indefinitely.

4. Facial asymmetry from excessive weakening of facial muscles contiguous to the orbicularis oculi, that is, the zygomaticus major and minor muscles
5. Exposure keratopathy from excessive weakening of the orbicularis oculi muscle, with lagophthalmos and corneal drying

To date, no long-term changes in muscle fiber size or permanent muscle fiber atrophy has been demonstrated in biopsied human muscle after multiple toxin injections over several years (22).

Duration of Action of Repetitive Injections

The duration of action of BTX for the treatment of hemifacial spasm is distinctly longer than in therapy for other forms of blepharospasm (Fig. 16). The duration of action is very similar to that seen in patients with aberrant regeneration of the facial nerve who are treated with BTX (25). The average duration of effect is 5.5 months (Table 1). The duration of effect can vary among individuals, and patients are often asked to come back when the symptoms are returning. It is often helpful to let the patients make their own judgments in this respect.

Sensitization, with decreasing effectiveness, after repeated injections is theoretically possible for patients with hemifacial spasm. Antibody formation has been demonstrated with large-dose applications, as in therapy for torticollis, and with intermediate doses such as those used to treat Meige syndrome. Because the dose requirement is lower for the treatment of hemifacial spasm, the risk of sensitization is probably considerably less. The incidence of sensitization and the long-term impact of this phenomenon still are subjects of active investigation. Sensitization has occurred in one patient treated for blepharospasm.

CONCLUSION

In summary, hemifacial spasm is a disorder of the facial nerve characterized by intermittent synchronous involuntary contractions of facial muscles. The condition not only impairs vision but is also cosmetically disfiguring and impairs interpersonal communica-

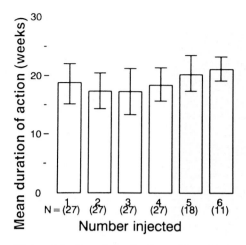

Figure 16   Duration of effect of botulinum toxin therapy for hemifacial spasm. N = number sampled.

tion. Although microvascular decompression of the facial nerve can be effective, most patients will prefer therapy with BTX injections. The injections need to be given periodically and indefinitely, usually at 4- to 6-month intervals. There have been no long-term adverse effects of repeated BTX injections for this condition over 7 to 8 years of clinical studies.

REFERENCES

1. Jannetta PJ, Abbasy M, Maroon JC, Ramos FM, Albin MS. Etiology and differential microsurgical treatment of hemifacial spasm. J Neurosurg 1977; 47:321.
2. Nelson VK. Electrophysiology of the facial nerve in hemifacial spasm: ectopic/ephaptic excitation. Muscle Nerve 1985; 8:545.
3. Dujonvy M, Osgoow CP, Faille R, Bennett HM, Kerber C. Posterior fossa AVM producing hemifacial spasm. Angiology 1979; 30:424.
4. Davis WE, Luterman BF, Pulliam MW, Templer JW. Hemifacial spasm caused by choles-teatoma. Am J Otol 1981; 2:272.
5. Wirtshaffer J. Incidence of intracranial lesions in patients with hemifacial spasm. Presented at the American Academy of Ophthalmology, 1987.
6. Walsh FB, Hoyt WF. Textbook of clinical neuro-ophthalmology. 3d ed. Baltimore: Williams & Wilkins, 1969.
7. Tolosa ES. Clinical features of Meige's disease (idiopathic orofacial dystonia): a report of 17 cases. Arch Neurol 1981; 38:147.
8. Marsden CD. Blepharospasm–oromandibular dystonia (Brueghel's syndrome). J Neurol Neurosurg Psychiatry 1976; 39:1204.
9. Meige H. Les convulsions de la face, une forme clinique de la convulsion faciale, bilatéral et médiane. Rev Neurol (Paris) 1910; 70:437.
10. Jankovic J. Etiology and differential diagnosis of blepharospasm and oromandibular dystonia. Adv Neurol 1988; 49:103.
11. Scott AB, Kennedy RA, Stubbs HA. Botulinum A toxin injection as a treatment for blepharospasm. Arch Ophthalmol 1985; 103:374.
12. Elston JS, Russell RW. Effect of treatment with botulinum toxin on neurogenic blepharospasm. Br Med J 1985; 290:1857.

13. Townsend D, Borodic G. Botulinum toxin for facial spastic disease. In: Hornblass A, ed. Textbook of oculoplastic surgery. Baltimore: Williams & Wilkins, 1988.
14. Dutton JJ, Buckley EG. Long term results and complications of botulinum toxin in the treatment of blepharospasm. Ophthalmology 1988; 95:1529–1534.
15. Borodic GE, Cozzolino D. Blepharospasm and its treatment, with emphasis on the use of botulinum toxin. Plast Reconstr Surg 1989; 83:546–554.
16. Savino PJ, Sergott RC, Bosley TM, Schatz NT. Hemifacial spasm treated with botulinum toxin injections. Arch Ophthalmol 1985; 103:1305–1306.
17. Borodic GE, Pearce LB, Cheney M, Metson R, Brownstone D, Townsend D, McKenna M. Botulinum A toxin for the treatment of aberrant facial nerve regeneration. Plast Reconstr Surg 1993; 91(6):1042–1045.
18. Scott AB, Suzuki D. Systemic toxicity of botulinum toxin by intramuscular injection in the monkey. Mov Disord 1988; 3:333–335.
19. Frueh BR, Nelson CC, Kapustiak JF, Musch DC. The effects of omitting the lower eyelid in blepharospasm treatment. Am J Ophthalmol 1988; 106:45–47.
20. Borodic GE, Joseph M, Fay L, Cozzolino D, Ferrante R. Botulinum A toxin for the treatment of spasmodic torticollis. Dysphagia and regional toxin spread. Head Neck 1990; 12:392–398.
21. Borodic GE, Weigner A, Ferrante R, Young R. Orbicularis oculi innervation zone and implications for botulinum A toxin therapy for blepharospasm. Ophthalm Plast Reconstr Surg 1991; 7:54–59.
22. Borodic GE, Ferrante R. Histologic effects of repeated botulinum toxin over many years in human orbicularis oculi muscle. J Clin Neuro-Ophthalmol 1992; 12:121–127.
23. Borodic GE, Pearce LB, Joseph M. Cranial cervical dystonias, multiple vs single injection strategies, a clinical study. Head Neck 1992; 14:33–37.
24. Borodic GE, Cheney M, McKenna M. Contralateral injection of botulinum toxin to achieve facial dynamic symmetry for the treatment of hemifacial spasm. Plast Reconstr Surg 1992; 90:972–977.
25. Borodic, GE. Botulinum A toxin application for expressionistic ptosis overcorrection after frontalis sling procedures. Ophthalm Plast Reconstr Surg 1992; 8:137–142.
26. Clark RT, Berris C. Botulinum toxin for facial asymmetry caused by facial nerve paralysis. Plast Reconstr Surg 1989; 84:353–355.

25

Management of Hemifacial Spasm with Botulinum A Toxin

Albert W. Biglan
University of Pittsburgh School of Medicine, Pittsburgh, Pennsylvania

Sang-Jin Kim
Keimyung University, Taegu, South Korea

INTRODUCTION

Hemifacial spasm is an acquired condition characterized by unilateral hyperactivity of the facial nerve, which causes paroxysmal contraction of the muscles innervated by this cranial nerve (Fig. 1, left). Between spasms, the facial musculature functions normally or may be slightly weak. The usual onset of hemifacial spasm is during the fifth or sixth decade of life, and this disorder can cause social disability as well as economic hardship. In many cases, hyperactivity of the facial nerve is due to nerve irritation, which in turn is caused by compression of the facial nerve by the posterior inferior cerebellar artery on the nerve where the nerve exits the brain stem. Diagnostic evaluation of symptoms of hemifacial spasm should include neuroradiological imaging, because such symptoms can be caused by tumors (1–3).

Mild forms of hemifacial spasm are managed with sedation or carbamazepine (4). For more severe forms, a microsurgical procedure for decompression of the facial nerve, the Jannetta procedure, may be recommended. This procedure is successful in curing 90% of patients with symptomatic hemifacial spasm (5). Recently, botulinum toxin type A (BTX-A) has been used to control facial spasm (Fig. 1, right) in patients who decline the Jannetta procedure or who have had this operation but still have residual facial muscle spasm (6,7).

INDICATIONS AND CONTRAINDICATIONS FOR TREATMENT WITH BOTULINUM TOXIN TYPE A

Patients for whom treatment of hemifacial spasm with BTX-A may be indicated include those in whom medical therapy has failed to relieve spasm, those with residual facial muscle spasm following a facial nerve decompression procedure, and those who are too ill

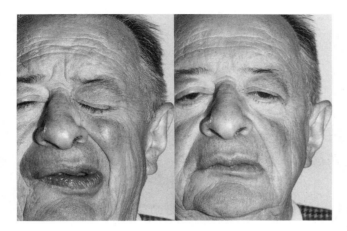

Figure 1   (Left) Moderate (+3) hemifacial spasm involving the left side of a patient's face. (Right) Same patient 2 weeks after treatment with botulinum toxin type A.

to undergo a neurosurgical procedure. In addition, some patients, especially more elderly patients, may refuse to have the neurosurgical decompression procedure and elect to control their spasm with periodic injections of BTX-A.

There are few contraindications for treatment of hemifacial spasm with BTX-A. Treatment should be withheld until a thorough investigation has been conducted to exclude a tumor or other treatable condition as the cause of symptoms. Young patients may be encouraged to consider the more definitive facial nerve decompression procedure, because it offers a permanent cure rather than the temporary control of the spasm offered by BTX-A. Patients who produce antibodies, and those who have had prior treatment with botulinum toxin and had a poor or absent response, should be offered other forms of therapy.

PROCEDURE FOR TREATING HEMIFACIAL SPASM WITH BOTULINUM TOXIN TYPE A

Injections of botulinum toxin are administered in an office setting. The patient is examined for the severity of the facial muscle spasm, and this is graded on a scale of +1 (mild) to +4 (severe). Photographs or videotape recordings of facial muscle activity may be obtained to document the degree of spasm. Neuroradiological imaging is recommended to help evaluate integrity of the seventh cranial nerve, its nucleus, and its efferent pathways.

After the patient has given informed consent to treatment with BTX-A, preparations are made for the injections. A 100-U vial of freeze-dried toxin is reconstituted with 2 ml of nonpreserved 0.9% saline solution to yield toxin in a concentration of 5 U/0.1 ml. The initial treatment dose is calculated on the basis of the severity and location of the patient's spasm. To bring out the spasm, the patient is asked to forcibly close the eyes and grimace. When the patient relaxes the facial muscles after this maneuver, the spasm will become evident.

Before injection of toxin, the patient's skin is cleansed with isopropyl alcohol. Typically, injections of toxin are given into (1) the central portion of the pretarsal

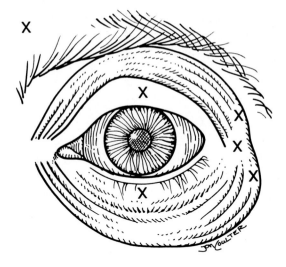

Figure 2 Schematic diagram showing the locations for botulinum toxin type A treatment of the orbicularis oculi, procerus, and corrugator muscles.

orbicularis muscle of the upper eyelid (5 U) (Fig. 2 and Fig. 3, top) (2) the lower eyelid (3 U) (Fig. 2 and Fig. 3, top), (3) the reflection of the orbicularis oculi muscle lateral to the orbital rim (10–15 U), (Fig. 3, bottom), and (4) the procerus and corrugator muscle group (Fig. 2), and the mentalis muscle (5 U each) (Fig. 4). The zygomaticus major muscle can be treated near its origin by injection of 5 U of toxin. Treatment of the orbicularis oris muscle is not recommended, because treatment will prevent this muscle from forming a watertight seal to keep fluids in the mouth.

Between 24 and 48 hours after initial injections of BTX-A an effect of the toxin will be evident. At 1 week the maximum effect of the treatment will be observed, and it is recommended that the patient's response to the injections be evaluated at this time. If spasm persists at the 1-week evaluation, another 5 U of toxin may be injected directly into the offending muscle group. Patients whose spasm is satisfactorily controlled by the initial injections are discharged after this 1-week visit until they require additional injections. This is usually 5 to 6 months after the initial treatment session.

When additional injections of toxin are required, a maintenance dose is calculated by adding the number of units of toxin given to each muscle group. This totaled maintenance dose is the dose that is administered for subsequent treatments. If side effects of toxin injection occur, the dose injected into the affected muscles at second or subsequent treatment sessions is reduced.

TREATMENT RESULTS

We performed a retrospective study of the effect of treatment of hemifacial spasm with BTX-A. Thirty-six patients were treated with toxin, either because a Jannetta procedure had provided only partial relief of their symptoms or because they had declined this neurosurgical procedure.

Sixteen of the 36 patients were men, and in 18 patients the right side of the face was affected. The mean age of the patients at the time of initial evaluation was 62.9 years

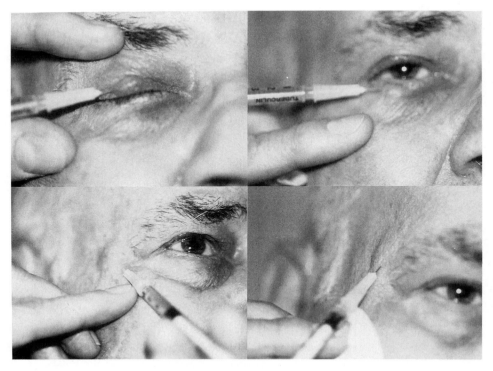

Figure 3 (Top) Botulinum toxin type A (BTX-A) is injected into the pretarsal orbicularis muscle of the upper and lower eyelids. (Bottom) The lateral reflection of the orbicularis oculi muscle is infiltrated with 15 units of BTX-A.

(range 23 to 85 years). The mean age at onset of symptoms was 55.6 years (range 17 to 84 years). The mean duration of symptoms before treatment was 7 years (range 1 to 25 years). Three patients had hemifacial spasm associated with a tumor (two acoustic neuromas and one "brain tumor" of unknown cytologic composition).

In this study group, 15 of 36 patients underwent a Jannetta procedure. Nine patients had the procedure before the BTX-A treatment and had incomplete relief of their hemifacial spasm following surgery; the other six patients requested a Jannetta procedure after they had started BTX-A treatments, either because it was the only option during a period when botulinum toxin was unavailable or because they were unwilling to continue long-term treatment with the toxin.

During the 7-year study period, the 36 patients received a mean of 3.77 treatments (range 1 to 11) with BTX-A. The number of treatments each patient required was related to the length of time for which the patient was under our care and to the severity of spasms at the first visit. The duration of symptoms had no influence on patients' responsiveness to treatment.

A maintenance dose was calculated for each patient as the total number of units of toxin needed to relieve the spasm. For 26 patients the maintenance dose level was the initial dose, for nine patients the maintenance dose was reached in the second session, and for one patient four treatment sessions were required to establish the maintenance dose.

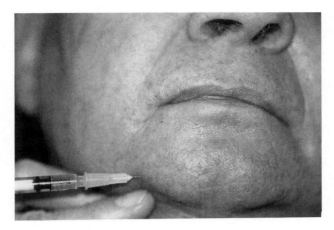

Figure 4 Spasm that involves the chin is treated with injection of 5 units of botulinum toxin type A into the mentalis muscle group.

The mean maintenance dose of BTX-A was 40.7 U (range 19–80 U), and the mean interval between treatments, once the maintenance dose was determined, was 5.6 months.

All patients showed some response to treatment with BTX-A. Two patients appeared to show a decreased effect following treatment, and one of these patients has subsequently been found to have antibodies to the toxin. This patient with antibodies was treated with 45 U followed by three additional 10-U treatments. Although toxin finally achieved control of this patient's spasm, she elected to proceed with neurosurgical decompression. The other patient's spasm could be controlled only by increasing his maintenance dose of BTX-A from 55 U to 80 U.

COMPLICATIONS AND THEIR MANAGEMENT

Although we have not noted hypersensitivity to BTX-A in our patients, some problems did occur that were related to temporary weakness in the muscles that had been injected with toxin. Of the 14 patients in this series who developed a complication, 12 had received 40 U or more of toxin. Complications, which lasted no more than 3 months, consisted of exposure keratitis with tearing (eight patients), biting the cheek or lip (three patients), and transient blepharoptosis and diplopia (one patient each). Complications were related to the treatment location and the amount of toxin injected at each visit.

Exposure Keratitis

Lagophthalmos may occur if too much BTX-A is injected into the orbicularis oculi muscle. The orbicularis oculi muscle is responsible for eyelid closure, and when this muscle is weakened excessively the eyelids cannot close unless external force is applied. Thus, spontaneous blinking or casual attempts at eyelid closure will result in incomplete eyelid closure, which in turn leads to exposure keratitis and drying of the cornea. This may cause irritation of the eye and in some cases infection. If exposure keratitis occurs, application once or twice each day of an ocular petrolatum or mineral oil lubricant such as

Lacrilube or Duratears is recommended. Because these ointments blur vision, we usually advise managing dry eye with artificial tear solutions during waking hours.

Facial Distortions

Injection of more than 7 U of toxin into the zygomaticus major group will cause loss of the nasolabial fold and drooping of the angle of the mouth, which alters facial expression undesirably. Weakening these muscles can also lead the patient to bite the inside of the cheek or lip, causing pain and possibly oral problems. If there is severe spasm of the zygomaticus muscle group, injection of 5 U into the zygomaticus major muscle, near its origin, will relieve spasm sufficiently for the patient to be comfortable.

Ptosis

If more than 10 U of toxin were injected into the pretarsal orbicularis muscle of the upper eyelid, ptosis of the eyelid occurred. Blepharoptosis will occur when the toxin diffuses behind the orbital septum and weakens the levator palpebrae superioris muscle, which is very sensitive to the toxin. Blepharoptosis is transient and will usually resolve in 4 to 6 weeks. Ptosis that is caused by the injection will disappear completely within 3 months.

Bruising

Another complication of BTX-A injection is mild bruising around the injection sites. This usually will disappear within a week. If the patient is taking aspirin or another anti-coagulant medication, discontinuing the anticoagulant 2 days before injection of BTX-A will reduce the amount of bruising caused by the injection.

Production of Antibodies

Some patients appear to form antibodies to BTX-A. The preliminary results of a study we conducted of patients who received as many as 33 injections for hemifacial spasm or other conditions with facial and cervical dystonia show that 67% of patients treated with BTX-A demonstrate some degree of antibody production 4 days following an injection. To date, however, we have not been able to find a correlation between the patient's response to the injection and the production of antibodies. Perhaps antibodies are biologically inactive, or the toxin may bind to the myoneural junction before interacting with the antibodies. Additional investigations are being conducted into the degree and clinical significance of antibody production.

CONCLUSION

Periodic injections of BTX-A are a satisfactory alternative for controlling hemifacial spasm in patients who have residual spasm following a Jannetta procedure or who decline neurosurgical treatment. Repeat injections are required approximately every 5 or 6 months. Most patients do not become resistant to treatments, and injections of toxin can maintain long-term control of the spasm even after eight or nine treatments. Transient complications do occur and are related to excessive paralysis of the orbicularis oculi muscle, causing lagophthalmos, or to weakening of the zygomaticus muscle group or the orbicularis oris muscles, causing difficulties in chewing and loss of a nasolabial crease.

REFERENCES

1. Jannetta PJ. Microvascular decompression for hemifacial spasm. In: May M, ed. The facial nerve. New York: Thieme, 1986:499–508.
2. Schloss MD, Bebear JP. Hemifacial spasm: importance of a complete investigation. J Otolaryngol 1976;5:319–330.
3. Jankovic J, Patel SC. Blepharospasm associated with brainstem lesions. Neurology 1983;33:1237–1240.
4. Alexander GE, Moses H. Carbamazepine for hemifacial spasm. Neurology 1982;32:286–287.
5. Jannetta PJ, Abbasy M, Maroon JC, et al. Etiology and definitive microsurgical treatment of hemifacial spasm: operative techniques and results in 47 patients. J Neurosurg 1977;47: 321–328.
6. Savino PJ, Sergott RC, Bosley TM, et al. Hemifacial spasm treated with botulinum A toxin injection. Arch Ophthalmol 1985;103:1305–1306.
7. Biglan AW, May M, Bowes RA. Management of facial spasm with clostridium botulinum toxin, type A (Oculinum). Arch Otolaryngol 1988;114:1407–1412.

26

Botulinum Toxin for Facial-Oral-Mandibular Spasms and Bruxism

Alfredo Berardelli, Bruno Mercuri, and Alberto Priori
La Sapienza University, Rome, Italy

INTRODUCTION

Hemifacial spasm (HFS) is a condition characterized by involuntary, paroxysmal tonic and clonic muscle twitches on one side of the face. Occasionally, the patient has a history of a lesion of the facial nerve or Bell's palsy (symptomatic type), but most patients have no prior neurological disturbances (cryptogenic type). Familial cases have also been described (1). Hemifacial spasm is a very disabling disease because severely affected patients can be functionally blind and because "these spasmodic innervations are peculiarly deforming—the nose is pulled to one side, the teeth bared in a snarl, the eye closed in a sinister wink" (2) (Fig. 1). Although in the cryptogenic forms no lesions can be demonstrated, some authors believe that HFS is caused by compression or irritation of the facial nerve by an aberrant artery at the point where the nerve exits the brain stem (3). Detailed pathophysiological studies suggest that HFS is due to a nerve abnormality peripheral to the facial nucleus and that the responsible mechanisms are ectopic excitation, ephaptic transmission, or lateral spread of impulses (3,4). However, another possible explanation is hyperexcitability of the facial nucleus (5).

Anticonvulsant drugs (phenytoin, carbamazepine, clonazepam) only occasionally give relief (6,7), and surgical decompression of the facial nerve (8,9), although useful, can lead to severe complications.

In 1973, Scott et al. (10) proposed botulinum toxin (BTX) injection as a specific treatment for strabismus. Subsequently, BTX was used in treating patients with HFS (11–23) (Table 1).

Here we present the results of BTX treatment of patients with HFS studied in the Movement Disorder Center of Rome since 1985. To discuss the use of BTX for other cranial muscles spasms, we also describe the results obtained in two patients with masticatory muscle involvement, one with cranial oromandibular dystonia and the other

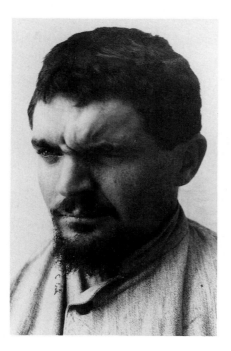

Figure 1 A case of hemifacial spasm observed in our Institute in 1916 (from the photographic collection of Prof. G. Mingazzini).

with hemimasticatory spasm, a rare condition secondary to trigeminal neuropathy (24). Our review will also discuss results reported by others in a group of patients with bruxism (25).

MATERIALS AND METHODS

All patients gave their informed consent, and the study was approved by the local ethical committee.

Patients with Hemifacial Spasm

A group of 57 patients (mean age 60.3 years, range 26–82) with HFS were treated in the Movement Disorder Center of Rome. In nine of these the spasm was secondary to a facial nerve palsy, and in the others it was considered cryptogenic. All the patients showed involuntary twitches of the orbicularis oculi muscle and of the lower facial muscles. The degree of the muscle spasm in the orbicularis oculi muscle was evaluated with Marsden and Schachter's rating scale (26) for involuntary movements, a clinical scale that assigns patients a score ranging from 0 to 8 according to their disability. The intensity of lower facial spasms was graded in three levels (absent, mild, severe). Each patient was seen before treatment, 3 to 4 weeks after treatment, and again 3 to 5 months afterward, always by the same physician. The following parameters were assessed in each patient: (1) basal disability score; (2) mean score obtained after treatment (i.e., the mean of the scores after each injection); (3) best score obtained after treatment (this value was obtained by taking

Table 1 Reports on Treatment with Botulinum Toxin in Patients with Hemifacial Spasm

Authors	Year	No. of patients
Frueh	1984	3
Tsoy	1985	5
Schorr	1985	5
Mauriello	1985	11
Savino	1985	15
Elston	1986	6
Brin	1987	4
Geller	1989	3
Jankovic	1990	18
Elston	1990	73
Berardelli	1990	12
Berardelli	1993	63

into account the best scores among the different injections performed); (4) time to onset of benefit as reported by the patients; and (5) mean duration of benefit.

Injections were repeated several times, and for some patients this treatment started in 1985. The effect of repeated BTX injections on the duration of benefit was studied in 37 of the 51 patients. These patients received four or more injections during the study period. Statistical significance was determined by the paired t-test and analysis of variance. Probability values less than 0.005 were considered significant. All results are reported as mean $\pm$ standard deviation.

Patients with Masticatory Spasms

Case 1

A 50-year-old woman had begun to experience, at the age of 44 years, involuntary twitches of the right temporalis and masseter muscles. The spasms occurred many times a day, spontaneously or triggered by chewing and speaking or other voluntary movements of the mouth and jaw. This patient also had localized scleroderma of the face.

Case 2

A 26-year-old man with torticollis and oromandibular dystonia had severe bilateral masseter muscle contractions. These caused an impairment of masticatory function and difficulty in opening the mouth.

In both patients the intensity of masticatory muscle spasms was graded in three levels (absent, mild, severe).

Botulinum Toxin Injections

The content of each vial of botulinum type A toxin (Oculinum, Allergan, 100 U) was diluted in 2 ml of saline solution (1 ml = 50 U). In patients with HFS the usual total dose was 0.2 to 0.4 ml (10–20 U). This was divided for injection at 3–4 sites into the orbicularis oculi muscle. Some patients received a total of 30–40 U. In patients with involuntary twitches of the lower facial muscles, 0.05–0.2 ml (2.5–10 U) of BTX were usually injected into the orbicularis oris or buccinator muscle or both. Some patients also had injections into the mentalis, levator anguli oris, and platysma muscles. In the platysma muscle the dose was usually higher. In the patient affected by oromandibular dystonia and hemimasticatory spasm, the toxin (50 U) was injected into the affected masseter muscle.

RESULTS

Hemifacial Spasm

In the 57 patients with HFS the mean disability score before treatment was 6.4 ± 1.2. After BTX treatment, the mean score was 1.5 ± 1.6 (77% of benefit) and the best score obtained was 0.6 ± 1.3, with a percentage of improvement reaching 91%. The mean onset of benefit was 4.8 ± 3.7 days. The mean duration of clinical improvement was 12 ± 5 weeks. Botulinum toxin treatment resulted in a similar degree of improvement in patients with cryptogenic and symptomatic HSF. The only difference between the two groups was that in the symptomatic patients clinical benefit was reached with a dosage of 10–15 U of toxin, whereas cryptogenic patients required 15–20 U to achieve the same clinical benefit.

Before treatment, the spasms in the lower facial muscles were of moderate to severe intensity. After treatment, all the patients reported a reduction in the frequency and intensity of the spasm; in some cases the improvement was mild, whereas in others the muscle spasms were totally abolished. The duration of the benefit varied from 8 to 15 weeks.

The effect of repeated injections in the orbicularis oculi muscle on the duration of the benefit was studied in 37 of 52 patients with HFS. Only five of these appeared to derive longer-lasting benefit.

Transient side effects occurred in 18 of the 57 patients with HFS (31%) and consisted of mild ptosis, diplopia, and weakness of the lower facial muscles, usually without significant functional impairment.

Masticatory Spasms

In the two patients with masticatory spasms, the injection of toxin markedly reduced the frequency and intensity of the spasm, with a good functional improvement. The benefit lasted for 12 weeks in the first patient and 13 weeks in the other. The two patients with masticatory spasm had no side effects.

DISCUSSION

The results obtained in our 57 patients show that BTX therapy is useful in relieving muscle twitches in patients with hemifacial spasm.

Mauriello (14) and Savino et al. (15) reported the effects of BTX therapy in 11 and 15 patients with hemifacial spasm, respectively. In Mauriello's patients the mean duration of benefit was 12 weeks (14). Elston in 1986 observed similar findings in six patients with HFS (16). Two of these also had injections in the lower facial muscles. Although treatment reduced the spasm, it also caused a mild, transient facial muscle weakness. Brin et al. (17) reported the effects of BTX injections in the orbicularis oculi and buccinator muscles in four patients with HFS. All of them had substantial relief of the spasms, which lasted from 10 to 12 weeks. Repeated injections provided a similar degree of benefit.

Geller et al. (18) also reported an improvement in three patients with HFS, and the benefit had a mean duration of 12 weeks. Jankovic et al. (19) reported a reduction (92%) in spasm and in facial twitching in 13 patients with hemifacial spasm. Elston (20) reviewed the results obtained in a series of 73 patients with hemifacial spasm studied in two centers in London. In 75% of the patients the abnormal movements were reduced; the improvement lasted for an average of 15 weeks.

In our series of patients with HFS, the mean and the maximum percentages of improvement were 77% and 91%, respectively, and the mean duration of clinical benefit was 12 weeks. Botulinum toxin treatment produced similar benefit in patients with symptomatic and cryptogenic hemifacial spasm. The degree and duration of benefit achieved were similar to findings reported by other authors.

A comparison between the effect of BTX in patients with HFS and in those with blepharospasm (see section on dystonia) shows a similar degree of benefit. Jankovic et al. (19) noted that patients with HFS have longer-lasting improvement than those with focal dystonia and proposed that the longer duration of improvement may be due to the subclinical denervation present in patients with HFS.

In our patients with HFS, the side effects were minor and consisted of transient ptosis and weakness in the lower facial muscles. These complications were also seen in the other two large series of patients studied (19,20). In comparison with patients with blepharospasm studied in our Movement Disorders Center (22), we noted that patients with HFS more frequently had weakness in the lower facial muscles. Patients with HFS are probably more susceptible to local weakness because of subclinical denervation of facial muscles.

The finding that in patients with HFS the effect of BTX is due to the weakness of the muscle is supported by the observation that the spasm is diminished only when the muscles are weak. Geller et al. (18) have studied the electrophysiological features of patients with HFS after treatment with BTX. They observed that transmission of excitation from the zygomatic branch to the mandibular branch of the facial nerve and vice versa was unaltered and that spontaneous generation of activity was still present even when BTX injection had clinically improved the spasm. Muscle responses were decreased in amplitude, the decrease reflecting the reduced number of activated muscle fibers. The authors concluded that the effect of BTX is related to the production of muscle weakness.

Finally, we will now comment on the use of BTX in patients with spasms in the masticatory muscles and patients with bruxism. Bilateral masticatory spasm is a common finding in patients with oromandibular dystonia, and BTX injection produces a clinical benefit, as shown by the case here reported (also see chapter 27). Isolated unilateral contraction of the masticatory muscles is an uncommon type of involuntary movement. In this condition the spasms are painful, and drug therapy gives no relief. In the first patient we treated for this condition, BTX injection was very effective and substantially reduced the frequency and intensity of the spasms. Bruxism is an involuntary rhythmic chewing-like jaw movements with grinding of the teeth, occurring at night. Although the etiology is usually psychological, drug treatments and organic lesions may be responsible (27–30). Bruxism can be relieved by intraoral occlusal splints, which suppress the tooth grinding (29). However, some preliminary results have shown that patients with bruxism have a reduction in the involuntary movements after injection of BTX in the masseter and temporalis muscles (25).

In conclusion, BTX injection is an efficacious and safe treatment for patients with HFS and for patients with masticatory muscle spasms. The usefulness of BTX in patients with bruxism still needs to be determined.

ACKNOWLEDGMENT

The authors are indebted to Diana Brusoni for typing the manuscript.

REFERENCES

1. Carter JB, Patrinely JR, Jankovic J, McCrary JA, Boniuk M. Familial hemifacial spasm. Arch Ophthalmol 1990; 108:249–250.
2. Wilson SAK. In: Bruce AN, ed. Neurology. 2nd ed. Vol.3. London: Butterworth and Co., 1955, 1937.
3. Nielsen VK. Pathophysiology of hemifacial spasm. I. Ephaptic transmission and ectopic excitation. Neurology 1984; 34:418–426.
4. Nielsen VK. Electrophysiology of the facial nerve in hemifacial spasm: ectopic/ephaptic excitation. Muscle Nerve 1985;8:545–555.
5. Ferguson JH. Hemifacial spasm and the facial nucleus. Ann Neurol 1978;4:97–103.
6. Alexander GE, Moses H. Carbamazepine for hemifacial spasm. Neurology 1982;32:286–287.
7. Herzberg L. Management of hemifacial spasm with clonazepam. Neurology 1985;35:1676–1677.
8. Nielsen VK, Jannetta PJ. Pathophysiology of hemifacial spasm. III. Effects of facial nerve decompression. Neurology 1984;34:891–897.
9. Jannetta PJ, Abbassy M, Maroon JC, et al. Etiology and definitive microsurgical treatment of hemifacial spasm: operative techniques and results in 47 patients. J Neurosurg 1987;47:321–328.
10. Scott AB. Botulinum toxin injection of eye muscles to correct strabismus. Trans Am Ophthalmol Soc 1981;79:734–770.
11. Frueh BR, Felt DP, Wojno TH, Musch DC. Treatment of blepharospasm with botulinum toxin. Arch Ophthalmol 1984;102:1464–1468.
12. Tsoy EA, Buckley EG, Dutton JJ. Treatment of blepharospasm with botulinum toxicity. Am J Ophthalmol 1985;99:176–179.
13. Schorr N, Seiff S, Kopelman J. The use of botulinum toxin in blepharospasm. Am J Ophthalmol 1985;99:542–546.
14. Mauriello JA. Blepharospasm, Meige's syndrome, and hemifacial spasm: Treatment with botulinum toxin. Neurology 1985;35:1499–1450.
15. Savino P, Sergott R, Bosley T, Schatz N. Hemifacial spasm treated with botulinum A toxin injection. Arch Ophthalmol 1985;103:1305–1306.
16. Elston JS. Botulinum toxin treatment of hemifacial spasm. J Neurol Neurosurg Psychiatry 1986;49:827–829.
17. Brin MF, Fahn S, Moskowitz C, et al. Localized injections of botulinum toxin for the treatment of focal dystonia and hemifacial spasm. Mov Disord 1987;2:237–254.
18. Geller BD, Hallett M, Ravits J. Botulinum toxin therapy in hemifacial spasm: clinical and electrophysiological studies. Muscle Nerve 1989;12:716–722.
19. Jankovic J, Schwartz K, Donovan DT. Botulinum toxin treatment of cranial-cervical dystonia, spasmodic dysphonia, other focal dystonias and hemifacial spasm. J Neurol Neurosurg Psychiatry 1990;53:633–639.
20. Elston JS. Botulinum toxin A in clinical medicine. J Physiol (Paris) 1990;84:285–289.
21. Berardelli A, Carta A, Stocchi F, Formica A, Agnoli A, Manfredi M. Botulinum toxin injection in patients with blepharospasm, torticollis and hemifacial spasm. Ital J Neurol Sci 1990;11:589–593.
22. Berardelli A, Formica A, Mercuir B, et al. Botulinum toxin treatment in patients with focal dystonia and hemifacial spasm. A multicenter study of the Italian Movement Disorder Study Group. Ital J Neurol Sci 1993;14:361–367.
23. Jankovic J, Brin MF. Therapeutic uses of botulinum toxin. N Engl J Med 1991;324:1186–1194.

24. Kaufman MD. Masticatory spasm in facial hemiatrophy. Ann Neurol 1980;7:585–587.
25. Wooten MP, Jankovic J. Bruxism in cranial cervical dystonia. Neurology, 1990;40(suppl 1): 142.
26. Marsden CD, Schachter M. Assessment of extrapyramidal disorders. Br J Clin Pharmacol 1981;11:129–151.
27. Glaros AG, Ros SM. Bruxism: a critical review. Psychol Bull 1977;34:767–778.
28. Magee KR. Bruxism related to levodopa therapy. JAMA 1970;214–247.
29. Pollack IA, Cwik V. Bruxism following cerebellar hemorrhage. Neurology 1989;39:1262.
30. Tison F, Louvet-Grendas C, Henry P, Lagueny A, Gaujard E. Permanent bruxism is a manifestation of the oculo-facial syndrome related to systemic Whipple's disease. Mov Disord 1992;7:82–85.

STRABISMUS

27

Clinical Use of Botulinum Toxin: Clinical Trials for Strabismus

Elbert H. Magoon
Canton Eye Center, Inc., Canton, Ohio

INDICATIONS AND CONTRAINDICATIONS

Botulinum toxin (BTX) treatment for strabismus is usually an alternative to traditional incisional strabismus surgery, but it has several unique uses when surgery is otherwise inappropriate. These include treatment during acute nerve palsy, acute Graves' disease with diplopia, and other situations where surgery is contraindicated. It can also be used preoperatively to enhance the power of surgery or postoperatively to improve a poor surgical result.

For nonparalytic horizontal strabismus, BTX is a very reasonable alternative to incisional surgery. It is very good at improving small angles of strabismus (under 20 prism diopters) and quite effective in improving moderate-size strabismus of 20 to 40 prism diopters. Large-angle strabismus of greater than 40 prism diopters can be treated but may require multiple injections,and results are usually less satisfactory than with traditional surgery. Relative contraindications include a complete long-standing paralysis or severe restrictive strabismus.

There are special situations where BTX therapy may be used in conjunction with strabismus surgery. This includes treatment after a poor surgical result in the immediate postoperative situation, which has been termed postoperative rescue. It is also possible to increase the power of a surgical result by the preoperative or intraoperative injection in association with surgery. This method is used, for example, in transposition surgery for nerve palsies, where it permits avoidance of operating on more than two rectus muscles and may prevent the complication of anterior segment ischemia.

Botulinum toxin can be used diagnostically, and the methods devised by Dr. A.B. Scott for its injection can also be used for diagnostic or therapeutic delivery of other drugs such as lidocaine (1) or bupivacaine (2).

Treatment of infants and children is a special indication. As will be seen below, our data suggest that they can be treated with BTX as effectively as adults and that injection may even offer some special advantages over incisional surgery.

METHODS

The technique involves placement of the BTX by injection directly into the extraocular muscle. Topical proparacaine drops alone provide adequate anesthesia without sedation. The toxin is injected into the appropriate muscle with a special needle on a tuberculin-type syringe. An electrode tip on the needle transmits the electromyographic response of the muscle to an amplifier. This amplifier provides audio feedback to the surgeon to assist in guiding needle placement. Insertion of the needle through the conjunctiva is painless. Advancement of the needle in the extraocular muscle and the injection of 0.1 ml BTX is only moderately uncomfortable. The procedure takes only a few minutes. This can be readily accomplished with most adults and is more frightening than painful. Some of the procedures described for older children in the next paragraph are occasionally used with apprehensive adults.

Most older children can tolerate the procedure with no sedation, but the patient's trust is required. The surgeon demonstrates to the child that the eye is numb from the drops, and carries out progressively more threatening maneuvers to demonstrate this to the child, touching the eye first with a cotton-tipped swab, then with a forceps, then with a small needle. Infants younger than 1 year of age can generally be restrained in an office setting and given the injection with no sedation, but this is not easy.

Children aged 1 to 6 years are usually given ketamine intravenously, 0.5 mg/kg body weight. This is much less than the usual anesthetic dose and provides a suitable hypnotic state, which may be augmented by a dark, quiet environment and hypnotic words from the surgeon or anesthesiologist. Other sedative and anesthetic agents decree the extraocular muscle's electromyographic response and are therefore unsuitable, but ketamine increases the electromyographic response and has been effective. Sedative management has been without complications in our patients.

RESULTS

Our work was done entirely under Dr. Scott's FDA protocol. Our individual results are less important than our participation in the pooled data from other investigators that helped form the basis of Dr. Scott's report to the FDA and of subsequent FDA approval. Figure 1 and Table 1 summarize those data (3).

Our data (4) on horizontal strabismus in adults treated by one surgeon are summarized in Table 2. Only patients with substantial follow-up of more than 1 year are included, and the results from this surgeon were comparable to the aggregate results of all the investigators as seen in Table 3.

Table 4 shows the chance of achieving correction of 10 prism diopters or less for the 55 esotropes and 75 exotropes in our study grouped by size of initial deviation. It shows a higher likelihood of satisfactory correction with one injection for smaller deviations. Nevertheless, Fig. 1 shows a greater total magnitude of correction for larger deviations.

In 1985 we reported 25 patients treated with 33 injections for vertical strabismus (5). Our subsequent experience supports the therapy as being effective if there is not substantial paralysis or restriction.

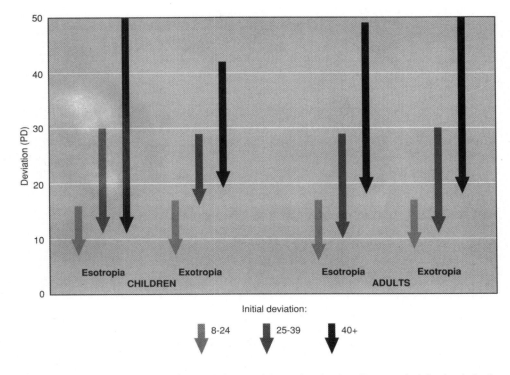

Figure 1 Initial and final deviation a minimum of 6 months after botulinum toxin injection in both children and adults.

Working with Dr. Scott, we showed that children and infants can achieve results comparable to those in adults (6). In one study with Dr. Scott, 82 children aged 13 years or younger were given injections of BTX for horizontal strabismus. Improvement was achieved in all but one patient. Reinjection was necessary in 85% of patients, but there were no systemic complications. Side effects included transient ptosis and hypertropia, but these typically resolved. One hundred thirty-eight injections were given: 92 in the hospital, 27 in the office without sedation (cooperative older children),and 19 to infants restrained in the office. The preinjection average deviation was 31.06 prism diopters. After injection, at last follow-up examination, 32 patients had straight eyes, 11 were undercorrected by 0 to 5 prism diopters, and 28 were undercorrected by more than 5 prism diopters. The postinjection deviation at the time of the most recent follow-up averaged 4.08 prism diopters. Of special interest is the treatment of infants. Babies under the age of 1 year are able to be treated with restraint and no sedation, using only topical anesthetic. During the postinjection paralysis, infants are almost always able to use the eyes together at least part of the time, as evidenced by head turn to place the eyes in the position of least deviation.

Babies can be treated earlier than is typical for incisional surgery. As the temporary overcorrection permits perfect alignment of the eyes with the head turn, it is conceivable that BTX therapy could have some advantage over traditional surgery. This observation has been important to the old argument over whether infantile strabismus is caused by sensory (or fusional) abnormalities or by a mechanical failure of eye alignment such as

Table 1 The Effect of Botulinum Toxin Injection on Strabismus in Adults[a]

	Number of patients	Average deviation			Final deviation ≤ 10 PD	
		Preinjection	Postinjection	% change	n	% of patients
Esotropia						
By number of injections						
1 injection	225	28 PD	9 PD	69	151	67
> 1 injection	159	32 PD	14 PD	58	68	43
All patients	384	30 PD	11 PD	65	219	57
By initial deviation						
0–10 PD	9	—	—	—	8	89
10–24 PD	132	17 PD	6 PD	62	95	72
25–39 PD	142	29 PD	10 PD	65	81	57
40+ PD	101	49 PD	18 PD	62	35	35
All patients	384	30 PD	11 PD	63	219	56
Exotropia						
By number of injections						
1 injection	139	28 PD	11 PD	61	83	60
> 1 injection	154	34 PD	13 PD	61	72	47
All patients	293	31 PD	12 PD	61	155	53
By initial deviation						
0–10 PD	6	—	—	—	6	100
10–24 PD	93	17 PD	8 PD	53	62	67
25–39 PD	112	30 PD	11 PD	64	60	54
40+ PD	82	50 PD	18 PD	64	27	33
All patients	293	32 PD	12 PD	60	155	52

[a]Results in 677 patients (aged 12–90 years) with follow-up of 6–83 months (average 17 months). Reduction rate of strabismus is broken down by number of injections and by initial deviation as measured in prism diopters (PD).

Table 2 Comparison of Average Results Grouped by Size of Initial Deviation

Group averaged (PD)	Number of patients	Average pretreatment deviation (PD)	Average posttreatment deviation (PD)	Average percent correction
0–24 ESO	20	16.9	7.75	48.75
25–39	17	29.18	8.5	68.88
≥ 40 ESO	18	47.5	24.1	48.67
0–24 EXO	16	17.9	8.56	42.88
25–39 EXO	25	30.12	11.0	63.16
≥ 40 EXO	34	53.53	19.29	63.35

PD = prism diopters; ESO = esotropia; EXO = exotropia.

Table 3 Comparison of Scott Grouped Data with Present Study

	Esotropia	Exotropia
Number of patients	384/55	293/75
Deviation before	30/31	31/38
Deviation after	11/13	12/14
Follow-up (months)	17/32	17/34

374

Table 4 Chance of Achieving Correction of 10 Prism Diopters or Less

	N	(%)
0–24 PD ESO	15/20	(75)
25–39 PD ESO	11/17	(65)
≥ 40 PD ESO	5/18	(28)
0–24 PD EXO	10/16	(63)
25–39 PD EXO	11/25	(44)
≥ PD EXO	14/34	(41)

tight medial rectus muscles. It supports the latter view, suggesting infantile esotropes do start with the normal potential for fusion but that it is lost because the eyes are not aligned during early critical periods of development.

We have studied the sensory and motor differences between BTX-treated esotropes and surgically treated esotropes with inconclusive results.

Another study, considering the stability of alignment change, compared the follow-up results of 85 children treated in the early 1980s (7). There was a shorter follow-up range of 6 to 24 months as of the last examination in 1984 versus a longer follow-up range of 2 to 5½ years as of the last examination before March of 1988. Fifty esotropes meeting the 2-year criteria for follow-up had an average deviation of 35 prism diopters before and 5 prism diopters after treatment. Twelve exotropes averaged 30 prism diopters before and 5 prism diopters after treatment (Table 5). No long-term complications were discovered. The results are similar to those of the shorter follow-up and suggest BTX is effective in creating a 2- to 5-year stable improvement for strabismic children.

DIRECTIONS FOR FUTURE RESEARCH

Highest priority for research should be given to *optimal* treatment of infantile strabismus with BTX surgery or both. Appropriate dosage schedule, timing of injection, timing of initial intervention, and long-term results should be studied. I see no question of the safety

Table 5 Comparison of Short- and Longer-Term Follow-up Results

Follow-up	N	Average phoria[a] (PD) Before	After	% residual[b]	% correction[c]
Esotropes					
6 mo–2 yr	55	31.95	4.98	0.156	0.844
2–5.5 yr	50	35.09	5.2	0.148	0.852
Exotropes					
6 mo–2 yr	15	33.0	6.8	0.206	0.794
2–5.5 yr	12	30.42	5.17	0.170	0.830

[a]All numbers calculated as plus, i.e., overcorrections make after-measurements higher (worse) even though they represent more effect.
[b][Average deviation after] ÷ [average deviation before] = % residual misalignment.
[c]100 − % residual = % correction.
PD = prism diopters.

and effectiveness for injections of children. The FDA's decision to approve BTX for use in patients over 12 years of age should, I believe, be rectified to include all ages, and no more research is necessary to that end.

Comparisons between BTX treatment and strabismus surgery would be of some interest. There have been no controlled studies. I am not certain they are very important, because we do know the characteristics of each approach. I would have some trouble trying to persuade patients to accept a random draw of one or the other, because the two approaches are so different and we know so much about each.

Dr. Scott has begun work with antitoxin to BTX. This may prove very helpful. Other toxins may have characteristics complementary to BTX, and work with them should be pursued.

A very high priority is research on ways to educate physicians to use the toxin. I would argue that every patient should be given the option of having BTX instead of incisional strabismus surgery. Clearly this has not been widely done. A great majority of patients with acute sixth nerve palsy should have treatment with BTX, and this is not being done. Indeed, education of practitioners in the use of this new technology is so important that its dissemination may be our most important research priority at this time.

REFERENCES

1. Magoon EH, Cruciger MP, Scott AB, and Jampolsky A. Diagnostic injection of Xylocaine into extraocular muscles. Ophthalmology 1982;89:489–491.
2. Magoon EH, Erzurum S. Eye alignment change from bupivacaine injection of eye muscles. Invest Ophthalmol Vis Sci 1986;27(suppl):1.
3. Scott AB. Botulinum toxin treatment of strabismus. Focal Points; Vol. VII, Module 12; 1989.
4. Magoon EH, Kalra H. Long term efficacy of botulinum treatment for adult horizontal strabismus. Presented at the American Academy of Ophthalmology Annual Meeting, November 1990.
5. Magoon EH, Dakoske C. Botulinum toxin injection for vertical strabismus. Am Orthoptic J 1985;35:48–52.
6. Magoon EH, Scott AB. Botulinum toxin chemodenervation in infants and children, an alternative to incisional strabismus surgery. J Pediatr 1987;110:719–722.
7. Magoon EH. Chemodenervation of strabismic children: a 2 to 5 year follow-up study compared with shorter follow-up. Ophthalmology 1989;96:931–934.

28

Strabismus: Other Therapies

Oscar A. Cruz
Cardinal Glennon Children's Hospital, St. Louis University School of Medicine, St. Louis, Missouri

John T. Flynn
University of Miami School of Medicine, Miami, Florida

INTRODUCTION

Strabismus is a group of disorders affecting ocular motility, of undetermined etiology, that result in a misalignment of the visual axes. Strabismus primarily affects infants and children up to adolescence. Manifest strabismus (-tropia) occurs in nearly 2% of American children aged 1 to 3 years and nearly 5% of school-age children and adolescents 12 to 17 years old. Latent strabismus (-phoria) is relatively common, and occurs in over 3% of toddlers and in approximately 16% of American school-age children and adolescents (1). Strabismus can be acquired by adults as a result of trauma, neurological disease, endocrinopathy, or cardiovascular disease, or as a latent deviation from childhood that has become manifest.

The signs and symptoms of strabismus are dependent on when the strabismus has presented itself. The most obvious sign if a deviation of the visual axis of one or the other eye. In children, there is usually a conspicuous lack of symptoms. Suppression of vision in the deviated eye can be alternating (in which case visual function is preserved in each eye) or monolateral (in which case the development of amblyopia in the habitually deviated eye will occur). In adults, the symptoms of strabismus are quite distressing to the patient.These patients often have diplopia (two images of a single object) or visual confusion (two objects located in the same place in space).

Simple inspection of a patient is not always sufficient for diagnosis of a manifest ocular deviation. The "cover test" (alternate cover) is used for detection. In patients without strabismus each eye is aligned with the fixation object. Therefore, covering either eye will not elicit a fixation movement of the fellow eye. In strabismus patients one eye is not aligned with the fixation object; therefore, if the fixating eye is covered, the deviating eye takes up fixation and a rapid fixation movement results. When the deviating eye is covered, there is no movement of the fixating eye, since this eye is already aligned with the fixation object. Consequently, each eye must be covered while one is observing the fellow eye to determine whether a deviation is present (2).

The quantitative measure of strabismus is the prism diopter. The prism diopter is the unit of measurement of an ophthalmic prism. A prism is defined as having the power of 1 prism diopter when it displaces the visual axis by 1 cm at a distance of 1 m. Since prisms or their equivalents are used to measure the relative position of the eyes, the term "prism diopter" has acquired a broader meaning and is used clinically to specify ocular deviations. In the prism cover test the cover is placed alternately over each eye several times to dissociate the eyes and to bring out the maximal deviation (alternate cover test). The just-uncovered eye makes a movement of redress opposite the direction of the deviation. This movement of redress is compensated for by using prisms of increasing power until the movement stops. The prism power is equivalent to the amount of the deviation. This test must be carried out fixating with each eye at 33 cm (near deviation) and at 6 m (distance deviation). This is a quick test for the measurement of heterotropia and heterophoria. No subjective factors other than attention and cooperation are required, and patient participation is minimal (2). For infants and uncooperative patients, the Hirschberg test or the prism reflex test of Krimsky is more useful. In the Hirschberg test, the deviation of the corneal light reflex (from a penlight or hand-held light) from the center of the pupil is estimated. Each 1 mm of decentration of the corneal reflection corresponds to 7° (approximately 15 prism diopters) of ocular deviation. In the prism reflex test of Krimsky, prisms of increasing power are placed before the *fixating* eye until the light reflex is centered in the deviating eye. The prism with sufficient power to achieve centration of the light reflex indicates the magnitude of the deviation. The examiner must sit directly in front of the deviating eye to avoid false readings (2).

A deviation of the visual axis is the most common sign in all neuromuscular anomalies of the eyes, except for supranuclear disorders.

Heterotropia is a manifest deviation (present at all times) of the visual axis that is not kept under control by the fusion mechanism. A "phoria" is a latent deviation that is controlled by the fusion mechanism so that under normal binocular conditions the eyes remained aligned.

In an esodeviation (convergent) or inward deviation of the cornea, the eye is rotated nasalward (Fig. 1). An exodeviation (divergent) is an outward deviation (Fig. 2). Hyperphoria or hypertropia occurs if one visual line is higher than the other and is usually defined by the elevated eye (Fig. 3). The terms "hypophoria" and "hypotropia" are also occasionally used to indicate which eye is fixating. For instance, in right hypertropia the (lower) left eye is the one fixating, whereas in right hypotropia the (higher) left eye is fixating.

Strabismus can also be classified according to variation of the deviation with gaze position. In comitant strabismus, the deviation does not vary with direction of gaze or fixating eye (the deviation is the same in all fields of gaze). In incomitant strabismus, the deviation does vary with different directions of gaze. Incomitance is usually caused by paralytic (innervational) strabismus or by restrictive (mechanical) strabismus.

Many therapies are used in the treatment of strabismus. The treatment chosen usually depends on the underlying mechanism responsible for the strabismus. The armamentarium includes spectacles, occlusion therapy (patching), prisms, miotic drops, orthoptic exercises, and finally eye muscle surgery. A brief discussion of each of these therapies and their role follows.

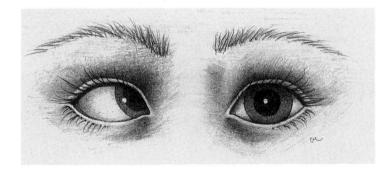

Figure 1 Right esotropia.

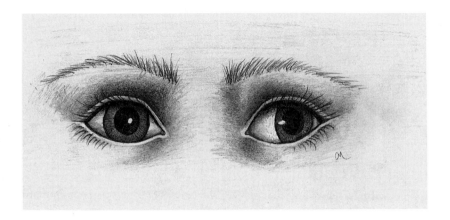

Figure 2 Left exotropia.

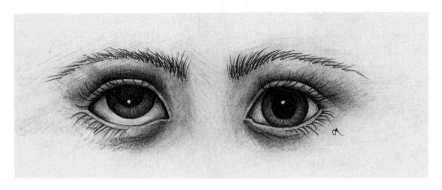

Figure 3 Right hypertropia with left eye fixation.

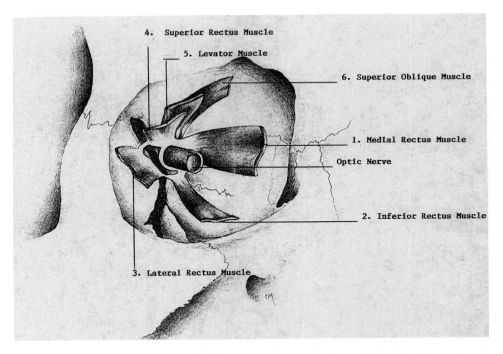

Figure 4   The annulus of Zinn within the right orbit. The inferior oblique muscle is not shown.

ANATOMY

A brief description of the anatomy and function for the extraocular muscles is important for the understanding of strabismus.

   There are three pairs of extraocular muscles in each orbit: a pair of horizontal rectus muscles, a pair of vertical rectus muscles, and a pair of oblique muscles. The origins of the four rectus muscles, the superior oblique muscle, and the levator muscle (principal elevator of the upper lid) are at the tip of the orbital pyramids arranged in a more or less circular formation, the annulus of Zinn (Fig. 4). The inferior oblique muscle originates from the periosteum of the maxillary bone. The rectus muscles attach themselves with broad, thin tendons to the sclera at varying distances from the corneal limbus in a spiral (spiral of Tillaux). The medial, superior, and inferior rectus muscles and the inferior oblique muscle are all innervated by the oculomotor nerve. The lateral rectus muscle is innervated by the abducens nerve. The superior oblique muscle differs from the other five extraocular muscle in that the trochlear nerve (its innervation) enters the muscle from the outer (orbital) surface rather that the bulbar surface (within the cone formed by the muscles).

EXTRAOCULAR MUSCLE PHYSIOLOGY AND KINETICS

The primary position of the eye is defined as that in which the eye is directed straight ahead with the head also being straight. The primary action of a muscle is considered the major effect on the position of the eye when the muscle contracts while the eye is in the primary position. The secondary and tertiary actions of a muscle are the additional effects on the position of the eye in the primary position. The globe usually can be moved about 50° in each direction from the primary position. However, under normal viewing circumstances, the eyes move only about 15–20° from the primary position before head movement occurs.

The rotations of the single eye are termed duction movements. Rotations around the vertical axis (horizontal excursions of the globe) are called adduction (movement nasalward) and abduction (movement templeward). Rotations around the horizontal axis (vertical excursions of the globe) are termed elevation or sursumduction and depression or deorsumduction. These four movements are the cardinal movements of the eye. A combination of the horizontal and vertical excursions moves the globe into various oblique positions in the directions up and right, up and left, down and right, and down and left.

Rotations around the anteroposterior axis of the glove, known as cycloductions, rotate the upper pole of the cornea templeward (excycloduction) or nasalward (incycloduction).

The horizontal rectus muscles are the medial rectus and the lateral rectus muscles. They have only horizontal actions, with the medial rectus being an adductor and the lateral rectus being an abductor.

The vertical rectus muscles are the superior rectus and inferior rectus muscles. The superior rectus muscle's primary action is elevation; secondary actions are adduction and incycloduction. The inferior rectus muscle's primary action is depression; secondary actions are adduction and excycloduction. The superior oblique muscle's primary action is incycloduction; secondary actions are depression and abduction. The inferior oblique muscle's primary action is excycloduction; secondary actions are elevation and abduction.

One must keep in mind that the vertical rectus muscles are the main movers from vertical gaze in all gaze position. In adduction (of 51°) the oblique muscles are nearly pure vertical rotators. Use of this fact is important in testing the ductions of the oblique muscles.

THERAPIES

Spectacles

Uncorrected hypermetropia (farsightedness) produces a blurred retinal image. Increased accommodative effort to produce and/or maintain a clear image on the retina may result in an esodeviation.

Accommodation is closely linked with the convergence mechanism. Increased central demands of accommodation will call for an increase of convergence innervation (accommodative convergence). Thus, uncorrected hypermetropia may lead to esophoria or esotropia unless the increase of accommodative convergence is offset by the fusion mechanism. Such esodeviation is eliminated by the prescription of hyperopic correction if the strabismus is purely refractional in nature (2). If glasses are worn but do not reduce the deviation to 10 prism diopters or less (which would permit the reestablishment of sensory binocular vision), surgical correction of the residual deviation is needed.

Miotic Therapy

The therapeutic effect of miotics is based on the facilitation of accommodation. In the treatment of accommodative esotropia, miotics reduce the accommodative effort, and less accommodative convergence occurs. Miotics are often helpful in differentiating between nonaccommodative esotropia and accommodative esotropia in estotropic infants. Failure to respond to miotics is a consistent feature of nonaccommodative esotropia.

Treatment with miotics is not without untoward side effects. Of major importance is the lowering of cholinesterase in the red blood cells, which causes a potential risk when a general anesthetic is given. Since cholinesterase is required for hydrolysis of succinylcholine, these patients may develop prolonged respiratory paralysis (4). The development of iris cysts occurs in some children using miotics, but these usually regress spontaneously after therapy is discontinued (5).

Occlusion for Amblyopia

Strabismic amblyopia is characterized by a unilateral reduction of central visual acuity in a strabismic patient resulting from long-continued fixation by the dominant eye coupled with suppression of the images in the deviated eye.

Clinical observation of strabismic infants suggests a prevalence of amblyopia of 40% at the time the strabismus is documented by a visit to an ophthalmologist (6). Children are most sensitive to amblyopia during the first 2 to 3 years of life. There is a limited period of susceptibility (sensitive period) for the development of amblyopia. Clinicians are well aware that amblyopia rarely develops after 6 to 8 years of age (7). Recent animal studies suggest that there may be multiple sensitive periods for different parts of the visual system and different visual functions (8). Psychophysical studies in humans with a history of strabismus imply that binocular vision is highly vulnerable during the first 18 months of life, and remains susceptible until at least age 7 years (9).

Amblyopia therapy takes priority over strabismus surgery; such surgery should probably be delayed until amblyopia has been treated and maximum central visual acuity obtained.

The first line of amblyopia therapy is occlusion of the sound eye. Occlusion forces the patient to use the amblyopic eye, and opaque occlusion ensures total reliance on the amblyopic eye.

Preferential looking and visual evoked potential studies have shown that the optotype or grating acuity difference between eyes of strabismic infants and young children can be manipulated rapidly and dramatically with occlusion therapy (10).

Occlusion of the sound eye may be instituted at any age, but the final level of visual acuity obtainable is often dependent on the age at which treatment is begun.

Table 1 Action of the Extraocular Muscles from the Primary Position

Muscle[a]	Primary	Secondary	Tertiary
Medial rectus	Adduction	—	—
Lateral rectus	Abduction	—	—
Inferior rectus	Depression	Excycloduction	Adduction
Superior rectus	Elevation	Incycloduction	Adduction
Inferior oblique	Excycloduction	Elevation	Abduction
Superior oblique	Incycloduction	Depression	Abduction

[a]The superior muscles are incycloductors; the inferior muscles are excycloductors. The vertical rectus muscles are adductors; the oblique muscles are abductors.
Source: Ref. 3.

Full-time occlusion is best instituted in early infancy. The younger the patient is, the more rapid the improvement in visual acuity will be and the better the ultimate prognosis. If acuity is improving, treatment should be continued until a plateau is reached and maintained for about 3 to 6 months (11,12).

Prisms

The many disadvantages of glass prisms limit their role in the treatment of strabismus. When a glass prism of high power is needed, excessive weight, disturbing reflections, aberrations, and cosmetically unacceptable appearance become a problem. Necessary changes of corrections are associated with excessive costs. Most of these problems were obviated by membrane fresnel prisms. These prisms, which are simply pasted to the back surface of spectacle lenses, are readily exchangeable and light, produce relatively less aberration, and are available in powers up to 30 prism diopters.

Prisms are used primarily in the treatment of nystagmus, comitant vertical hypertropia, paralytic strabismus, and convergence insufficiency. They are most effective in treating comitant restrictive strabismus. In thyroid ophthalmopathy, many patients with small deviations (albeit rarely comitant) are free of diplopia and avoid surgery.

In the treatment of nystagmus, prisms are used for two purposes: to improve visual acuity and to eliminate an anomalous head posture. Prisms base-out are prescribed to decrease the amplitude of nystagmus by stimulating fusional convergence (13). In the long-term treatment of an anomalous head posture, surgery is a more effective and practical approach.

Prisms are usually better tolerated when distributed between the two eyes and the prescription should be based on the minimal prismatic power that provides comfortable single binocular vision.

Orthoptic Therapy

Orthoptic therapy may aid patients who have symptomatic heterophorias. Orthoptic techniques and exercises can effect a significant response in enlarging fusional complitudes and improving alignment control and symptoms in patients with exophorias. Convergence insufficiency (exophoria greatest at near) is best treated in this manner. Patients with convergence insufficiency often suffer symptoms of ocular fatigue, discomfort, and headaches (asthenopia) when performing sustained near work. Orthoptic therapy is also employed to make patients aware of physiological diplopia in circumstances where elimination of suppression is the goal (3).

Surgery

Surgery is the mainstay in the treatment of strabismus. Although this is not intended as an instructional text on strabismus surgery, the basic tenets and techniques of surgery will be addressed.

Principles of Surgical Treatment of Strabismus

The primary goal is to eliminate the deviation of the visual axes. Surgery is performed for both cosmetic and functional reasons (i.e., to restore single binocular vision). If some degree of fusion can be achieved, this helps to maintain ocular alignment. Alignment of the visual axis can restore stereopsis in some patients. Elimination of diplopia is often a surgical goal in patients with adult-onset strabismus. Elimination of an abnormal head position is an indication for surgery, especially in patients with paralytic strabismus.

Surgery cannot directly affect the innervation reaching the eyes. The effect of surgery is mechanical, since the position of the globe in the orbit is changed.

Weakening the action of a muscle surgically (recession) is more effective in reducing deviation than is strengthening its action (resection).

The most common procedure to weaken the action of a muscle is a recession. In a recession, the muscle is disinserted from its position on the globe and then secured by sutures to a predetermined location on the sclera more posterior than its original insertion. The effect of a recession is due to a complex interaction of factors. The loss of rotational force (torque), the loss of contractile force caused by muscle length reduction, and the surgery itself, which removes (cuts) many supporting structures, all contribute to the effect of a recession. A rectus recession always has its greatest effect in the field of action of the muscle.

To strengthen or enhance the effect of a muscle or tendon, the resection technique is the most common method used. Resections increase the action of a muscle, as reflected in a length-tension curve, but tightening the muscle also produces a leash effect. This leash can cause a restriction of ocular rotation in the direction away from the muscle, causing large resections to have the greatest effect in the opposite field of gaze. Absorbable sutures are placed at a predetermined distance posterior to the muscle insertion, the muscle is removed from the globe, the muscle anterior to the position of the sutures is excised (resected), and the muscle is reattached to the globe at or near the original insertion. This technique is commonly used on any of the rectus muscles. It is rarely used to strengthen either of the oblique muscles. In terms of prism diopters of correction per millimeter of change, a resection is less effective than a recession.

A muscle's function can also be augmented by advancing the insertion nearer the limbus. The technique is commonly used for rectus muscles if the muscle has been previously recessed. Advancing a muscle anterior to its original anatomical insertion is rarely done, because the muscle will become visible under the conjunctiva. A tuck of the superior oblique tendon can improve its function and is often employed to enhance its effect. This procedure is usually limited to the superior oblique muscle (14).

There are a number of other procedures used to weaken the effect of a muscle or tendon. They usually have either specific indications or are specific to a certain muscle. A disinsertion is a severing of a muscle or tendon from the globe at its insertion. It is used by some surgeons as the standard weakening procedure for the inferior oblique muscle. This technique is rarely performed on rectus muscles. Cutting across a muscle (myotomy) or excising a portion of its tendon (myectomy) is used by some surgeons to weaken the inferior oblique muscle. This technique is not used for rectus muscles. An incision partially through a muscle margin (marginal myotomy) is sometimes used to weaken a muscle. A marginal myotomy entails actually weakening the muscle by reducing the number of contractle elements without changing its arc of contact to globe. This procedure is highly effective in further reducing the action of an already maximally recessed rectus muscle or when the muscle cannot be recessed because of other anatomical factors (extremely thin sclera, prior retinal detachment surgery, etc.). Cutting across the tendon (tenotomy) or removing a portion of the tendon (tenectomy) is the most commonly used procedure to weaken the superior oblique muscle. Denervation and extirpation is an inferior oblique muscle weakening procedure reserved for severe overaction or when reoperation is required after overaction recurs. Posterior fixation suture is a weakening procedure for the rectus muscle that weakens the muscle selectively in its field of action by decreasing the mechanical advantage of the muscle acting on the globe. This is accomplished by suturing the muscle to the sclera behind the equator and thus creating a new functional insertion, posterior to the anatomical insertion. One of the most common indications for posterior fixation suture is the treatment of incomitant strabismus in patients who are orthotropic in primary position but have diplopia in peripheral positions of gaze (15).

One technique that has had renewed interest is the use of adjustable sutures (16). The most important indication for an adjustable suture technique is complicated strabismus, including paralytic strabismus, large-angle strabismus, reoperations and thyroid myopathy. In this surgery, the effect of surgery can be augmented or decreased during the immediate postoperative period by pulling on or loosening the sutures, which are then permanently tied under topical anesthesia. The adjustment phase is performed when the patient is fully awake after the local anesthesias has worn off and when muscle function has returned to normal. While some strabismus surgeons do not find the immediate postoperative position of the globe to help in assessing the final result, we believe that adjustable sutures surgery is of great value in reoperations and restrictive strabismus and should be offered as an option to cooperative, willing adults. The possibility of correcting a large overcorrection or undercorrection of the first postoperative day is reassuring to the surgeon and the patient.

Anesthesia

The globe and adnexa can be completely anesthetized locally; therefore, every adult should be informed of this possibility and given the option of local or general anesthesia. Children and patients undergoing multiple reoperations or surgery on the muscles of both eyes should have general anesthesia, with infrequent exceptions.

Complications arising from either local retrobulbar anesthesia or general anesthesia during muscle surgery are extremely rare. Malignant hyperthermia, a rare life-threatening complication of general anesthesia, does occur more commonly in children with neuromuscular anomalies, including strabismus. A common complication is due to the oculocardiac reflex. Bradycardia caused by vagal stimulation results from pulling on a muscle, especially the medial rectus muscle. This reaction is transient, and normal cardiac rhythm is usually restored after the pull on a muscle is relaxed. Patients in whom this reflex is marked or prolonged become poor candidates for adjustable suture surgery (17).

REFERENCES

1. American Academy of Ophthalmology. Comprehensive pediatric eye evaluation, preferred practice pattern. San Francisco: American Academy of Ophthalmology, 1992.
2. Von Noorden GK. Quantitative diagnosis of strabismus. In: Atlas of strabismus. 4th ed. St. Louis, C.V. Mosby, 1983.
3. Von Noorden GK. Theory and management of strabismus. In: Binocular vision and ocular motility. 4th ed. St. Louis, C.V. Mosby, 1990.
4. Ellis PP, Esterdahl, M. Echothiophate iodide therapy in children: effect on blood cholinesterase levels. Arch Ophthalmol 1967;77:598.
5. Abraham SV. The use of echothiophate-phenyl-ephrine formulation (echophenyloine-B3) in the treatment of convergent strabismus and amblyopia special emphasis on iris cysts. J Pediatr Ophthalmol 1964;1:68.

6.   Costenbader FD. Infantile esotropia. Trans Am Ophthalmol Soc 1961;59:397.
7.   Von Noorden GK. New clinical aspects of stimulus deprivation amblyopia. Am J Ophthalmol 1981;92:416–421.
8.   Harwerth RS, Smith EL III, Duncan GC, et al. Multiple sensitive periods in the development of the primate visual system. Science 1987;232:235–238.
9.   Hohmann A, Creutzfeldt OD. Squint and the development of binocularity in humans. Nature 1975;254:613–614.
10. Odom JV, Hoyt CS, Marg E. Eye patching and visual evoked potential acuity in children four months to eight years old. Am J Optomet Physiol Opt 1982;59:706–717.
11. American Academy of Ophthalmology. Amblyopia, preferred practice pattern. San Francisco: American Academy of Ophthalmology, 1992.
12. Parks MM, Wheeler MB. Concomitant esodeviations. In: Tasman W, Jaeger EA, eds. Duane's clinical ophthalmology. Vol. 1. Philadelphia: J.B. Lippincott, 1989.
13. Dell'Osso, LF. Improving visual acuity in congenital nystagmus. In: Smith JL, Glaser J, eds. Neurophthalmology. Vol. 7. St. Louis: C.V. Mosby, 1973:98.
14. Helveston EM. Surgery of the superior oblique muscle. In: Symposium on strabismus. St. Louis, C.V. Mosby, 1979:150–153.
15. Reinecke RD. Muscle surgery. In: Tasman W, Jaeger EA, eds. Duane's clinical ophthalmology. Rev. ed. Vol. 5. Philadelphia: Harper and Row, 1991.
16. Kraft SP, Jacobson ME. Techniques of adjustable suture strabismus surgery. Ophthalm Surg 1990; 114:633–640.
17. Eustis HS, Elsworth CC, Smith DR. Vagal responses to adjustable sutures in strabismus correction. Am J Ophthalmol 1992;114:307–310.

29

Management of Acute and Chronic VI Nerve Palsy

Arthur L. Rosenbaum
Jules Stein Eye Institute, Los Angeles, California

ACUTE VI NERVE PALSY

Rationale for Treatment

Acute VI nerve palsy may be caused by a variety of insults, including cerebral trauma, diabetes, and viral illness. The patient notices the abrupt onset of diplopia. Surgical correction of the esotropia caused by weakness of the lateral rectus muscle is a therapeutic option usually reserved for those patients who do not spontaneously recover within the first 6 months. During this 6-month period, the patient may be incapacitated by diplopia and secondary medial rectus contraction may occur, because of the unopposed action of the paretic lateral rectus muscle.

Botulinum toxin (BTX) injection of the ipsilateral medial recuts muscle may allow the patient an area of single binocular vision during this potential recovery period and prevent contraction of the medial rectus muscle. Thus, surgery may be avoided in some cases if this medial rectus contraction can be prevented.

Clinical Trials

Metz and Mazow (1) reported 34 patients with acute VI nerve palsy who were treated with BTX and compared with a control group of 52 patient with acute VI nerve palsy not treated with BTX. In the treatment group, BTX injection occurred within 3 months of the onset of the palsy.

In the control group of patients with unilateral VI nerve palsy, 30% recovered spontaneously and 70% maintained an esotropic deviation large enough to require therapy. In the group of seven patients with bilateral VI nerve palsy, 42% recovered spontaneously and 58% required surgery.

In the treatment group, 90% demonstrated single binocular vision alone or with a small prismatic correction in their glasses, and 10% required surgery. Of the 11 patients with bilateral VI nerve palsy undergoing treatment, 36% recovered and 64% required surgery. In the patients with unilateral palsy who recovered completely, reduced abduction was noted in only 17%.

It should be noted that in this study, the patients were not randomized into control and treated groups. The control group consisted of patients who refused BTX therapy or who developed a VI nerve palsy before the advent of this treatment.

Complications included transient ptosis (32%) and transient vertical deviation (32%). No cases of permanently induced overcorrection, scleral perforation, or systemic complication occurred.

Wagner and Frohman (2) reported on eight patients with acquired VI nerve palsy who were treated with BTX to the antagonist medial rectus muscle. After a mean follow-up period of 20.6 months, seven were diplopia-free with excellent rotations, and five had complete resolution of the esotropia and diplopia and almost complete recovery of abduction. One patient had 6 prism diopters of residual esotropia, while another required surgery. One patient was lost to follow-up.

The preliminary results of a randomized prospective trial of BTX in acute VI nerve palsy were recently reported. Twenty-three patients with acute VI nerve palsy entered the study. Ten patients treated with BTX within the first 4 months following the onset of the palsy were compared with 13 controls who were not injected. In the treatment group, 2.5 U of BTX in a volume of 0.1 ml of sterile saline was injected into the ipsilateral medial rectus muscle, utilizing electromyographic control. Seventy-four percent of the total group recovered completely within 4 months following treatment. No significant difference could be found between the recovery rates of the treated and the untreated group. The authors report that the average size of the field of single binocular vision for the injected group showed no change after injection. Subjective reasons given for the improved responses included reduction in head posture and less frequent diplopia (3).

In a short report, the authors have updated this series to include 23 injected patients and 19 controls, and they still report that there is no evidence of any difference between the two groups in ultimate outcome (4).

Complications included one case of transient induced vertical strabismus.

CHRONIC VI NERVE PALSY

Rationale for Treatment

Six months following the onset of acute VI nerve palsy, the chance for significant spontaneous recovery is greatly diminished. At this point, therapy is aimed at a permanent correction of the esotropia and development of a large useful area of single binocular vision near the primary position.

In a discussion of treatment options for chronic VI nerve palsy, it is important to differentiate partial VI nerve palsy from paresis. For clarification, I will use the term "VI nerve paresis" to describe a situation in which the function of the VI nerve has been significantly compromised but some significant lateral rectus function remains. The term "VI Nerve palsy" denotes a situation in which a conclusion is reached that all effective lateral rectus function has ceased. Modern management of chronic VI nerve palsy requires this differentiation because therapeutic alternatives appropriate for paresis may be completely inappropriate or even harmful in the case of VI nerve palsy.

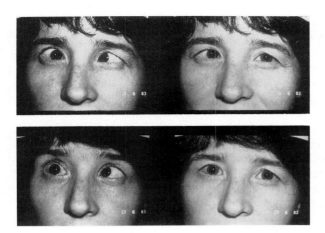

Figure 1 Top: patient with right sixth nerve palsy before treatment. Attempted right gaze with the left eye fixing (left) and right esotropia in the primary position (right). Bottom: one week after full right superior rectus and right inferior rectus transposition. Attempted right gaze with the left eye fixing (right); note marked improvement in abduction of the right eye. There is a small residual right esotropia in primary position (left).

Thus, the clinician is faced with the need to define the extent of residual rectus function in a patient with chronic VI nerve palsy, before deciding on a definitive treatment strategy.

In the past, most clinicians relied simply on the observation of residual abduction rotational movement of the globe as an indication of lateral rectus function. If the globe could not be abducted beyond the midline, a conclusion was reached that no residual

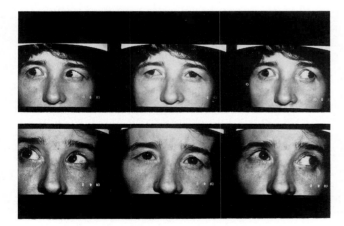

Figure 2 Top: patient with acquired sixth nerve palsy 1 week after botulinum toxin injection, 5 U, into the right medial rectus. Note full abduction of right eye, large right exotropia (center), and palsy of medial rectus muscle due to botulinum toxin injection (right). Bottom: Same patient 2 months later. In primary position she is orthotropic. Excellent abduction and adduction of the right globe are demonstrated. She has 50° of binocular diplopia-free field.

lateral rectus function was present. If there was substantial abduction rotation beyond the midline, one concluded that significant lateral rectus function remained. However, contracture of the ipsilateral medial rectus may prevent the eye from abducting beyond the midline, even though some residual rectus function may be present.

It is important for the surgeon to be comfortable with certain clinical tests that may indicate residual lateral rectus function. The observation of a floating or extremely slow saccadic movement in saccades generated between adduction and the primary position is a reliable indication that little or no lateral rectus function remains. This may be confirmed by actual measurement of horizontal saccadic velocities by conventional electro-oculographic techniques. A force generation test will indicate that little or no force is being generated by the affected lateral rectus muscle in cases of VI nerve palsy. Cases of VI nerve paresis will demonstrate definite force generation, even though the force generated may be reduced to a normal functioning lateral rectus muscle.

Botulinum toxin injection of the medial rectus muscle was used to confirm the presence of partial lateral rectus function in 12 patients requiring surgery for VI nerve palsy. In these cases, a single injection of BTX in the ipsilateral rectus muscle eliminated the medial rectus contracture. Following injection, the degree of abduction was observed. If the patient was able to abduct the eye beyond the midline, the diagnosis of VI nerve paresis was made. If no abduction was made beyond the midline following medial rectus injection, the diagnosis of VI nerve palsy was established (5).

This is an interesting new test that may be helpful in distinguishing paresis from palsy. However, this would delay definitive surgical correction for at least 4 to 8 weeks or until the effect of BTX has spontaneously worn off. Perhaps the same information could be obtained with local injection of lidocaine, which would paralyze the medial rectus for a few hours and permit observation of the abducted rotation.

In patients with VI nerve paresis, conventional strabismus surgery utilizing medial rectus recession and lateral rectus resection, using adjustable suture techniques, is the procedure of choice. A central field of single binocular vision can be obtained in 92% of such patients (6).

However, if conventional recess-resect surgery is performed on the horizontal rectus muscles in patients with VI nerve palsy, undercorrection frequently occurs and the degree of abduction rotation is usually poor. Frequently, this group of patients requires further surgery, and in one study the frequency of further surgery was 50%. In addition to requiring additional surgery, these patients demonstrated a smaller area of single binocular field (4).

In patients with true chronic VI nerve palsy, surgical options include various vertical rectus muscle transposition procedures combined with medial rectus recession. However, these procedures require disinsertion of three rectus muscles in the same eye, which increases the chance of anterior segment ischemia, a serious complication following strabismus surgery.

A combination of strabismus surgery involving two rectus muscles and BTX injection into the ipsilateral medial rectus may permit the attainment of a large area of single binocular vision, elimination of the esotropia, and surgery on only two instead of three rectus muscles.

Clinical Trials

Rosenbaum et al. (7) report on 10 adult patients with acquired VI nerve palsy who were treated a minimum of 8 months following onset. All patients underwent total transposition of the superior and inferior rectus muscle insertions to the area of the lateral rectus insertion, accompanied by BTX injection of the ipsilateral medial rectus muscle.

These patients developed a mean diplopia-free field of 51°, with a diplopia-free field in the abducted field of 20°. Preoperatively, most patients had no area of diplopia-free field and wore a patch to avoid diplopia. One patient eventually required additional surgery.

These results should be compared with those of conventional Jensen procedure transposition, combined with medial rectus recession, which was able to achieve a mean diplopia-free field of 41°.

Fitzsimons et al. (8) studied 11 patients with unilateral and 11 patients with bilateral chronic VI nerve palsy who were treated with injection of BTX to the contracted medial rectus muscle, followed by vertical rectus muscle transposition surgery. Botulinum toxin treatment of the medial rectus occurred 11 days before transposition surgery.

Eight patients with unilateral VI nerve palsy had not been treated previously and showed an average reduction of 42 prism diopters of esotropia 3 months following the combination of surgery and toxin injection. Two patients demonstrated a persistent induced vertical deviation, and further surgery was required in 5 cases, either for residual esotropia or for face turn.

Ten patients with bilateral VI nerve palsy showed a mean correction of 55 prism diopters 3 months following surgery and injection in both eyes. Induced vertical deviations were present in five patients, and further surgery was required in seven patients. One patient developed a large exotropia and required further surgery.

These authors have recently updated their series to include 59 patients with chronic VI nerve palsy treated with BTX injection to the ipsilateral medial rectus muscle and full vertical rectus muscle transposition. The expanded data confirmed the value of this technique in 33 patients with unilateral VI nerve palsy treated with combined medial rectus injection and vertical rectus muscle transposition. Thirty-three percent required further horizontal muscle surgery as a second procedure, usually consisting of bilateral medial rectus muscle recession utilizing adjustable suture techniques. Eighty-four percent achieved a centrally placed field of single binocular vision with an average size of the field of 59°.

Of patients with bilateral VI nerve palsy, 83% required further surgery for the horizontal deviation, with an average total number of operations of 2.8. Fifty percent achieved a central field of single binocular vision (9).

Complications following combined medial rectus muscle injection with BTX and vertical rectus muscle transposition are infrequent. Partial ptosis occurs in approximately 15% of patients. Occasionally, a vertical strabismic deviation occurs that may require surgery or prism correction. Recently, we have described an adjustable suture technique for the vertical rectus muscle transposition component of this procedure that should significantly reduce the incidence of induced vertical deviations.

Minimal signs of anterior segment ischemia have been demonstrated in a few patients (4,10).

Kraft and Allan (11) treated seven patients with total chronic VI nerve palsy a minimum of 12 months following onset. Six cases were unilateral and one case bilateral. The medial rectus muscle was injected with toxin, and a Jensen muscle transposition procedure was performed 2 to 3 weeks later. This combination led to a mean shift of horizontal strabismus angle of 54 prism diopters in the unilateral cases and 92 prism diopters in the bilateral cases.

Side effects included transient ptosis in five cases and a temporary vertical tropia in five cases. In all cases, the side effects were transient.

Scott and Kraft (12) treated 17 patients with lateral rectus paresis solely by injection of BTX to the antagonist medial rectus muscle to eliminate its contracture. Three cases were bilateral and 14 cases were unilateral. Twelve patients had moderate to marked medial rectus contracture, as determined by positive forced duction testing. The medial rectus contracture was successfully released in 11 of 12 cases. Several patients required strabismus surgery, but usually surgery on only two muscles was required.

In a group of four patients who were injected within 8 weeks of the onset of a complete lateral rectus palsy, and before the onset of medial rectus contracture, the lateral rectus paresis fully recovered. Orthophoria was present in the primary position, and no patient required surgery.

SUMMARY

In conclusion, BTX therapy appears to be helpful in the treatment of both acute and chronic VI nerve palsy. In patients with acute VI nerve palsy, BTX injection into the ipsilateral medial rectus muscle may provide a prompt return of binocular single vision and relief from diplopia within a few days following injection. This will allow a patient to avoid wearing a patch, and even to drive, if the field of single binocular vision is near the primary position.

One unanswered question is the determination of the optimal time for injection following the onset of acute VI nerve palsy. Many patients spontaneously recover, and some investigators feel that a few weeks, or even a month, should elapse before injection in order to avoid treating those patients who quickly recover. This may be especially important for patients who develop VI nerve palsy secondary to diabetes, since such a high percentage of these patients experience spontaneous resolution. On the other hand, injection seems to reduce the length of morbidity, even if spontaneous recovery occurs.

Botulinum toxin therapy in conjunction with full tendon transposition of the ipsilateral superior and inferior rectus muscles seems to be the most effective treatment for chronic VI nerve palsy. Surgery is required on only two rectus muscles, and a large area of single binocular vision may be obtained. Some cases will require a second surgical procedure to recess the ipsilateral medial rectus muscle, because the above-described combined therapy leaves a residual face turn and small to moderate angle of esotropia. However, this can easily be performed as a surgical procedure several months later, reducing the risk of anterior segment ischemia, since three rectus muscles will not be undergoing surgery at the same time.

The optimal dose of BTX for the treatment of acute and chronic VI nerve palsies remains somewhat unclear. The studies from great Britain all have used 2.5 U of toxin, while the United States experience has been with 5.0 U. If undercorrection occurs, is a second BTX injection helpful?

Complications have been infrequent, but they include induced vertical deviations resulting from BTX leakage to the superior and inferior rectus muscles, and ptosis.

Finally, very little information is available concerning the use of BTX in children with acute VI nerve palsies. These patients may be prone to develop amblyopia and lose some degree of binocular fusion ability secondary to VI nerve palsy. Thus, BTX injection may allow a rapid return of single binocular vision and fusion. However, using this drug in children requires general anesthesia and ketamine. In many children, the VI nerve palsy is secondary to a viral infection, and resolution improvement is common.

REFERENCES

1. Metz HS, Mazow ML. Botulinum toxin treatment of acute VI and III nerve palsy. Graefes Arch Clin Exp Ophthalmol 1988;226:141–144.
2. Wagner RS, Frohman LP. Long-term results: botulinum for VI nerve palsy. J Pediatr Ophthalmol Strabism 1989;26:106–108.
3. Cooper K, Lee JP, MacEwen C, Jones S. Botulinum toxin A injection for VI nerve palsy, a preliminary report. In: Tillson, ed., Transactions of the VII International Orthoptic Congress. 1991;336–340.
4. Lee JP. Modern management of VI nerve palsy. Austral N Zeal J Ophthalmol 1992;20:41–46.
5. Riordan EP, Lee JP. Botulinum toxin in partially recovered VI nerve palsy. Trans Eur Strabismol Assoc 1991;147–151.
6. Riordan EP, Lee JP. Botulinum toxin in unrecovered VI nerve palsy. Transactions of the European Strabismological Association, ed. Kaufmann, 1991;153–158.
7. Rosenbaum AL, Kushner BJ, Kirschen DL. Vertical rectus muscle transposition and botulinum toxin to the medial rectus for abducens palsy. Arch Ophthalmol 1989;107:820–823.
8. Fitzsimons R, Lee JP, Elston J. Treatment of VI nerve palsy in adults with combined botulinum toxin, chemodenervation, and surgery. Ophthalmology 1988;95:1535–1542.
9. Rosenbaum AL. Comment on Rosenbaum AL, Kushner JB, Kirschen D. Vertical rectus muscle transposition and botulinum toxin (Oculinum) to medial rectus for abducens palsy. Arch Ophthalmol 1991;109:1346.
10. Keech RV, Morris RJ, Ruben JB, Scott WE. Anterior segment ischemia following vertical muscle transposition and botulinum toxin injection. Arch Ophthalmol 1990;108:176.
11. Kraft S, Allan O. The use of botulinum toxin in the management of VI nerve palsy. Am Orthop J 1989;39:89–97.
12. Scott AB, Kraft SP. Botulinum toxin injection: the management of lateral rectus paresis. Ophthalmology 1985;92:676–683.

SPEECH AND VOICE DISORDERS

30

Clinical Aspects of Speech Motor Compromise

David B. Rosenfield
Baylor College of Medicine, Houston, Texas

INTRODUCTION

Language is the set of symbols (semantics, syntax, phonology) that we use in communication. This chapter addresses a subset of language: speech. Speech, a priori, is motor output. In particular, attention is focused on clinical syndromes of speech compromise that might prompt chemodenervation modes of therapy. However, first one needs to understand the basic neurophysiological substrate and mechanisms underlying disruption of speech motor production.

WHAT IS SPEECH?

"Speech" refers only to the actual output of sound. Thus, people can have speech-motor compromise (e.g., dysarthria, dysophonia, dysfluency) and not be aphasic (1). There are three basic components to speech motor output: articulation, respiration, and phonation. All of these motor control systems mutually interact and have inputs and outputs from multiple levels of the neuraxis. As with other types of motor compromise, these speech-related motor control systems can be rendered unstable and dysfunctional by disease (1–5).

There are many types of speech motor compromise. The expansive nosology of neurological disease can afflict any of the components of the speech motor control system. For various reasons, this nosology is less frequently applied to speech neuromotor disorders than to other realms of neurological disturbance, with the result that patients' symptoms and signs themselves often become the appellation of the disease. Thus, patients who yell at a concert and become hoarse are often labeled as having "voice abuse." Likewise, "stuttering," "aphonia," "dysphonia," "vocal strain," and other terms are sometimes presented as naming the disease process itself, whereas in essence they denote the symptom or sign and not the disease.

Other difficulties arise in evaluating speech disorders. First, one must recognize that what causes a problem need not be that which maintains the problem. Thus, an organic or psychogenic disturbance can cause a person to speak abnormally. The disturbance can disappear while the speech deficit remains, transiently or permanently. A common example is a patient who has an upper respiratory infection, develops hoarse sound output, and maintains that symptom following resolution of the primary ailment. That patient may have learned improper coping strategies in trying to phonate in the presence of damaged laryngeal tissue. Whether this relates to functional issues, poor vocal hygiene, disrupted cerebral "engrams," or end organ trauma-induced dystonia are all relevant questions. However, it should be recognized that the maintenance of the disrupted sound may not reflect the original pathology.

Similarly, one must query whether some patients with vocal tremor who develop dystonic-type phonatory output may have as their primary problem their neuromotor reaction to the underlying tremor, as opposed to the tremor being itself the direct nidus for the dystonic output of their sound. In this setting, one can query why some patients with vocal tremor fail to develop speech disruption other than the vocal tremor, whereas others develop strained/strangled speech output (further discussed below) (3,4,6–12).

Indeed, patients afflicted with speech-motor compromise often engage in counterproductive maneuvers as they attempt to speak appropriately. This can be seen in some of the above-described vocal tremor patients as well as in stutterers. Thus, a stutterer may thrust his tongue against the roof of his mouth in an effort to say "top," whereas he should let the tongue relax and fall. A dysphonic patient may bear down and strain in an attempt to phonate, whereas he should try a much softer "glottal attack." What feels right for the patient is oftentimes incorrect. This is frequently a focal point of speech therapy.

Another issue apparent in considering patients afflicted with speech-motor compromise is that one can have "disease" and not have any lesion. This issue holds for many disorders of movement and is herein only briefly discussed. Speech-motor output depends on multiple loops of inputs and outputs to cerebral processing. Disturbances of timing can disrupt output, and these disturbances need not be associated with anything "broken." A system can become underdamped and oscillate (e.g., tremor), become overdamped and dystonic (i.e., dystonia), exponentiate or act appropriately.(13) A single patient can have dystonia at times and tremor at others, all with nothing actually being destroyed in the central nervous system axis. McCulloch and Pitts pioneered this approach, recognizing "emergent properties" of the central nervous system. These emergent properties are not properties of individual neurons but, rather, appear only when neurons conjoin one another in a circuit. (An analogy is the ringing of a public address system: although the individual components can all function normally, an instability—e.g., ringing—can occur; the ringing is a property of the system, and not of any individual component.) Further, the instability can occur in the same system for different reasons at different times (14–19).

In order to know how to evaluate a patient's speech complaints, one must know how to evaluate clinically speech symptoms and signs. This requires a basic understanding of the clinical aspects of how a speech signal is produced. Following this discussion, one can address the symptoms and signs of clinical syndromes, focusing on relevant dysarthrias, some "classical" movement disorders, spasmodic dysphonia, and dysfluency.

CLINICAL ASPECTS OF SPEECH-MOTOR PRODUCTION

Normal speech production requires the dynamic interaction and coordination of sensory-motor control loops of different muscle groups: the respiratory, laryngeal, and articulator systems. These, in turn, interact with the "cognitive" system, which provides language, reasoning, and monitors as well as selects the words to be said (15). Any movement disorder that affects any of these motor systems can alter speech output (3–6).

Vocal folds (vocal cords) consist of striated muscles and articulatory joints (20). There are several vocal fold muscles, all but one of which are adductors. Each of these muscles contributes to vocal fold movement, and each has a separate effect on the level, length, thickness, and edge of the folds and the distribution of mass within the muscle (body) and mucosa of the folds (Table 1) (21). These factors all alter sound wave production (21–23).

Production of sound (phonation) requires appropriate stiffness/slackness of laryngeal vocal folds, an appropriate opening between the folds, and a specific volume and velocity of air moving through that opening. The volume and velocity of the air are altered by changes in subglottic (below the vocal folds) pressure, and by supraglottic contractions, which include movements of the pharynx and supralaryngeal articulators. A narrow but specific range of values exists for these three variables to produce phonation. Compromise of any of them (e.g., tremor, dystonia, weakness) can alter sound output (24). The spectrum of sound produced by the glottal source (larynx) is then filtered by the rostal air cavity and is altered by movement, normal or other (6,22,23).

From a clinical perspective, compromise in the sound source can produce dysphonia and articulator compromise can produce slurred speech. "Dysarthria," a term implying difficulty with articulation only, refers to defects in phonation as well as resonance. Whereas phonation primarily requires good strength, speed, and coordination of the laryngeal and respiratory systems and articulation requires similar interaction of the labial-lingual-mandibular tissue, resonation depends on velopharyngeal function, a weak palate causing hypernasal speech.

SYMPTOMS AND SIGNS

Organically induced speech motor disturbances usually have a gradual onset, unless they result from an ischemic episode or hemorrhage. Psychogenic disturbances usually present with an abrupt onset. Neurological disruption involving speech motor production is seldom associated with episodes of true normality. Although patients may say that at times their speech is normal, careful questioning reveals that the speech is more normal (e.g., less abnormal) at times but is not truly normal. Patients who do have intermittent periods of true normality are more likely to have a psychogenic disturbance (7,25–27).

Speech motor output is a finely controlled motor system and, as such, is sensitive to one's emotional milieu. Augmentation of speech disturbance when the patient is under stress is not a helpful clue in differentiating organic from nonorganic disease (3–7,27).

Most speech motor disruptions are not associated with laryngeal pain. When pain is present, the examiner should suspect focal laryngeal pathology or acid reflux involving the vocal folds. When patients complain of a strained or strangled sensation, with or without pain, one should then consider spasmodic dysphonia. As commented above, the sensation of tightness and strain may reflect the patient's coping strategies in dealing with

Table 1 Effect of Laryngeal Muscles on Vocal Fold Function

	CT	VOC	LCA	IA	PCA
Position	Paramedian	*Adduct*	*Adduct*	*Adduct*	*Abduct*
Level	Lower	Lower	*Lower*	0	*Elevate*
Length	*Elongate*	*Shorten*	Elongate	(Shorten)	*Elongate*
Thickness	*Thin*	*Thicken*	Thin	(Thicken)	Thin
Edge	*Sharpen*	*Round*	Sharpen	0	Round
Muscle (body)	*Stiffen*	*Stiffen*	Stiffen	(Slacken)	Stiffen
Mucosa (cover and transition)	*Stiffen*	*Slacken*	Stiffen	(Slacken)	Stiffen

0 = no effect; ( ) = slightly; italics = markedly; CT = cricothyroid muscle; VOC = Vocalis muscle; LCA = lateral cricoarytenoid muscle; IA = interarytenid muscle; PCA = posterior cricoarytenoid muscle. *Source:* Ref. 21.

the underlying sound production deficit. It can but does not necessarily imply a focal cervical or laryngeal dystonia. Were the patient to speak without these maneuvers, he might produce several glottal stops (staccatolike catches) and more obvious phonation tremor (3–7).

Many patients with neurolaryngeal motor control difficulty can speak at one pitch but not at another, illustrating that they have less interference from the movement disturbance at particular vocal fold tensions. This can result in speaking at a higher pitch, which in turn can cause strain. Singing is normally performed at a pitch higher than the pitch for normal speech and therefore can be spared in some speech motor disturbances. Intactness of singing does not mandate a psychogenic disturbance (3–7).

Subglottic pressure and laryngeal muscle tension required for sound production in laughter and crying are different from those required for normal speech output. If a patient has normal laughter and crying in the presence of abnormal speech production, one should suspect functional aphonia, voice abuse, or voice misuse as well as spasmodic dysphonia (3–7,26,27).

Some persons complain of a weak voice and tremor when anxious. This is probably due to accentuation of physiological tremor. This can cause cessation of speech output and may well account for the expression "scared speechless." In actuality, the patient is scared *voiceless*. The tremor results in transglottal aerodynamic changes such that appropriate oscillation does not occur. The majority of people who maintain this aphonia have it for functional reasons (6,25,27,28).

Patients with psychogenic aphonia may not complain of strain or strangle and are often able to cough and to laugh normally. Aphonia with preserved cough and laugh does not mandate a psychogenic disorder. To diagnose definitively functional aphonia, one needs evidence of a conversion reaction. One can have a functional disorder and not meet these criteria, but it is difficult to be certain about the diagnosis (25,29).

Patients who complain of a hoarse or raspy voice, without strain or strangle, can have vocal abuse (e.g., screaming at a sporting event) or voice misuse (e.g., lecturing to a class all day and developing hoarseness). Oftentimes, these patients improve considerably with voice rest (6).

GENERAL SPEECH MOTOR EXAMINATION

Evaluate the resting posture of the head and neck for tremor. Tremor of the thyroid cartilage usually suggests associated vocalfold tremor. If the head turns to one side, consider spasmodic torticollis. Tremor and torticollis are both associated with spasmodic dysphonia (3,7,9). Vocal fold tremor can produce phonatory tremor and can result in compensatory straining, thereby producing a nontremor type of speech pattern. Asking the patient to produce sound in a slow, easy mode can bring out the underlying tremor. Obviously, tremor or dystonia noted elsewhere on examination should raise suspicion of a movement disorder affecting the speech neuromotor apparatus (3–9,26).

The palate should elevate normally and symmetrically. The soft palate may oscillate in synchrony with essential tremor. Myoclonic movements of the soft palate at rest and during phonation occur in palatal myoclonus (6,7,26).

If there is a question of soft palate weakness, place a mirror under the nares while the patient repeats non-nasal sounds (nasal sounds are /m/, /n/, and /ng/); corresponding non-nasal sounds are /b/, /d/, /g/). Normally, the soft palate and pharynx close the nasal passages during non-nasal sound production and the mirror does not fog, demonstrating no evidence of nasal airway leakage. Uttering these sounds in the presence of ve-lopharyngeal insufficiency prompts air leakage through the nasal airway and clouds the mirror (6,7,26,30).

The most frequent cause of hypernasal speech and nasal air emission is vagal damage, at or above the level of the pharyngeal branches. Unilateral damage produces mild hypernasality, whereas bilateral damage causes more pronounced hypernasal symptoms. Patients with myasthenia or myopathy can have palate weakness resulting in hypernasal speech (6,7,31,32).

The second most common cause of hypernasal speech is bilateral upper motor neuron corticobulbar damage. In this instance, spasticity allegedly slows the movement of velopharyngeal closure, interfering with the synchrony of the soft palate and pharynx during speech. The velum is symmetric and the gag reflex may be hyperactive (6,7,31,32).

Patients with hyponasal speech (/m/ becomes /b/; /n/ becomes /d/; /ng/ becomes /g/) seldom have central nervous system disease. Common causes include rhinitis, enlarged adenoids, deviated nasal septum, and nasopharyngeal tumor (6,7,31,32).

A normal tongue can offer good pressure against the interior of the cheek. Fasciculations, atrophy, and anteroposterior furrows suggest lower motor neuron compromise. Unilateral XII nerve compromise causes deviation to the afflicted side upon attempted protrusion, but seldom causes major compromise of speech output. Bilateral involvement produces severe dysarthria, causing distortion of virtually all lingual consonants (/l/, /rf/) (6,7,31,32).

Lips should pucker well and, as for the muscles of the cheeks, be able to apply air pressure against pursed lips. Unilateral lower motor neuron facial weakness causes the mouth to droop and the cheek to bulge when one produces plosive sounds (/p/, /b/). The intact opposite side usually offers sufficient compression of the lips so that the deficit is mild. Bilateral facial nerve damage cause the lips to bulge considerably with plosive sound production, thus making the deficit more pronounced. Weakness of the lower lip can result in compromise of labiodental fricatives (/f/, /v/) (6,7,31,32).

Compromise of the motor division of the V nerve causes mandibular weakness, compromising tongue and lower lip approximation of the upper lip, teeth, and hard palate.

Unilateral lesions do not usually compromise speech, but bilateral lesions render virtually all speech sounds distorted and near-unintelligible. An increased jaw jerk suggests bilateral upper motor neuron damage above the pons (6,7,31,32).

A patient's contextual speech provides valuable data on respiration, phonation, resonance, articulation, and prosody. Damage to the recurrent laryngeal branch of the vagus nerve results in short phrases, diminished volume, and mild inhalation stridor. In some cases, the voice is hoarse. A higher vagal lesion, resulting in palate dysfunction, adds a component of hypernasality to speech. Multiple lower motor neuron cranial nerve deficits cause breathiness, diminished volume, hypernasality, nasal emission of air, inhalation stridor, short phrases, imprecise consonants, monopitch, and monoloudness (7,31,32).

Bilateral corticobulbar tract lesions cause spasticity, resulting in a slowed rate of speech and a harsh, strained, strangled output. Consonants are imprecise, pitch can be low (in some cases the patients strain, making the pitch high) and monotonous, and phrases are short with altered stress, monoloudness, breathiness, distorted vowels, effortful grunts at the end of phrases, hypernasality, and pitch breaks (7,31,32).

Cerebellar lesions can cause abnormalities in contextual speech, resulting in irregular random breaks in articulation, vowel distortions, excesses in stress, prolongation of sounds, increased intervals between words, varying harshness, and decreased rate (26,31,32).

Hypokinetic dysarthria (Table 2), akin to that noted in Parkinson's disease, results in short rushes of speech, increased rate, monopitch, decreased volume, monoloudness, altered stress, breathiness, imprecise consonants, harshness, low pitch, variations in rate, inappropriate silences, and palilalia (26,31–34).

Hyperkinetic dysarthria (Table 2) refers to dysarthria associated with hyperkinetic movement disturbance. It is associated with different findings, depending on the underlying cause. More salient findings are variable rate, inappropriate silences, imprecise consonants, irregular articulatory breakdowns, distorted vowels, harshness, strain of strangle, and monopitch (26,31,32).

It is often difficult to perceive precisely the underlying deficits in contextual speech. One can obtain a good clinical measure of the speech deficit by assessing repetitive utterance of the individual sounds /pa/, /ta/, and /ka/. The /p/ sound depends on good orbicularis oris power (VII nerve). The crispness of the /ta/ sound depends on adequate power in the tip of the tongue (XII), and the clarity of /ka/ reflects appropriate power and tone in the posterior tongue, as well as the palate (IX, X, and XII nerves). Also, all these sounds depend on appropriate mandibular power. The sounds should be crisp, with normal volume, and the rate should be regular and fast. A slow but rhythmic rate implies bilateral upper motor neuron compromise. An irregularly irregular rhythm implies cerebellar disease. Air wastage through the nares suggests palate weakness. The speech motor system is further assessed by evaluating laryngeal and velopharyngeal dysfunction (see Table 2) (26,31,32).

One must recognize that although these maneuvers screen the neuraxis for deficits in speech production, the perceptual-acoustic-physiological relationships are far more complex. Thus, despite a certain homogeneity of perceptual dimensions for any particular type of dysarthria, a wide variety of movement and motor control problems can exist for any member of that group. Etiological relationships have yet to be established between perceptual-acoustic dimensions or neurological signs (e.g., flaccidity, rigidity, spasticity) and their associated motor control problems (5,8,35,36).

In many instances, a laryngologist should examine the larynx. This is especially important if a patient complains of pain, phonation is defective, or a neurological ailment is not suspected. Laryngologists do not always focus on whether tremor, dystonia, or dyskinesia is present, at rest as well as during phonation. This should be emphasized when consultation is requested. The best mode of observing laryngeal movements is with a nasopharyngeal fiberoptoscope, thus allowing examination of the vocal folds at rest as well as during speech (6,37).

There are multiple causes of unilateral and bilateral vagus damage, each of which causes visible displacement of the vocal fold(s) to the paramedian (abducted) position (6). Vagal compromise rostral to the takeoff of its superior laryngeal branch causes paralysis of the vocal fold, placing the fold in a more abducted position, resulting in a wider glottis than that seen with lower lesions affecting only the recurrent laryngeal branch. Therefore, dysphonia is worse when the vagus lesion is above the takeoff of the superior laryngeal nerve than when it is not. Bilateral vocal cord paralysis results in more pronounced dysphonia than does unilateral vocal cord paralysis. Bilateral lesions above the takeoff of the superior laryngeal nerve, at the brain stem level, render the patient almost totally aphonic. An even more rostral lesion of the vagus, in the brain stem, above the takeoff of the pharyngeal branch, causes soft palate paralysis as well as vocal fold paralysis, resulting in hypernasality and nasal emission. Thus, soft palate paralysis in addition to laryngeal compromise raises suspicion of a high vagal lesion or a brain stem lesion that is affecting vagal lower motor neuron output (6,31,32).

One assesses phonation by asking the patient to sustain the vowel /a/ as long as possible (Table 2). The sound should be steady and clear, with good volume. Flaccid laryngeal muscles produce a breathy sound and decreased volume. Unilateral vocal cord weakness produces a voice less breathy but more hoarse than does bilateral vocal cord paralysis (6,31,32). Diplophonia (two tones simultaneously produced) is common in unilateral vocal cord paralysis because of the different vibration frequencies for each fold (38,39). Some patients with bilateral recurrent laryngeal nerve damage develop paralysis of the vocal cords in the midline. When this happens, the voice may be deceptively normal but the compromise of the abductors prevents opening of the glottis during inhalation, resulting in inspiratory stridor (26,31,32).

Strained/strangled hoarseness with vowel prolongation may indicate hyperadduction of the vocal cords. This can result from increased tone (upper motor neuron lesions or dystonia) or may reflect the patient's coping strategy for trying to overcome the speech deficit produced by an underlying tremor, intermittent movement disturbance, or mild weakness. Existence of a pseudobulbar cry strongly suggests bilateral upper motor neuron tract damage (6,26).

Tremor on vowel prolongation suggests essential phonatory tremor. Nonlaryngeal muscles usually manifest tremor in this disorder. Vocal cord tremor is usually fairly obvious on indirect laryngoscopy and may be present only during phonation or only at rest. Sometimes, the tremor cycle is associated with voice arrest (glottal stop), a finding more commonly associated with symptoms of spasmodic dysphonia (3–6,26–28,37).

Interruption of vowel prolongation is also observed in palatal-pharyngeal-laryngeal myoclonus. These interruptions, as opposed to those seen with essential phonatory tremor, are usually not associated with a rise and fall in pitch during contextual speech. Instead, the tone is steady between the interruptions. Further, the rate of volume prolongation interruption is usually one to four per second, as opposed to four to eight per second

Table 2 Differential Diagnosis of Dysarthria

Disease	Laryngeal phonatory function	Velopharyngeal function	Oral function
Myopathy/myositis	Hoarse, breathy, diplophonia, low volume	Hypernasal, nasal emission	All vowels and consonants may be compromised depending on which muscles are involved
Myasthenia gravis	Similar to above but may be intermittent; improves with rest	Similar to above but may be intermittent; improves with rest	Similar to above but may be intermittent; improves with rest
XII nerve lesion	Normal	Normal	Weak tongue, atrophy, fasciculations; drooling; imprecise vowels and lingual consonants
X nerve lesion	Hoarse, breathy, low volume, diplophonia	Hypernasal, nasal emission, if lesion is above pharyngeal branch	Normal
VII nerve lesion	Normal	Normal	Weak orbicularis oris; imprecise vowels and labial consonants
V nerve lesion	Normal	Normal	Weak mandibular muscles; imprecise vowels/consonants
Multiple cranial nerves	Breathiness, decreased volume, inhalation stridor, monopitch	Hypernasal, nasal emission	Imprecise vowels/consonants
Bilateral corticobulbar tract	Vocal fold hyperadduction, strained, strangled, harsh, variable pitch, monopitch	Hypernasal	Imprecise consonants, slow rate, increased gag, drooling

	Phonation	Resonance	Articulation
Amyotrophic lateral sclerosis	Strained, harsh, wet, gurgly quality; flutter during vowel prolongation	Hypernasal, nasal emission	Slow articulation, imprecise consonants, short phrases, vowel distortion
Parkinson's disease	Weak, monopitch, low volume, hoarse	Normal	Accelerated rate, repetitive dysfluencies, imprecise consonants
Cerebellar disease	Tremor, variations of loudness, or near normal	Normal	Irregular articulatory breakdowns, imprecise consonants, sometimes excessive and equal stress on all syllables of words
Hyperkinetic dysarthria–chorea	Sudden pitch and loudness alterations, phonatory arrest, strained harshness	Normal	Sudden alterations in precision of vowels and consonants
Hyperkinetic dysarthria–dystonia	Slow alterations of pitch and loudness, phonatory arrest, strained harshness	Normal	Slow alterations in consonants/ vowel precision
Hyperkinetic dysarthria– palatal-pharyngeal-laryngeal myoclonus	Rhythmic contractions of intrinsic-extrinsic pharyngeal muscles (1–4/sec)	Rhythmic contractions (1–4/sec)	Normal or imprecise vowels/ consonants
Hyperkinetic dysarthria–phonatory tremor	Rhythmic alterations of pitch and loudness, adductor phonatory arrests, compensatory strain or strangle	Normal	Near normal
Hyperkinetic dysarthria– Gilles de la Tourette's syndrome	Grunt, bark, squeaks, throat clearing, gurgling, moaning	Snorting, sniffing	Whistling, clicking, lip smacking, spitting, unintelligible sounds, echolalia, coprolalia; can have dysfluencies

Source: Adapted from Ref. 6, after Ref. 26.

for essential tremor. Also, laryngeal myoclonic movements are observed at rest as movements of the larynx under the skin of the neck, as well as with indirect laryngoscopy (26,40).

If a patient's cough is a weak explosive sound, the patient may have vocal cord adductor weakness. The sound of the cough is usually minimally compromised in unilateral vocal cord paralysis from recurrent laryngeal nerve damage but is very compromised (reduced) with a higher unilateral vagal lesion above the takeoff of the superior laryngeal nerve. Bilateral vagal lesions at this level cause a very defective or absent cough and are frequently associated with aspiration (26).

The examiner should have the patient produce a prolonged /a/ sound and repetitive /pa/, /ta/, and /ka/. Again, the /a/ vocalization provides good assessment of laryngeal phonation. Careful listening to repetitive utterance of /pa/, /ta/, and /ka/ offers good assessment of articulator function, as well as hypernasality and hyponasality. Just as rapid finger tapping can suggest cerebellar dysfunction (irregular tapping) or upper motor neuron compromise (slow but steady rate, regular rhythm), the repetitive utterance of these speech sounds can likewise suggest similar compromise (e.g., irregular rate with cerebellar disturbance; slow but rhythmic output with upper motor neuron compromise; see Table 2) (6,7,31,32).

INVESTIGATION

Most dysarthric patients require a detailed investigation, focused on determining the cause of their disturbance. The history and examination help determine the type of dysfunction, whether it is due to brain, brain stem, nerve, neuromuscular junction, or muscle damage (Table 2). Individuals with speech disorder due to muscle damage should have a complete evaluation for myositis, myopathy, and myasthenia; the most frequent causes of abnormality are polymyositis and hypothyroidism. If a nerve lesion is suspect, attention should focus on collagen vascular disease, toxic neuropathy, and tumors/neoplasm compressing the nerve. If lower motor neuron vagal dysfunction is present, a chest X-ray and a computed tomographic (CT) scan from the base of the skull through lower portions of the thyroid gland are required. If other evidence of central nervous system dysfunction is present, full neuroimaging studies may be required (3,7,31,32).

CLINICAL SYNDROMES

Movement disorders can afflict speech motor output by interfering with respiration, phonation, articulation, or any combination of these. Again, the patient's symptoms are compounded by how he or she tries to overcome the deficit. Tactics can range from speaking very softly to straining. Most investigators classify movement disorders as being either bradykinetic or hyperkinetic. Bradykinetic disturbances primarily involve parkinsonism and can also include chorea. Hyperkinetic disturbances can include tremor, dystonia, myoclonus, tics (Tourette's syndrome), chorea, and stereotypy. The common signs of these disorders are noted in Table 2 (6,26,31,32).

Parkinson's disease (PD) is often associated with poor presentation of air to the vocal apparatus and is further compromised by slow movement of speech-related muscles. An exemplar of hypokinetic dysarthria, PD dysphonia is characterized by decreased loudness with monopitch, monoloudness, and rather flat prosody (e.g., rhythm of speech). The volume is decreased and often decreases further at the end of a breath. Speech is produced in short rushes with inappropriate silences between words and syllables. The range of articulation for lingual and labial sounds is decreased. Laryngoscopy usually reveals vocal cord bowing with a midcord opening of the glottis on phonation. Vocal cord motion is slow and there may be salivary pooling of secretions on top of the vocal folds (6,31–34).

An increasing corps of investigators have focused on speech deficits in PD, addressing why an allegedly hypokinetic motor disturbance is characterized by "short rushes" of speech and a faster than average speaking rate (26). Although the term "hypokinetic dysarthria" appears to imply a physiological basis in the labiomotor system (e.g., decreased displacement amplitude and reduced velocity)(41–45), not all elements of speech motor output in PD patients are slowed. The extent to which the underlying hypokinesia contributes to the perception of dysarthria in PD patients depends on the demands of the task.

Caligiuri notes that an important task variable that differentially affects speech control in PD is speaking rate (46). Reviewing the literature, he notes that displacement amplitude, velocity, acceleration, and movement time of articulators all vary with speaking rate. Movement time always decreases and articulatory amplitude usually increases as speaking rate increases. If displacement amplitude and movement time decrease, velocity may not change as speaking rate increases. Velocity of displacement remains relatively constant despite changes in speaking rate, provided there are parallel changes in movement time and displacement amplitude (46).

Just as the articulatory kinematics of PD are complex and still not totally understood, so, too, are there disagreements regarding language and cognitive capabilities in PD patients. Several reports describe difficulty in performing tasks of lexical and sentence disambiguation, confrontation naming, generative naming, and syntactic judgments. Others find no consistent difference in vocabulary; PD patients sometimes use fewer words than controls in some situations but more words in other circumstances (reviewed by Lieberman et al [47]). Deficits reflecting syntax appear to be more consistent: differences in the syntactic complexity of the spontaneous speech in PD patients as well as increases in the number and duration of the short hesitation pauses that occur in the flow of speech have been reported (48,49). Using voice onset time (VOT) as a measure of time elapsing between the onset of phonation and the burst that occurs on the release of a stop consonant (voiced sounds such as /b/, /d/, and /g/ have a short VOT and unvoiced sounds such as /p/, /t/ and /k/ have a long VOT), Lieberman et al. (47) observed abnormalities in PD patients and posited prefrontal subcortical compromise as a correlate of their speech deficit.

Dystonia, a common exemplar of hyperkinetic dysarthria, is also addressed in Table 2. Many consider spasmodic dysphonia to be a type of dystonia and, as such, this disorder has received considerable attention.

SPASMODIC DYSPHONIA

Spasmodic dysphonia (SD) is a speech motor disturbance characterized by strained/strangled phonation with staccato-like catches in sound output (50). In 1871, Traube used the term "spastic dysphonia" to describe a patient with nervous hoarseness (51). Fraenkel subsequently described this speech abnormality as mogiphonia, noting that it had a slow mode of onset and was associated with laryngeal discomfort, spastic constriction of the throat muscles, and vocal fatigue (52). In 1968, Aronson et al. (50) popularized the disorder, reviewing it in detail. At that time, there were 122 cases in the literature, including 34 of their own cases. Aronson (53,54) later described two major types of SD: an adductor type that resulted from irregular hyperadduction of the vocal cords, and an abductor type associated with intermittent inappropriate abduction of the vocal cords. The first type is characterized by jerky or choppy breaks in phonation, staccato-like catches, strain, strangle, harsh voice, and monopitch. The sounds are usually jerky, effortful, and strained and are often associated with laryngeal discomfort, particularly strain. Severe, focal laryngeal pain is rare (27,28,55,56).

The second type of SD, the abductor type, is characterized by a breathy, effortful voice quality with sudden termination of voicing that results in aphonic whispered segments of speech. Volume is reduced and a tremor component to the sound output is often present. Further, speech intelligibility is usually decreased. It is not known whether the abductor SD patients have too much tone in their abductor muscle (posterior cricoarytenoid) or too little activity in their adductors (5,54–66).

The interruption of phonatory airflow in SD patients presumably results from intermittent spasmodic hyperadduction of the vocal folds. As noted earlier, a thorough history of the patient's complaints should be taken. Physical examination is similar to that for the dysarthrias discussed above, with special emphasis on listening for phonatory tremor and querying the presence or absence of underlying movement disorder. The diagnosis of adductor SD is not certain unless the patient complains of strain and strangle during speech production. If these symptoms are absent, the physician should suspect voice misuse or abuse, disturbances that relate to poor voice habits and vocal hygiene (5,27,29).

There has been increasing attention to SD. It is not clear what is the exact cause (cause being defined as necessary and sufficient conditions) of the disordered speech, but meaningful correlates have been observed.

In 1982 Marsden and Sheehy (67) noticed a relationship between oromandibular dystonia, torsion dystonia, and spasmodic dysphonias. Reviewing Critchley's case reports from 1939 (68), they found that the first patient had SD as well as tremor of the left arm and torticollis; a third patient had SD and tremor of the jaw. In their series, Marsden and Sheehy noted multiple presentations of the voice disturbances in these patients and queried whether isolated dysphonia could be the singular manifestation of a dystonia. Golper et al. (69) analyzed patients with oromandibular dystonia and noted that many had involvement of the platysma, soft palate, tongue, pharynx, and respiratory muscles. They observed that patients with speech motor compromise had voice stoppages, phonatory inhalation, strained/strangled voice, and vocal tremor. These authors contend that most of these signs were suggestive of dystonia. Schaefer (61) analyzed 28 patients with dysphonia, describing associated laryngeal tremor as well as velar, labial, and mandibular spasms. Two of his patients also had hand tremor. Further, two-thirds had dysphagia or complained of a lump in their throat. One-half of his patients had neck pain. He made an analogy between dysphonia and spasmodic torticollis. Rosenfield et al. (7) diagnosed oromandibular dystonia in 25 of 100 patients with SD. Twenty-two of these also had essential tremor.

In 1985, Blitzer et al. (70) described a dysphonia similar to that in patients with generalized and multifocal dystonia. Clinical and electromyographic studies suggested to them that most patients clinically diagnosed as having dysphonia had a form of cranial dystonia. They noted that, as with other forms of cranial dystonia, most patients presented in adulthood, spasms were poorly controlled by the patient,and symptoms were exacerbated by stress. They investigated a large group of dystonic patients, contending that laryngeal dystonia can present focally or in association with other dystonic movements (3,70).

Primary dystonia is usually action-induced. The symptom is enhanced with the use of the affected body part, which often appears normal at rest. Primary dystonia is observed in patients who have no history of neurological disease or exposure to drugs known to cause dystonia. Findings of neurological examination, aside from the dystonia, are normal, as are diagnostic studies. Patients who have these abnormalities are classified as having secondary dystonia (70). Primary dystonia includes familial and nonfamilial (sporadic) disorders.

Of 2556 cases of dystonia registered at the Dystonia Clinical Research Center at Columbia-Presbyterian Medical Center, New York City, 562 (22%) had vocal involvement. Of these 562 patients, 464 (82.5%) had primary dystonia and 98 (17.5%) had secondary dystonia. Of the group with primary dystonia, 273 (59%) were women and 191 (41%) were men. Of those with primary laryngeal involvement, 15% had involvement of other parts of their body. Twenty percent of patients with primary laryngeal dystonia had a family history of dystonia (3).

Several authors have described tremor activity in SD patients (7,50,61,70–74). Blitzer et al. (70) noted that almost 25% had an irregular tremor of 4–8 Hz on phonation. Aronson and Hartman (56) studied this tremor more closely in patients with dysphonia and noted that it was similar to that patients with essential tremor. They also noted that several patients had synchronous pharyngeal, lingual, velar, mandibular, facial, thoracic, or diaphragmatic tremor. Ludlow et al. (74) also noted a vocal tremor that affected vocal amplitude and discussed the relationship between essential tremor and SD. In a recent videoendoscopic study of 38 patients with SD, Woodson et al. (75) noted tremor of the larynx or pharynx in 29 patients. Rosenfield et al. (7) found essential tremor in 71 of 100 patients with SD, involving the larynx or pharynx in 59 subjects. These subjects were referred to a neurologically oriented speech clinic and were not culled from a base of dystonics.

During the evaluation of SD, patients should be put through vocal tasks to permit observation for tremor, hyperadduction, and inappropriate abduction as well. The hyperadduction can produce only a slight opening of the posterior commisure, cause closure of the false vocal folds, narrow the anteroposterior dimension of the glottis because of tipping of the arytenoids anteriorly, or present as complete apposition of the arytenoids against the petiole of the epiglottis (75). the laryngostroboscope can be helpful in defining tremor and in better demonstrating the hyperadduction (75).

In patients with the abductor form of SD, laryngostroboscopic examination demonstrates synchronous and untimely abduction of the true vocal folds, revealing a very wide glottic chink. These spasms are usually triggered by consonants, especially when located at the beginning of a word. Patients are usually worse on the telephone or when under stress. For adductor SD patients, laughing, yawning, and humming are normal; occasionally, singing is also normal, especially during the early periods of the illness and at higher pitches (7,50,54,71–73,75,76).

Hansonet et al. (5) performed a kinematic analysis of video-documented laryngeal examinations in SD patients. They discuss the relative imbalances and instabilities in tonic contraction among the intrinsic laryngeal muscles that interfere with the postural stability of the vocal folds for phonation. Commenting on the considerable variety in the regularity or irregularity and other characteristics of phonatory postural instability of the vocal processes, they note that the common result is spasmodic disruption of phonation. They believe that the relative balance of abductor versus adductor perceptual symptoms results from the relative balance of muscle tone between adductor and abductor muscle fibers and contend that kinematic data do not suggest that adductor and abductor symptoms in SD result from different basic pathophysiologies. They also address some adaptive strategies that patients have learned in order to compensate for the underlying deficits (5).

Blitzer et al. (72,73) address two other types of SD, in addition to the adductor and abductor variations. They contend that some patients have "compensatory abductor dysphonia," produced by intentionally not contracting their vocal folds in order to prevent the spasms and thus avoid the broken speech pattern of adductor SD. Thus, these patients have a breathy voice. The other type is "compensatory adductor dysphonia," which is very rare, and is observed in patients who tightly contract their vocal folds in an effort to prevent the breathiness underlying their primary abductor dystonic compromise (72,73). This is only conjecture. All one can observe is the actual performed movement. One can not definitely posit which patient moves the folds intentionally, as part of a (learned?) coping strategy, and which patient does not.

Blitzer and Brin (3,73) note that of their 562 patients with laryngeal dystonia, 512 (90%) had adductor vocal involvement, 50 (9%) had abductor vocal involvement, and three had adductor breathing dystonia (paradoxical movement of the vocal folds during respiration, causing inspiratory stridor). The average age at onset was 38 years for men as well as women for the adductor form of laryngeal dystonia. The average age at onset for the abductor group was 38 years for men and 36 years for women. The three patients with laryngeal adductor breathing dystonia were 27, 55, and 56 years old at the onset of their symptoms. The average age of all patients with laryngeal dystonia was 38 years, and that of patients with concurrent dystonia of another body part (229 patients) was 31 years.

In another recent study, 100 SD patients were evaluated by a neurologist, otolaryngologists, and speech-language pathologists. All but three had indirect laryngoscopy, usually performed with a flexible nasopharyngoscope. Of these 100 patients, 71 had underlying essential tremor (mean age men/women 60/45 years), 25 had oromandibular dystonia (mean age men/women 58/48), 12 were hypothyroid, and 27 were considered to have either a focal laryngeal dystonia or a functional disturbance (mean age men/women 49/43). Six patients had intermittent breathy dysphonia (ie, abductor type of SD; mean age men/women 43/38) (7).

Laryngeal electromyography (EMG), in one series of SD patients, revealed that 23% of the patients had an irregular tremor (4–8Hz), whereas only 6% had a regular tremor (similar to essential tremor). Seventeen percent of the patients had enlarged motor unit potentials, while 4% had small potentials and 6% had reduced number of motor units, the significance of which is not clear (73). Schaeffer et al. (77) performed EMG analysis and queried vagal nerve involvement. When the EMG signal is simultaneously analyzed with a voice spectrogram, a greater than normal delay in onset of sound production is observed, especially in the adductor type (78). Watson et al. (79) noted that EMG abnormalities were confined to kinesiologic abnormalities of muscle activation. Ludlow et al. (80) observed elevated levels of activity in the thyroarytenoid and cricothyroid muscles, during phonation as well as during breathing. Detecting such kinesiological abnormalities requires complicated analysis techniques and offers minimal practical use for routine diagnostic investigation.

There has been considerable discussion over how to classify SD patients, different investigators opting for different modes of treatment as well as different models (3–

7,25,56–65). This volume addresses the various strategies in therapy. From a strictly clinical standpoint, certain issues are important.

We do not currently know enough about SD to discuss its cause as being organic or psychogenic—it may well be both. As noted in earlier discussion, it may be that some patients (e.g., those with tremor or oromandibular dystonia) elect particular strategies to overcome their underlying motor disorder and, in this setting, develop SD. Certainly, a large percentage of SD patients have associated organic neurological disease (3–7). However, the associated movement disturbances of the laryngeal muscles have never been proved to be the necessary and sufficient conditions to cause SD. However, no psychiatric form of therapy has been found to be efficacious in curing SD. Ginsberg evaluated 11 surgically treated SD patients and found that the illness did not appear to be a somatoform disorder. They noted, however, that stress may play a role in its expression and that there may be secondary depression and anxiety (87).

As discussed in this volume, different investigators focus on different muscles as the culprit for the majority of symptoms in SD. Recalling the content of Table 1, each laryngeal muscle has a separate effect on the edge of the vocal fold as well as the distribution of mass within the muscle, in addition to altering the position of the vocal fold (21). The interactions are most complex, and there is not yet a large corpus of hard clinical data that permits dissection of one subgroup of SD patients from another in terms of which separate laryngeal muscles are affected. Blitzer and Brin (73) advocate bilateral vocal fold injection of botulinum toxin into vocal muscles in adductor SD and opt for bilateral posterior cricoarytenoid injection in abductor SD. Ludlow et al. (82) selected 10 abductor SD patients with spasmodic bursts of cricothyroid activity during speech and injected these muscles bilaterally with botulinum toxin. They noted group improvements for sentence duration, and some individual patients improved in the proportion of their speech that was voiced and in the duration of the voiceless consonants (82). Continued investigation needs to be done to learn more about the role of each of the laryngeal muscles in disturbed speech output, dysphonic and other. Then, speech scientists will be better able to treat the causal elements of SD.

After diagnosing the syndrome of SD, one must decide what studies are indicated for the individual patient. The studies should reflect the *postulated* cause. Thus, if an SD patient has tremor, the investigation should be appropriate to ascertaining the cause of tremor. Similarly, if dystonia is considered, a full dystonia evaluation is warranted.

DYSFLUENCY

Stuttering is a disturbance of human speech production manifested as repetitions, lengthening, and inappropriate pauses in the generation of consonants, vowels, and words. The accompanying pauses, lengthening, and repetitions, all of which give a choppy quality to the stutterer's speech, are referred to as *dysfluencies*. Pauses associated with muscular tension in the lips, face, and jaw are often referred to as *stuttering blocks* (83,84).

The stutterer's speech consists of sounds that are improperly patterned in time. There are a number of definitions, but most agree that the stuttered dysfluency is the response to an underlying problem and is not the nidus of the deficit itself. Years ago, especially in England, *stuttering* was differentiated from *stammering*. Stutterers repeated the sound until they achieved their target (e.g, p-p-p-pipe), whereas stammerers held on to the sound until the target was produced (e.g., p-----ipe). Most investigators and clinicians do not differentiate stuttering from stammering, primarily because stutterers can readily switch from one coping strategy to the other, just as many tic patients can opt for different strategies to hide a tic. Much of what the stutterer does, in an effort to produce the intended word/sound, is a secondary symptom. Thus, the grimacing, closing of eyes, and other accessory muscle activity that accompanies stuttered output is not akin to a true dystonia. Indeed, these are the features of stuttering that are most readily treated by a speech-language pathologist (2,14,20,83,84).

Stuttering is found in all cultures and in all languages. It is mentioned on Mesopotamian clay tablets, in Egyptian hieroglyphics, and in the Old Testament and the Holy Koran. It is a global disturbance, afflicting 1% of the world adult population and 4% of children. There is a higher concordance of stuttering among identical than among fraternal twins, suggesting a strong genetic component. Stuttering is two to four times more common in the male than in the female population. Stutterers do not stutter in all of their speech output. The majority of their output is fluently produced. The dysfluencies that they do produce are not randomly situated. Most of the dysfluencies occur at the beginning of sentences and phrases. Stutterers are fluent when they sing. Other fluency-evolving maneuvers, although not always as potent as singing, are speaking very slowly, stretching out all sounds, repetitive reading of the same passage, the number of dysfluencies decreasing with successive reading of the passage (known as adaptation), and presenting loud white noise to the stutterer's ears, so that he cannot hear his speech output. No psychiatric therapy has cured stuttering. Stutterers are more dysfluent when under stress, just as all patients afflicted with motor control disturbance usually worsen with stress (2,83,85,86).

As noted earlier, fluent speech requires the dynamic interaction and coordination of four neural systems. The three sensory-motor control loops (respiratory, laryngeal, and articulator) interact with the fourth component (the cognitive system), which provides language and selects the words to be said (14,15). Many authors discuss a stuttering event in terms of a breakdown in the dynamic coordination of these systems. Van Riper presents stuttered events as due to disruption of timing of the motor sequences between sound, syllable, and word production (87). Adams discusses disrupted motor timing during stuttered dysfluencies in each of the three sensory-motor systems (88). Perkins et al. present a discoordination hypothesis involving mistiming between systems (89). These authors systematically varied the interaction between the three sensory-motor systems by using three different speaking modes (normal voice, whispering, and articulation without phonation). The number of stuttered dysfluencies decreased significantly during whispering, and dysfluencies were virtually absent during silent articulation. As the amount of coordinated interaction required between the three sensory motor systems decreased, fluency increased. Thus, a stuttered event is a discoordination or mistiming between these systems. Using control theory, Nudelman et al. (14,15,90,91) model the stuttered event as an instability in a multiloop speech motor control system, commenting on the specific necessary and sufficient conditions that render the system unstable. They discuss how their model accounts for the clinical findings in stutterers.

In 1972, Rosenfield (92) reported a heretofore fluent adult who became dysfluent, without aphasia, following cerebral compromise. There is an expanding corpus of reports pertaining to previously fluent patients who become dysfluent following cerebral injury. In a recent review of this literature, the authors note that the lesions can be anterior or posterior, right or left, cortical or subcortical, unilateral or bilateral (93). Acquired stuttering (AS), as opposed to the above-mentioned developmental stuttering (DS), does not suggest a particular lesion location. Further, although AS patients are dysfluent, they are different from DS patients (Table 4). The age at onset, location of dysfluencies, affect, and response to fluency-evolving maneuvers are very different. Singing, repetitive reading of the same passage, interference from loud white noise, and having the patient speak extremely slowly are potent fluency-enhancing maneuvers for DS patients but are almost totally ineffective for the AS patients. Further, AS patients have dysfluencies scattered throughout the sentence, as opposed to DS patients, whose dysfluencies are primarily at the beginning of words and phrases. Also, AS patients are usually not emotionally distraught over their altered speech output. Their production of dysfluencies is usually not associated with embarrassment or objective indices of embarrassment, such as avoiding looking at the examiner. It is not known what role psychogenic factors play in the patients rendered dysfluent as a result of cerebral lesions (Table 3) (93).

Cluttering is another dysfluent disturbance of speech motor output. Clutterers produce abnormal speech characterized by excessive speed, repetitions, drawling, interjections, disturbed prosody, monotony, and sometimes inconsistent articulatory disturbances (Table 4). Some believe that clutterers have grammatical difficulties, hyperactivity, poor concentration, and compromise in thought process integration (94). There may be omission of sounds, syllables, and whole words, as well as the inversion of the order of sounds, or the repetition of the initial sounds, as well as a prolongation of several sounds in the word. Although the rate of speech may not always be severely increased, the listener usually has the sensation that it is. A major difference between clutterers and stutterers is that the former are usually not concerned about their speech deficits and are often irritated when others point them out (94).

Palilalia is another type of dysfluency. Palilalics compulsively repeat phases or words with reiteration at increasing speed and a frequent decrescendo of phonatory volume (Table 4). This disturbance is usually noted in Parkinson's disease and can also occur in pseudobulbar palsy (26,95).

Table 3 Features of Developmental Stuttering (DS) Compared with Acquired Stuttering (AS)

Feature	DS	AS
Age at onset	Childhood	Adulthood
Gender prevalence	Males predominate	Male = female
Location of dysfluencies in sentences	Beginning of sentence	Throughout sentence
Location of dysfluencies in words	Beginning	I,M,F
Periods of normality	Never	Never
Affect	Anxious	Seldom anxious
Severity	Varies	Seldom mild
Singing	Fluent	Dysfluent
Slowed speech	Fluent	Dysfluent
Loud, white noise	Fluent	Dysfluent
Adaptation	More fluent	No change
"Lesion"	No	Sometimes

I = initial position of word; M = middle position of word; F = final position of word.
Source: After Ref. 93.

Table 4 Differential Diagnosis of Dysfluency

Feature	Developmental stuttering	Acquired stuttering	Cluttering	Palilalia
Locus of lesion	Unknown	Usually cortical, but subcortical cases reported	Unknown	Basal ganglia; bilateral frontal cortex
Cause	Unknown	Vascular, metabolic, tumor	Unknown	Parkinson's disease, postencephalitis, syphilis
Duration	80% of children outgrow, adults have worse prognosis	Unilateral—good prognosis; bilateral—poor prognosis	Varies	Progressive
Locus of dysfluency	Beginning of sentence or phrase	Frequently scattered through sentence	Varies	Throughout sentence
Volume	Normal	Normal	Normal	Decreases at end of phrase
Response to singing	Fluent	Many improved somewhat, but not totally fluent	Varies	No change
Onset	Subacute	Subacute or acute	Gradual	Gradual
Adaptation effect	Promotes fluency	No effect	Varies	No effect
Reaction to dysfluencies	Anxious	Not anxious	Not concerned	Sometimes anxious
Metronome pacing	Promotes fluency	Little effect	Usually promotes fluency	Transiently promotes fluency

Source: Adapted from Ref. 6.

For stutterers and clutterers findings of neurological examination usually are normal. Palilalics may have stigmata of Parkinson's disease. Patients with AS can have any type of neurological deficit, but the lesions, if any are found, are usually small. Patients with DS and clutterers with no other complaints do not require any particular neurological investigation. The evaluation for AS should involve investigation for an underlying organic cause, including neuroimaging of the brain, electroencephalography, and other studies relating to acquired dysfunction, concentrating on tumor, vascular disease, and toxic and metabolic disturbances. Palilalics should have a thorough examination for basal ganglia disturbance, possible stroke, and tumor. Clutterers frequently warrant neuropsychological assessment to rule out any underlying learning disturbance (6).

CONCLUSION

There is a considerably expanding corpus of knowledge of speech motor disruption. This becomes especially pronounced as neurologists, otolaryngologists, speech-language pathologists, speech scientists, neurophysiologists, engineers, and others with an interest in neuroscience delve into the problems associated with disrupted speech motor output. This chapter attempts to sponsor basic clinical skills for those applying chemodenervation therapies. The problems are complicated, and it is hoped our expanded data from the use of this therapy will further expand our understanding of the mechanisms of speech output and how it can be compromised, and of how compromise can be treated.

ACKNOWLEDGMENTS

This work was sponsored by the M.R. Bauer and the Benjamin-Jeremiah-Gideon-Abigail-Rebekah-Maida Lowin Medical Research Foundations.

REFERENCES

1. Alexander MP, Benson DF. The aphasias and related disturbances. In: Joint RJ, ed. Clinical neurology. Vol. 1. Philadelphia: J.B. Lippincott, 1991.
2. Rosenfield DB. Scientific approaches to stuttering. CRC Crit Rev Clin Neurobiol 1984;1:117–139.
3. Blitzer A, Brin M. The dystonic larynx. J Voice 1992;6:294–297.
4. Swenson MR, Zwirner P, Murray T, Woodson GE. Medical evaluation of patients with spasmodic dysphonia. J Voice 1992;6:320–324.
5. Hanson DG, Logemann JA, Hain T. Differential diagnosis of spasmodic dysphonia: a kinematic perspective. J Voice 1992;6:325–337.
6. Rosenfield DB, Barroso AB. Dysarthria, dysfluency and dysphagia. In: Bradley WG, Daroff RB, Fenichel GM, Marsden CD, eds. Neurology in clinical practice. Stoneham, Massachusetts: Butterworth, 1991:129–141.
7. Rosenfield DB, Donovan DT, Sulek M, Viswanath NS, Inbody GP, Nudelman HB. Neurologic aspects of spasmodic dysphonia. J Otolaryngol 1990;19:231–236.
8. Tomoda H, Shibasaki M, Kuwoda Y, Shin T. Voice tremor: disregulation of voluntary expiratory muscles. Nuerology 1987;37:117–122.
9. Brown JR, Simonson J. Organic voice tremor: a tremor of phonation. Neurology 1963;13:520–525.
10. Hachinski VC, Thomsen IV, Buch NH. The nature of primary vocal tremor. Can J Neurol Sci 1975;2:195–197.

11. Critchley M. Observations on essential (heredofamilial) tremor. Brain 1949;72:113–139.

12. Massey EW, Paulson G. Essential vocal tremor: response to therapy. Neurology 1982;32:A113.

13. Stein RB, Oguztoreli MN. Reflex involvement in the generation and control of tremor and clonus. In: Desmedt JE, ed. Physiological tremors, pathological tremors and clonus, Progress in clinical neurophysiology, vol. 5. Basel, New York: Karger, 1978:28–50.

14. Nudelman HB, Herbrich KE, Hoyt BD, Rosenfield DB. A neuroscience approach to stuttering. In: Peters HFM, Halstijn W, Starkweather CW, eds. Speech motor control in stuttering. Amsterdam: Elsevier, 1991:157–162.

15. Nudelman HB, Herbrich KE, Hoyt BD, Rosenfield DB. Phonatory response times of stutterers and fluent speakers to frequency-modulated tones. J Acoust Soc Am 1992;92: 1882–1888.

16. Perekel DM. Logical neurons: The enigmatic legacy of Warren McCulloch. Trends Neurosi 1988;11:9–12.

17. McCulloch WS, Pitts WM. A logical calculus of the ideas immanent in nervous activity. Bull Math Biophys 1943;5:115–133.

18. McCulloch WS. Embodiments of the mind. Boston: MIT Press, 1965.

19. McCulloch WS. Mechanization of thought processes: proceedings of a symposium held at the National Physical Laboratory. Vol. 11. London: Her Majesty's Stationery Office, 1959: 611–634.

20. Rosenfield DB, Miller RH, Sessions RB, Patten BM. Morphologic and histochemical characteristics of laryngeal muscle. Arch Otolaryngol 1982;108:662–666.

21. Hirano M. Clinical examination of voice. New York: Springer-Verlag, 1981:7.

22. Wyke BD, Kirchner JA. Neurology of the larynx. In: Hinchcliffe R, Harrison D, eds. Scientific foundation of otolaryngology. London: William Heinemann Medical Books, 1976:546–574.

23. Borden GJ, Harris KS. Speech science primer: physiology, acoustics, and perception of speech. Baltimore: Williams & Wilkins, 1980.

24. Stevens KN, Klatt DH. Current models of sound sources for speech. In: Wyke B, ed. Ventilatory and phonatory control systems: an international symposium. Oxford: Oxford University Press, 1974:279–292.

25. Aronson AE, Peterson HW, Litin EM. Voice symptomatology in functional dysphonia and aphonia. J Speech Hearing Disord 1964;29:367–380.

26. Aronson AE. Motor speech signs of neurologic disease. In: Darby DK, ed. Speech evolution in medicine. New York: Grune & Stratton, 1981:159–180.

27. Rosenfield DB. Spasmodic dysphonia. In: Jankovic J, Tolosa E, eds. Facial dyskinesias. Advances in neurology, vol. 49. New York: Raven Press, 1988:317–327.

28. Rosenfield DB. Spasmodic dysphonia. In: Fahn S, Marsden CO, Calne DB, eds. Dystonia 2. Advances in neurology, vol. 50. New York: Raven Press, 1988:537–545.

29. Luchsinger R, Arnold GE. Voice-speech-language clinical commicalogy: physiology and pathology. Belmont, California: Wadsworth, 1965;324–333.

30. Rosenfield DB, Viswanath NS, Herbrich KE, Nudelman HB. Evaluation of the speech motor control system in amyotrophic lateral sclerosis. J Voice 1991;5:224–230.

31. Darley FL, Aronson AE, Brown JR. Differential diagnostic patterns of dysarthria. J Speech Hearing Res 1969;12:246–269.

32. Darley FL, Aronson AE, Brown JR. Motor speech disorders. Philadelphia: W.B. Saunders, 1975.

33. Ramig LO, Scherer RC. Speech therapy for neurologic disorders of the larynx. In: Blitzer A, Brin M, Sasaki C, Fahn S, Harris K, eds. Neurologic disorders of the larynx. New York: Thieme Medical Publishers, 1992:163–181.

34. Ramig LO. The role of phonation in speech intelligibility: a review and preliminary data from

patients with Parkinson's disease. In: Kent R, ed. Intelligibility in speech disorders. Amsterdam: John Benjamins, 1991:119–155.

35. Netsell R. A neurobiologic view of speech production and the dysarthrias. San Diego: College Hill Press, 1986:33–52.
36. Neilson PD, O'Dwyer N. Pathophysiology of dysarthrias in cerebral palsy. J Neurol Neurosurg Psychiatry 1981;44:1013–1019.
37. Woodson GE, Zwirner P, Murray T, Swensen MR. Functional assessment of patients with spasmodic dysphonia. J Voice 1992;6:338–343.
38. Kiritani S, Imagawa H, Hirose H. Observation of pathological vocal fold vibration using a high-speed digital image-recording system. Ann Bull RILP 1990;24:1–6.
39. Hirose H, Kiritani S, Imagawa H. Clinical application of high-speed digital imaging of vocal fold vibration. Vocal fold physiology: acoustical, perceptual, and physiological aspects of voice mechanisms. San Diego: Singular Publishing Group, 1991.
40. Doody RS, Rosenfield DB. Spasmodic dysphonia associated with palatal myoclonus. Ear Nose Throat J 1991;69:829–832.
41. Leanderson R, Meyerson BA, Perrson A. Lip muscle function in parkinsonian dysarthria. Acta Oto-Laryngologica 1971;74:350–357.
42. Nakano KK, Zubick H, Tyler HR. Speech defects of parkinsonian patients: effects of levodopa therapy on speech intelligibility. Neurology 1973;23:133–137.
43. Hirose H, Kiritani S, Ushijima T, Sawashima M. Patterns of dysarthric movements in patients with parkinsonism. Folia Phoniatrica 1981;33:204–215.
44. Hunker CJ, Barlow SM, Abbs JH. The relationship between parkinsonian rigidity and hypokinesia in the orofacial system: A quantitative analysis. Neurology 1982;32:749–754.
45. Caligiuri MP. Labial kinematics during speech in patients with parkinsonian rigidity. Brain 1987;110:1033–1044.
46. Caligiuri MP. The influence of speaking rate on articulatory hypokinesis in parkinsonian dysarthria. Brain Lung 1989;36:493–502.
47. Lieberman P, Kako E, Friedman J, Tajachman G, Feldman LS, Kimenez EB. Speech production, syntax comprehension and cognitive deficits: Parkinson's disease. Brain Lung 1992;43:169–189.
48. Illes J. Neurolinguistic features of spontaneous language production dissociate three forms of neurodegenerative disease: Alzheimer's, Huntington's, and Parkinson's. Brain Lung 1989;37:628–642.
49. Illes J, Metler EJ, Hanson WR, Iritani S. Language production in Parkinson's disease: acoustic and linguistic considerations. Brain Lung 1988;33:146–160.
50. Aronson AE, Brown JR, Litin EN. Spastic dysphonia: II. Comparison with essential (voice) tremor and other neurologic and psychogenic dysphonias. J Speech Hearing Disord 1968;33:219–231.
51. Traube L. Spastiche Form der nervosen Heiserkeit. Gesammelte Beitr Pathol Physiol 1871;2:677.
52. Fraenkel B. Ueber die Beschaeftigungsschwaeche der Stimme: Mogiphonic. Dtsch Med Wschr 1887;13:121–123.
53. Aronson AE. Clinical voice disorders. New York: Thieme-Stratton, 1980.
54. Aronson A. Audio seminars in speech pathology. Psychogenic voice disorder. Philadelphia: W.B. Saunders, 1973.
55. Aminoff MJ, Dedo HH, Izdebski K. Clinical aspects of spasmodic dysphonia. J Neurol Neurosurg Psychiatry 1978;41:361–365.
56. Aronson AE, Hartman DE. Adductor spastic dysphonia as a sign of essential (voice) tremor. J Speech Hearing Res 1981;46:52–58.
57. Zwitman DH. Bilateral cord dysfunctions: abductor type spastic dysphonia. J Speech Hearing Disord 1979;44:373–378.

58. Woodson GE, Zwirner P, Murray T, Swenson M. Use of flexible fiberoptic laryngoscopy to assess patients with spasmodic dysphonia. J Voice 1991;5:85–91.
59. Watson B, Schaefer S, Freeman F, Dembowski J, Kondraske G, Roark R. Laryngeal electromyography activity in adductor and abductor spasmodic dysphonia. J Speech Hearing Res 1991;34:473–482.
60. Pool KD, Freeman FJ, Finitzo T, Havashi MM, Chapman SB, Devous MD Sr, Close LG, Kondraske GV, Mendelson D, Schaeffer SD, et al. Heterogeneity in spasmodic dysphonia. Neurology and voice findings. Arch Neurol 1991;48:305–309.
61. Schaefer SD. Neuropathology of spasmodic dysphonia. Laryngoscope 1983;93:1183–1204.
62. Blitzer A, Lovelace R, Mitchell F, Fahn S, Fink M. Electromyographic findings in focal laryngeal dystonia (spastic dysphonia). Ann Otol Rhinol Laryngol 1985;94:591–594.
63. Shipp T, Izdebski K, Reed C, Morrisey P. Intrinsic laryngeal muscle activity in spastic dysphonia patients. J Speech Hearing Disord 1985;50:54–59.
64. Ludlow CL, Connor NP. Dynamic aspects of phonatory control in spasmodic dysphonia. Journal Speech Hearing Res 1987;30:197–206.
65. Rosenfield DB, Nudelman HB. Neurologic signs of spasmodic dysphonia—response to Drs. Aronson and Hartman (letter). J Otolaryngol 1991;20:148–149.
66. Aronson AE, Brown JR, Litin EM, Pearson JS. Spastic dysphonia. I. Voice, neurologic, and psychiatric aspects. Journal Speech Hearing Disord 1968;33:203–218.
67. Marsden CD, Sheehy MP. Dysphonia, Meige disease and tortion dystonia. Neurology 1982;32:1202–1203.
68. Critchley M. Dysphonia ("inspiratory speech"). Brain 1939;62:96–103.
69. Golper LAC, Nutt JG, Rau MT, Coleman RO. Focal cranial dystonia. J Speech Hearing Disord 1983;48:128–134.
70. Blitzer A, Lovelace RE, Brin MF, Fahn S. Electromyographic findings in focal laryngeal dystonia (dysphonia). Ann Otol Rhinol Laryngol 1985;94:591–594.
71. Fahn S, Marsden CD, Calne D. Classification and investigation of dystonia. In: Marsden CD, Fahn S, eds. Movement disorders 2. London: Butterworths, 1987:332–358.
72. Blitzer A, Brin MF, Fahn S, Lovelace RE. Clinical and laboratory characteristics of laryngeal dystonia: a study of 110 cases. Laryngoscope 1988;98:636–640.
73. Blitzer A, Brin MF. Laryngeal dystonia: a series with botulinum toxin therapy. Ann Otol Rhinol Laryngol 1991;100:85–90.
74. Ludlow CL, Naunton RF, Bassich CJ. Procedures for the selection of spastic dysphonia patients for recurrent laryngeal nerve section. Otol Head Neck Surg 1984;92:24–31.
75. Woodson GE, Zwirner P, Murray T, et al. Use of flexible laryngoscopy to classify patients with spasmodic dysphonia. J Voice 1991;5:85–91.
76. Cannito MP, Johnson P. Spastic dysphonia: A continuum disorder. J Commun Disord 1981;14:215–223.
77. Schaefer SD, Watson B, Freeman F, et al. Vocal tract electromyographic abnormalities in spasmodic dysphonia: a preliminary report. Trans Am Laryngol Assoc 1987;108:187–196.
78. Ludlow CL. Treatment of speech and voice disorders with botulinum toxin. JAMA 1990;264:2671–2675.
79. Watson B, Schaefer S, Freeman FJ, Dembousti J, Kondraske G, Roarke R. Laryngeal electromyographic activity in adductor and abductor spasmodic dysphonia. J Speech Hearing Res 1991;34:473–482.
80. Ludlow CL, Hallett M, Sedory SE, Fujita M, Naunton RF. The pathophysiology of spasmodic dysphonia and its modification by botulinum toxin. In: Beradelli A, Benecke R, Manfredi M, Masden CA. Movement disturbances II. London: Academic Press, 1990: 273–288.
81. Ginsberg BI, Wallack JJ, Srain JJ, Biller HF. Defining the psychiatric role in spastic dysphonia. Gen Hosp Psychiatry 1988;10:132–137.
82. Ludlow CL, Naunton RF, Tevada S, Anderson BJ. Successful treatment of selected cases in

abductor spasmodic dysphonics using botulinum toxin injection. Otolaryngol Head Neck Surg 1991;104:849–855.

83. Bloodstein O. An handbook on stuttering. Chicago: National Easter Seals Society, 1987.
84. Alfonso PJ. Subject definition and selection criteria for stuttering research in adult subjects. In: Cooper JA, ed. Research needs in stuttering: road blocks in future directions. ASHA report 18. Rockville, MD: American Speech-Language Hearing Association, 1990:15–24.
85. Porfert AR, Rosenfield DB. Prevalence of stuttering. J Neurol Neurosurg Psychiatry 1978;41:954–956.
86. Rosenfield DB, Boller F. Stuttering. In: Vinken PJ, Bruyn GW, Klawans HL, eds. Handbook of clinical neurology. Vol. 2. Amsterdam: Elsevier, 1985:169–173.
87. Van Riper C. The nature of stuttering. Englewood Cliffs, NJ: Prentice-Hall, 1974.
88. Adams MA. A physiologic and aerodynamic interpretation of fluent and stuttered speech. J Fluency Disord 1974;1:35–47.
89. Perkins W, Rudas J, Johnson L, Bell J. Stuttering discoordination of phonation with articulation and respiration. J Speech Hearing Res 1976;19:509–522.
90. Nudelman HB, Hoyt B, Herbrich KE, Rosenfield DB. A neuroscience model of stuttering. Journal Fluency Disord 1989;14:399–427.
91. Nudelman HB, Herbrich KE, Hoyt B, Rosenfield DB. Dynamic characteristics of vocal frequency functioning in stutterers and non-stutterers. In: P Peters H, Hulstijn W, eds. Speech motor dynamics in stuttering. Vienna, New York: Springer-Verlag, 1987:161–169.
92. Rosenfield DB. Stuttering and cerebral ischemia. N Engl J Med 1972;287:991.
93. Rosenfield DB, Viswanath NS, Callis-Landrum L, DiDanato R, Nudelman HB. Patients with acquired dysfluencies: what they tell us about developmental stuttering. In: Peters HFM, Halstijn W, Starkweather CW, eds. Speech motor control in stuttering. Elsevier, 1991: 227–284.
94. Boller F. Cluttering. In: Thopoulous M, ed. Neurogenetic directory: special edition. Handbook of clinical neurology, vol. 43. Amsterdam: Elsevier, 1982:220–221.
95. Boller F, Albert M, Denes F. Palilalia. Br J Disord Comm 1975;10:92–97.

31

Acoustic, Aerodynamic, and Videoendoscopic Assessment of Unilateral Thyroarytenoid Muscle Injection with Botulinum Toxin for Spasmodic Dysphonia

Gayle E. Woodson and Thomas Murry
University of Tennessee, Memphis College of Medicine, Memphis, Tennessee

Petra Zwirner
Georg August University, Göttingen, Göttingen, Germany

Michael R. Swenson
University of California, San Diego Medical Center, San Diego, California

INTRODUCTION

Spasmodic dysphonia (SD) is an idiopathic disorder in which the voice is impaired by uncontrolled contractions of laryngeal muscles. In recent years, at the University of California, San Diego (UCSD), we have used botulinum toxin (BTX) to treat more than 120 patients with adductor SD, using unilateral injection in about two-thirds of the cases. Complications have been limited to temporary problems with vocal breathiness, mild dysphagia, or aspiration. There have been no serious or permanent sequelae. The treatment has been extremely effective in that all patients have had elimination or significant reduction of excessive glottic closure, with remarkable improvement in vocal function. Few, however, have achieved a totally normal voice. Vocal smoothness is often achieved at the expense of vocal power, and sometimes the spasms cannot be completely eliminated without increasing the dose to a level that produces the unacceptable side effects of breathiness and aspiration.

Even though BTX does not cure spasmodic dysphonia, it is clearly the most satisfactory therapy currently available. Clinical research is needed to determine the factors limiting improvement, to determine the role of adjunctive speech therapy, and to develop treatment protocols that will maximize benefits and diminish side effects. Progress in such research will require the use of objective parameters that can be compared over time and between patients. Our group has measured a number of variables over the course of treatment in our patients, and we have identified some parameters that are useful in quantifying abnormal vocal function and response to treatment in patients with SD.

Generally speaking, experienced clinicians can easily recognize the signs and symptoms of dystonias including spasmodic dysphonia; however, objective and quantitative assessment is a complex problem. Clinical recognition of a sound or an observed movement is a subjective judgment. On the other hand, objective measures are relevant and valid only if they correlate with perceptually recognized features of the disorder. A parameter shown to be abnormal in patients with any disease may not bear any relation to pathological function or may remain abnormal after treatment has resulted in significant symptomatic improvement. The situation is further complicated by the fact that in dystonias, symptoms vary considerably over time, during different tasks, and in different situations. Many patients are more symptomatic when under stress. The testing environment is artificial and may be stressful, and its relevance to everyday life situations may be minimal.

In the specific case of SD, muscle spasms occur in intrinsic laryngeal muscle and can be visually observed only with special endoscopic equipment. Because of the difficulty in observing pathologic function inside the vocal tract, spasmodic dysphonia was until recent years believed to be a psychiatric problem. Quantification of this abnormal movement is extremely difficult. On the other hand, the voice that is produced by the patient can be recorded and objectively analyzed. Airflow and pressure can also be physically measured. Finally, careful analysis of endoscopically acquired video recordings can be used to assess laryngeal movements.

ACOUSTIC ANALYSIS

Most methods of diagnosing spasmodic dysphonia and other vocal disorders, as well as assessing response to treatment, are based on the sound of the voice. Acoustic signals are easy to record, and quantitative analysis is fairly straightforward. However, the resulting data give little insight into pathophysiology. It is also true that analysis of sound alone may not actually reflect the handicap experienced by the patient, as symptoms may be more related to the degree of effort required to speak than to the quality of the voice produced. The difficulty, both physical and emotional, experienced by the patient in his attempts to communicate cannot be directly measured. Further, to obtain quantitative indicators of function that can be objectively analyzed by statistical methods, it is necessary to employ direct physical measurements during controlled phonatory tasks. The validity of such objective measures, obtained in arbitrary situations, can be established only by demonstrating correlation with the dysfunction experienced by the patient in everyday speech, as assessed by more subjective means.

The speech of patients with SD has been described as strained and strangled, effortful, choked, laborious, and jerky, with overpressure, hard glottal attacks, and voice stoppages, and this characteristic voice is easily recognized by most clinicians who work in this field. However, the same vocal qualities can be recognized in many patients with neurological diseases such as Parkinsonism, cerebellar ataxia, Huntington's disease, and essential tremor (1). Since acoustic changes are not sufficiently specific to separate spasmodic dysphonia from other neurological voice disorders, they should be regarded as indicators of function, rather than diagnostic tests.

Notwithstanding these qualifying statements, our studies of clinical validity demonstrate that several acoustic measurements, listed in Table 1, are quite useful in documenting the severity of SD and in monitoring response to treatment. The methods and results of several studies are summarized below.

Table 1 Acoustic Changes with Botulinum Toxin Treatment of Spasmodic Dysphonia

Parameter	Before treatment	One month later
F_0	Normal	No change
SD F_0	Elevated	Significantly improved
SN ratio	Decreased	Significantly improved
Shimmer	Increased	No significant change
Jitter	Increased	No significant change
Voice break factor	>1 abnormal	Significantly improved

F_0 = fundamental frequency; SD F_0 = standard deviation of fundamental frequency; SN = signal-to-noise.
Source: Adapted from Ref. 4.

Standardized recordings were made of sustained vowel vocalizations by 19 patients, before and after unilateral treatments with BTX (15 to 30 U) (2). Recordings were made in a soundproof room with a constant mouth-to-microphone distance. Subjects were asked to take a deep breath and sustain the vowel /a/ at a comfortable intensity and pitch for as long as possible. Similar recordings were made of 11 normal control subjects in two sessions 2 weeks apart. The acoustic signals were digitized and analyzed using C-speech software to determine five acoustic parameters: fundamental frequency, standard deviation of fundamental frequency, jitter (frequency perturbation), shimmer (amplitude perturbation), and signal-to-noise ratio. Two other measurements were obtained, maximum phonation time and the number of phonatory breaks in a sustained vowel. We defined a phonatory break as a signal stop with a length longer than two cycles. We divided the number of voice breaks by the maximum phonation time, in seconds, to derive a new parameter, the voice break factor.

Spasmodic dysphonia patients differed significantly from control subjects in every acoustic parameter except fundamental frequency. Standard deviation of the fundamental frequency, an indicator of pitch instability, was a mean of 12.1 in patients, versus 2.0 in controls. Mean jitter and shimmer were 0.28 msec and 16.6%, respectively, for patients, and 0.028 msec and 2.4% for controls. Mean signal-to-noise ratio was 12.6 for patients and 21 for controls. All SD patients had voice breaks, with a mean voice break factor of 1.16, while normal subjects had no voice breaks at all.

At 1 week after injection, patients were all greatly improved symptomatically. However, only standard deviation of the fundamental frequency and voice break factor were significantly improved, to 5.7 and 1.16, respectively. Jitter and shimmer were still very abnormal, and variability between subjects was quite large. It was apparent that either BTX did not alter the pathophysiology of jitter and shimmer in these patients, or that any resulting improvement was overshadowed by the effects of vocal fold weakness.

Our clinical experience has indicated that many patients develop symptoms of mild glottal incompetence during the 2 or 3 days after injection, with breathiness, occasional diplophonia, and even mild aspiration. These problems most often resolve within 1 to 2 weeks, suggesting that data collected at 1 week may not be a good indicator of eventual outcome. To document this phenomenon, and to study the more long-term effects of therapy, we conducted a subsequent study of acoustic changes not only at 1 week, but also at 1 month after injection (3). Eleven patients with adductor SD were studied, before and after unilateral injection of BTX. The acoustic results at 1 week in these 11 patients were, in general, consistent with those of the 19 patients mentioned above. Four weeks after therapy, acoustic analysis indicated further voice improvement, particularly for the signal-to-noise ratio, which became significantly better, improving from 14.5 before and 14.6 after 1 week, to 17.9 1 month after treatment. However, all acoustic characteristics were still significantly different when compared with those of the normal control subjects.

AERODYNAMIC MEASURES

The pathophysiology of SD results in significant aberrations of air flow and pressure during speech. Measurement of pressure is technically difficult, but it is an easy task to measure phonatory air flow, most commonly by having a subject vocalize into a mask coupled to a pneumotachygraph. One can choose to study mean air flow during a sustained vowel, or to analyze the AC changes that correspond to the acoustic signal. Because the voice is unstable in SD, it is quite difficult to get meaningful data from the AC signal, and mean air flow is much more useful.

In adductor SD, mean phonatory air flow is decreased, and sudden drops in air flow can be observed. After successful BTX therapy, mean air flow increases and sudden drops either are abolished or become less frequent and less severe. Maximal benefit is attained when the dose of BTX is just sufficient to increase air flow to a normal level. Further BTX results in excessive vocal fold weakness and, consequently, vocal breathiness. In contrast, air flow is above normal in most cases of abductor spasmodic dysphonia, and bursts of air flow can indicate a component of abductor spasm in a patient who clinically appears to have only adductor spasm. Control of adductor spasms can occasionally unmask a latent abductor component, with disappointing functional results. Identification of abductor spasms before injection can serve as an indicator to use a more conservative initial dose of toxin in adductor muscles.

We obtained standardized air flow recordings of the vowel /a/ before and after treatment in the same 11 patients reported in the second study described above (3). Mean air flow rates were determined during the steady-state portion of the phonation. The SD patients had mean phonatory air flow rates 20–75% below normal values before BTX injection, with an overall mean value of 107.2 cc/sec. Mean airflow in the normal controls was 177–187 cc/sec. One week after BTX injection, air flow rates ranged from 140 cc/sec to values in excess of 400 cc/sec, with an overall mean of 357.8. At 1 month after injection, mean air flow was closer to normal, at 230.6 cc/sec. The changes in phonatory airflow parallel the symptoms of glottal incompetence, which are most pronounced at 1 week, and largely resolve by 1 month.

Measurement of the maximum phonation time (MPT) for a sustained vowel is an indirect measure of glottic competence. If the vocal folds are not close enough together, excessive air flow is required for phonation, and patients run out of air quickly. The result is a short MPT. In a condition of increased laryngeal resistance, such as SD, one would expect a prolonged MPT. In fact, we have found that MPT per se is not useful in assessing patients with SD, as this parameter varies significantly with different levels of sound pressure, pitch, and quality of the vowel utilized. A standardized procedure can reduce the variability of MPT. However, laryngeal control is so severely impaired in patients with SD that the recommendations for standardization cannot be implemented. Further, MPT is also influenced by respiratory and psychological factors, as well as compensatory speech strategies that can be unique to each patient. In our studies, MPT showed no consistent or significant difference after treatment; it was increased in 42% of patients and decreased in the other 58%. We did find the MPT to be useful, however, in calculating the voice break factor (number of voice breaks dividend by the MPT), as described in the section on acoustic analysis.

There are very few data regarding subglottic pressure measurement in SD. In studies of voice physiology and pathology, estimation of subglottic pressures during phonation is most commonly accomplished by noninvasive measures, extrapolating from oral pressure at a point in time when the vocal folds are determined to be *open*. This technique has not been validated in the population of patients with SD and would most likely be inaccurate, because of the instability of pressure and flow, and also because the maximum subglottic pressure is actually generated during glottal spasm, when the vocal folds are *closed*. Direct measurement of subglottic pressure requires placement of a catheter in the trachea, either percutaneously or transglottally. The former approach impairs glottic function, and the latter carries a risk of bleeding.

An alternative approach is to measure intraesophageal pressure, which correlates approximately with subglottic pressure during phonation. In one of the earliest reports of the use of BTX for spasmodic dysphonia, pressure was measured by means of an intraesophageal transducer, before and after treatment (5). The two reported patients had very severe spasmodic dysphonia that significantly impaired communication. Before treatment, the first patient generated 23–23 cm H_2O of intrathoracic pressure during phonation. After injection of 30 U of BTX into the left thyroarytenoid muscle, his voice was much improved and less effortful, and intrathoracic pressure during phonation was only 5 cm H_2O. The second patient, who was nearly aphonic, generated 75 cm H_2O during attempted phonation, and also had episodes of airway obstruction due to laryngospasm. After injections of 20 U of BTX, phonatory intrathoracic pressure dropped from 75 cm H_2O to 3.5 cm H_2O. In both patients, pressure generation during Valsalva maneuver was also markedly reduced, indicating that the observed drop in glottal resistance was due to peripheral weakness, and not a specific phonatory effect.

The intraesophageal transducer is not generally used in assessing vocal function, because of patient discomfort and the risks associated with transnasal placement of an esophageal catheter. Development of a practical and accurate means of determining subglottic pressure in these patients would be extremely useful, both in measuring the degree of effort required to initiate phonation and in determining the significance of abnormal phonatory airflow. For example, a reduced phonatory effort may be due to increased laryngeal resistance (elevated subglottic pressure) resulting from laryngeal spasm, or to decreased force of expiration (diminished subglottic pressure). The latter situation could result from dystonia or dyskinesia of respiratory muscles, or from a voluntary disease in breath support during phonation.

VIDEOENDOSCOPY

We have studied the use of videoendoscopy in patients with SD, and have found analysis of recordings to be quite useful in diagnosis and assessment, as well as in studying the pathophysiology of the disorder and its response to BTX therapy (6). First, we studied untreated patients to identify abnormal parameters that might correlate with subjective severity. Then we evaluated patients before and after treatment with BTX, to track the changes in these parameters and determine their correlation with clinical improvement.

We analyzed recordings before treatment of 38 patients diagnosed as having spasmodic dysphonia. Patients recited a standardized sequence of utterances: counting one through ten, sustaining "i" and "ah," saying "Pay Paul a penny" and "We mow our lawn all year,'' and singing ''Mary had a little lamb.'' We developed a visual scoring scale to characterize specific elements of laryngeal dysfunction, including excessive phonatory activation of intrinsic laryngeal muscles, abnormal activation of extrinsic laryngeal muscles, tremor, and spasmodic movements unrelated to phonation.

In each category, one to two parameters were identified and rated on a four-point scale, with 0 as normal and 3 as most abnormal. Parameters indicating intrinsic laryngeal muscle hyperactivity included excessive adduction of the arytenoids, abduction of the vocal folds during phonation, and rigidity of the vocal folds. Abductor and adductor forms of dysphonia, sometimes mixed, have previously been described, but we also have observed rigidity limiting phonation without excessive closure or sudden opening. This may be because of simultaneous activation of the adductors and the posterior cricoarytenoid. Parameters used to assess extrinsic laryngeal muscle hyperfunction were false cord adduction and compression of the larynx in the sagittal dimension. If the full width of true vocal folds visible during exhalation also was visible during phonation, the rating was 0 or normal. If up to one-third was covered, the score was 1; covering of one-third to two-thirds was rated 2; and total covering of the true vocal folds was rated 3. Tremor was scored independently for presence and severity during phonation and respiration. Spasmodic laryngeal abductions and adductions unassociated with phonation were noted and scored.

Of the 38 patients, 37 had some evidence of excessive glottic closure. The only exception was a subject with abductor spasms. In three patients, events of excessive glottic closure were attributed to a sudden increase in the amplitude of a vocal tremor, rather than isolated spasmodic closure. Extrinsic laryngeal muscle hyperfunction was extremely common, occurring in 33 patients. Tremor was also frequent, occurring during phonation in 28 subjects and during quiet expiration in 19 (total incidence of 29). Spasmodic movements unassociated with phonation were observed in 14 patients.

To determine the clinical significance of each category of observed dysfunction, we compared the mean video ratings in each category to overall functional status, as determined by the following criteria. If the speech disturbance was annoying but not disabling, level I was assigned. A patient with a definite speech handicap who could nonetheless continue to function in job and social roles was rated at level II. Severe speech problems causing career change or restriction of social interaction were rated at level III.

The score of each category of endoscopically observed category of dysfunction increased with the clinical level of functional impairment, but these trends were not statistically significant. A significant interaction could be demonstrated only for the total score of all categories of endoscopic parameters.

In an additional analysis, recordings were made in 17 patients before and 1 month after unilateral BTX injection and analyzed by blinded observers. Assessment of vocal fold motion indicated that BTX therapy was extremely effective in controlling excessive glottic adduction, as this parameter was normalized or significantly improved in all subjects, and the mean score for this parameter decreased significantly. Mean tremor score also decreased significantly, but not all patients were improved. The mean scores for extrinsic laryngeal hyperfunction were not different before and after therapy, and in fact, three patients had a significant increase in false fold closure and anterior-posterior compression after treatment.

It appears that although excessive activation of intrinsic laryngeal muscles is a central feature of SD, it is by no means the only speech abnormality that contributes to overall dysfunction. Most patients also have hyperfunction of extrinsic laryngeal muscles or laryngeal tremor. Although unilateral BTX injection is highly effective in reducing excessive glottic closure and improving phonatory air flow, it is somewhat less effective in controlling tremor and does not significantly affect hyperfunction of extrinsic laryngeal muscles. It is possible that these problems may account for some of the persisting vocal problems and acoustic perturbation after therapy. Addressing these problems could result in successful rehabilitation of patients with SD.

Satisfactory therapy for extrinsic muscle hyperfunction might be attained by injecting additional muscles with BTX or by speech therapy techniques, depending on the pathophysiology of dysfunction. If the extrinsic laryngeal muscle dysfunction is due to a regional dystonia, then it would probably respond to local injection of BTX. The exact muscles involved in hyperfunctional dysphonia have never been conclusively identified, but all candidates are much larger than intrinsic laryngeal muscles and would presumably require a larger dose of toxin for effect. It is also possible that the abnormal activation of extrinsic laryngeal muscles may be a result of psychiatric causes or functional adaptation and therefore responsive to speech therapy.

The lack of consistency of unilateral toxin treatment in relieving vocal tremor suggests that there may be different types of tremor, some of which do not respond to toxin. Alternatively, tremor reduction could require a bilateral toxin effect, in which case the effect of a unilateral injection would be dependent on the diffusion of the toxin to the opposite side of the larynx. This could vary with dosage and patient factors. Further study is required to resolve this issue.

UNILATERAL VERSUS BILATERAL INJECTION

It has been observed that the total dose of BTX required for improvement of SD is smaller when the drug is deposited bilaterally rather than in only one side of the larynx (7). Although some patients respond better to unilateral injection, others perform best after bilateral injection. The mechanism of action of bilateral and unilateral injection appears to differ. Ludlow et al. found that unilateral injection only reduced symptoms significantly only when the vocal fold movement was visibly reduced (8). Bilateral injection, however, is capable of producing significant improvement with doses so small that no impairment of vocal fold motion can be observed. Although symptom improvement can be achieved with a total dose about five times lower than that required for results with unilateral injection, the incidence of breathiness and aspiration in our patients appears to be significantly higher at 1–2 weeks after bilateral injection. This was confirmed by objective findings of a greater increase in airflow and phonatory instability at 1 week in bilaterally injected patients (9). At one month, however, symptoms of glottal incompetence improve and there is little discernable difference between the two groups.

SUMMARY

Our studies have defined some specific voice effects of unilateral BTX injection as a treatment for spasmodic dysphonia: elimination of voice breaks, stabilization of the fundamental frequency, and increase in phonatory airflow. These parameters are very useful in confirming the diagnosis, planning treatments, and documenting response to therapy. The parameters will also be of value to measure function in research protocols for optimizing response to BTX and exploring new ways of managing this devastating disease.

REFERENCES

1. Zwirner P, Murry T, Woodson G. Phonatory function of neurologically impaired patients. J Commun Disord 1991;24:287–300.
2. Zwirner P, Murry T, Swenson M, Woodson.G. Acoustic changes in spasmodic dysphonia after botulinum toxin injection. J Voice 1991;5:78–84.
3. Zwirner P, Murry T, Swenson M, Woodson G. Effects of botulinum toxin therapy in patients with adductor spasmodic dysphonia: acoustic, aerodynamic and videoendoscopic findings. Laryngoscope 1992;102:400–406.
4. Zwirner P, Murry T, Woodson GE. Bilateral vs unilateral botulinum toxin treatment of spasmodic dysphonia. Submitted for publication.
5. Miller RH, Woodson GE, Jankovic J. Botulinum toxin injection of the vocal fold for spasmodic dysphonia. Arch Otolaryngol 1987;113:603–605.
6. Woodson GE, Zwirner P, Murry T, Swenson M. Use of flexible fiberoptic laryngoscopy to classify patients with spasmodic dysphonia. J Voice 1991;5:85–91.
7. Blitzer A, Brin MF, Fahn S, Lovelace RE. Localized injections of botulinum toxin for the treatment of focal laryngeal dystonia (spastic dysphonia). Laryngoscope 1988;98:193–197.
8. Ludlow CL, Naunton RF, Sedory MA, Schultz MA, Hallett M. Effects of botulinum toxin injections on speech in adductor spasmodic dysphonia. Neurology 1988;38:1220–1225.
9. Woodson GE, Zwirner P, Murry T, Swenson M. Functional assessment of patients with spasmodic dysphonia. J Voice 1992;6:338–343.

32

Oromandibular Dystonia: Treatment of 96 Patients with Botulinum Toxin Type A

Mitchell F. Brin, Andrew Blitzer, Susan Herman, and Celia Stewart
Columbia University College of Physicians and Surgeons, New York, New York

INTRODUCTION

Oromandibular dystonia (OMD) is dystonia involving the masticatory, lower facial, and tongue muscles and producing spasms and jaw deviation. In the early sixteenth century, Brueghel often painted faces with open mouths and contracted facial muscles, postulated to have had OMD (1). In 1899, Gowers (2) described conditions producing tonic and clonic jaw contractions. The differential diagnosis of tonic spasms included tetanus, trauma, hysteria, brain stem lesions, and hypothermia. Convulsions, rigors, paralysis agitans, facial pain, and chorea were recognized as causes of clonic spasms.

Just after the turn of the century, Meige (3) reported a syndrome of spasms of the eyelids in addition to contractions of the pharyngeal, jaw, and tongue muscles. Characteristic of dystonia, these spasms were often provoked by voluntary action (talking, eating), or lessened by humming, singing, yawning, or voluntarily opening the mouth. Some of the patients with Meige's syndrome developed other signs of dystonia, including torticollis or writer's cramp. In 1976, Marsden (4) concluded that blepharospasm and oromandibular dystonia were within the spectrum of adult-onset segmental torsion dystonia. Other reviews have supported this assertion (5–15).

The etiology and differential diagnosis of OMD are similar to those of other focal or segmental dystonias (16). Because the condition is uncommon, misdiagnosis is widespread. Sustained or repetitive muscle contractions associated with bruxism typically occur in sleep (17), a time when most classical movement disorders such as OMD are not present. Most patients are initially diagnosed as having temporomandibular joint disorder (TMD) and treated with a variety of appliances (5,18), usually to no avail. Nevertheless, dental appliances may be useful for treating some cases of orofacial dyskinesias, and some of these patients are thought to have OMD (19). The true incidence of benefit from

Table 1 Muscles Affecting Jaw and Tongue Movement

Muscle	Primary and secondary functions
Masseter	Jaw closing
Temporalis	Jaw closing; anterior fibers assist in jaw opening, deviation, and protrusion
Internal pterygoid	Jaw closing
Digastric (anterior and posterior)	Jaw opening
External pterygoid	Jaw opening, deviation to opposite side, and protrusion
Genioglossus	Tongue protrusion, passive jaw opening
Hyoglossus	Tongue protrusion, passive jaw opening
Genihyoid	Jaw opening
Mylohyoid	Elevation of hyoid, jaw opening

physical methods is not known; most patients present themselves to a referral center only after conservative therapies in the community have failed.

On the basis of clinical phenomenology, patients can be classified as having predominantly jaw-closing (JC), jaw-opening (JO), or jaw-deviation dystonia. Many patients with jaw deviation also have jaw opening, and these cases are classified as primarily jaw-opening in the discussion that follows. The muscles controlling these movements are listed in Table 1.

Drug therapy has been the mainstay of treatment, with anticholinergics, benzodiazepines (20–22) or baclofen (23) being most effective. The combination of the dopamine-depleting agent tetrabenazine with lithium carbonate is quite helpful in managing patients (24). We and others have reported success in managing OMD with local injections of botulinum toxin type A (BTX-A) (18,25–29).

TECHNICAL CONSIDERATIONS

Treatment of jaw dystonia requires a detailed knowledge of the local anatomy and management of potential complications of therapy. In most cases, we recommend that patients be evaluated by a neurologist, otolaryngologist, and speech-language pathologist. In selected cases where there are signs or symptoms of TMD, including joint pain or click or restricted jaw mobility, an evaluation by a TMD specialist may be appropriate. We have seen cases in which OMD and TMD coexist and a coordinated treatment approach is required.

All pterygoid muscle injections are performed with electromyographic (EMG) guidance, as these muscles are not easily palpated by examination. We use EMG for the other jaw muscles to improve precision and accuracy and aid in injecting regions of active contraction. This is particularly important when performing follow-up injections. Gestures, such as opening the mouth when injecting the lateral pterygoid muscle, or comparing opening the mouth with protruding the tongue when injecting the digastric muscle, are helpful to target the toxin injection.

We use two rating scales to assess function (Table 2). Although both scales are easy to administer, the linear 0–100% scale is preferred by patients and provided a comprehensive data set for this report. We have previously demonstrated a close relationship between our original four-point scale and the linear scale (25). Patients appear to be more comfortable

Table 2 Global Clinical Rating Scales[a]

Ask the patient to use the following two scales: "For the area of the body being treated, how would you rate your current condition?"

Scale 1: Disability Rating Scale

0 = *Normal*
1 = *Mild* discomfort or functional impairment
2 = *Mild to moderate* discomfort or functional impairment
3 = *Moderate* discomfort or functional impairment
4 = *Moderate to severe* discomfort or functional impairment
5 = *Severe* discomfort or functional impairment
6 = *Completely disabled or incapacitated*

Scale 2: Percent of Normal Function Rating Scale

0% = Fully disabled, no useful function
100% = Normal

[a]See Ref. 30.

with the latter linear continuous scale than with a scale of discrete points. Evaluation of the outcome of treatment is complicated by the observation that patients tend to show a greater degree of peak improvement or function with subsequent treatments, until a plateau of effect is reached. Therefore, we describe the initial function as compared with the plateaued or peak function for each patient. These results are then averaged and reported.

RESULTS

The demographic features of patients treated are outlined in Table 3. It is intriguing that all of the jaw-deviation patients were women. However, this may be a chance finding with the limited number of patients in this group. If one pools all patients with lateral pterygoid involvement (i.e., the jaw-opening and jaw-deviation groups), the percentage of female patients is 75.6%, and this is not significantly different than the figure for cases involving jaw-closing muscles. Secondary causes of jaw dystonia included tardive dystonia (9), peripheral trauma (4), head injury (2), metabolic causes (2), perinatal anoxia (1), encephalitis (1), and other symptomatic causes of dystonia (7).

Table 3 Demographic Characteristics of Patients with Oromandibular Dystonia Treated with Botulinum Toxin

Deviation	N	% Female	Age at onset of dystonia (years)	% Idiopathic
Jaw closing	51	74.5	43.5 ± 2.7	70.6
Jaw opening	40	67.5	44.0 ± 3.1	75.0
Jaw deviation	5	100	46.6 ± 6.7	80.0
All patients	96	72.9	43.9 ± 2.0	72.9

Table 4 Doses of Botulinum Toxin Type A in Jaw Muscles[a]

Muscle	Dose (U)	
	Median ± SD	Range
Masseter	24.5 ± 17.7	2.0–100.0
Temporalis	18.5 ± 11.9	2.0–75.0
Medial pterygoid	16.3 ± 8.1	5.0–40.0
Lateral pterygoid	15.9 ± 8.7	2.5–60.0
Anterior digastric	9.8 ± 4.6	3.75–30.0

[a]Units are for Oculinum/BOTOX (Allergan Pharmaceuticals, Irvine, California) (30).

At the beginning of our treatment program in 1984, there were no published guidelines for using BTX-A to treat focal dystonias. In general, our approach was empiric, beginning with small doses and titrating to the needs of the patient, selecting the muscles that on clinical examination had the greatest spasm, and drawing on our previous experience. Injections are currently performed on an ambulatory basis, except for patients who have severe jaw-closing dystonia and require parenteral feedings until treatment permits resumption of oral feeding.

Doses of botulinum toxin used are outlined in Table 4. After a careful examination, the dose is adjusted, taking into account the force of contractions, mass of muscle, and weight of the patient. Toxin is usually diluted to a concentration of 25 U/ml. Toxin is distributed over 3–5 sites into each muscle. Typically, the initial treatment is inadequate to provide substantial relief, and an additional treatment is administered in 2–4 weeks. However, after the initiation phase of treatment, we discourage "boosters" because of our concern about antibody development.

Results of injections are summarized in Table 5. The improvement in function is statistically significant for all three groups treated (Fig. 1). The duration of benefit was approximately 3 months, being longest for the patients with jaw-closing dystonia and shortest in the jaw-deviation group.

Side effects were uncommon (Table 6). Although there were 14 instances of dysphagia, only one was severe, requiring a change of diet. Most cases involved jaw-opening muscles, particularly the digastrics. One patient with jaw-closing dystonia had a marked weakness of jaw closing, requiring an elastic bandage wrapped around his jaw to assist eating. Injection of the pterygoid muscles occasionally caused rhinolalia or nasal regurgitation. One patient with severe jaw-opening dystonia was treated aggressively and developed antibodies to BTX-A.

Table 5 Results of Injections

Deviation	% Function pre-BTX-A	% Function post-BTX-A	% Change post–pre	*p* value (post–pre)	Duration of benefit (weeks)
Jaw closing	29.6 ± 2.7	72.0 ± 4.4	45.0 ± 4.6	0.0001	14.6 ± 2.1
Jaw opening	30.8 ± 4.0	73.8 ± 4.2	43.9 ± 4.7	0.0001	11.8 ± 2.1
Jaw deviation	38.8 ± 9.2	75.8 ± 12.2	37.0 ± 7.2	0.014	10.8 ± 5.0

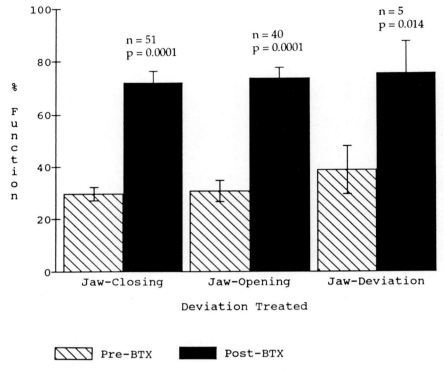

Figure 1 Percent of normal function in patients with oromandibular dystonia before and after treatment with botulinum toxin type A.

CONCLUSION

The management of OMD has been revolutionized by the introduction of BTX-A as a form of interventional neurology (31). Patients with OMD benefit from local injections of BTX-A into the inappropriately contracting muscles. In most cases of focal disease, patients discontinued alternative pharmacotherapy and have continued to benefit with repeated injections every 3–4 months; however, an occasional patient will derive benefit for up to 1 year (jaw-closing), 38 weeks (jaw-opening), or 25 weeks (jaw-deviation).

Our results are consistent with those reported by other investigators (27–29). Our doses administered are smaller than Jankovic's (28); adverse effects are less common in our series. We postulate that we can administer a lower dose of toxin with significant benefit because we employ EMG guidance to target actively contracting muscle. Use of this technique may be more important on follow-up, when islands of muscle wasting may be present.

Intraoral injections should be performed by a physician trained in the anatomy and physiology of the oral cavity and in an environment equipped to manage complications.

ACKNOWLEDGMENTS

Supported in part by NIH Grants NS-26656, NS-24778, DC-01139, CA-13696, and RR-00645, and the Dystonia Medical Research Foundation.

Table 6 Adverse Effects

Deviation	N	Total number of treatment visits	Visits with adverse effects[a] (% visits)	Patients with adverse effects (% group)
Jaw closing	51	290	12 (4.1)	6 (11.8)
Jaw opening	40	172	17 (9.9)	7 (17.5)
Jaw deviation	5	19	0	0

No. of episodes	Complaint

Jaw-Closing Dystonia

No. of episodes	Complaint
2	Weakened chewing
2	Marked soreness, pain at injection site
2	Hematoma, facial swelling
2	Headache/scalp tenderness
1	Rash
1	Enhanced lower facial spasms
1	Lower facial drooping
1	Jaw tremor
1	Swelling of knuckles
1	Dysphagia

Jaw-Opening Dystonia

No. of episodes	Complaint
13	Dysphagia
2	Nasal speech
1	Breathy voice
1	Painful chewing
1	Nasal regurgitation
1	Dysarthria
1	Clogged ears
1	Blocking antibody formation

[a]Some visits had multiple adverse effects.

REFERENCES

1. Parkes D, Schachter M. Meige, Brueghel or Blake. Neurology 1981; 31:498.
2. Gowers WR. Manual of diseases of the nervous system, 3rd ed. London: Churchill, 1899:200.
3. Meige H. Les convulsions de la face: une forme clinique de convulsions faciales, bilaterale et mediane. Rev Neurol (Paris) 1910; 21:437–443.
4. Marsden CD. Blepharospasm-oromandibular dystonia syndrome (Brueghel's syndrome). A variant of adult-onset torsion dystonia? J Neurol Neurosurg Psychiatry 1976; 39:1204–1209.
5. Thompson PD, Obeso JA, Delgado G, Gallego J, Marsden CD. Focal dystonia of the jaw and the differential diagnosis of unilateral jaw and masticatory spasm. J Neurol Neurosurg Psychiatry 1986; 49:651–656.
6. Jankovic J. Blepharospasm and oromandibular-laryngeal-cervical dystonia: a controlled trial of botulinum A toxin therapy. Adv Neurol 1988; 50:583–591.
7. Tolosa E, Marti MJ. Blepharospasm-oromandibular dystonia syndrome (Meige's syndrome): clinical aspects. Adv Neurol 1988; 49:73–84.

8. Tolosa E, Kulisevsky J, Fahn S. Meige syndrome: primary and secondary forms. Adv Neurol 1988; 50:509–515.

9. Tolosa ES. Clinical features of Meige's disease (idiopathic orofacial dystonia). A report of 17 cases. Arch Neurol 1981; 38:147–151.

10. Jankovic J, Ford J. Blepharospasm and orofacial-cervical dystonia: clinical and pharmacological findings in 100 patients. Ann Neurol 1983; 13:402–411.

11. Berardelli A, Rothwell J, Day B, Marsden C. Pathophysiology of blepharospasm and oromandibular dystonia. Brain 1985; 108:593–608.

12. Nutt JG, Hammerstad JP. Blepharospasm and oromandibular dystonia (Meige's syndrome) in sisters. Ann Neurol 1981; 9:189–191.

13. Marsden CD. Problems of adult-onset idiopathic torsion dystonia and other isolated dyskinesias in adult life. Adv Neurol 1976; 14:259–276.

14. Defazio G, Lamberti P, Lepore V, Livrea P, Ferrari E. Facial dystonia: clinical features, prognosis and pharmacology in 31 patients. Ital J Neurol Sci 1989; 10:553–560.

15. Jordan DR, Patrinely JR, Anderson RL, Thiese SM. Essential blepharospasm and related dystonias. Surv Ophthalmol 1989; 34:123–132.

16. Brin MF. Advances in dystonia: genetics and treatment with botulinum toxin. In: Smith B, Adelman G, eds. Neuroscience year, supplement to the encyclopedia of neuroscience. Boston: Birkhauser, 1992:56–58.

17. Dyken ME, Rodnitzky RL. Periodic, aperiodic, and rhythmic motor disorders of sleep. Neurology 1992; 42 (Suppl 6):68–74.

18. Blitzer A, Brin MF, Greene PE, Fahn S. Botulinum toxin injection for the treatment of oromandibular dystonia. Ann Otol Rhinol Laryngol 1989; 98:93–97.

19. Sutcher HD, Underwood RB, Beatty RA, Sugar O. Orofacial dyskinesia: a dental dimension. JAMA 1971; 216:1459–1463.

20. Klawans HL, Tanner CM. Cholinergic pharmacology of blepharospasm with oromandibular dystonia (Meige's syndrome). Adv Neurol 1988; 49:443–449.

21. Gimenez Roldan S, Mateo D, Orbe M, Munoz Blanco JL, Hipola D. Acute pharmacologic tests in cranial dystonia. Adv Neurol 1988; 49:451–465.

22. Greene P, Shale H, Fahn S. Analysis of open-label trials in torsion dystonia using high dosages of anticholinergics and other drugs. Mov Disord 1988; 3:46–60.

23. Gollomp SM, Fahn S, Burke RE, Reches A, Ilson J. Therapeutic trials in Meige syndrome. Adv Neurol 1983; 37:207–213.

24. Jankovic J, Orman J. Tetrabenazine therapy of dystonia, chorea, tics, and other dyskensias. Neurology 1988; 38:391–394.

25. Brin MF, Fahn S, Moskowitz C, et al. Localized injections of botulinum toxin for the treatment of focal dystonia and hemifacial spasm. Mov Disord 1987; 2:237–254.

26. Brin MF, Blitzer A, Greene PE, Fahn S. Botulinum toxin for the treatment of oromandibulolingual (OMD) dystonia. Neurology 1989; (Suppl 1):294 (abstract).

27. Lagueny A, Deliac MM, Julien J, Demotes Mainard J, Ferrer X. Jaw closing spasm—a form of focal dystonia? An electrophysiological study. J Neurol Neurosurg Psychiatry 1989; 52:652–655.

28. Jankovic J, Schwartz K, Donovan DT. Botulinum toxin treatment of cranial-cervical dystonia, spasmodic dysphonia, other focal dystonias and hemifacial spasm. J Neurol Neurosurg Psychiatry 1990; 53:633–639.

29. Hermanowicz NM, Rontal MM, Rontal EM, Truong D. Treatment of oromandibular dystonia with botulinum toxin. No Journal Found 1991.

30. Brin MF, Blitzer A. Botulinum toxin: dangerous terminology errors (letter). JR Soc Med 1993; 86:494.

31. Brin MF. Interventional neurology: treatment of neurological conditions with local injections of botulinum toxin. Arch Neurobiol 1991; 54(Suppl 3):7–23.

33

Botulinum Toxin Injection for Adductor Spasmodic Dysphonia

Christy L. Ludlow, Karen Rhew, and Eric Anthony Nash
National Institute on Deafness and Other Communication Disorders, National Institutes of Health, Bethesda, Maryland

CHARACTERISTICS OF ADDUCTOR SPASMODIC DYSPHONIA

Speech Symptoms

Adductor spasmodic dysphonia (SD) is an idiopathic voice disorder typically beginning between 30 and 50 years of age. Symptom onset is usually gradual, beginning with uncontrolled voice breaks, hoarseness, and increased effort associated with speaking. The symptoms typically progress over 1 to 2 years and then remain chronic. Patients report that onset may have been associated with an upper respiratory infection, a stressful period in their life, or no apparent cause. The speech is characterized by pitch or voice breaks during vowels, difficulties initiating voice (1), and a harsh, strained, effortful voice quality (2). This disorder can be distinguished from abductor spasmodic dysphonia, which is characterized by a breathy voice quality and prolongation of voiceless consonants (s, p, t, k, f, h, th).

Before 1960, SD was thought to be a psychogenic voice disorder. Aronson et al. (3,4) noted that many SD patients have movement disorders and suggested that this might be a neurological disorder. More recently, the disorder is considered a focal dystonia involving the laryngeal musculature (5). The two types of SD, adductor and abductor, are believed to be due to hypertonia in different sets of laryngeal muscles. The purpose of this chapter is to describe some of our experiences and results in treating patients with adductor SD using botulinum toxin (BTX).

Movement Abnormalities

To identify the movement abnormalities producing speech symptoms in adductor SD, fiberoptic nasolaryngoscopy is used to view the vocal folds during speech (6). Pitch and voice breaks are associated with vocal fold hyperadduction or squeezing either on voice onset or during vowels. This hyperadduction of the vocal folds disrupts the air flow through the folds, stopping vocal fold vibration, thus resulting in voice interruptions or breaks. When hyperadduction is less severe, voicing may not be disrupted but a rapid change in voice pitch may occur. These voice and pitch breaks are most easily heard during sentences with all voiced sounds, that is vowels, liquids (r and l sounds), and semivowel sounds (such as y and w). In some patients, overadductions also occur at speech onset, resulting in harsh glottal attacks. Some patients also have a harsh, strained voice quality, usually because of continuous vocal fold hyperadduction. This hyperadduction may also impair voice quality by involving the ventricular or false folds above the vocal folds. On fiberoptic examination, the ventricular folds may hyperadduct, obscuring views of the vocal folds during phonation.

In some patients, a focal vocal fold tremor may accompany adductor SD (7). The tremor becomes most evident on prolonged vowels and usually results in voice or pitch breaks at a regular rate of 4–15 Hz (8). Our experiences in using BTX in patients with focal vocal tremor are reported in chapter 37.

Muscle Activation Abnormalities

Adductor SD derives its name from the voice and pitch breaks occurring in association with spasms in the thyroarytenoid muscle during speech (9,10). In one study, the activation levels of both the thyroarytenoid and the cricothyroid muscles were heightened in adductor SD in comparison with controls during quiet respiration. This finding suggests that a constant hypertonia may be present in at least two pairs of laryngeal muscles (10). Additional quantitative studies are needed to compare activation levels of both intrinsic and extrinsic laryngeal muscles in patients with adductor SD and in normal subjects. Although the thyroarytenoid muscle is affected in adductor SD, two other adductor muscles may also be affected, the interarytenoid and the lateral cricoarytenoid. Because both are less accessible via percutaneous electromyography than the thyroarytenoid, they have not been studied extensively in this disorder. Individual differences in response to treatment may depend on the extent of involvement of muscles other than the thyroarytenoid in patients with adductor SD.

PATIENT SELECTION FOR TREATMENT: DIFFERENTIAL DIAGNOSIS

Because BTX injection could possibly have long-term detrimental effects on the laryngeal muscles, it is important to use this treatment only for neurogenic SD and not for patients whose voice disorders should be treated with less invasive methods such as voice therapy. Difficulties with differential diagnosis pose a dilemma in selecting patients for treatment with BTX. Patients with adductor SD may have other focal dystonias in addition to adductor SD, such as torticollis, suggesting a neurological disorder. However, the absence of such other disorders does not preclude adductor SD. In such cases only the speech symptoms can be used to determine the type of voice disorder. None of the voice and speech symptoms used for identifying adductor SD are pathognomonic for the disorder. As described above, adductor SD patients typically have spasmodic voice and pitch breaks on vowels and use considerable effort while talking. Other voice disorders can have similar symptoms, however. Patients with muscular tension dysphonia often have constant hoarse, effortful phonation with vocal fold hyperadduction (11). Muscular tension dysphonia is a hyperfunctional voice disorder that responds well to voice therapy aimed at improved voicing techniques, relaxation, change in head position, and changes in lifestyle. Many patients with very severe forms of adductor SD, however, can have severe constant hyperadduction similar to muscular tension dysphonia.

Other patients can have voice symptoms similar to adductor SD but may have a psychogenic disorder, possibly due to some unresolved psychological conflict (12–18). In our series, over 60% of patients with adductor SD report symptom onset following a stressful period or event in their lives such as a divorce, death in the family, or loss of employment. A positive history of stress during symptom onset, therefore, is not useful in discriminating those patients with a psychogenic disorder. The psychogenic etiology of a voice disorder can be certain only when a patient has a permanent dramatic spontaneous resolution of the voice abnormality. Some have suggested that when patients have constant hoarseness during voicing without intermittent voice or pitch breaks and are free of any structural abnormalities such as nodules, polyps, vocal fold paralysis, etc., the disorder may be psychogenic rather than neurogenic (11). When speech symptoms are not diagnostic, a trial of voice therapy may be helpful. Those patients whose symptoms reverse entirely in a few sessions of voice therapy are likely to have a psychogenic disorder. Unfortunately, the response of such patients to BTX injection has not been studied systematically at this time.

Because speech disorders can alter personal identity and self-esteem, many adductor SD patients appear to have some psychological component to their disorder. Feelings of anxiety, depression, and inadequacy may be present (19). Cannito (19) found that many SD patients are extremely anxious about their disorder, and are often overwhelmed, depressed, and narcissistic about it. These psychological problems usually resolve spontaneously following successful treatment with BTX.

Because objective criteria for differential diagnosis between muscular tension dysphonia (functional dysphonia), psychogenic dysphonia, and SD are currently unavailable, examination by a team including an otolaryngologist and a speech pathologist is recommended. If a psychogenic etiology is suspected, a neurologist and a psychiatrist should be consulted.

PERCUTANEOUS INJECTION TECHNIQUE

The first approaches used for injecting BTX into the thyroarytenoid muscles in adductor SD were percutaneous, that is, entering the larynx through the cricothyroid membrane. A Teflon-coated hypodermic 27-gauge 1½-inch needle is connected to one pole of a physiological signal amplifier with a reference electrode placed on the side of the neck. The tip and the hub are bare, allowing the needle to act as a monopolar electrode. A ground is usually placed on the patient's back. We use the same approach to the thyroarytenoid as described by Hirano and Ohala (20) for laryngeal electromyography. The external landmarks of the cricoid cartilage, the thyroid cartilage, and the cricothyroid space are identified by palpation. After the skin is cleaned with alcohol, a small subcutaneous injection of lidocaine is placed over the cricothyroid membrane. The injection needle is inserted 2–8 mm to the side of the midline through the cricothyroid membrane and angled superiorly and laterally toward the inferior edge of the vocal fold. An oscilloscope is used to visually monitor the electromyographic signal while listening to the signal via an acoustic amplifier. If the needle is in the glottic space or too close to the edge of the fold, voice will be heard in the EMG signal and seen on the monitor as a 100- to 200-Hz complex waveform in the EMG signal. In such instances, the needle needs to be directed more laterally. Similarly, if the needle is placed too far laterally the vibration of the thyroid cartilage during voicing will be seen and heard in the EMG signal. If the needle is too far inferior the lateral cricoarytenoid muscle pattern is found: increased activity during expiration and bursts at phonation onset and offset, without sustained activity during prolonged phonation. Thyroarytenoid verification patterns include sustained activity during prolonged vowel production and high activation during effort closure of the vocal folds. No predominant pattern appears in the thyroarytenoid muscle in association with respiration; thyroarytenoid motor units fire during inspiration and expiration (21).

Although this is the standard electromyographic approach used for gaining access to the thyroarytenoid muscle, it is not without problems. Once through the cricothyroid membrane, the needle must be sharply angled superiorly to reach the thyroarytenoid muscle. Depending on the angle of the needle and the variation in laryngeal anatomy among patients, the lateral cricoarytenoid or the portion of the cricothyroid that passes through the cricothyroid space and inserts just inside the inferior rim of the thyroid cartilage may be reached. The thyroarytenoid, lateral cricoarytenoid, and cricothyroid muscles are contiguous in the inferior posterior region of the vocal fold. This difficulty is compounded by the usual practice of using a monopolar electrode for BTX injection. The monopolar electrode has a wide recording field, making it impossible to determine which of the three muscles the needle tip is in. Another potential source of variability in treatment is diffusion of the toxin beyond the injection site (22). The peroral (23) and endoscopic (24) approaches to the thyroarytenoid from above the vocal fold are more likely to result in injections into the major belly of the thyroarytenoid alone, as long as the depth of insertion is not too great.

Unilateral Injections: Doses

Some centers initially used unilateral injections of BTX because of concern that bilateral weakening of the vocal folds would result in aspiration or airway problems (25,26). The left thyroarytenoid was usually selected because of the longer course of the recurrent laryngeal nerve on that side, making it more vulnerable to accidental injury in the neck or chest. Dosages ranged from 15 to 35 U. Injection at more than one site was used to increase diffusion throughout the muscle because of the even dispersion of the end plates in this muscle (27) and to prevent the accumulation of excessive fluid in one location. In our clinic, the patient is initially injected with 15 U. If adequate symptom reduction is not achieved and vocal fold movement is not significantly reduced on the injected side at 2 weeks, a second treatment of 15–20 U is administered in the same thyroarytenoid. During our first year of treating patients with this technique, a few patients were given a third injection of 30 U, resulting in a maximum total treatment of 60 U. We now use smaller doses, only occasionally administering a second injection of 15 U in the same vocal fold. The considerable variation in doses used among centers (28) may relate to differences in individual patient responses and physician experience and skill in administering the injections. Further, when patients come from a great distance, some physicians may be more likely to use larger initial dosages to eliminate the need for additional injections.

In comparing unilateral and bilateral injections, each injection type has advantages and disadvantages. The unilateral injection has the advantage that only one side of the larynx is treated, so that the potentially harmful effects of needle injury on the muscle and BTX denervation are confined to one side of the larynx. Further, the dose of a unilateral injection can be increased with less potential risk of aspiration or airway problems, because the uninjected vocal fold can compensate for the opposite weakened one. The

Table 1 Outcome Following Unilateral or Bilateral Botulinum Toxin Injection in Adductor Spasmodic Dysphonia

Measures	Unilateral[a]		Bilateral[b]	
	Mean	(SD)	Mean	(SD)
Amount/muscle (U)	19.9	(12.9)	4.2	(4.25)
Total dose (U)	19.9	(13.0)	9.5	(9.6)
Dysphagia (days)	6.1	(10.4)	7.4	(11.7)
Breathiness (days)	13.7	(22.5)	12.2	(15.9)
Best effect (days)	90.9	(67.8)	87.9	(66.1)
Symptom return (days)	131.0	(88.0)	120.0	(77.1)

[a]79 patients, 265 injections.
[b]42 patients, 238 injections.
SD = standard deviation.

disadvantage of this injection technique is that it requires more toxin, an average of 20 U per patient, in contrast with 9 U per patient with the bilateral injection technique (Table 1).

Bilateral Injection Dosages

The bilateral injection approach was first used by Brin and Blitzer (29) and is currently the most frequently used technique. Between 1.25 and 3.5 U of BTX are injected into each vocal fold, depending on symptom severity. The clear advantage is lower cost because less toxin is used per patient. Although considerable attention has been given to the effects of repeated denervation by BTX on muscle anatomy, very little, if any, attention has been given to the potential effects of repeated needle trauma over many years (30–33). Muscle fibrosis and scarring on both sides of the larynx as a result of bilateral injections could have long-term detrimental effects on voice and airway protection. Significant changes have been reported in muscle biopsies of the orbicularis oculi in patients treated for blepharospasm (30). Study of patients receiving repeated injections over many years is needed to determine the long-term effects. The other disadvantage of the bilateral approach is that if the initial injection is not effective, there is more risk that additional doses may cause excessive bilateral vocal fold weakness, causing problems with aspiration. One solution is to give the second injection in only one vocal fold, using a large dose of 10 U.

EFFECTS OF BOTULINUM TOXIN INJECTIONS IN ADDUCTOR SPASMODIC DYSPHONIA

Duration of Benefit

Patients in our treatment program are asked to keep a daily chart on their symptoms. Reinjection is not offered until at least 5 months have elapsed and symptoms have returned. Patients are asked to rate their symptoms relative to pretreatment levels on a daily basis. The scale is from +3 to −3, with 0 being their pretreatment level. If their symptoms improve relative to pretreatment levels, they are told to assign a rating from

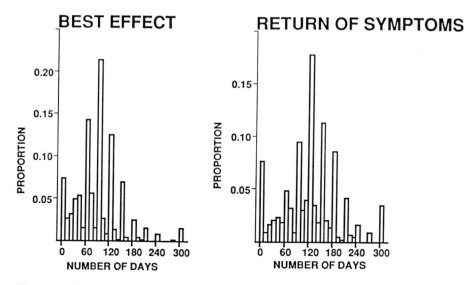

Figure 1 Frequency histograms showing the distribution of patient responses for the duration in days of their best effect following injection and the number of days before the return of symptoms. Includes the data from 503 injections.

+1 (some improvement) to +3 (excellent improvement). If symptoms or side effects are worse than before treatment, they are asked to rate them from −1 (somewhat worse) to −3 (dramatically worse). This rating scale was used by patients to rate breaks, hoarseness, effort, swallowing difficulties, and breathiness.

These daily ratings are used to determine the number of days a patient had breathiness and dysphagia by counting the number of days after injection that the patient had negative scores in each category. The duration of best effect is determined by the number of days the patient remained at the highest rating, 2 or 3. Time before the return of symptoms is the total number of days before a patient's ratings return to 0 for 3 days consecutively. Although this rating process is highly subjective, it provides an indication of the patients' response to treatment, an important measure of treatment effects.

Occasionally patients have reported voice changes within 5 hours after injection. The majority, however, have benefits beginning within 2 to 3 days after injection. The benefit can continue to increase up to 7 days following injection. Over the next few weeks, the side effects continue to decrease, while the benefits remain stable for the next few months (Table 1). No significant differences were found between unilateral and bilateral injection types in the duration of the best effect and the total number of days before the return of symptoms (Table 1). The highest proportion of patients reported a return of symptoms by 120 days, and symptoms had fully returned by 240 days in almost all patients (Fig. 1).

Side Effects

Within 3 days most patients report a significant reduction in the effort they require to produce speech. Although this effect cannot be objectively measured, it is the most significant benefit of BTX injections for adductor SD and is usually the first noticed by patients. Swallowing difficulties appear early, usually within 3 days in about 60% of

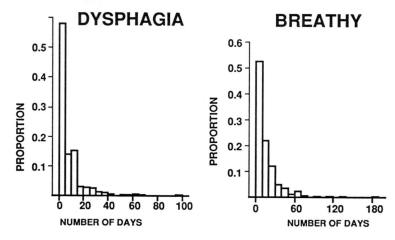

Figure 2 Frequency histograms showing the distribution of patient responses for the duration in days of dysphagia following injection and the duration in days of breathiness following injection. Includes the data from 503 injections.

patients, and are due to a slower speed of swallowing (34). These difficulties mostly affect liquids and only rarely affect solids. Patients are instructed to use a straw to reduce the amount of liquid taken for each swallow, to swallow carefully, and to change head posture by holding the head down while swallowing. Swallowing problems usually resolve within 3 to 7 days (Table 1).

Breathiness affects 65% of patients, starting 3 days following injection and lasting up to 2 weeks. Once this breathiness has resolved, the improvement in the voice becomes greatest around 3 weeks and lasts between 2 and 5 months (Table 1). During this time, the voice becomes smoother, with few or no breaks. In general, vocal quality is good, although the pitch may be somewhat higher.

In our series of 415 injections, 200 bilateral and 215 unilateral, the side effects are similar for the two types (Table 1). Breathiness was reported following 69% of bilateral and 62% of unilateral injections, while some dysphagia occurred following 62% of bilateral and 60% of unilateral injections. The breathiness was gone by 30 days and dysphagia had resolved by 15 days in most patients (Fig. 2).

Repeated Treatment

Since we began treatment with BTX in 1985, we have been following a group of patients who have received up to 15 repeated bilateral injections and another group receiving up to 10 unilateral injections. The doses have remained stable after the first few treatments, when a patient's individual effective dose was being determined (Fig. 3). No differences have been found between bilateral and unilateral injections with repeated treatments. Thus, the combined data for unilateral and bilateral injections over the first 8 treatments are plotted in Figs. 4, 5, and 6. The mean duration of the patients' best effect, usually characterized by an absence of symptoms, has steadily decreased, while the mean number of days to return of symptoms has also tended to decrease with repeated treatment (Fig. 4). The duration of dysphagia has steadily decreased with repeated treatment in only the bilateral-injection group (Kruskal-Wallis $F = 9.973$, $p = 0.02$), although breathi-

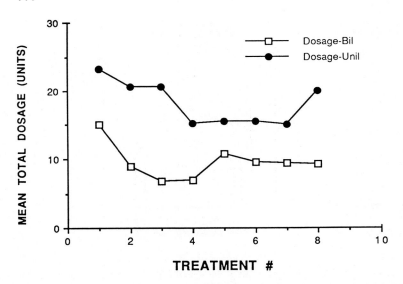

Figure 3 The mean doses used for repeated treatments for bilateral injections (filled circles) and for unilateral injections (open squares).

ness has tended to increase with repeated treatment (Fig. 5). Patients were asked to compare the severity of their symptoms before their first injection with the severity of their symptoms when these had returned after treatment. This provides an estimate of whether symptoms return to their original baseline levels after the effect of a treatment has worn off. Between 20% and 50% of the patients report that when their symptoms return 5

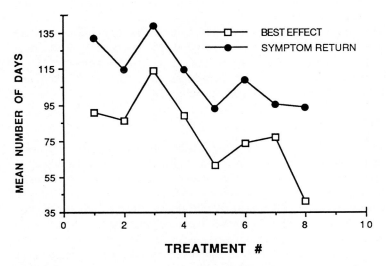

Figure 4 The mean duration in days of best effect for repeated treatments (open squares) and the mean duration in days before return of symptoms (filled circles). Includes data for both bilateral and unilateral injections.

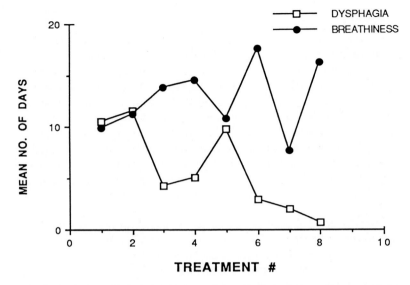

Figure 5 The mean duration in days of dysphagia for repeated treatments (open squares) and the mean duration in days of breathiness (filled circles). Includes data for both bilateral and unilateral injections.

or more months following a treatment, they are less severe than before the initial BTX injection. This phenomenon has remained stable with repeated treatment (Fig. 6), although a small proportion of patients thought their symptoms were somewhat worse.

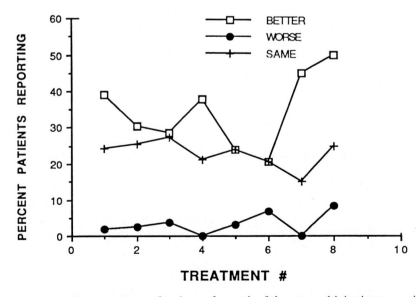

Figure 6 The percentage of patients after each of the repeated injections reporting that with the return of symptoms, their symptoms were better (open squares), or worse (filled circles) than or the same (plus signs) as before any injection.

Treatment Difficulties

Some patients have not responded well to the standard methods of BTX treatment described above. These patients required repeated injections before improvement was achieved. Among 265 unilateral treatments, 11 patients required more than two injections to achieve some benefit. Three of these patients had previously had surgical procedures for SD, such as type III thyroplasty (35) in two and unilateral recurrent nerve section (36) in another. Some of the other SD patients requiring further injections had particularly severe SD symptoms; one had severe head tremor, and another had a constant hoarseness that was never improved, although her spasms were reduced. These patients required an average total dose of 58 U to get some benefit and had an average of 54 days of symptom control or best benefit and 89 days before return of symptoms. Duration of dysphagia was 12 days and duration of breathiness was 17 days. The benefits to these patients, therefore, were less than usual, although they received an increased number of injections and a larger total dosage. Eight of these patients subsequently returned for repeated treatment and were effectively treated with one or two injections starting at a higher dose.

Similarly, in 10 of the 238 bilateral treatments, more than two injections were required to achieve some benefit. Two of these patients had undergone a type III thyroplasty, and three had had a recurrent nerve section. Three of the 10, two of whom had had surgery, were among those who were also treated at another time with unilateral injections and required more than two treatments with that approach as well. The third patient previously had contact ulcers and vocal fold stripping resulting in a constant strained hoarseness in addition to SD. In these difficult-to-treat bilaterally injected patients, the mean total amount used per muscle was 12 U, with a total dose of 41 U. On the third injection in these patients, one side was selected for a unilateral injection of between 5 and 12 U. Following treatment, these patients had an average of 9 days of dysphagia, breathiness for 12 days, a mean duration of best benefit of 33 days, and return of symptoms in 45 days.

Many of these difficult-to-treat patients had had surgical procedures (thyroplasty or nerve section) that interfered with the ability to treat them without using exceptional doses. When these patients did evidence some benefit, the benefit was relatively short-lived and the voice changes less dramatic.

Treatment Failures

Eight patients with symptoms of adductor SD have not shown any improvement following treatment with BTX injection. One man had been to several other centers, previously had a nerve section, and had a more complex disorder also involving the pharyngeal and oral-lingual musculature. Injections into both laryngeal and oral-lingual muscles produced no change in his voice and speech symptoms. A second patient had a recurrent nerve section with secondary vocal fold atrophy and glottal incompetence. He continued to have spasmodic activity on the unoperated side of the larynx and was unable to benefit from a small BTX injection, which only aggravated his symptoms. Two patients were treated several times with both the unilateral and the bilateral approach and failed to respond to either treatment. No vocal fold movement reduction was achievable, although large doses were used. Antibody testing was negative in one. The other has refused testing.

The four other nonresponders had a suspected psychogenic component to their voice disorder. One was inconsistent in her symptoms, having a normal voice at times on the telephone, but being severely impaired in our clinic. Another had a complete remission of his symptoms after an emotional confrontation with a family member. A third had a dramatic voice improvement following injection of saline but very little improvement, if any, following injection of BTX. A fourth had a severely marked tremor which started within hours of the patient's being physically attacked and had no improvement following multiple treatment attempts.

Spontaneous Remission of Symptoms

Over the last 5 years, 16 patients have demonstrated long-term relief of symptoms for periods of over 2 years. All were treated with BTX, and their initial symptoms ranged from mild to very severe. In some, symptoms never returned after a treatment. In others, symptoms started to return and then remitted gradually over several months. Several of these patients have returned regularly for follow-up examinations, allowing us to assess the degree to which they are symptom-free. No difference in the past history, previous exposure to voice therapy or psychological counseling, duration of symptoms, etc., could distinguish between those with symptom remission and others returning at regular intervals for treatment (37).

Of these 16 patients, seven have been symptom-free for over 3 years. Two of these seven patients had relatively mild symptoms of short duration, only 1 year, when they were first treated. The other 5 had moderate to severe symptoms on initial evaluation. Of these five, two required at least three injections to benefit from their first treatment. One patient received intensive voice therapy following injection and believes that his frequent work on voice therapy, combined with BTX treatment, contributed to his success. Another reported that after her second treatment the improvement in her voice allowed her to resolve several other stressful difficulties in her life. Although she continues to have some very mild symptoms, she no longer needs treatment.

The other nine of the 16 patients have had some degree of symptom return, but their symptoms are very mild and they no longer feel the need for treatment. They all say that their disorder no longer disturbs them and that they are satisfied with their current voice.

Unfortunately, there is no study of a large group of untreated patients with adductor SD for an equivalent 7-year period to determine whether spontaneous remission would occur without BTX injection. One report has found a remission rate of 14% in a group of untreated adductor SD patients (38). This rate is similar to ours and may represent a natural outcome of the disorder in a small proportion of patients.

CONCLUSIONS

Our experience thus far in using BTX injection for adductor SD has suggested that the unilateral and bilateral injections have similar benefits and side effects. The major advantage of the bilateral injection approach is that smaller amounts of toxin are used. The advantage of the unilateral approach is that the potential for needle injury is confined to one side of the larynx. Our results have demonstrated that patients with previous surgical procedures, such as thyroplasty or recurrent nerve section, can benefit from treatment, but that their benefit is of lesser degree and shorter duration than that of patients who have not had surgical procedures.

FUTURE DIRECTIONS

Our experiences with BTX have identified several issues that need to be addressed.

First, diagnostic criteria are needed to identify patients with neurogenic SD and differentiate them from patients with voice disorders that do not require treatment with BTX, such as muscular tension dysphonia, hyperfunctional voice, or psychogenic dysphonia.

Second, careful study is needed to determine the effects of repeated needle insertions independent of the effects of BTX denervation in the laryngeal muscles.

Third, our results suggest that the length of benefit may diminish with repeated treatment in adductor SD. Changes occurring in the central nervous system in response to repeated muscle denervation may alter the pathophysiology of the disorder (10,39,40). With continued treatment, a patient's disorder may adapt to peripheral changes and become increasingly resistant to treatment.

Fourth, a subgroup of patients was difficult to treat. Investigations are needed to determine whether such patients have a different pathophysiology, or whether they have additional disorders making them resistant to treatment.

Finally, the potential of some patients for spontaneous remission from adductor SD needs to be further investigated. Because ours is an experimental program and return of symptoms was required before reinjection, we were able to identify such patients. In a typical clinical practice, however, reinjection is often given more frequently in an effort to maintain patients in a symptom-free state. It is conceivable that some patients might be reinjected unnecessarily under these circumstances.

REFERENCES

1. Ludlow CL, Connor NP. Dynamic aspects of phonatory control in spasmodic dysphonia. J Speech Hearing Res 1987;30:197–206.
2. Aronson AE. Clinical voice disorders: an interdisciplinary approach. New York: Thieme-Stratton, 1980.
3. Aronson AE, Brown JR, Litin EM, Pearson JS. Spastic dysphonia: II. Comparison with essential (voice) tremor and other neurologic and psychogenic dysphonias. J Speech Hearing Disord 1968;33:219–231.
4. Aronson AE, Brown JR, Litin EM, Pearson JS. Spastic dysphonia I. Voice, neurologic, and psychiatric aspects. J Speech Hearing Disord 1968;33:203–218.
5. Blitzer A, Brin MF, Fahn S, Lovelace RE. Clinical and laboratory characteristics of focal laryngeal dystonia: study of 110 cases. Laryngoscope 1988;98:636–640.
6. Parnes SM, Lavorato AS, Myers EN. Study of spastic dysphonia using videofiberoptic laryngoscopy. Ann Otol 1978;87:322–326.
7. Aronson AE, Hartman DE. Adductor spastic dysphonia as a sign of essential (voice) tremor. J Speech Hearing Disord 1981;46:52–58.
8. Koda J, Ludlow CL. An evaluation of laryngeal muscle activation in patients with voice tremor. Ann Otol Rhinol Laryngol 1992;107:684-696.
9. Shipp T, Izdebski K, Reed C, Morrissey P. Intrinsic laryngeal muscle activity in a spastic dysphonic patient. J Speech Hearing Disord 1985;50:54–59.
10. Ludlow CL, Hallett M, Sedory SE, Fujita M, Naunton RF. The pathophysiology of spasmodic dysphonia and its modification by botulinum toxin. In: Berardelli A, Benecke R, Manfredi
    M, Marsden CD, eds. Motor disturbances. 2nd ed. Orlando, Florida: Academic Press, 1990:274–288.
11. Morrison MD, Nichol H, Rammage RA. Diagnostic criteria in functional dysphonia. Laryngoscope 1986;94:1–8.
12. Aronson AE, Peterson HW, Litin EM. Psychiatric symptomatology in functional dysphonia. and aphonia J Speech Hearing Disord 1966;31:115–127.
13. Elias A, Raven R, Butxher P, Littlejohns DW. Speech therapy for psychogenic voice disorder; a survey of current practice and training. Br J Disord Commun 1989;24:61–76.

14. Hartman DE, Daily WW, Morin KN. A case of superior laryngeal nerve paresis and psychogenic dysphonia. J Speech Hearing Disord 1989;54:526–529.
15. Kinzl J, Biebl W, Rauchegger H. Functional aphonia. A conversion symptom as defensive mechanism against anxiety. Psychother Psychosom 1988;49:31–36.
16. Sapir S, Aronson AE. The relationship between psychopathology and speech and language disorders in neurologic patients. J Speech Hearing Disord 1990;55:503–509.
17. Aronson AE. Importance of the psychosocial interview in the diagnosis and treatment of ''functional'' voice disorders. J Voice 1990;4:287–289.
18. Ginsberg VI, Wallach JJ, Strain JJ, Biller HF. Defining the psychiatric role in spastic dysphonia. General Hospital Psychiatry 1988;10:132–137.
19. Cannito MP. Emotional considerations in spasmodic dysphonia: psychometric quantification. J Commun Disord 1991;24:313–329.
20. Hirano M, Ohala J. Use of hooked-wire electrodes for electromyography of the intrinsic laryngeal muscles. J Speech Hearing Res 1969;12:362–373.
21. Chanaud CM, Ludlow CL. Single motor unit activity of human intrinsic laryngeal muscles during respiration. Ann Otol Rhinol Laryngol 1992;101:832–840.
22. Shaari CM, George E, Wu BL, Biller HF, Sanders I. Quantifying the spread of botulinum toxin through muscle fascia. Laryngoscope 1991;101:960–964.
23. Ford CN, Bless DM, Lowery JD. Indirect laryngoscopic approach for injection of botulinum toxin in spasmodic dysphonia. Otolaryngol Head Neck Surg 1990;103:5:1:752–758.
24. Rhew K, Ludlow CL. Endoscopic technique for injection of botulinum toxin through the flexible nasolaryngoscope. Otolaryngol Head Neck Surg 1992;107:239.
25. Miller RH, Woodson GE, Jankovic J. Botulinum toxin injection of the vocal fold for spasmodic dysphonia. Arch Otolaryngol Head Neck Surg 1987;113;603–605.
26. Ludlow CL, Naunton RF, Sedory SE, Schulz GM, Hallett M. Effects of botulinum toxin injection on speech in spasmodic dysphonia. Neurology 1988;30:1220–1225.
27. Rosen M, Malmgren LT, Gacek RR. Three-dimensional computer reconstruction of the distribution of neuromuscular junctions in the thyroarytenoid muscle. Ann Otol Rhinol Laryngol 1983;92:424–429.
28. Consensus Statement. Clinical Use of Botulinum Toxin. NIH Consensus Development Conference Consensus Statement 1990;8:1–20.
29. Brin MF, Fahn S, Moskowitz C, et al. Localized injections of botulinum toxin for the treatment of focal dystonial and hemifacial spasm. Mov Disord 1987;2:4:237–254.
30. Alderson K, Holds JB, Anderson RL. Botulinum-induced alteration of nerve-muscle interactions in the human orbicularis oculi following treatment for blepharospasm. Neurology 1991;41:1800–1805.
31. Harris CP, Alderson K, Nebeker J, Holds JB, Anderson RL. Histologic features of human orbicularis oculi treated with botulinum A toxin. Arch Ophthalmol 1991;109:393–395.
32. Holds JB, Alderson K, Fogg SG, Anderson RL. Motor nerve sprouting in human orbicularis muscle after botulinum A injection. Invest Ophthalmol Vis Sci 1990;31:964–967.
33. Borodic GE, Ferrante R. Effects of repeated botulinum toxin injections on orbicularis oculi muscle. J Clin Neuro-ophthalmol 1992;12:121–127.
34. Sedory SE, Ludlow CL. The effects of botulinum toxin injection on swallowing in spasmodic dysphonia. ASHA J 1989;31:164.
35. Tucker HM. Laryngeal framework surgery in the management of spasmodic dysphonia: preliminary report. Ann Otol Rhinol Laryngol 1989;98:52–54.
36. Dedo HH, Izdebski K. Intermediate results of 306 recurrent laryngeal nerve sections for spastic dysphonia. Laryngoscope 1983;93:9–16.
37. Ludlow CL, Bagley JA, Yin SG, Koda J, Rhew K. A comparison of different injection techniques in the treatment of spasmodic dysphonia with botulinum toxin. J Voice 1992;6:380-386.

38. Chevrie-Muller C, Arabia-Guidet C, Pfauwadel MC. Can one recover from spasmodic dysphonia? Br J Disord Commun 1987;22:2:117–128.
39. Ludlow CL, Baker M, Naunton RF, Hallett M. Intrinsic laryngeal muscle activation in spasmodic dysphonia. In: Benecke R, Conrad B, Marsden CD, eds. Motor disturbances. Orlando, Florida: Academic Press, 1987:119–130.
40. Ludlow CL, Schulz GM. Physiological changes following treatment of speech and voice disorders with botulinum toxin. In: DasGupta BR, ed. Botulinum and tetanus neurotoxins: neurotransmission and biomedical aspects. New York: Plenum Press, 1992; in press.

34

The Evaluation and Management of Abductor Laryngeal Dystonia

Andrew Blitzer and Mitchell F. Brin
Columbia University College of Physicians and Surgeons, New York, New York

INTRODUCTION

Laryngeal dystonia (LD) or spasmodic dysphonia (SD) is a speech disorder characterized by breaks in speech fluency. In 1871, Traube (1) coined the term "spastic dysphonia" when describing a patient with nervous hoarseness. Schnitzler (2) used the terms "spastic aphonia" and "phonic laryngeal spasm" to describe such patients. His writings on "spastic aphonia" may have been the earliest descriptions of abductor spasmodic dysphonia. In 1899, Gowers (3) described phonic paralysis as a condition in which the vocal cords could not be brought together during speech. Aronson (4,5) linked both as variations of spasmodic dysphonia and identified two subtypes: the *adductor* type, in which there is irregular hyperadduction of the vocal folds producing a strain-strangle, choked voice quality with abrupt initiation and termination of voicing resulting in short breaks in phonation and speech produced with great effort; and the *abductor* type, which is a whispering dysphonia due to intermittent abduction of the vocal folds with a reduction of loudness and aphonic segments of speech. Aronson describes "a voice in which normal or hoarse voice is suddenly interrupted by brief moments of breathy or whispered (unphonated) segments." The voice may begin as nonspecific hoarseness and over a period of days or weeks develop intermittent breathy breaks (4).

There is a small group of patients who demonstrate a mixed abductor-adductor type of voice, with an admixture of breathy breaks and tight, harsh sounds (4). Cannito and Johnson (6) proposed that both conditions exist in all patients, with a variable expression depending on the amount of adductor or abductor activity.

CLINICAL CHARACTERISTICS

There may be profound disability in patients with abductor LD. Telephone calls and stress exacerbate the disorder and make the speech pattern more unintelligible (4,7–9). Speech therapy and relaxation therapy have not been found to provide any long-term benefit, but they may help to moderate the symptoms. Pharmacotherapy also has not shown any long-term benefits. Our group reported early benefit in some patients with anticholinergics (7–9), but in most of the cases the early success was not maintained or was inadequate to improve the quality of life.

Fiberoptic laryngoscopic examination of patients with abductor LD has shown "a synchronous and untimely abduction of the true vocal folds exposing an extremely wide glottic chink" (4,9–11). The opening spasms seem to be triggered by consonant sounds, particularly when they are in the initial position in words. Patients often have a normal laugh, normal yawn, and normal humming and occasionally a normal singing voice. It was our belief that successful treatment would necessarily have to weaken the posterior cricoarytenoid (PCA) muscle(s), thereby reducing the ability of the muscle to produce spasms (7–9).

Localized injections of botulinum toxin (BTX) into the thyroarytenoid muscle(s) have been shown by our group and others to be very effective therapy for adductor LD (7–9,12–15). We have to date treated nearly 600 adductor LD patients, who recovered to average of 90% of normal function. The injections could be given comfortably via a percutaneous route in an ambulatory setting. The side effects of such injections were minimal. The effect of the injections lasted an average of 4 months (8,15).

DEVELOPMENT OF BOTULINUM TOXIN THERAPY FOR ABDUCTOR LARYNGEAL DYSTONIA

We were initially reluctant to inject BTX into the PCA muscle because of the potential for airway compromise. A severely disabled abductor dysphonia patient urged us to treat his PCA muscle to help correct his spasms, even if it necessitated a tracheostomy. One of the authors (AB) attempted to inject his PCA muscle via direct laryngoscopy without electromyographic (EMG) control. With a poor response, and an uncomfortable patient, we developed a percutaneous technique using EMG guidance. The patient's larynx is manually rotated, and a Teflon-coated hollow EMG recording needle is place through the skin, posterior to the thyroid lamina, until it reaches the cricoid cartilage. This directly impales the PCA. The patient is then asked to sniff, producing maximum PCA activity as observed on the EMG. Botulinum toxin is injected when the needle is in an area of brisk electrical activity. Our technique evolved with increased experience, good results, and a lack of complications (Figs. 1–4)

CURRENT EXPERIENCE WITH BOTULINUM TOXIN FOR ABDUCTOR LARYNGEAL DYSTONIA

Over the past 4 years we have treated 56 patients with abductor LD. We begin by weakening one PCA muscle with an injection of 3.75 U (Oculinum units) in 0.15 ml. After 1 week, a fiberoptic laryngoscopy is performed to observe the vocal cord function. In approximately 25% of our patients, weakening or paralyzing just one PCA muscle allowed for significant voice improvement. The other patients may have little or no benefit, despite production of an abductor paresis or paralysis with a unilaterally medialized vocal cord. These patients need additional toxin injections. For those who still have abduction on the treated side, an additional 2.5–3.75 U are given to paralyze the PCA. If the PCA is already paralyzed, and the voice is not improved, conservative serial doses of

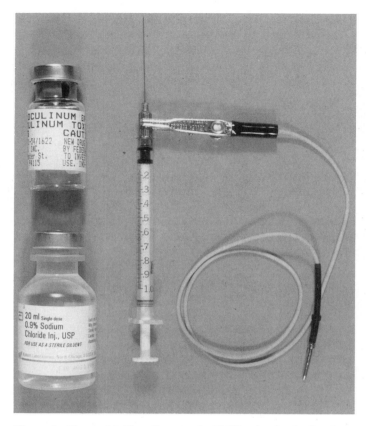

Figure 1 Freeze dried botulinum toxin (BTX); a bottle of saline for reconstitution; and a 27-gauge electromyographic injection needle used for local injections of BTX after it is placed into the posterior cricoarytenoid muscle.

0.675–2.5 U in 0.1 ml are given into the contralateral PCA. No further injections are given if there has been stridor or if the glottic chink has been significantly narrowed. When both of the patient's PCA muscles have been treated and are weakened, and there is narrowing of the glottic chink, and to patients with significant tremor, we give 2.5 U of BTX in 0.1 ml into the cricothyroid muscle. Several patients additionally have needed a combination of BTX injections of the PCA and type I thyroplasty.

The results of these injections are in scored several ways. One score uses a subjective rating scale that we have employed for 8½ years with out adductor LD patients. The patients, the doctors, and the speech therapists score the patient's voice for percentage of normal function. Videotapes of patients reading standard passages are also made on each visit. The most conservative rating is used (7,9,15).

In addition, we have developed and used a standardized vocal rating scale in which items are rated in from 1 = normal to 7 = very severe, where 2 = mild, 3 = mild/moderate, 4 = moderate, 5 = moderate/severe, and 6 = severe. The most significant items in evaluating abductor LD patients are the overall severity, breathy voice quality, aphonia, and tremor (9,13).

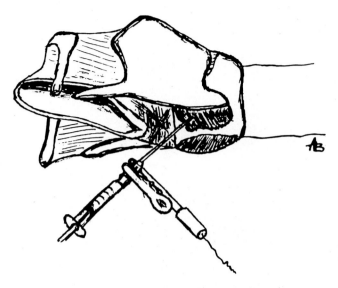

Figure 2 A diagram showing the rotation of the larynx with insertion of the electromyographic needle posterior to the posterior thyroid lamina impaling the posterior cricoarytenoid muscle overlying the cricoid cartilage.

PATIENT POPULATION

Over the past 9 years we have evaluated 93 patients who have been characterized as having abductor SD. Of these 93 patients, 47 were male (50.5%) and 46 were female (49.5%); 23 were Jewish (25%) and 70 were non-Jews (75%). There were 76 patients (82%) whose dystonia was characterized as primary, and 64 (69%) of the patients had focal involvement (including 12 with secondary dystonia). Of the 64 patients with focal dystonia, 34 were male (53%) and 30 were female (47%). The focal dystonia group was composed of 11 Jews (17%) and 53 non-Jews (83%). The age at onset of the primary focal LD ranged from 12 to 68 years, with an average of 39.6 years. In the adductor LD group, patients are 50% male and 50% female, with a mean age at onset of 38.8 years. There are 23% Jewish and 77% non-Jewish patients in a large series of adductor LD.

RESULTS

Of the 93 patients with abductor LD, we treated 56 with BTX; of these patients, 33 (59%) were male and 23 (41%) female. Of the group of 56 patients, 13 (23%) had only one PCA injected. Thirteen patients had both cricothyroid muscles injected as well as both PCAs. These were patients who, despite significant limitation of abduction, still had breathy breaks or tremor. These injections were based on work reported by Ludlow et al. (14), who reported hyperactivity of the cricothyroid (CT) muscles in patients with abductor spastic dysphonia. Ten patients in their series were found to have EMG bursts of the CT during voice breaks on speaking. They therefore postulated that these patients would benefit from BTX injection of the CT. They then gave these patients bilateral CT injections of 5–10 U/side. When assumed by spectrographic analysis of speech rate, percent

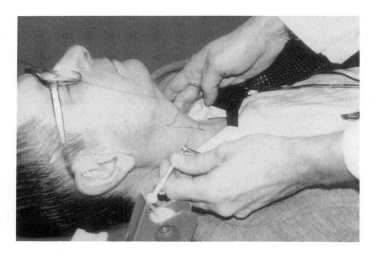

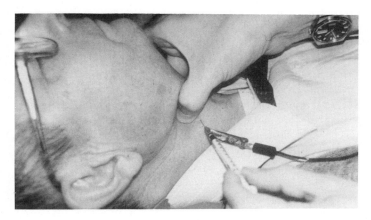

Figure 3 Photograph of the posterior cricoarytenoid muscle injection with electromyographic guidance.

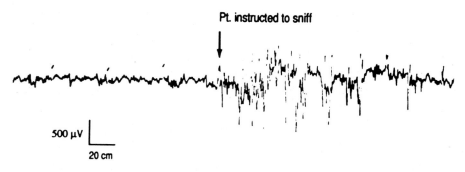

Figure 4 Electromyographic signal with needle in the posterior cricoarytenoid muscle with the patient maximally contracting the muscle with a sniff.

periodicity, and length of voiceless consonants, all patients had improvement. This treatment was not helpful in patients with only activation abnormalities of the PCA muscle.

Nine patients had a unilateral type I thyroplasty in addition to BTX injection to prevent significant abduction. This technique is based on the experience with one of our patients who was totally aphonic. Before BTX injections for abductor dysphonia, he was offered a type I thyroplasty in the belief that this would prevent a wide-open glottic chink on speaking and allow him to have some voicing. He had an initial success after surgery to about 70% of normal function. With time, however, his voice quality deteriorated. We postulated that the PCA became stronger with isometric contraction against the implant. With increasing strength, the breathiness became worse. When this occurred, we injected both of his PCA muscles with small amounts of toxin, which produced an improvement to 80% of normal function. With this experience, we treated eight additional patients who had limited benefit from bilateral PCA injections and CT injections with unilateral type I thyroplasty. All patients had improvement with this combination of treatment, with an overall improvement to 81% of normal function.

As assessed with our functional rating scale, the entire group of patients started with an average initial function of 31% (range 5–85%). The average best posttreatment function was 70% (range 40–95%). The average percent improvement was 39% (range 5–85%).

When this group of patients is subdivided further, most had only focal laryngeal abductor spasms, but eight had tremor, seven had segmental cranial or axial dystonic involvement, and three had combined tremor, segmental involvement, and/or respiratory involvement. The highest percent improvement was found in the group with focal spasms, with an average of 42.3% improvement and in the group with segmental cranial involvement, with 38% improvement. The worst percent improvement was found in the group with combined dystonic abnormalities, with only 30% improvement.

According to our standardized rating scale, the average pretreatment overall severity was 5, and the average posttreatment overall severity was 3; the average pretreatment severity of aphonia was 3.2, with an average posttreatment score of 1.8; the average pretreatment severity of breathy voice quality was 4.5, with an average posttreatment score of 1.8; and the average pretreatment severity of tremor was 2.2, with an average posttreatment score of 2.0.

The pre- and posttreatment overall severity when graphed shows a clear improvement in almost all of the cases (Figs. 5 and 6). Figure 7 shows the average pre- and posttreatment severity of tremor when graphed. Notice that several of the patients were worse after treatment. We believe that the tremor existed before but was visual and not voiced. With BTX treatment, PCA weakening occurs and the tremor becomes more audible. The quality of speech was still disabling in some cases. We believe this is due to an underlying unvoiced tremor that becomes apparent when there is increased phonation. In addition, we found a poor response to BTX in those abductor LD patients who had a combined disorder of segmental cranial or axial involvement, tremor, and/or respiratory involvement.

Since there is a variable response to toxin, we looked carefully at the preinjection factors that led to a better or worse result. From this analysis we devised a staging system for abductor LD patients (Table 1) in which stage I includes patients with focal symptoms; stage II those with segmental cranial or axial involvement; stage III those with tremor; and stage IV those who have tremor with segmental axial/cranial and/or respiratory dyssynchrony. This staging system will allow better pretreatment counseling of patients. They

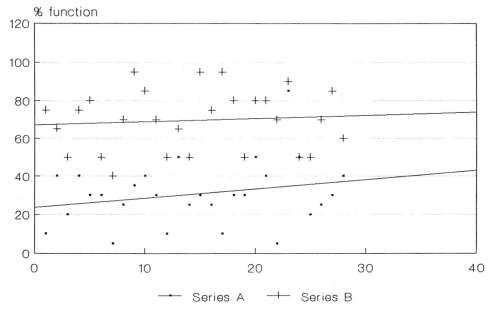

Figure 5 Graph of percent of normal function in patients with abductor laryngeal dystonia. Series A, pretreatment; series B, posttreatment.

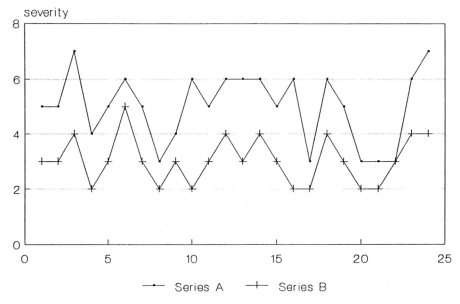

Figure 6 Graph of overall severity of abductor laryngeal dystonia on a scale of 0 as normal to 8 as most severe. Series A, pretreatment; series B, posttreatment.

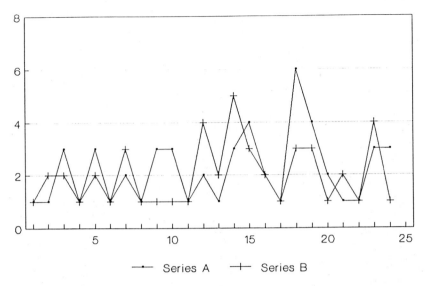

Figure 7 Graph of tremor in patients with abductor laryngeal dystonia on a scale of 0 as normal to 8 as most severe. Series A, pretreatment; series B, posttreatment.

can be prepared for the type of response expected and for the possibility that other injections or procedures may be necessary to achieve the most functional voice.

The adverse experiences have included 16 cases of exertional wheezing/stridor when going up stairs or jogging and 15 cases of mild dysphagia. The dysphagia is probably related to diffusion of some of the toxin out into the inferior constrictor muscle. These side effects have been transient, typically resolving within 1 week.

CONCLUSIONS

Our data indicate that abductor or "whispering" dysphonia is a form of laryngeal dystonia. We have found that abductor LD can be safely and effectively treated with either unilateral or bilateral posterior cricoarytenoid BTX injections using a percutaneous technique. In our series of 56 patients treated with BTX, the average improvement was to 70% of normal function. Several patients also needed cricothyroid injections and/or type I thyroplasty to maximize the benefit. Pretreatment signs of tremor, multifocal dystonic involvement, or respiratory involvement usually denoted a poorer functional result and/or a more extensive treatment course.

Table 1 Abductor Laryngeal Dystonia Staging System

Stage I:	Focal disease
Stage II:	Segmental cranial or axial
Stage III:	Tremor
Stage IV:	Tremor with segmental dystonia and/or respiratory dysynchrony

ACKNOWLEDGMENTS

Supported in part by NIH grants NS-26656, DC-01140, NS-24778, and CA-13696 and the Dystonia Medical Research Foundation.

REFERENCES

1. Traube L. Spastische Form der nervosen Heiserkeit. Gesammelte Beitr Pathol Physiol 1871;2:677.
2. Schnitzler J. Klinischer Atlas der Laryngologie nebst Anleitung zur Diagnose und Therapie der Krankheiten des Kehlkopfes und der Luftröhre. Vienna: Braumuller; 1895:215.
3. Gowers WR. Manual of diseases of the nervous system. London: Churchill; 1899:200.
4. Aronson A. Abductor spastic dysphonia. In: Aronson A, ed. Clinical voice disorders. 2d ed. New York: Thieme, 1985:187–197.
5. Aronson AE, Hartman DE. Adductor spastic dysphonia as a sign of essential tremor. J Speech Hearing Disord 1981;46:52–58.
6. Cannito MP, Johnson P. Spastic dysphonia: a continuum disorder. J Commun Disord 1981;14:215–223.
7. Blitzer A, Brin MF, Fahn S, Lovelace RE. Clinical and laboratory characteristics of laryngeal dystonia: a study of 110 cases. Laryngoscope 1988;98:636–640.
8. Blitzer A, Brin MF. Laryngeal dystonia: a series with botulinum toxin therapy. Ann Otol Rhinol Laryngol 1991;100:85–90.
9. Blitzer A, Brin MF, Stewart C, Fahn S. Abductor laryngeal dystonia: a series treated with botulinum toxin. Laryngoscope 1992;102:163–167.
10. Woodson GE, Zwirner P, Murray T, et al. Use of flexible laryngoscopy to classify patients with spasmodic dysphonia. J Voice 1991;5:85–91.
11. Parnes SM, Lavarato AS, Myers EN. Study of spastic dysphonia by video fiberoptic laryngoscopy. Ann Otol Rhinol Laryngol 1978;87:322–329.
12. Miller RH, Woodson GE, Jankovic J. Botulinum toxin injection of the vocal folds for spasmodic dysphonia. Arch Otolaryngol 1987;113:6035.
13. Ludlow CL, Naunton RF, Sedory SE, Schulz GM, Hallett M. Effect of botulinum toxin injections on speech in adductor spasmodic dysphonia. Neurology 1988;38:1200–1215.
14. Ludlow CL, Hallett M, Sevory SE, et al. The pathophysiology of spasmodic dysphonia and its modification by botulinum toxin. In: Berardelli A, Benecke R, eds. Motor disturbances II. London: Academic Press, 1990:274–288.
15. Brin MF, Blitzer A, Stewart C, Fahn S. Treatment of spasmodic dysphonia (laryngeal dystonia) with injections of botulinum toxin: review and technical aspects. In: Blitzer A, Brin MF, Sasaki CT, Fahn S, Harris K, eds. Neurological disorders of the larynx. New York: Thieme, 1992:214–229.

35

Indirect Laryngoscopic Approach for Injection of Botulinum Toxin in Spasmodic Dysphonia

Charles N. Ford

University of Wisconsin Clinical Science Center, Madison, Wisconsin

INTRODUCTION

Indirect laryngoscopy (IDL) is the most common method of visualization used by otolaryngologists for routine examination of the larynx. Using indirect visualization, the clinician can perform minor laryngeal surgical procedures including biopsies, excisions, and vocal fold injections. Medialization injections are best done with this approach because it allows for visual monitoring of contour changes with the vocal folds in a natural position and also permits incremental testing of the voice and intraoperative videostroboscopy in some cases. The advantage of visual monitoring by a technique familiar to all otolaryngologists makes this approach very useful for vocal fold injection of botulinum toxin (BTX). That portion of the vocal fold visible by IDL consists of the medial thyroarytenoid muscle (TAM), and it is the TAM that is the most common site of BTX injection for spasmodic dysphonia management. Indirect largyngoscopy allows one to direct the injection to specific regions of the muscle, varying both the anterior-to-posterior location and the depth of injection.

SELECTION OF INDIRECT LARYNGOSCOPIC PERORAL APPROACH

Injection of BTX is currently the treatment of choice for symptomatic relief of patients with spasmodic dysphonia (SD). Symptoms of adductor SD can usually be controlled by repeated injections of BTX into the TAM. Initial studies demonstrating the efficacy of BTX injections in controlling SD symptoms used relatively large BTX doses to produce paralysis of laryngeal muscles (1). Subsequent studies (2) achieved effective symptomatic relief with much smaller amounts of BTX. Since side effects of choking, aspiration, and phonatory breathiness appeared to be dose-related, we developed a protocol to determine

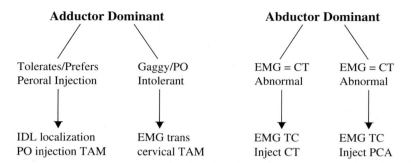

Figure 1 Algorithm that can be used in deciding the appropriate approach for injection.

the smallest effective dose. Using an IDL peroral approach we were able to direct the placement of BTX visually to produce therapeutic effects with lower doses than had been previously reported (3). In that study the minimal effective dose was titrated for each patient using incremental unilateral injections.

The IDL approach has a theoretical basis for use, in addition to the relative convenience of the technique. Rosen and his co-workers (4) studied the anatomical distribution of motor end plates in laryngeal muscles. Unlike other muscles, where the end plates are often clustered in a narrow band, motor end plates within the TAM were found to be diffusely distributed. As described elsewhere in this text, BTX acts at the myoneural junction. It seems appropriate to attempt to distribute the toxin to the greatest number of end plates in order to achieve maximum blockade with the smallest possible dose. One of the initial goals in using the IDL approach was to decrease dose-related side effects and increase the efficacy of BTX by precise placement in the TAM.

In our experience, the IDL approach is preferable to electromyography (EMG)-guided injections for all adductor SD patients who tolerate intraoral examinations without excessive gagginess. Two-thirds of the patients whom we have injected both ways prefer the peroral to the transcervical approach. We have also observed more postoperative edema and ecchymosis in the vocal folds of patients treated by cutaneous puncture with EMG guidance only.

An algorithm that can be helpful in deciding on the appropriate approach for injection is shown in Fig. 1.

TECHNIQUE

The IDL technique does not require EMG monitoring or expertise. The larynx is visualized with a regular laryngeal mirror while the patient assists by holding his or her tongue out with a gauze pad. The larynx is adequately anesthetized by dripping approximately 1 ml of 4% cocaine on the mucosal surfaces of the endolarynx. Satisfactory anesthesia can also be achieved with lidocaine or tetracaine, but cocaine is quicker and can be effective in smaller doses. A laryngeal injector device (5) (oro-tracheal injector, Xomed-Treace, Jacksonville, Florida) facilitates accurate dispensing and precise placement of the toxin in the vocal fold. The vocal fold is penetrated on the superior surface, and BTX is delivered to multiple sites on the anterior-to-posterior axis.

OUTCOMES

As with other techniques, results of peroral BTX injection are usually not evident for several days, although side effects may be noted sooner. In rare instances, patients note immediate improvement within minutes or hours of injection. This may be the result of altered proprioception from topical anesthesia or mechanical alteration of the vocal fold, and in some cases may indicate a psychogenic variant of SD. Typically, patients note a breathy dysphonia within 12–48 hr that they may describe as hoarseness. Within 1–2 weeks patients will notice less breathiness and increased smoothness, with loss of voice breaks.

For the group of patients with adductor-dominant SD, results have been excellent with relatively low doses (2.0–5.0 U) (3). A review of factors that might have an impact on response to IDL-administered BTX indicated that the specific diagnosis or type of SD was most important (6). The subjective rank-based outcome of patients with adductor SD was significantly better than for patients with either mixed or abductor SD. It also appeared that among patients with adductor SD, those with the most severe symptoms (as measured by vocal fold diadochokinetic performance) had the best outcomes. Prior BTX treatment seemed to have a favorable effect on outcome as measured by the duration of symptom-free interval after treatment; the duration of symptom relief increased with subsequent injections, with a mean increase of 4.4 weeks in this sample group. Our subsequent experience suggests that this may be a function of unilateral injection rather than IDL technique. In most of the patients showing increasing symptom-free intervals after treatment, the injections had been done unilaterally. Intolerance of peroral injection seemed to affect outcome adversely. Many of the patients who had problems with the IDL injection because of hyperactive gagging were subsequently treated with EMG trans-cutaneous injection and seemed to do better. In retrospect, it appears that technical factors may have played a role in outcome. Prior recurrent laryngeal nerve section did not adversely affect the results of patients injected by IDL. Patient age did not appear to influence response to treatment, nor did duration of symptoms before therapy. Analysis of a number of preoperative voice measures (maximum phonation time, air flow, frequency, intensity, jitter, shimmer, and signal-to-noise ratio) showed no correlation with postoperative outcome.

Objective assessment of treatment results is difficult because results are transient. Although we continue to study all patients initially and during treatment, most patients do not return when asymptomatic. They tend to return only when symptoms are returning; at that time they fail to exhibit their best posttreatment voices. Efficacy studies were limited to a group of 27 patients who returned for 1-month follow-up voice evaluation after initial treatment (7). No significant differences were noted for measures made during sustained vowel production. The posttreatment recordings of signal-to-noise ratio (SNR), jitter, shimmer, and standard deviation of fundamental frequency showed little change compared to those recorded before treatment. For example, in a comparison of pretreatment and postinjection SNR the mean change was 0.66 (SD 2.5880, $p = 0.1870$). The greatest differences attributed to BTX injection were noted during conversational speech and designated readings. Both the objective timing and the subjective distortion percentages measured from the connective speech samples taken from the first paragraph of the Rainbow Passage demonstrated significant differences. The mean time required to read the paragraph decreased by nearly 4.5 sec, while the percentage of words judged to be abnormal decreased by 41% and the percentage of words with voice breaks decreased by 26%. Perceptual judgments based on tape recordings of random pre-BTX and post-BTX samples indicated clearly improved voices in 80% of cases; 12% were questionable or caused judges to disagree, and 8% were judged worse. Most patients reported improved voices and responded to questionnaires filled out during examinations.

COMPLICATIONS

In treating more than 100 patients with IDL injection of BTX, we have had no major complications. Approximately 75% of patients describe some transient breathiness and occasional choking on liquids within a few days of injection; no patients have experienced serious airway problems or clinically significant aspiration episodes. Two patients suffered minimal abrasions and edema during our early studies when we were attempting to inject all patients with the IDL approach. Our subsequent study of patients treated with EMG-guided transcutaneous injections reveal this to be a much more common problem with the nonvisualized techniques. At this time we do not advocate IDL injection for hyperactive gaggers, and we have had no recent vocal fold injuries during IDL injection. One patient experienced hyperventilation during application of topical anesthetic to the larynx.

SUMMARY

The rationale for peroral injection is based on three assumptions: (1) This approach allows precise, visually controlled placement of BTX so that a diffuse field of motor end plates in the TAM can be affected with minimal dose; (2) patients are likely to prefer this technique because it is well tolerated by most and, if the dose is reduced, there is less likelihood of dose-related side effects such as breathiness and choking; and (3) it is a technique that relies on skills common to otolaryngologists and does not require EMG equipment or expertise. As with other procedures, it is important to select the proper patients for treatment.

For most adductor SD patients, IDL injection of BTX is the first line of chemolysis treatment. Gaggy patients and those with a low tolerance for indirect laryngoscopy and intraoral manipulation tend to do poorly with the peroral injection technique. It would appear that this approach is contraindicated for such patients as well as for those with SD of the nonadductor variety. In addition, we consider patients with allergy to local anesthetics and those with active laryngitis to be inappropriate candidates for peroral BTX injection.

REFERENCES

1. Miller RH, Woodson GE, Jankovic J. Botulinum toxin injection of the vocal fold for spasmodic dysphonia. Arch Otolaryngol Head Neck Surg 1987;113:603–605.
2. Blitzer A, Brin MF. Laryngeal dystonia: a series with botulinum toxin therapy. Ann Otol Rhinol Laryngol 1991;100:85–89.
3. Ford CN, Bless DM, Lowery JD. Indirect laryngoscopic approach for injection of botulinum toxin in spasmodic dysphonia. Otolaryngol Head Neck Surg 1990;103:752–758.
4. Rosen M, Malmgren LT, Gacek RR. Three-dimensional computer reconstruction of the distribution of neuromuscular junctions in the thyroarytenoid muscle. Ann Otol Rhinol Laryngol 1983;92:424–429.

5. Ford CN. A multipurpose laryngeal injector device. Otolaryngol Head Neck Surg 1990;103:135
   –137.
6. Ford CN. Indirect laryngoscopic approach for injection of botulinum toxin in spasmodic
   dysphonia (abstr). NIH CDC Abstracts 1990;8:131–133.
7. Ford CN, Bless DM, Patel NY. Botulinum toxin treatment of spasmodic dysphonia: techniques, indications, efficacy. J Voice 1992;6:in press.

36

Unilateral Injection of Botulinum Toxin in Spasmodic Dysphonia

Donald T. Donovan
Baylor College of Medicine and The Methodist Hospital, Houston, Texas

Kenneth Schwartz and Joseph Jankovic
Baylor College of Medicine, Houston, Texas

INTRODUCTION

Adductor spasmodic dysphonia is a voice disorder of unknown etiology characterized by frequent glottal stops and pitch breaks resulting in slow, effortful speech. Characteristically, patients have difficulty initiating phonation, and the voice sounds strained and strangled. It is most often the result of hyperadduction of the vocal folds (adductor spasmodic dysphonia), but breathy and whispering voice may result from abnormal separation of the vocal folds (abductor spasmodic dysphonia) (1,2). For many years spasmodic dysphonia was thought to be a psychogenic voice disturbance. However, current evidence suggests that adductor spasmodic dysphonia is the manifestation of an underlying neurological disorder (3,4). While it may present as a focal dystonia of the larynx without any other overt neurological signs or symptoms (5), it is often associated with laryngeal and pharyngeal tremors or is seen as one component of generalized craniofacial dystonia (Meige's syndrome) (3,6).

Multiple attempts to treat adductor spasmodic dysphonia with pharmacological agents, psychotherapy, hypnosis, voice therapy, and surgical procedures have met with limited success (7,8). In 1980, Scott proposed the use of botulinum toxin (BTX) as a therapeutic agent for the treatment of strabismus (9). It subsequently proved to be an effective modality in a multitude of neurological movement disorders, including cervical dystonia, oromandibular dystonia, torticollis, blepharospasm, hemifacial spasm, writer's cramp, and more recently hand tremor (10–14). In 1987, Miller et al. (12) reported injecting BTX in the larynx to treat two patients with severe adductor spasmodic dysphonia, with promising results. Extensive subsequent work at the same institution has demonstrated that BTX injections are very effective treatment for adductor spasmodic dysphonia.

A variety of injection techniques have been tried since the initial trial, but in our experience, the unilateral injection of BTX into the left thyroarytenoid muscle has proved to be the most consistently reliable, safe, and effective method of injection. Results are seen quickly, and patients are extremely gratified by the effect it has on their voice and their lives. In this chapter we will discuss the evaluation of the patient, the technique of unilateral injection, and the results that can be expected of this method of intervention in the treatment of various manifestations of adductor spasmodic dysphonia.

EVALUATION AND PATIENT SELECTION

All patients referred for evaluation and treatment undergo a complete neurological as well as otolaryngological head and neck examination. The laryngological evaluation includes laryngoscopy with an Olympus flexible fiberoptic nasopharyngolaryngoscope with video recordings. Video stroboscopy is also performed when the patient's voice condition permits. Stroboscopy is often not possible in patients with severe spasmodic dysphonia, because the frequent glottal stops interrupt the detection of fundamental frequency that is necessary for the strobe light to be activated. All patients should be assessed by a certified speech language pathologist for evaluation of vocal function and rehabilitation potential with speech therapy.

Proper selection of patients most suitable for injection depends on the speech and voice characteristics, the duration of symptoms, the severity of the condition, and failure to respond to alternative therapies. Persons in whom the diagnosis of spasmodic dysphonia is not confirmed by history, physical examination, and voice assessment and who do not have any appreciable form of dystonia are not offered injections. Patients whose symptoms are extremely mild or occur only intermittently should be given a trial of speech therapy. Patients who demonstrate hyperadduction of the vocal folds and involuntary contractions that result in glottal stops, pitch breaks, and decreased pitch range, with altered speech intelligibility, are considered candidates for BTX injections. Persons in whom previous therapies have failed and who are sufficiently motivated to undergo injections seem to obtain the best results from the treatment.

After complete assessment of the patient, the treatment options are discussed at length with the patient. The potential benefits as well as the risks, including the unknown long-term side effects that repeat injections may have on neuromuscular function and voice quality, should be communicated to the patient. After informed consent is obtained, the patient is prepared for the injection.

RATIONALE FOR UNILATERAL INJECTION

When the first injection of BTX for spasmodic dysphonia was done at our institution, no previous reports of laryngeal injections existed in the literature. Therefore, there were no guidelines to follow. Hence, the left thyroarytenoid muscle was chosen arbitrarily as a single injection site for the initial trials. The reasons for selection of this muscle for unilateral injection included the following: (1) if a complete paralysis of the muscle occurred there would be no risk of airway obstruction, which can be precipitated by a complete bilateral vocal cord paralysis of acute onset; (2) the nerve supply to the left thyroarytenoid muscle from the left recurrent laryngeal nerve has a much longer anatomic course in the chest and neck and statistically is more susceptible to injury or dysfunction at a future time, as a result of other medical problems such as carcinoma of the lung, thoracic aortic aneurysms, mitral valve enlargement, or cardiovascular thoracic surgery; (3) placement of the needle into the left side of the larynx is much easier for a right-handed physician standing on the patient's right side; and (4) if there were permanent long-term untoward sequelae from the BTX, only one muscle group would be damaged. As experience was gained, trials with unilateral right-sided injections, bilateral injections, and endoscopically guided direct needle placement into the left true vocal fold were performed. In our experience, the left unilateral injection proved to be the safest, easiest, and most predictable and effective method for delivery of BTX. Other investigators have clearly demonstrated acceptable efficacy of bilateral small-dose injections of BTX and multiple injections placed unilaterally, as well as endoscopically directed unilateral or bilateral injections (15–19). However, long-term follow-up of different methods of injection has not demonstrated any significant improvement in overall results over those obtained with single unilateral injections (15–19).

METHOD OF INJECTION

The unilateral injection of BTX into the left thyroarytenoid muscle is performed with a Teflon-coated needle and a 1-ml tuberculin syringe under laryngeal electromyographic (EMG) control. The details of the technique are as follows: Injections may be performed with the patient in a sitting or supine position. Most patients are more comfortable in a supine position. The procedure is described to the patient. The physician stands on patient's right side. The cricoid cartilage and cricothyroid membrane are identified by palpation. The skin of the neck overlying the cricoid cartilage is then anesthetized with 1% lidocaine solution. Usually less than 1 ml of lidocaine is necessary. Following this, standard recording electrodes are placed for simultaneous EMG recording. Any standard EMG equipment or appropriately integrated components may be used to record laryngeal muscle electrical activity.* The grounding recording electrode is placed over the clavicle, the negative electrode is placed in the region of the sternal notch, and the remaining positive electrode with an alligator clamp is used to contact the Teflon-coated needle. Before proceeding, however, the alligator clamp may be clipped to a positive electrode placed over the masseter muscle, and the patient may be asked to clench his or her teeth. Intense electrical activity seen on the oscilloscope confirms the integrity of the system before connection and placement of the actual injection needle. A modified 1½-inch 27-gauge Teflon-coated hypodermic needle is used to inject the BTX. (Fig. 1). A previously prepared solution of BTX with the appropriate dose is drawn up. In general, dilutions for laryngeal injections are 10 U/0.1 ml or 10 U/0.2 ml of injectable normal saline.

Once the dose has been selected and BTX drawn up, the syringe is attached to the needle and a positive electrode is clipped to the hub of the needle on its non-Teflon-coated metal portion. The needle is placed in the skin of the neck in the midline overlying the cricoid cartilage. The needle is then directed laterally and slightly superiorly until the cricothyroid membrane is encountered. The membrane is then pierced, with care taken to keep the needle tunneling submucosally and angling toward the left thyroarytenoid muscle. Passage through the cricothyroid membrane is usually discernible by slight increase and then sudden decrease in resistance to the pressure required to advance the needle. If the angle of insertion is too medial, the tip will pass through the subglottic

---

*Component parts consisting of recording electrodes, insulated wire connections, a preamplifier, an amplifier, and a Gould 260 Wave Form Processor with 1604 Digital Storage Oscillo Scope may be wired to detect electrical signals from thyroarytenoid muscles during the course of the procedure to permit proper identification of appropriate muscle groups.

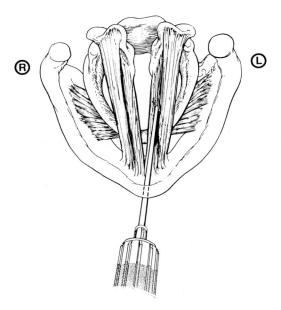

Figure 1 A Teflon-coated needle in the left thyroarytenoid muscle is directed through the cricothyroid membrane slightly superiorly and laterally. The alligator clamp and wire electrode is attached to stippled non-Teflon-coated portion of the needle.

mucosa and stimulate the patient's cough reflex or at least a sensation of need to clear the throat. If the needle is placed too lateral, the inner perichondrium of the thyroid cartilage will be encountered. This is usually associated with significant increase in discomfort or pain. It is always important to remember that anatomically the left thyroarytenoid muscle originates on the inner surface of the ipsilateral thyroid ala and that its fibers course posteriorly to insert in the muscular process of the ipsilateral arytenoid cartilage. The most superior aspect of the fibers of the muscle make up the vocalis muscle, to which is attached the vocal ligament that forms the image of vocal cord seen from the endo-laryngeal surface. Placement of the needle into the appropriate muscle is best accomplished by making individual passes in the direction of the muscle, with slight change in angulation of the needle beginning medially and working laterally (Fig. 1).

Once the muscle is located by palpation, the patient is asked to phonate the letter ''e.'' If the needle placement is in the thyroarytenoid muscle, intense electrical activity will be observed on the EMG monitor milliseconds before audible sound production is detected. The patient is asked to repeat phonation one or two more times to confirm the position of the needle by duplicating the appropriate electrical response. (Fig. 2A and B) When the position is confirmed, the BTX is slowly injected into the muscle. The needle is then withdrawn, the electrodes are removed, and the patient is observed for 5 to 10 min for any adverse effects from the procedure itself.

DOSES

The appropriate dose of BTX is the amount that achieves maximal response with minimal side effects. This will vary with each individual patient. Ten to 15 U is the most appropriate range for the initial injection. As there were no guidelines at the time of the

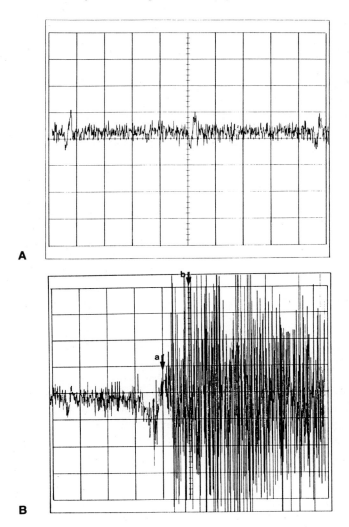

Figure 2 (A) Tracing recorded from needle placed in the left thyroarytenoid muscle during quiet respiration. Some background electrical activity is detected but no significant motor unit potentials are demonstrated. (B) The intense increase in electrical activity which is present during phonation of /i/. The electrical activity is visible (a) slightly before audibly perceptible sound production, (b), confirming the needle's location in appropriate musculature.

first laryngeal injections, 30 U of BTX was chosen at that time. This dose produces a dramatic voice response in most patients within 24 to 48 hours. However, it often makes the voice a little too breathy, and patients find themselves clearing their throats for 1–2 weeks following the injection. On examination, the patient demonstrates complete paralysis of the injected musculature. In an effort to decrease the length of time for which a patient experiences the side effects, the initial dose was gradually lowered.

Patients with uncomplicated adductor spasmodic dysphonia should receive an initial dose of 15 U. The dose at subsequent visits may be titrated on an individual basis. Patients who demonstrate a suboptimal response with no side effects may receive a larger dose in

5-U increments with each visit until maximal response with minimal side effects has been achieved. Patients who have excellent voice results without side effects or a reasonable response with undesirable side effects may receive a decreased dose in 2.5-U increments in an attempt to maximize the response and minimize the side effects by using the lowest dose possible. In our experience, as well as others', unilateral injections of less than 7.5 U have been ineffective in achieving sufficient paresis of left thyroarytenoid muscle to produce voice improvement for a satisfactory length of time (15). Conversely, no patients have required more than 30 U of BTX to attain a therapeutic response.

RESPONSE TO UNILATERAL INJECTIONS— ASSESSMENT OF RESPONSE

In general, there is detectable subjective and objective response to unilateral injection of BTX within 24–48 hr. There is occasionally a period of breathiness and mild hoarseness that lasts 10–14 days. Following resolution of side effects, the patient enjoys a maximally functional voice or peak effect period, which lasts an average of 4–6 months.

The response to BTX injection can be measured both subjectively and objectively. Objective measurements include videoendoscopic recordings, laryngeal EMG, and voice analysis of a number of parameters including fundamental frequency, frequency and pitch stability, vocal range, and aerodynamic assessments (15,20–22). Subjective measurements include patient and family assessment of voice changes, trained speech-pathological voice evaluation, and various psychosocial functional assessments. No single method of analysis is ideal for all patients, nor do all patients need to undergo comprehensive assessment including all available tests while receiving BTX injections. However, all patients should be followed by at least one method of objective and subjective evaluation.

Videoendoscopic evaluation of unilateral injection will demonstrate one of three general patterns: complete paralysis, paresis, or no visible diminution of muscular activity. In complete paralysis, the vocal fold will usually be in a paramedian position, slightly bowed, and incompletely approximated by the opposite vocal fold. The voice will be weak and breathy. The patient may have mild pooling of secretions in the posterior glottic chink. This finding is seen transiently after injection of higher doses of BTX. If the dose is excessive for an individual patient, this may last for a number of weeks. Alternatively, the patient may demonstrate paresis of the vocal fold with little or no motion; however, there will be good tone, no secretions, and good approximation from the contralateral vocal fold, which will result in a smooth functional voice. This is an optimal result on physical examination and should be the finding during the period of maximum voice improvement, if the improvement is to be attributed to BTX. The third possible finding is little or no diminution of motion of the injected musculature. This implies an ineffective injection. This may result from failure of the injection be taken up by the appropriate musculature, loss of potency of the toxin, or inadequate dose of BTX for an individual patient. All patients who have undesirable or unexpected voice, swallowing, or airway symptoms for an extended time should undergo repeat videolaryngoscopy.

Electromyographically, patients with adductor spasmodic dysphonia demonstrate a number of abnormalities. They may demonstrate increased amplitude of motor unit potentials, asynchronous activity similar to that seen in tremor disorders, or periodic bursts of activity. Some patients will have relatively normal patterns and amplitudes of electrical activity on phonation (20). Following a unilateral injection of BTX, these patients will have marked decrease in amplitude of motor unit potentials and occasional early denervation pattern of activity.

Spectrographic analysis of speech characteristics describing effects of BTX was first reported by Ludlow et al (15). They demonstrated significant reduction in pitch breaks, glottal stops, phonatory aperiodicity, and sentence time as a direct result of BTX administration. It was shown that only patients in whom some paresis of the vocal fold could be demonstrated had changes that could be documented spectrographically. Truong et al. (23) reported similar findings in a double-blind, controlled study confirming the changes to be a direct result of BTX treatment. Although speech volume is reduced, BTX does not appear to cause aphonia. (Fig. 3A and B)

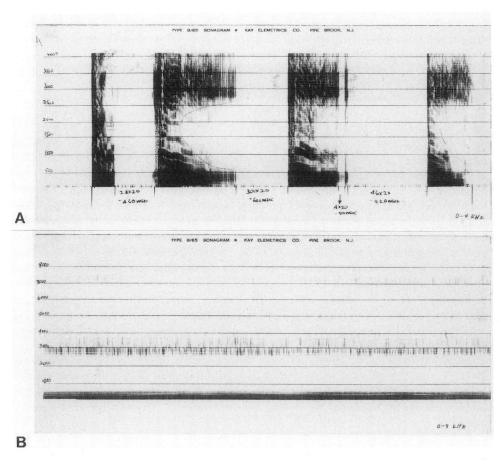

Figure 3 (A) Spectographic pattern with 300 Hz filtering of patient with severe spasmodic dysphonia (SD) phonating the letter /i/. The phonatory aperiodicity is demonstrated by loss of harmonics or lack of open space between the signals. The glottal stops are indicated by the break in the signal, and the intensity of the signal generated is signified by the intensity of the lines. (B) The spectrographic pattern of severe SD following unilateral injection of 30 U of botulinum toxin into left thyroarytenoid muscle. There is slight decrease in intensity of the signal but elimination of glottal stops and improvement in the periodicity.

Alterations in aerodynamic parameters of adductor spasmodic dysphonia have been demonstrated previously (24). Many patients exhibit irregular fluctuations of phonatory air flow and zero expiratory air flow levels intermittently. Some patients have an air flow pattern more consistent with tremor and a superimposed spasmodic pattern. Recently, unilateral injections of BTX have been shown to improve air flow control dramatically (22).

Subjectively, patients can be assessed in a number of ways. A series of rating scales that includes both patient assessment and evaluation by trained listeners is probably the most useful combination of methods. We have chosen a combination of assessments that includes functional impairment, maximum improvement or "peak effect," and global rating scale of functional improvement (14). This assessment can be obtained from (1) a daily diary in which patients are asked to record the degree of their laryngeal spasm and functional impairment; (2) audiocassette tape recordings of standard words and sentences that patients are asked to perform and return 6 to 8 weeks following their injection; and (3) review and rating of pre- and postinjection video recordings.

The severity of the dystonia is rated on a functional impairment scale (0–4) adapted from a scale used to monitor patients with other movement disorders (0 = no spasm; 1 = mild, barely noticeable; 2 = mild, without functional impairment; 3 = moderate spasm, moderate functional impairment; 4 = severe, incapacitating spasm). The peak effect is the maximum benefit obtained from the injection. The peak effect is rated on the 0–4 scale (0 = no effect; 1 = mild improvement; 2 = moderate improvement, but no change in function; 3 = moderate improvement in severity and function; 4 = marked improvement in severity and function). A global rating is used to measure the overall response and is defined as the peak effect score, minus 1 point if the injection was associated with mild to moderate complications, and minus 2 points if it was associated with severe or disabling complications. "Latency" is defined as the interval (in days) between the injection and the first sign of improvement following the injection. The maximum duration of improvement is the number of weeks during which the patients experienced the peak effect. The total duration is the entire period in weeks after the injection during which the patient notes any improvement.

Data for the first 51 patients treated at the Baylor College of Medicine departments of neurology and otorhinolaryngology confirms the effectiveness of this treatment. The results of 146 BTX injections in the first 51 patients treated over a 7-year period showed the population to be fairly representative of patients with adductor spasmodic dysphonia. There were 9 male and 42 female patients. The average age was 55 years, with a range of 28–85 years. The duration of their symptoms at the time of presentation was approximately 7 years. The criteria for unilateral injection of BTX were as outlined above. The average number of injections per patient has been three. Ninety-two percent of patient injections resulted in documented paresis of the left true vocal fold. The average duration of follow-up has been 2 ½ years.

The functional impairment associated with their spasmodic dysphonia was rated 3.63 ± 0.53 (range 1–4). Thus, this patient population had moderate to severe spasm causing significant impairment in daily function. The mean peak effect for all patients has been 3.31 ± 1.13 (range 0–4) with a global rating of 2.83 ± 1.18 (range 1–4) (Fig. 4). This suggests that most patients experienced moderate to marked improvement in severity and function. None of the patients without some paresis of the left thyroarytenoid muscle had improvement of their voice. Paresis was not achieved in 8% of patients. In unilateral injections, failure to produce some paresis results in little or no improvement in speech

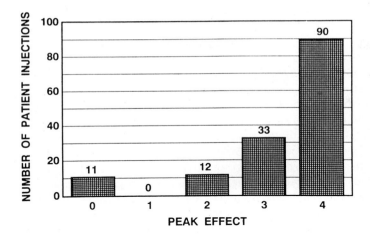

Figure 4 Graph showing the number of treatment visits producing high peak effect representing significant improvement in severity and function.

parameters measured (15). If those patients in whom no paresis was seen are excluded from the total, the average global rating is 3.0. The latency to response was approximately 2.47 ± 3.31 (range 0–14) days, and the duration of maximum response averaged 13.12 weeks ± 8.03 (range 0–54). The duration of total response (time for which patients perceived some positive effects of the injection) was 16.0 ± 9.5 (range 0–60) weeks.

COMPLICATIONS

No major life-threatening complications attributable to unilateral laryngeal injections of BTX have been reported. However, many patients experience some side effects associated with paresis of the left thyroarytenoid muscle. Symptoms patients encounter are mild dysphagia, hoarseness or breathiness of the voice, and occasional choking spells. In our experience approximately 18% of unilaterally injected patients experience some mild dysphagia characterized by throat clearing or sensation of mild choking on liquids. Twenty-eight percent have mild hoarseness, most frequently described as breathiness or loss of volume of the voice. Approximately 6% of patients feel their hoarseness or lack of volume was a significant disability in their daily function while it lasted. There were no cases of aspiration, fever, or pneumonia. All symptoms resolved as laryngeal muscle tone returned, on an average occurring in 30.87 ± 22.97 (range 3–98) days. Ludlow et al. (15) have demonstrated that there is an 80% reduction in speed of swallowing following unilateral BTX injection, as well as reduction in speech volume, but they likewise did not note any significant aspiration and had no instances of aphonia. The incidence and severity of mild dysphagia and breathiness of the voice appear to increase with higher doses (25–30 U), but lower doses result in a slight decrease in duration of peak effects.

VARIATIONS IN RESPONSE TO INJECTION

Spasmodic dysphonia is a complex speech disorder. People who develop voice characteristics of spasmodic dysphonia are not a homogeneous group of patients (2,3,23). In evaluation of response to BTX, three groups of patients have been identified. They may be categorized on the basis of videolaryngoscopic findings and associated neurological abnormalities. It is important to appreciate the differences in these subsets, as the response to therapy and the patient's perception of improvement and satisfaction with the results differ in each group. The first group consists of patients who have a focal dystonia manifested only by laryngeal spasmodic dysphonia. The second group has associated segmented cranial facial dystonias, e.g., blepharospasm, oromandibular spasm, cervical dystonia, or hemifacial spasm. The third group has a laryngeal dystonia with associated laryngeal or pharyngeal tremor contributing to their speech pattern.

Patients with an isolated laryngeal dystonia and those with other cranial facial dystonias demonstrate a hyperfunctional vocal mechanism with extreme overclosure of the glottis, strained and strangled voice quality, and very effortful speech with multiple glottal stops and pitch breaks. They tend to use the larynx more as a sphincter than a vocal instrument. Patients with associated cranial facial dystonias generally have the most difficulty in rendering any vocal sound and in communicating with others. Patients with an underlying laryngeal or pharyngeal tremor exhibit less intense spasm; nonetheless, they have significant trouble generating intelligible speech because of the modification of the speech signal by the tremor in the supraglottic and pharyngeal portion of the vocal tract.

In our experience, the group with focal laryngeal dystonia, which included 30% of all patients at the time of presentation, had moderately severe spasms with significant functional deficits. Functional impairment deficits rated 3.1 ± 1.5 (range 0–4). The peak effect of the treatment in this group was 3.8 ± 1.3 (range 1–4). The patients with severe laryngeal dystonia in association with other cranial facial dystonias had the most severe and incapacitating spasmodic dysphonia, as evidenced by their preinjection functional impairment rating of 3.5, representing severe incapacitating spasms. Peak effect in this group was 3.1 ± 0.7 (range 2–4). Duration of maximum response in both of these groups averaged 12.2 weeks, with some perceived response lasting 6 months. The patients with laryngeal dystonia and associated laryngeal or pharyngeal tremor had a peak effect of only 2.7 ± 0.9 (range 0–4). Thus, their perceived satisfaction and improvement of the spasm was less dramatic. Duration of the response was also less great, averaging only 8.8 weeks.

In patients with a significant hyperfunctional vocal mechanism, the paresis of the left true vocal fold appears to diminish not only activity on the injected side but muscle activity on the opposite side as well (22). Whether this is a direct effect of spread of toxin, which is unlikely, or the result of alteration of kinesthetic sensation and its effects on biofeedback loops within the central nervous system is unclear. In patients with intense overclosure and sphincteric laryngeal function, the decreased effort required to produce speech and the decreased time necessary to complete the speech signal (Fig. 5A and B) tend to have dramatic effects on the patient's and independent listener's perception of functional improvement.

The association of tremor with adductor dysphonia has been previously recognized (25,26). Patients with focal laryngeal adductor spasmodic dysphonia with associated tremor do not perceive as much improvement following injection. Direct visualization of the larynx demonstrates that BTX will eliminate the spasm and in many instances will diminish the tremor, but the effects on the tremor are not as complete or dramatic as they are in controlling the spasm. This results in a decreased perception of improvement on the part of the patient and the family, because the tremor continues to have some effect on the speech signal.

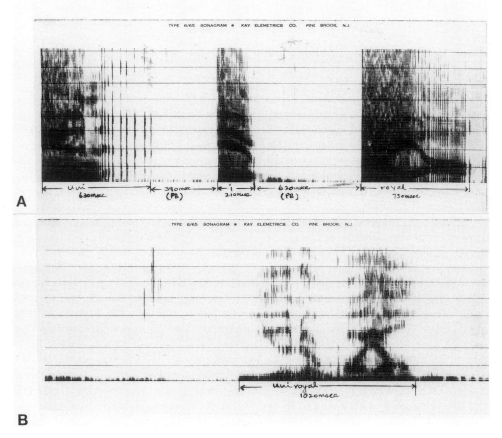

Figure 5 (A) The spectrographic pattern with 300 Hz filtering of a patient with severe spasmodic dysphonia saying the word "uniroyal." The aperiodicity, glottal stops, and pitch breaks are all evident. The total time required to vocalize this single word was 2580 msec. (B) The sound spectrograph with 300 Hz filtering of same patient saying "uniroyal," 24 hours following injection of 30 U of botulinum toxin. There has been elimination of glottal stops and pitch breaks and marked decrease in time required to deliver the speech signal, to 1020 msec.

The therapeutic response attributed to BTX is due to its ability to block neuromuscular transmission (27), although the apparent clinical effect in relieving laryngeal tension may extend beyond the injected musculature. Several clinical trials comparing BTX with placebo have clearly demonstrated that the toxin is responsible for therapeutic improvement in dystonia (13,23). Temporary paresis caused by the toxin prevents hyperadduction of the vocal folds and in most instances eliminates the glottal stops and pitch breaks. Interestingly, prevention of hyperadduction can be seen following either unilateral or bilateral injections (15,17). In addition, BTX treatment has been shown to be effective for patients in whom spasmodic dysphonia recurs after recurrent-laryngeal-nerve surgery

(28). To obtain clinical improvement with unilateral injections, however, requires slightly higher doses of the toxin (15).

ADVANTAGES AND DISADVANTAGES OF UNILATERAL INJECTION

Multiple approaches have been attempted to inject BTX into muscles most affected by spasm. Investigators have advocated single unilateral injections, multiple unilateral injections, small-dose bilateral injections, indirect laryngoscopic injections, and a point-touch technique eliminating the need for EMG confirmation of needle placement (12,15,17 –19). Each technique has its advocates, but each has advantages and disadvantages, and no one method may be ideal for every patient. However, unilateral injection of BTX into the left thyroarytenoid muscle under EMG control is clearly safe, effective, and reproducible.

Although this method does require additional equipment to monitor muscle electrical activity, there are numerous advantages. In the supine position it is extremely comfortable for the patient. Because there is no instrumentation of the nose or throat, there is no discomfort for the patient, and stimulation of the gag reflex, coughing, or choking is avoided. For patients with spasmodic dysphonia whose underlying disorder is a result of loss of fine motor control, manipulation of the nose and throat region can be extremely difficult to tolerate. While the unilateral injection does require a slightly higher total dose of toxin than is commonly used in bilateral injections, 10–15 U as compared with 5 U, it requires a single needle insertion and unilateral identification of only one muscle rather than two. Unilateral injections have a slightly longer duration of the maximum response, 12–16 weeks versus 8–12 weeks, and longer duration of overall response at 6 months or longer. Thus, unilateral injection allows a longer interval between repeat injections and is less time-consuming and expensive for the patient. At the recommended doses, almost all patients notice some improvement in a short time, which is important for many patients from a psychological standpoint. Finally, unilateral paralysis of a vocal cord will not result in any airway problems, whereas the inadvertent development of complete bilateral vocal cord paralysis could result in stridor and airway obstruction.

CONCLUSIONS

Patients with adductor spasmodic dysphonia can be categorized as having (1) focal laryngeal dystonia, (2) segmental cranial laryngeal dystonia, or (3) a combination of laryngeal and pharyngeal dystonia and tremor. Botulinum toxin injections provide improvement in the voice in over 90% of treatment sessions. Response occurs rapidly, within 1–3 days, and lasts 4–6 months. While repeat injections are required, on the average, every 4–6 months, patients are generally pleased because the treatment decreases phonatory breaks, improves pitch control, and eliminates the laryngeal discomfort and strain of vocalization and speech. Functional improvement is greatest in patients with hyperfunctional vocal mechanisms. The degree of improvement and level of satisfaction are more variable in patients with a tremor component. There do not appear to be any significant complications associated with unilateral injections. Although patients may have mild dysphagia and breathiness of voice for a few days following injections, these symptoms subside quickly and are rarely a problem for the patient. Unilateral injections may begin at 15 U of BTX injected into the left thyroarytenoid muscle under laryngeal

EMG control, and the dose should be titrated on subsequent visits, balancing effect and duration of response against the nature and duration of side effects. Delivery of BTX by this technique is an extremely safe, effective, and reliable method to treat adductor spasmodic dysphonia.

REFERENCES

1. Parnes SM, Lavarato AS, Myer EN. Study of spastic dysphonia by video fiberoptic laryngoscopy. Ann Otolaryngol 1978;87:322–326.
2. Ludlow CL, Connor NP. Dynamic aspects of phonatory control in spasmodic dysphonia. J Speech Hearing Res 1987;30:197–206.
3. Rosenfield DB, Donovan DT, Sulek M, et al. Neurologic aspects of spasmodic dysphonia. J Otolaryngol 1990;19:231–236.
4. Schaefer SD. Neuropathology of spasmodic dysphonia. Laryngoscope 1983;93:1183–1204.
5. Blitzer A, Brin MF, Fahn S, et al. Clinical and laboratory characteristics of focal laryngeal dystonia: study of 110 cases. Laryngoscope 1988;98:636–640.
6. Jankovic J, Fahn S. Dystonia syndromes. In Jankovic J, Tolosa E, eds. *Parkinson's disease and movement disorders*. Baltimore: Urban and Schwartzenberg, 1988:283–314.
7. Aronson AE, De Santo LW. Adductor spastic dysphonia: three years after recurrent laryngeal nerve resection. Laryngoscope 1983;93:1–8.
8. Aronson AE. Organic voice disorders: neurologic diseases adductor spastic dysphonia. In: *Clinical voice disorders*. New York: Thieme, 1990.
9. Scott AB. Botulinum toxin injections of eye muscles to correct strabismus. Trans Am Ophthalmalog Soc 1981;79:734–770.
10. Jankovic J, Brin MF. Therapeutic uses of botulinum toxin. N Engl J Med 1991;324;1186–1194.
11. Jankovic J, Schwartz K. Botulinum toxin injection for cervical dystonia. Neurology 1990;40:277–280.
12. Miller RH, Woodson GE, Jankovic J. Botulinum toxin injection of the vocal fold for spasmodic dysphonia. Arch Otolaryngol Head Neck Surg 1987;113:603–605.
13. Jankovic J, Orman J. Botulinum A toxin for cranial-cervical dystonia: a double-blind, placebo-controlled study. Neurology 1987;37:616–623.
14. Jankovic J, Schwartz K, Donovan DT. Botulinum toxin treatment of cranial-cervical dystonia, spasmodic dysphonia, other focal dystonias and hemifacial spasm. J Neurol Neurosurg Psychiatry 1990;53:633–639.
15. Ludlow CL, Naunton RF, Sedory SE, et al. Effects of botulinum toxin injections on speech in adductor spasmodic dysphonia. Neurology 1988;38:1220–1225.
16. Blitzer A, Brin MF, Fahn S, et al. Localized injections of botulinum toxin for the treatment of focal laryngeal dystonia (spastic dysphonia). Laryngoscope 1988;98:193–197.
17. Blitzer A, Brin MF. Laryngeal dystonia: a series with botulinum toxin therapy. Ann Otol Rhinol Laryngol 1991;100:85–89.
18. Ford CN, Bless DM, Lowery JD. Indirect laryngoscopic approach for injection of botulinum toxin in spasmodic dysphonia. Otolaryngol Head Neck Surg 1990;103:752–758.
19. Green DC, Berke GS, Gerratt BR. Point-touch technique of botulinum toxin injection for the treatment of spasmodic dysphonia. Ann Otol Rhinol Laryngol 1992;101:883–887.
20. Blitzer A, Lovelace RE, Brin MF, et al. Electromyographic findings in focal laryngeal dystonia (spastic dysphonia). Ann Otol Rhinol Laryngol 1985;94:591–594.
21. Hanson DG, Gerratt BR, Karin RR, et al. Glottographic measures of vocal fold vibration: an examination of laryngeal paralysis. Laryngoscope 1988;98:541–549.
22. Zwirner P, Murray T, Swenson M, et al. Effects of botulinum toxin therapy in patients with adductor spasmodic dysphonia: acoustic, aerodynamic, and videoendoscopic findings. Laryngoscope 1992;102:400–406.

23. Truong, DD, Rontal M, Rolnick M, et al. Double-blind controlled study of botulinum toxin in adductor spasmodic dysphonia. Laryngoscope 1991;101:630–634.
24. Davis PJ, Boone DR, Carroll RL, et al. Adductor spastic dysphonia: heterogeneity of physiologic and phonatory characteristics. Ann Otol Rhinol Laryngol 1988;97:179–185.
25. Aronson AE, Hartman DE. Adductor spastic dysphonia as a sign of essential tremor. J Speech Hearing Disord 1981;46:52–58.
26. Ludlow CL, Hallett M, Sedory SE, et al. The pathophysiology of spasmodic dysphonia and its modifiability by botulinum toxin. In: Berardelli A, Benecke R, Manfredi M, Marsden CD, eds. Motor disturbances II. London: Academic Press, 1990:273–288.
27. Sellin LC. The action of botulinum toxin at the neuromuscular junction. Med Biol 1981;59:11–20.
28. Ludlow CL, Naunton RF, Fujita M, et al. Spasmodic dysphonia: botulinum toxin injection after recurrent nerve surgery. Otolaryngol Head Neck Surg 1990;102:122–131.

37

Responses of Stutterers and Vocal Tremor Patients to Treatment with Botulinum Toxin

Sheila V. Stager and Christy L. Ludlow
National Institute on Deafness and Other Communication Disorders, National Institutes of Health, Bethesda, Maryland

INTRODUCTION

Botulinum toxin (BTX) injection into thyroarytenoid muscles is a successful treatment for patients with adductor spasmodic dysphonia (1–6), a focal dystonia of the laryngeal musculature(1). Although side effects such as swallowing problems and breathiness occur, patients continue to return for injections. This suggests that treatment benefits far outweigh side effects, even on subsequent injections (7).

Few attempts have been made to use BTX treatment for other voice and speech disorders thought not to be focal dystonias but demonstrating laryngeal muscle activation abnormalities (8–13). Two such disorders are chronic developmental stuttering and essential voice tremor. We have been injecting BTX into intrinsic laryngeal muscles of patients with both these disorders. This chapter reviews some of the rationale for using BTX to treat them and compares their reactions to this treatment with those of patients having adductor spasmodic dysphonia (ADDSD).

BACKGROUND ON STUTTERING

Stuttering is defined by the International Classification of Diseases as "disorders in the rhythm of speech, in which the individual knows precisely what he wishes to say, but at the time is unable to say it because of an involuntary, repetitive prolongation or cessation of the sound"(14). The diagnosis of stuttering is made when speech is characterized by repetitions and/or prolongations of sounds or inappropriately long silent periods during speech. Stutterers may also exhibit word or phrase repetition, word revision, insertions of filler words and sounds such as "you know" or "uh," and facial postures unusual for speech, such as closing the eyes, bobbing the head, or grimacing. All these behaviors interfere with the speaker's ability to communicate. Most stutterers also complain that the fear and anxiety accompanying speech are as much a part of the problem as these overt behaviors.

Stuttering is, in most cases, developmental. It may also occur as a conversion reaction (15) or be acquired as a result of neurological injury to unilateral subcortical pyramidal and extrapyramidal systems (16) or frontal and parietal regions (17). Onset of developmental stuttering generally occurs around the age of 4–5 years, and the disorder affects approximately 1% of the prepubescent population (18). Approximately 57–78% of stuttering children recover by age 16 (18). Stuttering is three times more prevalent in the male than in the female population. First-degree relatives of stutterers have a much higher risk of developing stuttering, especially male relatives of female stutterers, suggesting a genetic component to the disorder (18).

The cause of the intermittent breakdown in the control, timing, and coordination of the speech musculature in stuttering remains an enigma (19–21). Some aspects of stuttering are similar to other speech motor control disorders such as dysarthria, dystonia (22), and apraxia (17). With dysarthrias, stuttering shares slowing of movement initiation, exacerbation with stress, and improvement with increased task constraints (22) and with a slowed, rhythmically paced rate of speech. With dystonias, stuttering shares initiation difficulties, excessive muscle activation patterns, task-specificity, and improvement with massed practice (22). With apraxias, stuttering shares difficulty with initiation, difficulty with increased task complexity, and variability in whether a specific sound is produced correctly or fluently (17). The major difference between stuttering and other speech motor control disorders, however, is that the severity of stuttering symptoms is not consistent across time or speaking situations. Even a severe stutterer can have fluent periods, and most stutterers can speak fluently in certain situations.

Speech motor control performance has been assessed in stutterers through a variety of techniques (i.e., reaction time studies, perturbation studies, reflex studies). Stutterers are slower than control subjects on simple and complex phonatory reaction times tasks even when they are fluent (23,24). However, onset of muscle activity is not delayed in stutterers during reaction time tasks (25). During movement perturbation studies, stutterers are able to compensate normally for unanticipated loads delivered to the lower lip during fluent speech (26). However, muscle activity and displacement in response to loads are smaller in amplitude and later in time in comparison with nonstutterers. Studies of reflex activity in stutterers have demonstrated no hyperreflexia in nonspeech movements (26,27). Finally, kinematic studies of stutterers' speech have suggested that amplitudes and velocities of lip and jaw movements may be decreased (28) and that the sequencing of articulator movement may be different from that of control subjects (29).

Looking specifically at how speech is produced in stutterers, studies have focused on describing dysfluencies, in an attempt to find commonalities among the seemingly disparate symptoms of repetitions, prolongations, silent blocks, interjections, and vocalized pauses. Electromyographic (EMG) studies have reported the following abnormalities in muscles of the face, lip, jaw, and/or larynx during dysfluencies: (1) high levels of muscle activity during blocks (8,9,30–32); (2) inappropriate bursts of activity before and during periods of acoustic silence (9); (3) disruption of the normal reciprocity between abductor and adductor muscle groups during blocks (8,9); and (4) large rhythmic oscillations in lip, jaw, and neck muscles in the frequency range of 5–12 Hz (21). There are also some reports that muscles have reduced activity during dysfluencies (21,33). It should be noted that these muscle activation abnormalities could be due to the stutterer's attempts to control the speech musculature rather than to the intrusion of involuntary motor patterns during speech.

If high levels of muscle activity co-occur with dysfluencies, reducing muscle activity should be associated with improved fluency. Some researchers have compared levels of activity in stutterers in dysfluent and fluent speaking situations. Speaking in situations such as reading along with another speaker, pacing speech with a metronome, delaying auditory feedback, and speaking under masking noise improves fluency in stutterers (34). Reduced muscle activity has been reported for speech under these conditions in comparison with speech produced with dysfluencies (8). Biofeedback training to lower resting muscle activation levels before attempting speech has also been found to improve fluency (35,36). Thus, reduced activity seems to be associated with improved fluency. Because BTX is another agent that reduces muscle activity, it was hypothesized that its injection into laryngeal muscles would improve fluency.

An open trial of BTX injection into intrinsic laryngeal muscles of stutterers was initiated. The results (analyzed in 1988) for the first seven chronic adult stutterers were encouraging (2). Six of these seven subjects were severe stutterers who had previously received more traditional behavioral speech therapies but were unable to maintain their fluency following treatment. As a result of the injections, stutterers spoke faster, with longer periods of fluent speech. Significant decreases occurred in the numbers of word repetitions and interjections, but not in the numbers of sound prolongations and repetitions. The results, therefore, suggested that although stuttering frequency was not significantly reduced, other aspects of speech did improve. Although improvement has been demonstrated by objective measures, patients' subjective responses are equally important in determining the efficacy of this treatment. We now have data on 19 subjects over the last 6 years.

BACKGROUND ON VOCAL TREMOR

Voice tremor is defined as regular tremorous interruptions in the voice occurring at a frequency around 5 Hz (12). Some patients have voice tremor associated with spasmodic dysphonia (37–39), while others do not have spasmodic disruptions. Voice tremor is usually accompanied by tremor involving the head and/or hands (40–43). More rarely, it can be focal to the larynx alone (42,44). Clinically, a tremor component can be identified by asking the patient to prolong a vowel for at least 10 sec.

Unlike stuttering, both vocal tremor and ADDSD are adult-onset disorders (45). They may also occur as a conversion reaction (38,39,45). More women than men are affected by both tremor and ADDSD (45).

To understand more about tremor occurring in muscles used in respiration and phonation, patients with vocal tremor have been studied with electromyography. There has been some disagreement as to whether tremor was evidenced in intrinsic laryngeal muscles (11,13,46). This disagreement could relate to the lack of a consistent method of quantifying whether tremor was present or absent in the signal (12). When a quantification system was used, tremor was exhibited in over 80% of the thyroarytenoid recordings and at a lower percentage in the cricothryoid, posterior cricoarytenoid, and extrinsic laryngeal muscles (12). The high percentage of patients demonstrating tremor activity in the thyroarytenoid muscle suggested that thyroarytenoid BTX injections might be a reasonable treatment approach.

An open trial of BTX injection into the thyroarytenoid muscle of vocal tremor patients was initiated. The results (analyzed in 1989) with the first seven vocal tremor patients were encouraging (47). As a result of the injection, the amplitude of the tremor component, when measured in the acoustic signal, significantly decreased in six of the seven patients (47). Again, improvement has been demonstrated by objective measures, but the subjective impressions of the patients are also important. We now have data on 13 patients over the last 4 years.

BOTULINUM TOXIN INJECTIONS IN ADDUCTOR SPASMODIC DYSPHONIA, STUTTERING, AND VOCAL FOLD TREMOR

The purpose of the preceding discussion was to demonstrate that like ADDSD, stuttering and vocal tremor are associated with laryngeal muscle activation abnormalities and can be shown objectively to improve following BTX injection. Because of these factors, it was reasonable to suggest that vocal tremor patients and stutterers should also report benefit following BTX injection. To evaluate the benefit of thyroarytenoid muscle injections in these two other disorders, we collated patients' reports on the duration of symptom relief, side effects, and desire for reinjection to compare with reports obtained from patients with ADDSD.

We began evaluating the use of BTX in patients with ADDSD and stuttering in 1986 and in patients with vocal tremor in 1988. For comparison purposes, we evaluated patient responses to all open-trial, EMG-guided percutaneous unilateral or bilateral thyroarytenoid muscle injections in all three groups. All patients met the following criteria: (1) no psychogenic component to their disorder; (2) no other neurological conditions, such as blepharospasm, Meige's syndrome, torticollis, stroke, or trauma; (3) no other speech/language disorders; and (4) no previous medical procedures for their symptoms, including recurrent laryngeal nerve section or crush, thyroplasty, or vocal cord stripping. Within disorder classifications, the severity of symptoms ranged from mild to severe. In addition, most stuttering patients had received traditional behavioral therapies and reported no long-term benefit for their fluency. Only one was receiving speech therapy at the time of injection. Table 1 summarizes patient characteristics in the three groups.

Following every injection, patients were asked to fill out a rating sheet daily for several months. They were asked to rate the degree to which the side effects of breathy/hoarse voice and dysphagia affected them and the degree to which the injection changed their symptoms. Pitch and phonatory breaks were rated in ADDSD, voice shakiness and effort were rated in voice tremor, and number of dysfluencies or blocks, fear of speaking, and tension were rated in stutterers. A seven-point rating scale was used. Patients were told that a rating of 0 meant that their symptoms and side effects were unchanged from the day of injection (baseline). Negative scores (-1 to -3) were to be used if patients thought their symptoms or side effects were worse than at baseline, and positive scores ($+1$ to $+3$) if patients thought their symptoms or side effects were better than at baseline. Subjects were asked to keep daily logs until the ratings for all factors had returned to 0.

From these logs, we were able to determine the number of days that patients reported having the side effects of dysphagia and breathy/hoarse voice. The number of days on which the subjects reported the largest positive score for any symptom (meaning they felt they were benefiting from the injection) was considered the number of days of best effect. Once their symptom ratings started to decline, we were able to determine the number of days required for symptoms to return to 0, or baseline.

Table 1 Characteristics of the Three Patient Groups: Adductor Spasmodic Dysphonia (ADDSD), Vocal Tremor, and Stuttering

Group	No. of patients	% female	Mean age (yr)	Age range (yr)	No. of injections	% bilateral
ADDSD	101	65	47.4	22–77	303	44
Stuttering	19	21	35.4	18–56	23	30
Tremor	13	92	59.5	33–75	24	41

Comparisons of number of days of side effects and benefit between the three groups of patients had to take into account the fact that the data included both bilateral and unilateral injections. Significantly less toxin is injected with bilateral than with unilateral injections, but the number of days of benefit is equally great for the two injection types in ADDSD, and the duration of breathiness is somewhat shorter for bilateral than unilateral injections in men with ADDSD (7). A contingency table was computed to determine whether the distributions of bilateral and unilateral injections differed in the three groups, and no significant differences were found (Table 1). Thus, the data from both injection types were pooled.

The total number of injections received by patients in the three groups differed, because we started injecting ADDSD and stuttering patients in 1986 and did not start injecting patients with tremor until 1988. A Kruskal-Wallis analysis revealed a significant difference ($p = 0.02$) between the groups for the number of years since the first injection. Thus, a direct comparison between the three groups of the total number of injections was not valid. For this reason, we elected to analyze data for only the first two injections to determine whether there was differences in the number of days of side effects and number of days of benefits.

Because the amount of BTX injected did not differ among the three groups for the first two injections, Kruskal-Wallis analyses were conducted to examine group differences in outcome (Table 2). No significant differences were found among the three groups for the number of days of dysphagia or days of hoarseness. However, significant differences were found for the number of days of best effect and number of days needed to return to baseline.

The ADDSD and tremor patients were similar in the number of days of reported benefit and the duration before return to baseline. The stutterers, however, reported fewer days of benefit and fewer days to return to baseline in comparison with the other two groups. Laryngoscopic examination revealed that a decrease in vocal fold movement was achieved for all stutterers. These patients also did not exhibit fewer days of side effects as compared with the other two groups. Therefore, we cannot conclude that stutterers did not get adequate doses of BTX. We can only conclude that the difference in stutterers' responses to BTX lies in the nature of their disorder.

Another aspect of perceived benefit is the number of times patients returned for subsequent injection. A contingency table revealed significant differences among the three groups in the mean number of injections (Table 2). One could argue that this was an artifact related to the number of years since patients had been admitted. For example, a patient admitted in 1992 was eligible for only one injection, while a patient admitted in 1986 could have been eligible for up to 13 injections. Therefore, another approach was used to address this question. Each patient was categorized as having either one or many

Table 2 Injection Outcomes in the Three Patient Groups: Adductor Spasmodic Dysphonia (ADDSD), Vocal Tremor, and Stuttering

Group	Years injected	Mean no. of rounds	No. days dysphagia	No. days hoarse	No. days of best effect	No. days return to baseline
ADDSD	3.8	4	7.5	13.3	91.5	134.7
Stuttering	3.1	2	5.3	13.6	39.2	61.2
Tremor	2.8	3	8.6	11.9	80.9	123.4
Statistical comparison	K-W, 0.02	Chi-square, 0.009	K-W, NS	K-W, NS	K-W, 0.008	K-W, 0.006

K-W = Kruskal-Wallis; NS = not significant.

injections. A contingency table revealed that the three groups were significantly different ($p = 0.04$) in the distributions of patients receiving one or more injections (Table 3). About 40% of stutterers did not return for subsequent injections, as compared with about 10% of the ADDSD patients and 9% of the vocal tremor patients.

Not only did the percentage of subjects receiving only one injection differ, but the ADDSD patients and the stutterers had different reasons for not wanting to be reinjected. In the ADDSD group, one patient was admitted in 1992 and was waiting for a second injection; two patients reported side effects and no benefits (in one a vocal fold growth developed that may have affected his response); two patients went to another center after the first injection; and the remaining nine reported long-term effects (for at least 2 years) or return to normal voice following a single injection. Among the stutterers, two patients did not want to be reinjected because the side effects, breathiness in particular, outweighed their speech benefit. Four patients did not perceive that they benefited from injection. In summary, a majority of the ADDSD patients who received only one injection at our facility were pleased with the effects of BTX, while one-third of the stutterers were dissatisfied. In addition, some ADDSD patients have benefited from a single BTX injection for at least 2 years, while no stutterers or voice tremor patients have demonstrated long-term effects.

About 60% of stutterers did request more than one injection. The issue then becomes whether they have continued to request BTX injections. Of the 19 stutterers, only 2 (11%) currently use BTX as the primary means for managing their stuttering. This can be compared with the 98% of ADDSD patients and 100% of voice tremor patients who do so.

These figures suggest that BTX has little potential for long-term treatment of stuttering. However, before BTX is dismissed as a treatment, its outcome should be compared to the long-term benefits from other therapies. The results of BTX treatment should be compared with data on long-term outcomes for behavioral therapy. It should be kept in mind, however, that only stutterers who had failed to maintain fluency following traditional behavioral therapy were included in this study.

Behavioral therapy usually involves training stutterers to produce speech in a manner different from natural speech, by allowing some air to escape through the vocal folds before voice onset, slowing their speech rate, or exaggerating speech movements. While fluency initially improves with these techniques (48), stutterers often obtain little benefit or tend not to use such techniques over the long term.

In behavioral therapy, only one-third of stutterers report continued success with using techniques for 6 months, one-third return to pretreatment levels, and another third never

Table 3 Percentage of Patients Who Received One or More Injections in the Three Patient Groups: Adductor Spasmodic Dysphonia (ADDSD), Vocal Tremor, and Stuttering

Group	One injection	More injections
ADDSD	12	88
Stuttering	38	62
Tremor	0	100

Chi-square $= 6.48$, $p = 0.04$.

complete the therapy (49). Considering the possible population differences, BTX treatment was only somewhat less successful: one-third were dissatisfied following one injection, 55% stopped using BTX after a few injections because of perceived lack of benefit, and only 11% of stutterers continued to use BTX to manage fluency past 1 year.

One of the major reasons cited for failure of behavioral therapy is that speech following treatment is distinguishable from normal (50–54) and requires constant control. Stutterers seem to prefer stuttering over using altered speech patterns following behavioral therapy or having changes in their voice quality following BTX injection.

DISCUSSION

Injecting BTX into thyroarytenoid muscles of patients with ADDSD, vocal tremor, and stuttering resulted in different reports of perceived benefit for the three groups. The patients of all groups received a therapeutic dose of BTX and reported similar durations for the side effects of breathiness/hoarseness and dysphagia. However, the duration of best effect and the number of patients returning for multiple injections differed. Both the ADDSD and voice tremor patients were enthusiastic about the treatment. The duration of best effect was similar for both populations, and both groups were likely to return for reinjection. If an ADDSD patient received only one injection at our facility, this was not due to displeasure with the result of the injection. Stutterers, on the other hand, reported fewer days of benefit and did not always return for multiple injections. This patient population seemed disturbed by the side effects, which minimized their perception of any benefit.

We were not able to compare across patient groups the specific aspects of improvement, because they differed depending on the disorder. For example, pitch breaks occur in ADDSD, but not so much in tremor or stuttering. Blocks occur only in stuttering, and not in tremor or ADDSD. However, we can offer some observations on a few of the more specific factors.

One of the few factors that were reported by all patient groups was the amount of effort required for speech. A reduction of effort was noted by both ADDSD and tremor patients regardless of the quality of their voice. In fact, this seemed to be the greatest benefit from the patients' perspective, and they did not seem to worry about how they sounded to others. Stutterers reported the opposite. They did not spontaneously note reduced tension as a benefit. When asked, they acknowledged that their blocks might be reduced in effort, but they focused on how different their speech sounded from others', and from their own voice before injection.

One of the major factors that needs to be addressed in the treatment of stuttering is their fear of speaking, anxiety about using the telephone, etc. Subjects did not necessarily report that BTX injections reduced their fear of speaking. This would make this treatment ineffective in this group regardless of significant speech changes in the clinical setting.

These subjective results could be related to differences in patients' expectations of improvement as a result of the onset of these disorders. Patients with ADDSD or tremor had a normal voice for a long time before developing their voice disorder. Suddenly, they were unable to communicate with as much facility as before, and the impact of this must be devastating. For them, any treatment that eases their symptoms and allows them to communicate would be an improvement. Stutterers, on the other hand, have been stuttering all their life, and have learned, with varying degrees of success, to continue to communicate. Thus, improvement to them may mean how closely their speech approximates normalcy.

In conclusion, then, BTX injection does not seem to be beneficial in the treatment of stuttering. In contrast, voice tremor seems to be benefited by thyroarytenoid injections, and the duration of effect and long-term benefits seem to be similar to those of patients with ADDSD.

ACKNOWLEDGMENTS

The authors would like to acknowledge others who have contributed to this research: Jo Bagley, M.S., Mihoko Fujita, M.D., Junji Koda, M.D., Ralph Naunton, M.D., Eric Nash, M.D., Karen Rhew, M.D., Toshiyuki Yamashita, M.D., and Sheng-Guang Yin, M.D.

REFERENCES

1. Blitzer A, Brin MF. Laryngeal dystonia: a series with botulinum toxin therapy. Ann Otol Rhinol Laryngol 1991; 100:85–89.
2. Ludlow CL. Treatment of speech and voice disorders with botulinum toxin. JAMA 1990; 264:2671–2675.
3. Ford, CN, Bless DM, Lowery JD. Indirect laryngoscopic approach for injection of botulinum toxin in spasmodic dysphonia. Otolaryngol Head Neck Surg 1990;103:752–758.
4. Ludlow CL, Naunton RF, Sedory SE, Schulz GM, Hallet M. Effects of botulinum toxin injections on speech in adductor spasmodic dysphonia. Neurology 1988;38:1220–1225.
5. Truong DD, Rontal M, Rolnick M, Aronson AE, Mistura K. Double-blind controlled study of botulinum toxin in adductor spasmodic dysphonia. Laryngoscope 1991;101:630–634.
6. Jankovic J, Schwartz K, Donovan DT. Botulinum toxin treatment of cranial-cervical dystonia, spasmodic dysphonia, other focal dystonias and hemifacial spasm. J Neurol Neurosurg Psychiatry 1990;53:633–639.
7. Ludlow CL, Bagley JA, Yin SG, Koda J, Rhew K. A comparison of different injection techniques in the treatment of spasmodic dysphonia with botulinum toxin. J Voice 1992;6(4):380–386.
8. Freeman FJ, Ushijima T. Laryngeal muscle activity during stuttering. J Speech Hearing Res 1978;21:538–562.
9. Shapiro A. An electromyographic analysis of the fluent and dysfluent utterances of several types of stutterers. Fluency Disord 1980;5:203–231.
10. Conture EG, McCall GN, Brewer DW. Laryngeal behavior during stuttering. J Speech Hearing Res 1977;20:661–668.
11. Tomoda H, Shibasaki H, Kuroda Y, Shin T. Voice tremor; dysregulation of voluntary expiratory muscles. Neurology 1987;37:117–122.
12. Koda J, Ludlow CL. An evaluation of laryngeal muscle activation in patients with voice tremor. Ann Otol Rhinal Laryngol 1992;107(5):684–696.

13. Ardran G, Kinsbourne M, Rushworth G. Dysphonia due to tremor. J Neurol Neurosurg Psychiatry 1966;29:219–223.
14. World Health Organization. Manual of the international statistical classification of diseases, injuries, and causes of death. Geneva: World Health Organization, 1977:202.
15. Mahr G, Leith W. Psychogenic stuttering of adult onset. J Speech Hearing Res 1992;35:283–286.
16. Ludlow CL, Rosenberg J, Salazar A, Grafman J, Smutok M. Site of penetrating brain lesions causing chronic acquired stuttering. Ann Neurol 1987;22:60–66.
17. Rosenbeck J, Messert B, Collins M, Wertz RT. Stuttering following brain damage. Brain Lang 1978;6:82–96.
18. Andrews G, Craig A, Feyer A-M, Hoddinott S, Howie P, Neilson M. Stuttering: a review of research findings and theories circa 1982. J Speech Hearing Res 1983;48:226–246.
19. Kent RD. Stuttering as a temporal programming disorder. In: Curlee RF, Perkins WH, eds. The nature and treatment of stuttering: new directions. Boston: College Hill Press, 1984:283–302.
20. Mackay DG, MacDonald MC. Stuttering as a sequencing and timing disorder. In: Curlee RF, Perkins WH, eds. The nature and treatment of stuttering: new directions. Boston: College Hill Press, 1984:261–282.
21. Smith A. Neural drive to muscles in stuttering. J Speech Hearing Res 1989;32:252–264.
22. Ludlow CL. Measurement of speech motor control processes in stuttering. In: Peters HFM, Hulstijn W, Starkweather CW, eds. Speech motor control and stuttering. Amsterdam: Elsevier, 1991:479–491.
23. Watson BC, Alphonso PJ. Physiological bases of acoustic LRT in nonstutterers, mild stutterers and severe stutterers. J Speech Hearing Res 1987;30:434–447.
24. Peters HFM, Hulstijn W, Starkweather CW. Acoustic and physiological reaction times of stutterers and nonstutterers. J. Speech Hearing Res 1989;32:668–680.
25. Harbison DC, Porter RJ, Tobey EA. Shadowed and simple reaction times in stutterers and nonstutterers. J Acoust Soc Am 1989;86:1277–1284.
26. Caruso AJ, Gracco VL, Abbs JH. A speech motor control perspective on stuttering: preliminary observations. In: Peters HFM, Hulstijn W, eds. Speech motor dynamics in stuttering. New York: Springer-Verlag, 1984:245–258.
27. Smith A, Luschei ES. Assessment of oral-motor reflexes in stutterers and normal speakers: preliminary observations. J Speech Hearing Res 1983;26:322–328.
28. Zimmerman G. Articulatory dynamics of simple ''fluent'' utterances of stutterers and nonstutterers. J Speech Hearing Res 1980;23:95–107.
29. Caruso AJ, Abbs JH, Gracco VL. Kinematic analysis of multiple movement coordination during speech in stutterers. Brain 1988;111:439–455.
30. Fibiger S. Stuttering explained as a physiological tremor. Speech Trans Lab Quart Stat Rep 1971;2–3:1–24.
31. Kolotkin M. Manschreck R, O'Brien D. Electromyographic tension levels in stutterers and normal speakers. Perceptual and Motor Skills 1979;49:109–110.
32. Platt LJ, Basili A. Jaw tremor during stuttering block. J Commun Disord 1973;6:102–109.
33. McClean M, Goldsmith H, Cerf A. Lower-lip EMG and displacement during bilabial disfluencies in adult stutterers. J. Speech Hearing Res 1984;27:342–349.
34. Andrews G, Howie P, Dozsa M, Guitar B. Stuttering: speech pattern characteristics under fluency-evoking conditions. J Speech Hearing Res 1982;25:208–216.
35. Guitar B. Reduction of stuttering frequency using analog electromyographic feedback. J Speech Hearing Res 1975;18:672–685.
36. Hanna R, Wilfling F, McNeill B. A biofeedback treatment for stuttering. J. Speech Hearing Disord 1975;40:270–273.
37. Hartman DE, Vishwanat B. Spastic dysphonia and essential (voice) tremor treated with primidone. Arch Otolaryngol 1984;110:394–397.
38. Aronson AE, Brown JR, Litin EM, Pearson JS. Spastic dysphonia: II. Comparison with

essential (voice) tremor and other neurological and psychogenic dysphonias. J Speech Hearing Disord 1968;33:219–231.

39. Aronson AE, Hartman DE. Adductor spastic dysphonia as a sign of essential (voice) tremor. J Speech Hearing Disord 1981;46:52–58.

40. Lou JS, Jankovic J. Essential tremor: clinical correlates in 350 patients. Neurology 1991;42:234–238.

41. Findley LJ, Gresty MA. Head, facial and voice tremor, Adv Neurol 1988;49:239–253.

42. Brown JR, Simonson J. Organic voice tremor. Neurology 1963;13:520–525.

43. Massey EW, Paulson GW. Essential vocal tremor: clinical characteristics and response to therapy. South Med J 1985;78:316–317.

44. Hachinski VC, Thomsen IV, Buch NH. The nature of primary vocal tremor. Can J Neurol Sci 1975;2(3)195–197.

45. Aronson AE, Brown JR. Litin EM, Pearson JS. Spastic dysphonia. I. Voice, neurologic, and psychiatric aspects. J Speech Hearing Disord 1968;33:203–218.

46. Shipp T, Izdebski K, Reed C, Morrissey P. Intrinsic laryngeal muscle activity in a spastic dysphonic patient. J Speech Hearing Disord 1985;50:54–59.

47. Ludlow CL, Sedory SE, Fujita M, Naunton RF. Treatment of voice tremor with botulinum toxin injection (abstr). Neurology 1989;39:353.

48. Andrews G, Guitar B, Howie P. Meta-analysis of the effects of stuttering treatment. J Speech Hearing Disord 1980;45:287–307.

49. Martin RR. Introduction and perspective: review of published research. In: Boberg E, ed. Maintenance of fluency. New York: Elsevier North Holland, 1981:1–30.

50. Ingham RJ, Gow M, Costello J. Stuttering and speech naturalness: some additional data. J Speech Hearing Disord 1985;50:217–219.

51. Ingham RJ, Packman AC. Perceptual assessment of normalcy of speech following stuttering therapy. J Speech Hearing Res 1978;21:63–73.

52. Martin RR, Haroldson SK, Triden K. Stuttering and speech naturalness. J Speech Hearing Disord 1984;49:53–58.

53. Runyan CM, Adams MR. Perceptual study of the speech of "successfully therapeutized" stutterers. J Fluency Disord 1978;3:25–39.

54. Runyan CM, Adams MR. Unsophisticated judges' perceptual evaluations of the speech of "successfully treated" stutterers. J Fluency Disord 1979;4:29–38.

MISCELLANEOUS DISORDERS

38

Treatment of Tremors with Botulinum Toxin

Joseph Jankovic
Baylor College of Medicine, Houston, Texas

CLINICAL CHARACTERISTICS AND DIFFERENTIAL DIAGNOSIS OF TREMORS

Tremor is a rhythmic, oscillatory movement produced by alternating or synchronous contractions of antagonist muscles. It is the most common movement disorder, but only a small fraction of those who shake seek medical attention. Tremors can be classified according to their phenomenology, distribution, frequency, or etiology (1,2). Phenonemonologically, tremors are divided into two major categories: rest and action tremors. *Rest tremor* is present when the affected body part is fully supported and not actively contracting; it is absent during voluntary muscle contraction and during movement. *Action tremors* occur with voluntary contraction of muscles, and they can be further subdivided into postural, kinetic, task- or position-specific, and isometric tremors. *Postural tremor* is evident during maintenance of an antigravity posture, such as holding arms in an outstretched horizontal position in front of the body. *Kinetic tremor* can be seen when the voluntary movement starts (*initial tremor*), during the course of the movement (*dynamic tremor*), and as the affected body part approaches the target, e.g., while performing the finger-to-nose or the toe-to-finger maneuver (*terminal tremor*). *Task-specific tremors* occur only during, or are markedly exacerbated by, a certain task, such as writing (primary handwriting tremor), or speaking or singing (voice tremor). *Position-specific tremors* occur while holding a certain posture (e.g., the "wing-beating" position or holding a cup close to the mouth), or while standing (orthostatic tremor). *Isometric tremor* occurs during a voluntary contraction of muscles that is not accompanied by any appreciable change in the position of the body part. Tremors can also be classified according to their anatomical distribution, e.g., limbs, head, tongue, voice, and trunk. Because of the complexity of limb tremors, it is best to describe them according to the joint about which the oscillation is most evident, e.g., metacarpal-phalangeal joints, wrist, elbow, and ankle. In most tremors, the frequency ranges from 4 to 10 Hz. The "slow" tremors (frequency 1–3 Hz) are sometimes referred to as "myorhythmia" and are usually associated with brain stem pathology, while the "fast" tremors (frequency 11–20 Hz) often represent harmonics of other tremors. Some investigators believe that "orthostatic tremor" is simply a harmonic of essential tremor.

Parkinsonian disorders are responsible for the majority of rest tremors. Rest tremor typically consists of a 4- to 5-Hz alternating supination-pronation movement of the forearm sometimes accompanied by an adduction-abduction tremor of the thumb (the "pill-rolling" tremor). In addition to hand and arm tremors, there is often a foot flexion-extension and leg abduction-adduction tremor as well as a rhythmical jaw opening-closing movement and a lip and chin tremor. Head/neck oscillation is rarely seen in Parkinson's disease, unless there is coexistent essential tremor (3).

In addition to rest tremor, parkinsonian patients often also exhibit postural tremor; but the most common types of postural tremor are physiological and essential tremors. By definition, physiological tremor is not symptomatic. A variety of factors can exacerbate physiological tremor and make it not only symptomatic, but even disabling. Frequencies of physiological and enhanced physiological tremors are typically 8–12 Hz in the hands but may be as low as 6.5 Hz in other parts of the body. The amplitude of physiological (and essential) tremor may be enhanced by anxiety, stress, exercise, fatigue, thyrotoxicosis, hypoglycemia, hypothermia, pheochromocytoma, alcohol withdrawal, beta-adrenergic and dopaminergic drugs, lithium, valproate, neuroleptics, tricyclics, cyclosporine, pindolol, xanthines (caffeine, theophylline), and other toxins (e.g., dioxin).

Besides parkinsonian rest tremor, essential tremor is the most common type of tremor seen by neurologists. It has been estimated that there are more than a million cases of essential tremor in the United States (4). Although essential tremor is often termed "benign," in many instances it is functionally disabling, interfering with activities of daily living and one's livelihood. Patients with essential tremor often have difficulties with writing, eating, and pouring of liquids. When it affects the voice it may compromise speaking and singing. Furthermore, the tremor is often a source of embarrassment and may interfere with normal social interactions. Essential tremor is transmitted as an autosomal dominant trait with very high penetrance. The frequency of essential tremor ranges between 4 and 12 Hz, and there is an inverse relationship between frequency and amplitude (5). Essential tremor is most evident when the hands and arms are held against gravity (postural tremor). Some variants of essential tremor occur only during the performance of a specific activity (e.g., writing).

Patients with cerebellar outflow lesions usually exhibit a coarse postural and kinetic tremor, most evident during goal-directed movements (e.g., finger-to-nose). Lesions of the dentate nucleus or the superior cerebellar peduncle proximal to the decussation correlate with kinetic tremor ipsilateral to the side of the lesion, whereas lesions distal to the decussation result in kinetic tremor contralateral to the side of the lesion. Lesions in the cerebellar hemisphere tend to produce kinetic tremors with a variable frequency ranging from 5 to 11 Hz; high brain stem lesions are usually associated with tremor frequency in the range of 5–7 Hz, and lower brain stem lesions produce faster tremors, ranging from 8 to 11 Hz (6). In contrast, the frequency of classical midbrain (red nucleus) tremor is relatively slow, at 2–3 Hz (7).

PATHOPHYSIOLOGY OF TREMORS

Our understanding of the mechanisms involved in the generation of tremors has been facilitated by the development of neurophysiological and other quantitative techniques such as electromyographic (EMG) recordings and uniaxial and triaxial accelerometers, and by the application of computer technology to analyze the frequency spectra and other tremor-related physiological variables (8,9). There is a growing body of evidence supporting the notion that central oscillators are important in the generation of physiological and pathological tremors (10–12). Intracellular recordings have demonstrated that neurons in the inferior olive and other brain stem and subcortical nuclei have spontaneous oscillatory activity (11,12). Disinhibition of central oscillators in the basal ganglia and thalamus, as a result of nigrostriatal dopamine deficiency, is thought to contribute to the pathophysiology of parkinsonian rest tremor (10,11). Spinal proprioceptive reflexes may modify the spontaneous oscillatory activity (13,14). The frequency and amplitude characteristics of physiological tremor are largely determined by the mechanical properties of the limb, stretch reflexes, and the heart's mechanical activity (15). Mechanical loading, such as attaching weights around the wrist, decreases peak tremor frequency of physiological tremor (16). In contrast, tremor frequency remains constant and independent of load in patients with postural kinetic tremor and essential tremor (16,17). Cerebellar kinetic tremor is associated with error in timing and amplitude of the EMG activities of agonists and antagonists (18,19). The important role of peripheral reflex mechanisms in the pathogenesis of cerebellar kinetic tremor is supported by the observation that the character of the tremor can be altered by mechanical loading to the tremulous limb (20).

TREATMENT OF TREMORS

When designing protocols to study the effects of a therapeutic intervention on tremor-related functional impairment and on the mean amplitude (and frequency) of tremor, it is important to be constantly aware of the marked and intra- and interindividual and diurnal variations (21). Unified Tremor Rating Assessment (UTRA) is currently being evaluated and validated by the Tremor Investigation Group (TRIG). This rating scale is designed to assess functional disability caused by tremor. Recent studies have demonstrated that despite biomedical and technological advances, clinical rating scales can produce a more valid index of tremor-induced disability than various "quantitative techniques," including accelerometry and EMG (22,23).

The treatment of rest tremors is similar to that of parkinsonism and consists chiefly of anticholinergic and dopaminergic drugs (24). Although most rest tremors do not cause severe disability, some high-amplitude rest tremors may be quite embarrassing, annoying, and even exhausting. These tremors rarely improve with pharmacological therapy. In such medically intractable cases, ventral lateral thalamotomy may provide benefit by dramatically reducing the amplitude of the tremor (25–27). Although this procedure is effective in a majority of cases, the tremor recurs in about 20% of patients, and there is a considerable risk of contralateral hemiparesis, hemianesthesia, ataxia, speech disturbance, and other potential complications. These are compounded when the procedure is performed bilaterally. Tremor can be relieved not only by a thalamic lesion, but also by thalamic stimulation, perhaps through "jamming" of the low-frequency oscillatory inputs (28).

Using high-frequency ($\geq$ 100 Hz) stimulation, with the tip of a monopolar electrode implanted stereotactically in the ventral intermedial nucleus of the thalamus (Vim) contralateral to the disabling tremor, Benabid et al. (28) noted "complete relief" of contralateral tremor in 27 of 43 thalami stimulated (63%) and "major improvement" in 11 (23%). The series included 26 patients with Parkinson's disease and six with essential tremor; seven patients were previously treated with thalamotomy. Although thalamic stimulation is promising, its chronic effects are still unknown. Regrettably, thalamic stimulation does not appear to be useful in the treatment of predominantly kinetic and axial tremors. Stereotactically placed lesions in the external, posteroventral portion of the medial globus pallidum (GPi) or in the subthalamic nucleus were reported to result not only in marked improvement in tremor but also in bradykinesia (27,29–31). However, contralateral hemiparesis, hemiballism, and visual field defects are among several potential risks that must be considered before these procedures can be recommended for patients with drug-resistant tremors.

The treatment of postural tremor depends largely on its severity; many patients require nothing more than simple reassurance. Alcohol reduces the amplitude of essential tremor in about two-thirds of patients; some use it regularly for its "calming" effect and some use it prophylactically, for example before an important engagement where the presence of tremor could be a source of embarrassment (2). Although there is no evidence that patients with essential tremor have an increased risk of alcoholism, the regular use of alcohol to treat essential tremor is inadvisable and must be discouraged. Propranolol, a beta-adrenergic blocker, remains the most effective drug for the treatment of essential tremor and enhanced physiological tremors, although other beta blockers may also exert antitremor activity (32). A central mechanism of action has been suggested for this group of drugs, but some beta blockers exert potent antitremor activity even though they are not lipid-soluble and hence do not cross the blood-brain barrier. This suggests that the therapeutic effect of beta blockers may be mediated, at least in part, by the peripheral beta-adrenergic receptors (33). Propranolol and other beta blockers, however, may cause fatigability, sedation, depression, and sexual impotence, and these drugs should be avoided in the presence of congestive heart failure, chronic pulmonary obstructive disease, asthma, and insulin-dependent diabetes. The antitremor effect of primidone has been confirmed by several controlled and open trials (34,35). Primidone, however, can cause sedation, dizziness, and a variety of idiosyncratic reactions. The benzodiazepine drugs, such as lorazepam, clonazepam, and diazepam, and barbiturates also may have some ameliorating effects on essential tremor and its variants.

Kinetic tremors caused by cerebellar outflow lesions are usually resistant to pharmacological therapy, although carbamazepine and clonazepam may provide at least partial relief (36,37). Wrist weights, when applied before meals, may enable patients with severe kinetic tremor to feed themselves (20). A lesion or high-frequency stimulation of the Vim nucleus of the thalamus may offer a useful alternative to some patients with severe and disabling cerebellar tremor (28,38).

Despite advances in the pharmacological and surgical treatment of tremors, current antitremor therapies are not entirely satisfactory in all patients, and drug-induced side effects and surgical complications often limit their usefulness. There is a need for an effective therapy that would, without the risk of serious complications, control intractable tremor and improve the patient's ability to perform activities of daily living.

TREATMENT OF TREMORS WITH BOTULINUM TOXIN

Botulinum toxin (BTX) has been used in the treatment of a variety of dystonic and related conditions (39). The therapeutic effects are thought to be primarily due to its action at the neuromuscular junction. The heavy chain of the toxin binds to the presynaptic cholinergic terminal, and the light chain prevents the quantal release of acetylcholine from the presynaptic vesicle by cleaving synaptic protein SNAP-25 (40). This causes chemodenervation of the injected muscles. Discussion of the structure and mechanism of action of BTX is beyond the scope of this chapter; this topic is reviewed in chapters 1 and 2.

Dystonia is often accompanied by dystonic, essential, or both types of tremor (3,41,42). The coexistence of dystonia and tremor is particularly evident in patients with task-specific movement disorders, such as writer's cramp (43). During our 10-year experience with BTX treatment in more than a thousand patients with various forms of dystonia, we observed that patients with dystonia and coexistant tremor noted improvement not only in their abnormal dystonic movements and postures, but also in their tremor, when they were treated with BTX. Since tremor of any cause is produced by muscle contractions, we postulated that chemodenervation of the abnormally contracting muscles with BTX may be beneficial in the treatment of tremors (44).

In our original trial, we treated 51 patients with various disabling tremors with BTX (44). The tremors were classified as dystonic in 14, essential in 12, a combination of dystonic and essential in 22, parkinsonian in one, peripherally induced in one, and of midbrain origin in one. The average age of the patients was 55.8 years, and average duration of symptoms was 13.9 years (Table 1). During a total of 160 treatment visits, an average of 242 ± 75 U of BTX were injected per visit in cervical muscles of 42 patients with head tremor, and 95 ± 38 U in forearm muscles of 10 patients with hand tremor; one patient was injected in both. Patients with lateral (negation) oscillation of the head were injected in both splenius capitis muscles, and in one or both sternocleidomastoid muscles if there was an anterior-posterior (affirmation) component. Asymmetrical dosages or additional neck muscle injections were often required in patients with dystonic tremor. The muscles were identified by observation and palpation. Electromyography was not particularly helpful either for localizing the involved muscles or for guiding the injections. The total dose was distributed into four to six different sites anatomically related to those muscles involved in the production of the tremor: wrist extensors (predominantly extensor carpi radialis and ulnaris) and wrist flexors (predominantly flexor carpi radialis and ulnaris). In some patients we also injected more proximal muscles (e.g. biceps, triceps, deltoid) if the clinical examination indicated more widespread involvement. The doses in

Table 1 Botulinum Toxin in Tremor: Demographic Data (N = 51)

Sex (women)	30 (59%)
Age (yr)	55.8 ± 11.8 (19–80)
Age at onset (yr)	42.1 ± 13.7 (5–66)
Duration of tremor (yr)	13.9 ± 12.6 (1–52)
Severity of tremor	3.1 ± 0.8 (1–4)

Source: Ref. 44.

Table 2 Botulinum Toxin in Tremor: Results (N = 51)

Variable	Mean ± SD	(Min–max)
Peak effect	3.0 ± 1.2	(0–4)
Head tremor	3.0 ± 1.1	(0–4)
Hand tremor	2.0 ± 1.7	(0–4)
Essential tremor	3.4 ± 0.9	(1–4)
Dystonic tremor	3.5 ± 0.6	(2–4)
Combination tremor	3.0 ± 1.4	(0–4)
Latency of effect (days)	6.8 ± 7.2	(0–35)
Duration of total response (weeks)	12.5 ± 7.5	(0–36)
Duration of maximum response (weeks)	10.5 ± 6.4	(0–26)

Source: Ref. 44.

the opposing muscle groups varied, depending in part on whether there was evidence of coexistent dystonia.

The average peak effect, defined as the maximum benefit rated on a 0–4 scale, was 3.0. Thirty-five (67%) patients improved (peak effect ≥ 1) (Table 2). The average latency from injection to response was 6.8 days, and the average duration of maximum improvement was 10.5 weeks. Local complications, lasting an average of 20.6 days, were noted in 17 patients (40%) injected for head tremor, consisting chiefly of dysphagia in 12 (29%), transient neck weakness in four (10%), and local pain in two (5%) (table 3). Six patients (60%) with hand tremor had transient focal weakness. Electromyographic recordings showed decreased amplitude of EMG bursts after BTX treatment (Table 4) (Fig. 1). In addition to improvement in these quantitative measures, some patients noted improvement in their ability to perform daily activities, such as eating, dressing, and writing (Fig. 2).

Although the results of this original pilot study must be confirmed by a well-designed placebo-controlled trial, the results of our experience are encouraging enough to conclude that BTX is a promising new therapy for patients with intractable tremor. In another pilot study, all eight patients (seven with Parkinson's disease and one with essential tremor) reported some improvement (45). This ranged from mild to marked, with a mean of 2.6 on a 0–4 global rating scale. Only three patients showed more than 50% reduction in tremor severity on a clinical rating scale and by physiological measurements.

Table 3 Botulinum Toxin in Tremor: Complications

	Patients		Visits	
Any complication	23/51	(45.1%)	31/160	(19.4%)
Localized weakness	9/51	(17.6%)	12/160	(7.5%)
Hand	6/10	(60.0%)	8/20	(40.0%)
Neck	4/42	(9.5%)	24/141	(17.0%)
Dysphagia	12/42	(28.6%)	14/141	(9.9%)
Disabling complications	0		0	

Source: Ref. 44.

Table 4 Electromyographic Results (N = 14)

EMG Variable	Before treatment	After treatment
Amplitude $(\mu V)^a$	58.8 ± 52.0	12.3 ± 21.2
Frequency (Hz)	5.0 ± 0.7	4.5 ± 1.9
Burst duration (msec)	107.7 ± 33.1	76.9 ± 36.6
Interburst interval (msec)	83.8 ± 29.8	77.5 ± 32.3

[a]$p < 0.01$ (paired *t*-test).
Source: Ref. 44.

BEFORE BOTOX

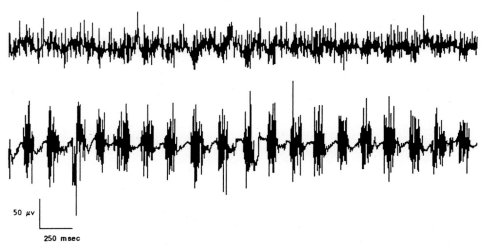

AFTER BOTOX

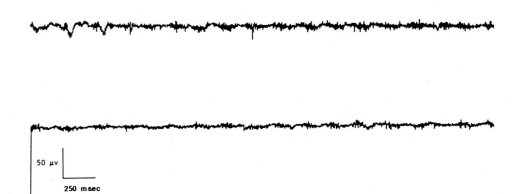

Figure 1 Electromyographic activity in forearm extensor (upper tracing) and flexor (lower tracing) muscles in a patient with essential tremor before and after treatment with botulinum toxin.

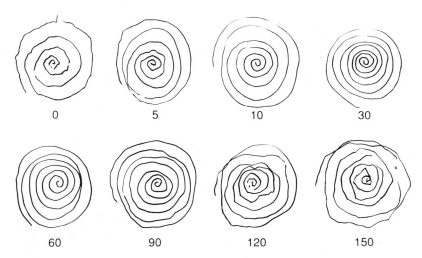

Figure 2 Tremulous drawing of a patient with essential tremor before botulinum toxin (BTX) injection. After 5 days there is an improvement in the drawing, which is maintained 10 through 90 days after treatment. The handwriting tremor subsequently recurs as the effects of BTX wear off.

The beneficial effects of BTX in voice tremor have been previously suggested, but not fully described (46). In their recent update on 13 patients treated with BTX for voice tremor, Stager and Ludlow (chapter 37) concluded that voice tremor, was as amenable to this treatment as was spasmodic dysphonia. Although some patients developed dysphagia and hoarseness, lasting on the average 8.6–11.9 days, most have noted improvement in their tremor for 2.7–4.1 months. In our own experience, however, we find that patients with voice tremor, either alone or in combination with spasmodic dysphonia, do not respond as well to BTX injections as do patients with isolated spasmodic dysphonia.

The encouraging results of these open trials should be confirmed by a controlled study. A double-blind, placebo-controlled trial of BTX in essential tremor of hands is currently being conducted in multiple centers. It is important to point out that, while controlled studies are needed, the design of such studies is not an easy task. The challenge is to design a controlled trial that allows for flexibility. This is critical in order to obtain optimal therapeutic result. In the treatment of tremor, the dose and the site of injection may change from one treatment to the next depending on the response to previous treatments (whether favorable or not) and on residual effects at the time of subsequent injection. Although the therapeutic effect demonstrated by a controlled trial may not be as robust as that indicated by open trials, the controlled trial may provide clues to which patients may be the best candidates and what method promises the best results. One advantage of this treatment over drugs is that it produces no systemic side effects, and its efficacy appears to be the same or similar irrespective of the etiology of the tremor. The disadvantage of this treatment are that it is usually applicable only in focal tremors, there is often an accompanying weakness, the effects are transient, and the treatment is quite costly. Future studies should examine which clinical variables, anatomical locations, etiologies, and methods of injection determine best the effects of BTX on tremor.

REFERENCES

1. Hallett, M. Classification and treatment of tremor. JAMA 1991;266:115–117.
2. Lou JS, Jankovic J. Tremors. In: Appel SH, ed. Current neurology. Vol. 11. Chicago: Mosby Year Book, 1991:199–232.
3. Lou JS, Jankovic J. Essential tremor: clinical correlates in 350 patients. Neurology 1991; 41:234–238.
4. Findley LJ, Koller WC. Essential tremor: a review. Neurology 1987;37:1194–1197.
5. Elble RJ, Higgins C, Hughes L. Longitudinal study of essential tremor. Neurology 1991;42:441–443.
6. Cole JD, Phillip HI, Sedgwick EM. Stability and tremor in the fingers associated with cerebellar hemisphere and hemisphere tract lesions in man. J Neurol Neurosurg Psychiatry 1988;51:1558–1568.
7. Sabra AF, Hallett M. Action tremor with alternating activity in antagonist muscles. Neurology 1984;34:151–156.
8. Elble RJ, Koller WC. The measurement and quantification of tremor. In: Tremor. Baltimore: Johns Hopkins University Press, 1990:10–36.
9. Gresty M, Buckwell D. Spectral analysis of tremor: understanding the results. J Neurol Neurosurg Psychiatry 1990;53:976–981.
10. Lamarre Y. Animal models of physiological, essential and parkinsonian-like tremors. In: Findley LJ, Capildeo R, eds. Movement disorders: tremor. New York: Oxford University Press, 1984:183–194.
11. Llinas RR. The intrinsic electrophysiological properties of mammalian neurons: insights into central nervous system functions. Science 1988;242:1654–1664.
12. Kepler TB, Marder E, Abbott LF. The effect of electrical coupling on the frequency of model neuronal oscillators. Science 1990;240:83–85.
13. Burne JA. Reflex origin of parkinsonian tremor. Exp Neurol 1987;97:327–339.
14. Logigian EL, Wierzbicka MM, Bruyninckx F, Wiegner AW, Shahani BT, Young RR. Motor unit synchronization in physiologic, enhanced physiologic and voluntary tremor in man. Ann Neurol 1988;23:242–250.
15. Marsden CD. Origins of normal and pathological tremor. In: Findley LJ, Capildeo R, eds. Movement disorders: tremor. New York: Oxford University Press, 1984:37–84.
16. Elble RJ. Physiologic and essential tremor. Neurology 1986;36:225–231.
17. Homberg V, Hefter H, Reiners K, Freund HJ. Differential effects of changes in mechanical limb properties on physiological and pathological tremor. J Neurol Neurosurg Psychiatry 1987;50:568–579.
18. Flament D, Hore J. Movement and electromyographic disorders associated with cerebellar dysmetria. J Neurophysiol 1986;55:1221–1233.
19. Hore J. Flament D. Evidence that a disordered servo-like mechanism contributes to tremor in movements during cerebellar dysfunction. J Neurophysiol. 1986;56:123–136.
20. Sanes JN, LeWitt PA, Mauritz K-H. Visual and mechanical control of postural and kinetic tremor in cerebellar system disorders. J Neurol Neurosurg Psychiatry 1988;51:934–943.
21. Van Hilten JJ, van Dijk JG, Dunnewold RJW, et al. Diurnal variation of essential and physiological tremor. J Neurol Neurosurg Psychiatry 1991;54:516–519.
22. Tolosa E, Fahn S. Clinical rating scale for tremor. In: Jankovic J, Tolosa E, eds. Parkinson's disease and movement disorders. 2d ed. Baltimore: Williams & Wilkins, 1993:271–280.
23. Findley LJ, Bain PG. Tremor assessment in clinical trials. 1993; J Neurol Neurosurg Psychiatry.
24. Jankovic J, Marsden CD. Therapeutic strategies in Parkinson's disease. In. Jankovic J, Tolosa E, eds. Parkinson's disease and movement disorders. 2d ed. Baltimore: Williams & Wilkins, 1993:115–144.

25. Burnett L, Jankovic J, Grossman RG. Thalamotomy in movement disorders: an update. Neurology 1992;42(suppl 3):198.

26. Fox MW, Ahlskog JE, Kelly PJ. Stereotactic ventrolateralis thalamotomy for medically refractory tremor in post-levodopa era Parkinson's disease patients. J Neurosurg 1991;75: 723–730.

27. Diederich N, Goetz CG, Stebbins GT, et al. Blinded evaluation confirms long-term asymmetric effect of unilateral thalamotomy on tremor in Parkinson's disease. Neurology 1992;42:1311–1314.

28. Benabid AL, Pollak P, Gervason C, et al. Long-term suppression of tremor by chronic stimulation of the ventral intermediate thalamic nucleus. Lancet 1991;1:403–406.

29. Laitinen LV, Bergenheim AT, Hariz MI. Leksell's posteroventral pallidotomy in the treatment of Parkinson's disease. J Neurosurg 1992;76:53–61.

30. Bergman H, Wichmann T, DeLong MR. Reversal of experimental parkinsonism by lesions of the subthalamic nucleus. Science 1990;249:1436–1438.

31. Aziz TZ, Peggs D, Sambrook MA, Crossman AR. Lesion of the subthalamic nucleus for the alleviation of 1-methyl-4-phenyl-1,2,3,6-tetrahydropyridine (MPTP)-induced parkinsonism in the primate. Mov Disord 1991;6:288–292.

32. Calzetti S, Sasso E, Baratti M, Fava R. Clinical and computer-based assessment of long-term efficacy of propranolol in essential tremor. Acta Neurol Scand 1990;81:392–396.

33. Guan X-M, Peroutka SJ. Basic mechanisms of action of drugs used in the treatment of essential tremor. Clin Neuropharmacol 1990;13:210–223.

34. Koller WC, Royse VL. Efficacy of primidone in essential tremor. Neurology 1986;36:121–124.

35. Sasso E, Perucca E, Fava R, Calzetti S. Quantitative comparison of barbiturates in essential hand and head tremor. Mov Disord 1991;6:65–68.

36. Trelles L, Trelles JO, Castro C. Successful treatment of two cases of intention tremor with clonazepam. Ann Neurol 1984;16:621.

37. Sechi GP, Zuddas M, Piredda M, et al. Treatment of cerebellar tremors with carbamazepine: a controlled trial with long term follow-up. Neurology 1989;39:1113–1115.

38. Nagaseki Y, Shibazaki T, Hirai T, et al. Long term follow-up results of selective VIM-thalamotomy. J Neurosurg 1986;65:296–302.

39. Jankovic J, Brin MF. Therapeutic uses of botulinum toxin. N Engl J Med 1991;324:1186–1194.

40. Blasi J, Chapman ER, Link E, et al. Botulinum neurotoxin A selectively cleaves the synaptic protein SNAP-25. Nature 1993;365:160–163.

41. Jankovic J, Fahn S: Dystonic syndromes. In: Jankovic J, Tolosa E, eds. Parkinson's disease and movement disorders. 2d ed. Baltimore: Williams & Wilkins, 1993; 337–374.

42. Jankovic J, Leder S, Warner D, Schwartz K. Cervical dystonia: clinical findings and associated movement disorders. Neurology 1991;41:1088–1091.

43. Rosenbaum F, Jankovic J. Task-specific focal dystonia and tremor: categorization of occupational movement disorders. Neurology 1988;38:522–527.

44. Jankovic J, Schwartz K. Botulinum toxin treatment of tremors. Neurology 1991;41:1185–1188.

45. Trosch R, Pullman SL. Botulinum A toxin injections for the treatment of hand tremors (abstr). Ann Neurol 1992;32:250.

46. Ludlow CL, Sedory SE, Fujita M, Naunton RF. Treatment of voice tremor with botulinum toxin injections (abstr). Neurology 1989;39:353.

39

Botulinum Toxin in the Treatment of Tics

Joseph Jankovic
Baylor College of Medicine, Houston, Texas

CLINICAL CHARACTERISTICS OF TICS AND TOURETTE'S SYNDROME

Motor tics consist of brief and intermittent abnormal movements occurring against a background of normal motor activity (1). Motor tics are often accompanied by abnormal sounds, called phonic or vocal tics. The term "phonic tic" is preferred because, in contrast to "vocal tic," it includes sounds produced by air moving through the nasal, oral, pharyngeal, laryngeal, and respiratory passages as well as sounds produced by the vocal cords. Tics may resemble normal mannerisms or gestures, but they are most frequently present in the setting of Tourette's syndrome (TS) or other movement disorders (1).

Both motor and phonic tics can be categorized as either simple or complex (1,2). Simple motor tics involve only one group of muscles, causing a brief, isolated, jerk-like movement such as an eye blink, nose twitch, head jerk, or shoulder shrug. Simple phonic tics consist of meaningless, inarticulate noises such as sniffing, throat clearing, grunting, squeaking, screaming, coughing, blowing, and sucking sounds. Complex motor tics are coordinated, sequenced movements resembling normal motor acts or gestures that are inappropriately intense and timed. Complex phonic tics include linguistically meaningful utterances and verbalizations, such as shouting of obscenities or profanities (coprolalia), repetition of someone else's words or phrases (echolalia), and repetition of one's own utterances or phrases (palilalia). The abnormal movements or sounds are often preceded by feelings or sensations, such as a "burning feeling" in the eye before an eye blink, a "tension or crick in the neck" relieved by stretching of the neck or jerking of the head, a "feeling of tightness or constriction" relieved by arm or leg extension, "nasal stuffiness" before a sniff, "dry or sore throat" before a grunt, "itching" before a shoulder shrug, and others. These premonitory symptoms are typically, albeit temporarily, relieved by the execution of the movements or sounds. They are sometimes referred to as sensory tics (3), but the term ''premonitory symptom'' may be more appropriate (2,4). Therefore, in addition to tics that are truly involuntary (nonsuppressible), there are semivoluntary tics that occur in response to these premonitory symptoms and seemingly voluntary (intentionally produced) tics that are easily suppressible (5).

Tics can be classified according to their duration, speed, and postural change into *clonic*, *tonic*, and *dystonic* types (2). Clonic tics are produced by abrupt and brief (< 100 msec) muscle contractions, whereas tonic and dystonic tics represent more sustained (> 300 msec) contractions. Tonic tics consist of isometric contractions of muscles without accompanying movement, such as limb or abdominal muscle tensing. Dystonic tics are manifested by twisting, squeezing, or other briefly sustained movements and abnormal postures (6). Dystonic tics include oculogyric deviations, blepharospasm, bruxism, mouth opening, torticollis, and rotatory movements of the shoulder. The previously described premonitory symptoms are more common and more intense with dystonic than with clonic tics. To further characterize clonic and dystonic tics, we studied 156 patients with TS; 89 (57%) exhibited dystonic tics, including oculogyric deviations (28%), blepharospasm (15%), and dystonic neck movements (7%) (6). Since there was no difference in clinical variables between patients with dystonic tics and those with only clonic tics, we concluded that, despite previous reports, the presence of dystonic tics should not be considered atypical or unusual in TS. Dystonic tics should be distinguished from persistent dystonia, typically seen in patients with idiopathic torsion dystonia. Clonic or dystonic tics are relatively rare in patients with torsion dystonia but may occur more frequently than in the general population. We reported nine patients with coexistent TS and persistent dystonia in whom tics began at a mean age of 9 years, while dystonia followed the onset of tics by an average of 22 (10–38) years (7). The possible association between tics and dystonia is also supported by certain overlapping clinical features, such as the presence of pain in some patients with tics and with dystonia, the suppressibility of both with volition and with sensory tricks (gestes antagonistes), the occasional presence of both movement disorders in the same family, and the response to botulinum toxin (BTX) (5,8).

The most common cause of tics, particularly when they begin in childhood, is TS. This genetically determined disorder is manifested by a broad spectrum of motor and behavioral disturbances (9–11). To aid in the diagnosis of TS, the Tourette Syndrome Association formulated the following criteria for definite TS: (1) both multiple motor and one or more phonic tics have been present at some time during the illness, although not necessarily concurrently; (2) the tics occur many times a day, nearly every day, or intermittently throughout a period of more than 1 year; (3) the anatomical location, number, frequency, type, complexity, or severity of tics changes over time; (4) onset is before age 21; (5) involuntary movements and noises cannot be explained by other medical conditions; and (6) motor and/or phonic tics must be witnessed by a reliable examiner directly at some point during the illness or be recorded by videotape or cinematography (1). Probable TS type 1 meets all the criteria except 3 and/or 4, and probable TS type 2 meets all the criteria except 1; it includes either single motor tic with phonic tics or multiple motor tics with possible phonic tics. Although the diagnostic criteria require that the onset be before the age of 21, in 96% of patients the disorder is manifested by age 11 (10). In 36–48% the initial symptom is eye blinking, followed by tics involving the face and head. Vocalizations have been reported as the initial symptom in 12–37% of patients, with throat clearing being the most common. During the course of the disease, nearly all patients exhibit tics involving the face or head, two-thirds have tics in the arms, and half have tics involving the trunk or legs. Coprolalia, perhaps the most recognizable symptom of TS, is present in fewer than half of all patients. Copropraxia and echolalia have been reported in about 30% of patients, echopraxia in about 25%, and palilalia in 10%. In addition to motor and phonic tics, patients with TS often exhibit a variety of behavioral symptoms, particularly attention deficit with hyperactivity (ADHD) and obsessive-compulsive disorder (OCD). These behavioral disorders appear to be an integral part of the syndrome, although only OCD has been thought to be genetically linked to TS (12).

PATHOPHYSIOLOGY OF TICS AND TOURETTE'S SYNDROME

Although the pathophysiological mechanisms of tics are still unknown, there is a growing body of evidence supporting a physiological rather than psychogenic origin (4,10–12). Despite the observation that some tics may be voluntary, physiological studies suggest that most tics do not involve motor pathways normally used for willed movements (13). The most intriguing hypothesis, supported partly by increased 3H-mazindol binding in TS brains, suggests that TS represents a developmental disorder resulting in dopaminergic hyperinnervation of the ventral striatum (14). This portion of the basal ganglia is anatomically and functionally related to the limbic system, and this link may explain the frequent association of tics and behavioral problems.

Finding the genetic marker, and ultimately the gene, has been one of the highest priorities in TS research during the past decade. Unfortunately, despite a concentrated effort by many investigators, the TS gene has thus far eluded this intensive search. Assuming that genetic heterogeneity is not an important factor in TS, over 90% of the genome has been already excluded, (15; Kidd, personal communication). Two genetic hypotheses have been proposed: (1) a sex-influenced autosomal dominant mode of inheritance and (2) a semidominant, semirecessive pattern of inheritance (12,16). The latter model takes into account the common observation that both parents of a TS child often exhibit TS or a forme fruste of TS (16). Finding a genetic marker and ultimately the gene will be helpful not only in improving our understanding of this complex neuro-behavioral disorder, but also in clarifying the epidemiology of TS. Because the clinical criteria are not well defined, the estimated prevalence rates for TS have been reported to range between 1/100 and 1/10,000 (11). If a careful family assessment, including examination of both parents and other relatives, is made and if certain behavioral symptoms, particularly ADHD, OCD, and poor impulse control, are accepted as probable manifestations of TS, then the true prevalence of TS may be close to 1% of the general population.

TREATMENT OF TICS AND TOURETTE'S SYNDROME

The broad range of neurological and behavioral manifestations of TS necessitates individualization of therapy; the treatment must be specifically tailored to the patient's needs (Table 1). Of the pharmacological agents used for tic suppression, we find fluphenazine most effective and least sedating; we rarely use haloperidol because it frequently causes troublesome sedation, depression, weight gain, and school phobia. While these side effects can also be seen with fluphenazine, they seem less frequent and less severe. If fluphenazine fails to control tics adequately, we switch to pimozide, molindone, or thiothixene, in that order. The most serious side effect of these drugs, other than hepatotoxicty (and cardiotoxicity with pimozide), is tardive dyskinesia. This iatrogenic

Table 1 Treatment Strategies in Tourette's Syndrome

Tics	OCD	ADHD
Fluphenazine	Imipramine	Clonidine
Pimozide	Clomipramine	Imipramine
Haloperidol	Fluoxetine	Desipramine
Thiothixene	Sertraline	Deprenyl
Trifluoperazine	Clonazepam	Naltrexone
Molindone	Carbamazepine	Methylphenidate
Nicotine	Trazodone	Dextroamphetamine
Clonazepam		
Clonidine	**Neurosurgery**	
Naltrexone		
Tetrabenazine		
Sulpiride		
Tiapride		
Flunarizine		
Clozapine		
Botulinum toxin		

OCD = obsessive-compulsive disorder; ADHD = attention deficit with hyperactivity.

disorder is only rarely persistent in children. However, tardive dystonia, a variant of tardive dyskinesia most commonly seen in young adults, may persist and occasionally progresses to a generalized and disabling dystonic disorder (17). Therefore, careful monitoring of patients is absolutely essential. The dosage should be reduced and the drug discontinued during periods of remission and during vacations. Clonazepam may also be useful, particularly in patients with severe clonic tics. Tetrabenazine, a monoamine-depleting and dopamine receptor–blocking agent, is a powerful anti-tic drug, although it may cause daytime sedation, nighttime insomnia, depression, and parkinsonism (18). This drug has a major advantage over other neuroleptics in that it does not cause tardive dyskinesia. Tetrabenazine is not readily available in the United States, but it can be obtained from England with a special permission and with an IND number.

The dopamine receptor–blocking drugs may not be effective or desirable when behavioral symptoms dominate the clinical syndrome. We use clonidine or desipramine in mild cases of ADHD and in an attempt to treat impulse control problems. Methylphenidate, although clearly effective in the treatment of ADHD, may exacerbate tics. In a pilot open trial, we found deprenyl to be effective in controlling the symptoms of ADHD without exacerbating tics (19). The use of deprenyl in ADHD is based on the knowledge that this monoamine oxidase B (MAO-B) inhibitor metabolizes to amphetamines and that MAO inhibitors have been found beneficial in the treatment of ADHD. In patients with disabling symptoms of OCD, the most effective drugs are imipramine, desipramine, clonazepam, fluoxetine, clomipramine, and sertraline (20). In patients with extremely severe and disabling OCD in whom optimal pharmacological therapy has failed, psychosurgery may be considered as a last resort (21).

Botulinum toxin is an effective treatment for a variety of disorders manifested by inappropriate muscle contractions (22,23), but its efficacy in the treatment of tics has not been previously documented. Ten male patients, aged 13 to 53 years, diagnosed with TS manifested by disabling focal tics were included in a pilot study (Table 2). Five patients

Table 2 Botulinum Toxin Injections for Tics

Patient no./ sex/age/ session	Site of injection	Dosage/ session (U)	Peak effect (0–4)	Duration (weeks)	Effect on premonitory symptoms	Complications
1/M/16/1	B, E	50	2.0	4		Ptosis
2	B, E	55	4.0	18		
3	B, E	55	3.0	16		
4	B, E	30	4.0	14		
2/M/17/1	Trapezii,	200	4.0	16	+ + +	
	Rhomboids	100	4.0	16	+ + +	
2	Trapezii,	200	4.0	16	+ + +	
	Rhomboids	100	4.0	16	+ + +	
3/M/20/1	Splenii	200	4.0	12	+ +	Neck weakness
2	Splenii	150	4.0	12	+ +	
3	Splenii	150	4.0	20	+ +	Neck pain
4	Splenii	150	4.0	20	+ +	Neck stiffness
5	Splenii	150	4.0	20	+ +	
4/M/53/1	B, F	40	4.0	20	+ +	
2	B, F	60	4.0	12	+ +	
3	B, F	60	4.0	16	+ +	
4	B, F	60	4.0	16	+ +	
	Masseters	45	4.0	16		
5	B, F	70	4.0	18	+ +	
	Masseters	80	4.0	18		
5/M/17/1	B, E	60	4.0	16	+ + +	
6/M/21/1	Splenii	200	3.0	6	+ +	Neck weakness
2	Splenii	200	3.0	14	+ +	
7/M/15/1	R Splenius	75	4.0	2	+ + +	Neck pain
	R Rhomboid	75	4.0	2	+ + +	
8/M/13/1	R Splenius	75	4.0	—	+ +	
	R Trapezius	100	4.0	—	+ +	
9/M/53/1	B, E	70	4.0	—	+ +	
10/M/17/1	B, E	70	2.0	—		

B = eyebrow; F = face; E = eyelids; M = male; R = right; U = mouse units; + = partial relief; + + = moderate to marked relief; + + + = complete abolishment of premonitory symptoms.

had frequent blinking and blepharospasm, rendering them "blind," and five other patients had severe, painful, and repetitive dystonic tics involving their neck or shoulder muscles. The doses used to inject involved muscles were similar to those in patients with dystonia. The smallest dose per treatment session, 30 U, was used in a patient with frequent blinking and blepharospasm; the highest dose per treatment session was 300 U in a patient with severe shrugging and rotation of shoulders.

The response to BTX treatment was assessed by a previously described 0–4 scale rating the "peak effect" (24). All 10 patients experienced moderate to marked improvement in their tics, usually within 2–7 days after injection (Table 2). Of the 29 treatment sessions, only two failed to produce improvement of sufficient magnitude to cause a significant reduction in disability. All others resulted in functional improvement as well as in reduction in the amplitude and frequency of the tics. While this motor and functional improvement was an expected outcome of the treatment, we were surprised to note that the majority of patients also had marked or complete resolution of the premonitory symptoms. All patients except one reported a build-up of "tension," "feeling," or "discomfort" before each or most of their tics. These symptoms were completely abolished in seven of 22 treatments (32%) and markedly relieved in the rest. When the effects of BTX treatment wore off, the premonitory symptoms and the tics returned. The observation that local muscle paralysis has an ameliorating effect on the premonitory symptoms underscores the importance of peripheral sensory input in the generation of motor tics. In patient 3, the tics remitted for 18 months after the last treatment. Before BTX treatment, the patient was never without the repetitive head extension for more than a few seconds (while awake). It is therefore unlikely that he would have achieved a spontaneous remission without the therapeutic intervention.

There were no serious complications, but transient ptosis was present in one patient after the initial treatment for eyelid tics; neck pain or stiffness occurred in three treatment sessions, and neck weakness resulted after two sessions (Table 2). The ptosis lasted 4 weeks; all other side effects resolved completely within 2 weeks after injection. The patients have continued to respond; this argues strongly against the presence of blocking antibodies.

CONCLUSION

This first study of BTX in the treatment of tics indicates that chemodenervation with BTX is a safe and effective treatment for patients with focal, particularly dystonic, tics. The treatment ameliorates not only the motor manifestations of tics, but also the premonitory sensory component. This latter observation supports the notion that sensory feedback mechanisms play an important role in the pathophysiology of tics. Further studies are needed to confirm our preliminary results and to define the role of BTX in the treatment of tics.

REFERENCES

1. Jankovic J. Diagnosis and classification of tics and Tourette's Syndrome. In: Chase T, Friedhoff A, Cohen DJ, eds. Tourette's syndrome. Advances in neurology, vol. 58. New York: Raven Press, 1992:7–14.
2. Jankovic J, Lang AE, Kurlan R. Diagnostic criteria for tics. Mov Disord 1994; in press.
3. Kurlan R, Lichter D, Hewitt D. Sensory tics in Tourette's syndrome. Neurology 1989;39:731–734.
4. Leckman JF, Pauls DL, Peterson BS, et al. Pathogenesis of Tourette's syndrome. Clues from the clinical phenotype and natural history. In: Chase T, Friedhoff A, Cohen DJ, eds. Tourette's syndrome. Advances in neurology, vol. 58. New York: Raven Press, 1992:15–24.
5. Lang AE. Clinical phenomenology of tic disorders: selected aspects. In: Chase T, Friedhoff A, Cohen DJ, eds. Tourette's syndrome. Advances in neurology, vol. 58. New York: Raven Press, 1992:25–32.
6. Jankovic J, Stone L. Dystonic tics in patients with Tourette's syndrome. Mov Disord 1991;6:248–252.
7. Stone L, Jankovic J. The coexistence of tics and dystonia. Arch Neurol 1991;48:862–865.
8. Jankovic J. Botulinum toxin in the treatment of tics associated with Tourette's syndrome. Neurology 1993;43(Suppl 2):A310 (*abstract*).
9. Jankovic J, Rohaidy H. Motor, behavioral and pharmacologic findings in Tourette's syndrome. Can J Neurol Sci 1987;14:541–546.

10. Robertson MM. The Gilles de la Tourette syndrome: the current status. Br J Psychiatry 1989;154:147–169.
11. Singer HS, Walkup JT. Tourette syndrome and other tic disorders. Diagnosis, pathophysiology, and treatment. Medicine 1991;70:15–32.
12. Pauls DL. Issues in genetic linkage studies of Tourette syndrome. Phenotypic spectrum and genetic model parameters. In: Chase T, Friedhoff A, Cohen DJ, eds. Tourette's syndrome. Advances in neurology, vol. 58. New York, Raven Press, 1992:151–157.
13. Obeso JA, Rothwell JC, Marsden CD. The neurophysiology of Tourette syndrome. In: Friedhoff AJ, Chase TN, eds. Gilles de la Tourette syndrome. Advances in neurology, vol. 35. New York: Raven Press, 1982:105–114.
14. Singer HS. Neurochemical analysis of postmortem cortical and striatal brain tissue in patients with Tourette syndrome. In: Chase T, Friedhoff A, Cohen DJ, eds. Tourette's syndrome. Advances in neurology, vol. 58. New York: Raven Press, 1992:135–144.
15. Pakstis AJ, Heutink P, Pauls DL, et al. Progress in the search for genetic linkage with Tourette syndrome: an exclusion map covering more than 50% of the autosomal genome. Am J Human Genet 1991;48:281–294.
16. Comings DE, Comings BG. Alternative hypotheses on the inheritance of Tourette syndrome. In: Chase T, Friedhoff A, Cohen DJ, eds. Tourette's syndrome. Advances in neurology, vol. 58. New York: Raven Press, 1992:189–200.
17. Singh S, Jankovic J. Tardive dystonia in patients with Tourette's syndrome. Mov Disord 1988;3:274–280.
18. Jankovic J, Orman J. Tetrabenazine therapy of dystonia, chorea, tics and other dyskinesias. Neurology 1988;38:391–394.
19. Jankovic J. Deprenyl in attention deficit associated with Tourette's syndrome. Arch Neurol, 1993;50:286–288.
20. Pigott TA, Pato MT, Bernstein S, et al. Controlled comparisons of clomipramine and fluoxetine in the treatment of obsessive-compulsive disorder. Arch Gen Psychiatry 1990;47:926–932.
21. Jenike MA, Baer L, Ballantine HT, et al. Cingulotomy for refractory obsessive-compulsive disorder. Arch Gen Psychiatry 1991;48:548–555.
22. Jankovic J, Brin MF. Therapeutic uses of botulinum toxin. N Engl J Med 1991;324:1186–1194.
23. Clarke CE. Therapeutic potential of botulinum toxin in neurological disorders. Q J Med 1992;82:197–205.
24. Jankovic J, Schwartz K, Donovan DT. Botulinum toxin treatment of cranial-cervical dystonia, spasmodic dysphonia, other focal dystonias and hemifacial spasm. J Neurol Neurosurg Psychiatry 1990;53:633–639.

40

Botulinum Toxin: Potential Role in the Management of Cerebral Palsy During Childhood

L. Andrew Koman, James F. Mooney III, and Beth Paterson Smith
Bowman Gray School of Medicine, Wake Forest University, Winston-Salem, North Carolina

INTRODUCTION

Neuromuscular blockade of spastic skeletal muscles has been used as an adjunct to the management of dynamic muscle imbalance in children and adults with cerebral palsy or following "closed head injury." (1,2) Percutaneous intramuscular injection of dilute (45%) alcohol into spastic muscles (1,3) and the topical application of alcohol or phenol on surgically exposed motor nerves (3–5) both have been used to decrease painful spasticity or to improve function by reversible neuromuscular blockade. However, the pain associated with these intramuscular injections and the need for surgical exposure for the topical application necessitate the use of local or general anesthesia in children, thereby increasing potential morbidity and cost. The potential of botulinum toxin (BTX) type A as a reversible neuromuscular blocking agent that can be injected intramuscularly without local or general anesthesias makes it an attractive modality for patients with spastic skeletal muscles.

Intramuscularly injected BTX has proven efficacy in specific ocular and facial dystonias involving small muscle groups, and its mechanism of action has been well described (6–12). Intramuscular injections of BTX for larger skeletal muscle dystonias (i.e., spasmodic torticollis, which involves the sternocleidomastoid, trapezius, and splenius muscles) have provided clinical palliation without significant side effects and without the need for anesthetics or sedation (13–18). Focal dystonias of the hand have been managed by intramuscularly injected BTX (19), and reports of using BTX in spastic upper extremities following cerebrovascular accidents (stroke) (20) and in the spastic adductor muscles of patients with multiple sclerosis (21) have been favorable. The purpose of this chapter is to describe our preliminary experience with BTX in the management of cerebral palsy in children and to discuss its potential value for this purpose.

CEREBRAL PALSY

Cerebral palsy, by definition, is a nonprogressive motion disorder secondary to a finite central nervous system insult in the perinatal period (arbitrarily defined as the initiation of gestation to the day before the child turns 2 years old). Thus, prenatal, natal, and postnatal events as diverse as forceps trauma, intracerebral bleeding, or infections involving the central nervous system may result in the variety of peripheral manifestations that collectively are called cerebral palsy. It is estimated that 5000 to 7000 new cases of cerebral palsy occur annually (Cerebral Palsy Facts and Figures (fact sheet), United Cerebral Palsy Association, Inc., August 9, 1986), and currently there are an estimated 500,000 to 700,000 cases of cerebral palsy in the United States.

In the past, classic "cerebral palsy" was often related causally to cerebral anoxia and/or kernicterus (maternal-fetal Rh incompatibility). With the advent of Rh screening and exchange transfusion, kernicterus has ceased to be a significant etiological factor in cerebral palsy. Because epidemiological studies have failed to document significant anoxic factors in the majority of children clinically diagnosed with cerebral palsy, it appears that as-yet-undefined environmental or genetic factors may be causally involved in the onset of cerebral palsy (22). Thus, the term "cerebral palsy," which is based on historical precedence, encompasses a variety of clinical entities that may well have few physiological or etiological factors in common.

Among the many known peripheral manifestations of cerebral palsy (Table 1), spastic "agonist" muscles, which create muscle imbalance across a joint by overpowering antagonist muscles, are amenable to neuromuscular blockade. Botulinum toxin, by the selective weakening/partial paralysis of overactive muscle, may reestablish that balance, thereby improving active range of motion and function. Botulinum toxin is effective only under the following circumstances: (1) a preinjection muscle imbalance is present, with identifiable and relatively stronger spastic agonist muscle(s); (2) the antagonist muscle(s) is sufficiently powerful for functional control if "agonists" are weakened sufficiently *or* is capable of appropriate hypertrophy and strengthening if allowed to perform through more appropriate range of joint motion; and (3) no fixed joint deformity is present. Because BTX works through restoration of muscle balance by selective paralysis, it has potential applications in dynamic joint deformity secondary to muscle spasticity in extremities with or without athetosis. Administration of BTX appears to affect extremity dysfunction secondary to spasticity independently of the underlying cause.

RATIONALE FOR USE OF BOTULINUM TOXIN IN CEREBRAL PALSY

Muscle imbalance secondary to spasticity may result in inappropriate joint positioning that interferes with extremity function or ambulation. The spasticity, with or without athetosis, may create a dynamic deformity sufficient to interfere with function (e.g., patient positioning, hygiene, independence of activities of daily living, sitting balance, and ambulation). The intramuscular administration of BTX has the potential to correct motor imbalance, thereby enhancing control of the extremities and improving functional position or gait.

The exaggerated and excessive contractions of spastic muscles initiated by abnormal stretch reflexes secondary to pyramidal or extrapyramidal lesions occur in specific patterns. These patterns result from spasticity on one side of a joint, with relative

Table 1 Peripheral Manifestations of Cerebral Palsy

Muscle
   Spasticity
   Rigidity
   Weakness
   Athetosis
Joint deformity
   Fixed contracture
   Dynamic deformity

hypotonia on the other side, and may vary from patient to patient. The most common patterns of spasticity in the upper extremity include internal rotation of the shoulder, flexion of the elbow, pronation of the forearm, wrist flexion, and finger flexion with the thumb in the palm. In the lower extremity, imbalance results most frequently in varying degrees of hip flexion and adduction deformity, knee flexion, and ankle plantar flexion. Over time, these sustained imbalances of spasticity-induced joint positioning result in further shortening of the spastic, or agonist, muscles and an increase in the resting length of the relatively hypotonic, or antagonist, muscle groups, with subsequent further weakening. These changes, in turn, result in further imbalances, which lead to joint contracture, and if full range of motion of a joint is not maintained by active motor power or passive assistance, fixed contracture and/or bony deformity will result.

In the absence of fixed deformity or rigid joint contracture, BTX can be used to restore across-joint muscle balance by diminishing the effects of spasticity in agonist muscles and thereby facilitating and improving function of the previously weakened antagonist muscles. Potential secondary gains are prevention of joint contracture or fixed deformity and alteration of the natural history of the specific motor deficit. This occurs by the selective creation of "weakness" in injected spastic muscles, reversing the across-joint imbalance. However, BTX cannot correct underlying etiological factors involved in spasticity or directly improve function or performance. Nor can it be effective if fixed deformity or rigid joint contracture is present.

ALTERNATIVE MANAGEMENT AND PERSPECTIVE

Multiple modalities and interventions have been used to deal with the spasticity and secondary deformities of cerebral palsy. These include oral pharmacological intervention, physical therapy, surgery (neurosurgical and/or orthopedic) (2,23–28), and neuromuscular blockage with alcohol or phenol (1,3,29). Unfortunately, alteration of spasticity by currently available oral pharmacological intervention has not been effective; oral doses sufficient to decrease tone result in excessive sedation or unacceptable side effects. The ability of physical therapy as an isolated entity to alter the natural history of cerebral palsy and provide long-term benefit has been difficult to document (27,28,30).

The optimal approach to managing the spasticity of cerebral palsy would be to weaken selected abnormal "target" muscles long enough to restore or improve joint or extremity balance by a technique that requires no anesthesia or sedation and will be neutralized over 3 to 6 months. Such therapy would provide short-term palliation or, by repeat injection, long-term alteration in the natural history of cerebral palsy and, in the child, might be used to postpone corrective surgery until growth would no longer affect the outcome. Unfortunately, neuromuscular blocking agents such as bupivacaine provide diagnostic information in a time frame too transient to provide true clinical palliation (3). Surgical procedures are, in general, irreversible. Thus, the advent of BTX as a reversible, target-specific neuromuscular blocking agent has great appeal and potential.

Background

In 1987, the department of orthopedic surgery at Wake Forest University undertook the first known clinical trials of BTX in cerebral palsy. Initial study goals were to determine the drug's efficacy in this specific pediatric patient population, safety considerations including side effects, the maximal duration of action, the optimal dosage, and appropriate injection techniques.

At the initiation of these trials, no clinical series of children with cerebral palsy had received BTX for the management of extremity deformity. The senior author (LAK) was aware of the observations following BTX injection in one child with cerebral palsy (personal communication, Dr. Alan Scott, Smith-Kettlewell Eye Research Institute, San Francisco, California). The studies described below were performed while BTX for any purpose was an investigational drug, and Food and Drug Administration (FDA) approval for these studies was beneath the mantle of Dr. Scott's FDA approval for its use in patients with cerebral palsy. All protocols were approved by the appropriate federal and local review boards, and informed consent was obtained from all involved parties.

Clinical Experience

Two types of preliminary clinical trial, an open drug trial and a double-blind, placebo-controlled feasibility trial, have been completed to determine the potential functional benefits of BTX injections in the clinical management of children with cerebral palsy. We present our experience in the use of BTX for trunk and lower extremity spasticity.

METHODS

The following were common to both protocols.

Injection Technique

In both trials, the BTX was injected directly into the "target" muscle(s) identified by clinical and/or electrodiagnostic evaluation. In the larger muscles of the lower extremity, electromyographic control was not used for needle placement. The "target" muscle was palpated under tension, and the area of the neuromuscular junction was estimated. Under appropriate sterile technique (sterile technique employed Betadine skin preparation, sterile gloves, needles, and syringes, and a "no-touch" injection protocol—i.e., skin site and needle point were not touched during the procedure), a 23-gauge needle was placed within the proximal muscle belly and a predetermined dose/dilution of BTX was injected after withdrawal sufficient to ensure nonvascular delivery (Figs. 1 and 2).

Dosage and Toxin Preparation

Dosage was based on a maximal total dose to the patient (6 U/kg) and an arbitrary division based on relative muscle mass and size (Table 2). The BTX, prepared at Smith-Kettlewell

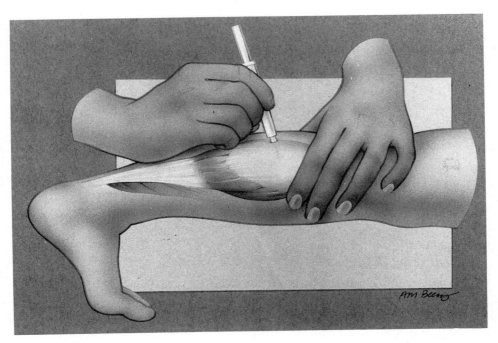

Figure 1 Insertion of 23-gauge needle into muscle belly of medial gastrocnemius in a child using a "no-touch" technique of the skin (after Betadine skin preparation) and the needle. The needle is inserted through the skin, and the fascia over the muscle is felt as a "pop." The position of the needle within the muscle belly can be sensed, and botulinum toxin is delivered in a fanlike pattern after negative pressure is applied to the syringe to ensure that the needle is extravascular. (Reproduced with permission from Mooney JF III, Koman LA, Smith BP. Neuromuscular blockade in the management of cerebral palsy. In: Ehrlich MG, ed. Advances in orthopedics, Mosby Yearbook Publ., St. Louis, 1993, pp. 337–344.)

Eye Institute, was supplied in vials in a frozen, crystallized form and was reconstituted with physiological saline. All doses in this pediatric population were based on weight.

Safety Considerations

Following injection, the parents or guardians of the patients were contacted daily by a telephone call from a registered nurse. These calls monitored the type and duration of side effects or beneficial effects that followed each injection and were continued until any reported side effects were resolved.

Evaluation

Patients in both groups were evaluated by a physician rating scale (Table 3), physician examinations, physical therapy examinations and global assessment, parent responses, and clinical gait analysis either from direct observation or from videotapes. Formal two-dimensional gait analysis was performed in the double-blind trial. Participants in the double-blind treatment protocol also received a Biodex computerized dynamometer evaluation to assess strength and endurance.

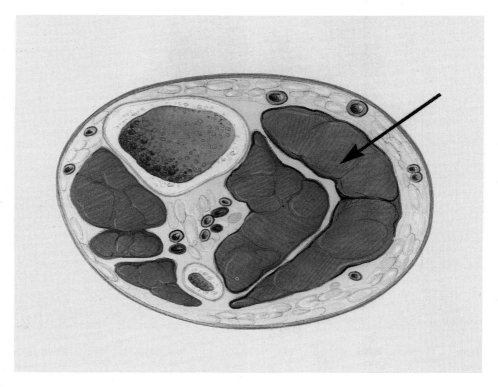

Figure 2 Cross-section showing needle placement in gatrocnemius.

Open Drug Trial

Entry into the open drug trial required (1) dynamic deformity predominantly secondary to spasticity, (2) dynamic deformity unresponsive to orthotics and physical therapy, and/or (3) surgical intervention as the only realistic alternative. The objectives of the open trial were to determine (1) the dose of BTX (units per kilogram of body weight) required to produce muscle weakness, (2) the duration of BTX-induced muscle weakness, (3) the

Table 2 Dose Based on Muscle Mass/Size

Muscle	Relative muscle mass value (U/kg)
Posterior tibial	0.5
Medial gastrocnemius[a]	1.0
Lateral gastrocnemius[a]	1.0
Peroneals	0.5
Paraspinal	1.0

[a]Initial injection of medial gastrocnemius and lateral gastrocnemius for dynamic equinus deformity would equal 2 $\times$ mass value $\times$ 1–2 U/kg body weight.

Table 3 Physician Rating Scale (PRS) for Gait
Analysis (Determined for Each Limb Injected)

Dynamic function (range of motion)	Score
1. Crouch	
Severe ($> 20°$ hip, knee, ankle)	0
Moderate ($5–20°$ hip, knee, ankle)	1
Mild ($< 5°$ hip, knee, ankle)	2
None	3
2. Equinus foot	
Constant (fixed contracture)	0
Constant (dynamic contracture)	1
Occasional heel contact	2
Heel-to-toe gait	3
3. Hind foot	
Varus at foot strike	0
Valgus at foot strike	1
Occasionally neutral at foot strike	2
Neutral at foot strike	3
4. Knee	
Recurvatum $> 5°$	0
Recurvatum $0–5°$	1
Neutral (no recurvatum)	2
5. Speed of gait	
Only slow	0
Variable (slow-fast)	1
6. Gait	
Toe-to-toe	0
Occasional heel-to-toe	1
Heel-to-toe	2

local side effects or potential systemic toxicity of BTX injections, and (4) the clinical value of BTX in the alleviation of muscle spasticity.

Patients in the open trial were divided into two groups: ambulatory (N = 7) and nonambulatory (N = 11) (Table 4). These 18 children received a total of 50 injections of BTX.

The seven ambulatory children (hemiplegia, N = 3; diplegia, N = 4) were injected with BTX in an attempt to improve gait. All had progressive dynamic equinovarus or equinovalgus foot/ankle deformities unresponsive to bracing or other forms of treatment. In the patients with equinovalgus deformities, BTX injections of 2–3 U/kg were divided between the medial gastrocnemius and the lateral gastrocnemius muscles. In the patients with equinovarus deformities, BTX was injected into the posterior tibialis muscle as well as the medial and lateral gastrocnemius muscles. Two weeks after the initial injections, each patient was evaluated, and in the absence of clinical weakness or improved ankle/foot dorsiflexion, an additional 1–2 U/kg of BTX was administered. Subsequent injections were administered at 3- to 5-month intervals if improvements in gait pattern or ankle/foot range of motion diminished. In order to evaluate the effect of BTX on ambulatory function, patients were evaluated with the physician rating scale (PRS), and the differences between the pretreatment PRS score and the maximal posttreatment PRS score were determined for all the treated legs.

The 11 nonambulatory children with cerebral palsy were evaluated to determine the effects of BTX on lower extremity and back spasticity. Diagnoses included spastic diplegia (N = 1), spastic quadriplegia (N = 6), spastic quadriplegia with athetosis (N = 3), and spastic quadriplegia with scoliosis (N = 1). Each patient was given BTX injections in the muscles of the lower extremities and/or back to decrease spasticity, to increase range of motion, to improve positioning, and to help prevent hip subluxation. The initial dose for four of the patients was 2 U of toxin/kg body weight; the remaining seven patients received higher initial doses (3–4.5 U/kg body weight) because of the higher estimated mass of the spastic muscles involved. These nonambulatory patients were evaluated at 2 to 3 weeks after injection. Criteria for reinjection included any of the following: (1) failure to achieve adequate reduction in ''target'' muscle tone; (2) failure to reach a clinically significant result; and (3) deterioration with increasing spasticity.

Results.   Following injections, the majority of patients exhibited moderate or marked improvements. All patients exhibited reduced spasticity and improved positioning. Clinical weakness of target muscles without weakening of nontarget muscles was achieved in all cases at doses of 1–3 U/kg for each muscle unit injected. Injections in one patient permitted bracing that had not been tolerated previously. Hip subluxation was reduced in two patients. Before receiving BTX injections, one patient had had difficulty sitting; after treatment with BTX, she was able to sit ''Indian style.'' Opisthotonic posturing was sufficiently reduced in two patients to enable them to sit in wheelchairs. Injections of BTX in the hip muscles of two patients resulted in increased range of motion, enabling them to be positioned more comfortably. Two patients with overactive hamstrings exhibited less scissoring following BTX injections. Another patient, who had severe paraspinal spasticity and pain due to a nonflexible scoliotic curve, reported an alleviation of pain as well as reduced spasticity after injection of BTX into the paralumbar muscles. However, the injections did not affect the degree of scoliotic curvature. One patient with significant equinovalgus deformity exhibited increased range of motion following BTX injection.

In the seven ambulatory patients, the average PRS score increased from 5.1 to 11.2, or an average total of 6.1.

Side Effects.   There were no significant side effects or adverse reactions in this group. Patients reported soreness of the injected muscles after one-third of the injections. Less commonly reported side effects included muscle cramping, tiredness, an unrelated rash on the arm, decreased bladder control, decreased head control for one day, fever, and crankiness in one patient each, and weakness in two patients.

Double-Blind Placebo-Controlled Feasibility Trial

Twelve ambulatory patients (aged 4 to 11 years; four with hemiplegia, eight with diplegia) were enrolled in this study (Table 4). Enrollment requirements included (1) cerebral palsy; (2) absence of other significant health problems; and (3) equinovarus or equinovalgus foot deformities associated with dynamic joint contracture that had not responded to standard physical therapy orthotics, or nonoperative forms of treatment. The goal of this trial was to determine the effects of two injections of BTX on lower-leg function over a 4- to 6-week treatment period.

Six patients were randomly assigned to receive the toxin and the other six to receive a placebo; all injections were given in a double-blind fashion. In the hemiplegic patients, only the affected leg was assessed and injected. In the diplegic patients, both legs were assessed and injected. For the first injection, each patient received a toxin dosage (or saline placebo) of 1 U/kg body weight for each leg—that is, hemiplegic patients received a total

Table 4 Summary of Botulinum Toxin Type A Drug Trial (1/88 Through 5/90)

Patient group	No. of patients	Age range (years)	Sex	Muscles injected	No. of injections	Dosage in units (average)	Time between injections in weeks (average)	Duration of treatment in months	Treatment outcome
Open trial									
Ambulatory	7	5–16	4 male 3 female	Medial and lateral gastrocnemius, posterior tibialis	23	28–200 (91)	2–57 (16)	7–26	Improved gait pattern
Nonambulatory	11	3–13	3 male 8 female	Paraspinal, upper leg, lower leg	27	10–111 (55)	2–29 (15)	7–23	Decreased spasticity, improved positioning, reduced pain
Double-blind trial									
Ambulatory	12	4–11	8 male 4 female	Medial and lateral gastrocnemius, posterior tibialis	24	16–185 (50) (12 placebo; 12 toxin)	2–3 (2)	1–1.75	Gait pattern as evaluated by PRS (see Table 5)
Follow-up	11	4–11	7 male 4 female	Medial and lateral gastrocnemius, posterior tibialis	28	16–100 (66)	3–53 (23)	5–22	Improved gait pattern

of 1 U/kg body weight, whereas diplegic patients received a total of 2 U/kg body weight. In equinovalgus extremities, injections were made into the medial and lateral gastrocnemius. In equinovarus extremities, the posterior tibialis muscle, as well as the medial and lateral gastrocnemius muscles, was injected. Two weeks after the first injection, each patient received a second injection at double the initial dose in the same injection sites. Lower-extremity function was assessed by physical therapy evaluation Biodex evaluation, PRS, and parent evaluation.

Results. Global physical therapy evaluations indicated no consistent pattern in overall clinical performance by summary score, thereby supporting the absence of systemic toxicity or effects. Computerized dynamometer assessment, an attempt to measure strength and endurance of the lower extremities before and after toxin injection, showed no consistent differences between the treatment groups and sufficient variability within the placebo group to suggest that this test is unreliable in this patient population. When the differences between the maximal post-treatment PRS score and the pretreatment PRS score were determined, patients receiving placebo had an average improvement of 2.3 in their score (from 5.3 to 7.6), whereas the patients receiving toxin had an average improvement of 3.1 after treatment (from 5.3 to 8.4). Two of the six patients in the placebo group (33%) showed an improvement in gait pattern as assessed by the PRS; five of the six patients in the toxin group (83%) showed an improvement (Table 5).

Before the double-blind code was broken, parents of four of the six children receiving BTX had reported that their child's gait had improved during the trial. One of the two children in whom no improvement was reported was found to have an element of fixed contracture, which would have made it difficult to detect improvement. Parents of two of the six children receiving placebo reported that their child improved during the trial; however, one of these two children had received unscheduled and excessive physical therapy during the trial, which probably was the cause of that short-term improvement.

Side-Effects and Adverse Reactions. Patients receiving placebo reported more side effects than those receiving toxin. The most common side effect in the placebo group was soreness of the injection site (N = 3); other side effects (occurring in one patient each) included fatigue, migraine headache, unsteadiness, and weak, wobbly knees. The only side effect reported by patients in the toxin group was soreness at the injection site in three of the six patients. There were no generalized or clinically significant systemic complications. The side effects were transient, generally lasting 1–2 days.

Following completion of the double-blind trial, all six patients who had received toxin during the trial and five of the six patients who had received placebo were entered into the open trial so that they could receive further toxin injections if necessary. The average difference between the pretreatment PRS score and the maximal post-treatment PRS score during the participation of these 11 patients in the open trial was 4.1 (an improvement from 5.4 to 9.5).

Table 5 Gait Pattern as Evaluated by Physician Rating Scale in Double-Blind, Placebo-Controlled Trial

	No change	Improvement
Placebo (N = 6)	67%	33%
Toxin (N = 6)	16%	83%

CONCLUSION

Results from these two trials suggested that BTX is potentially beneficial in the management of cerebral palsy. The trials determined that (1) the optimal target dose of BTX for large muscles (i.e., gastrocnemius) is 2–4 U/kg body weight; (2) BTX has a maximal effect for 3–6 months; (3) minor variations of injection sites within the muscle belly do not appear to affect the therapeutic benefit of BTX; (4) local side effects are negligible (and no systemic toxicity was observed); and (5) BTX has significant clinical potential in temporarily alleviating muscle spasticity.

Prospects for Long-Term Follow-Up

During the 29 months of these BTX studies, 46 patients received a total of 141 toxin injections. Among eight patients who were managed with a total of 33 serial injections for over 20 months (range 20–29 months), none showed evidence of systemic toxicity and all continued to respond to treatment. Five of these long-term patients were ambulatory children who received a total of 24 BTX injections. All continued to exhibit improved gait patterns due to reduced lower-extremity spasticity. Although the use of BTX may not remove the prospect of future surgical treatment for these patients, it has helped to delay surgery and has demonstrated the potential for moderate to long-term modification of the natural history of the lower-extremity dynamic deformities of cerebral palsy. These studies support the need for further evaluation of BTX in children with cerebral palsy. The variability of response to BTX demonstrated in this paper suggests that future prospective evaluation of BTX in children with cerebral palsy is mandatory *before* BTX is used generally in the management of cerebral palsy. Indications for the use of BTX in cerebral palsy require verification of short- and long-term efficacy beyond what is reported here.

REFERENCES

1. Carpenter EB, Seitz DG. Intramuscular alcohol as an aid in management of spastic cerebral palsy. Dev Med Child Neurol 1980;22:497–501.
2. Bleck EE. Orthopaedic management in cerebral palsy. Philadelphia: J.B. Lippincott, 1987.
3. Carpenter EB. Role of nerve blocks in the foot and ankle in cerebral palsy: therapeutic and diagnostic. Foot Ankle 1983;4:164–166.
4. Botte MJ, Keenan MAE. Percutaneous phenol blocks of the pectoralis major muscle to treat spastic deformities. J Hand Surg 1988;13A:147–149.
5. Braun RM, Hoffer MM, Mooney V, McKeever J, Roper B. Phenol nerve block in the treatment of acquired spastic hemiplegia in the upper limb. J Bone Joint Surg 1973;55A: 580–585.
6. Alpar AJ. Botulinum toxin and its uses in the treatment of ocular disorders. Am J Optom Physiol Opt 1987;64:79–82.
7. Arthurs B, Flanders M, Codère F, Gauthier S, Dresner S, Stone L. Treatment of blepharospasm with medication, surgery and type A botulinum toxin. Can J Ophthalmol 1987;22:24–28.
8. Carruthers J, Stubbs HA. Botulinum toxin for benign essential blepharospasm, hemifacial spasm and age-related lower eyelid entropion. Can J Neurol Sci 1987;14:42–45.
9. Dutton JJ, Buckley EG. Botulinum toxin in the management of blepharospasm. Arch Neurol 1986;43:380–382.
10. Elston JS. Botulinum toxin therapy for involuntary facial movement. Eye 1988;2:12–15.
11. Kraft SP, Lang AE. Cranial dystonia, blepharospasm and hemifacial spasm: clinical features and treatment, including the use of botulinum toxin. Can Med Assoc J 1988;139:837–844.

12.   Brin MF, Fahn S, Moskowitz C, et al. Localized injections of botulinum toxin for the treatment of focal dystonia and hemifacial spasm. Mov Disord 1987;2:237–254.

13.   Gelb DJ, Lowenstein DH, Aminoff MJ. Controlled trial of botulinum toxin injections in the treatment of spasmodic torticollis. Neurology 1989;39:80–84.

14.   Stell R, Thompson PD, Marsden CD. Botulinum toxin in spasmodic torticollis. J Neurol Neurosurg Psychiatry 1988;51:920–923.

15.   Tsui JKC, Calne DB. Botulinum toxin in cervical dystonia. Adv Neurol 1988;49:473–478.

16.   Tsui JKC, Eisen A, Calne DB. Botulinum toxin in spasmodic torticollis. Adv Neurol 1988;50:593–597.

17.   Tsui JKC, Eisen A, Stoessl AJ, Calne S, Calne DB. Double-blind study of botulinum toxin in spasmodic torticollis. Lancet 1986;2:245–247.

18.   Tsui JKC, Fross RD, Calne S, Calne DB. Local treatment of spasmodic torticollis with botulinum toxin. Can J Neurol Sci 1987;14:533–535.

19.   Cohen LG, Hallett M, Geller BD, Hochberg F. Treatment of focal dystonias of the hand with botulinum toxin injections. J Neurol Neurosurg Psychiatry 1989;52:355–363.

20.   Das TK, Park DM. Botulinum toxin in treating spasticity. Br J Clin Pract 1989;43:401–402.

21.   Tsui JKC, Snow B, Bhatt M, Varelas M, Hashimoto S, Calne DB. New applications of botulinum toxin in the lower limbs (abstr). Neurology 1990;40(suppl 1):382.

22.   Nelson KB, Ellenberg JH. Antecedents of cerebral palsy. Multivariate analysis of risk. N Engl J Med 1986;315:81–86.

23.   Barabas G, Taft LT. The early signs and differential diagnosis of cerebral palsy. Pediatr Ann 1986;15:203–214.

24.   Albright AL, Cervi A, Singletary J. Intrathecal baclofen for spasticity in cerebral palsy, JAMA 1991;265:1418–1422.

25.   Diamond M. Rehabilitation strategies for the child with cerebral palsy. Pediatr Ann 1986;15:230–236.

26.   Peacock WJ, Arens LJ, Berman B. Cerebral palsy spasticity. Selective posterior rhizotomy. Pediatr Neurosci 1987;13:61–66.

27.   Piper MC, Kunos VI, Willis DM, Mazer BL, Ramsay M, Silver KM. Early physical therapy effects on the high-risk infant: a randomized controlled trial. Pediatrics 1986;78:216–224.

28.   Wright T, Nicholson J. Physiotherapy for the spastic child: an evaluation. Dev Med Child Neurol 1973;15:146–163.

29.   Tardieu G, Tardieu C, Hariga J, Gagnard L. Treatment of spasticity by injection of dilute alcohol at the motor point or by epidural route. Clinical extension of an experiment on the decerebrate cat. Dev Med Child Neurol 1968;10:555–568.

30.   Palmer FB, Shapiro BK, Wachtel RC, et al. The effects of physical therapy on cerebral palsy. A controlled trial in infants with spastic diplegia. N Engl J Med 1988;318:803–808.

41

Clinical Trials for Spasticity

Joseph King Ching Tsui
University of British Columbia, Vancouver, British Columbia, Canada

Christopher F. O'Brien
*Colorado Neurological Institute and University of Colorado Health Sciences Center,
Englewood, Colorado*

INTRODUCTION

Botulinum toxin (BTX) has been extensively employed in treating ophthalmological disorders, different forms of focal dystonia, and hemifacial spasm (see other chapters of this book). Sufficient data are available demonstrating safety and efficacy in these conditions. In diseases associated with increased muscular activity, patients may suffer from pain, deformity, and disability. Intramuscular injections of BTX would be a logical approach to provide symptomatic relief. Spasticity is one such condition.

SPASTICITY

Spasticity is a major factor in the day-to-day management of patients with a variety of chronic neurological conditions. Problems stemming from spasticity include pain, restricted range of motion, clonus, overwhelming muscle antagonism, and intermittent spasms. Spasticity may also result in poor hygienic care and causes difficulty in fitting braces.

Physiotherapy plays a major role in the management of spasticity. Treatments currently available for spasticity include oral medications, surgical procedures, and intrathecal infusion of baclofen. Oral medications may fail to reduce spasticity significantly, and side effects include sedation and generalized weakness (Young and Delwade, 1981a, 1981b; Rice, 1987). Nerve root sections, myotomy, and tenotomy carry surgical risks and are disfiguring, and recurrence of spasticity is unpredictable. Intrathecal infusion of baclofen requires complex procedures and close monitoring (Penn et al., 1989).

The success of BTX injections for dystonia has been described in other chapters of this book. Dystonia is believed to be caused by abnormality in the neural pathways in the basal ganglia, resulting in abnormal muscular activities. Involuntary and inappropriate muscle contractions may be spontaneous or precipitated by specific actions. Spasticity is caused by interruption of the pyramidal pathways producing increased gamma motor neuron activity due to the release of descending inhibition. It is accompanied by increased muscle tone and enhanced stretch reflexes. There is unidirectional velocity-dependent resistance to passive movements. The final common pathway for both conditions is excessive involuntary contraction of muscles. Injections of BTX should help in both situations. Conditions with spasticity that may potentially be helped by BTX include post-stroke states, cerebral palsy, selected cases of multiple sclerosis (Snow et al., 1990), destrusor-sphincter dyssynergia (bladder sphincter dysfunction) (Dykstra and Sidi, 1990), and post-traumatic spasticity. The application of BTX in these conditions can best be regarded as investigational. At present, controlled clinical trials of BTX therapy in this broad range of conditions with spasticity are needed to establish its efficacy and safety.

CLINICAL TRIALS

Study Designs

Patient Selection

In initial studies, it is important to assess the safety and efficacy of BTX in involuntarily contracting muscles with spasticity. Enrollment of patients suffering from the same disease with a uniform pattern of spasticity will facilitate data analysis. The following are prerequisites for inclusion into studies:

Failed medical treatment—patients should have tried various forms of medical therapy with no benefits or intolerable side effects.
Absence of contactures—contractures produce persistent joint deformity that will not respond to weakening of muscles induced by BTX.
Absence of excessive wasting of the muscles to be injected—it is difficult to estimate the optimum amount of BTX to be injected into muscles with grossly reduced muscle bulk. Patients with anterior horn cell diseases or coexisting myasthenic syndromes should be avoided.
Minimal or no previous surgical intervention—previous surgical intervention may distort regional anatomy, and identification of the appropriate muscles to be treated may be difficult.

Evaluation should be performed by a neurologist skilled in the assessment of spasticity. The goals for functional improvement should be clearly defined. These may include criteria such as fitment of ankle-foot orthoses, improved gait, decreased leg adductor pain, facilitation of hygienic care, and improved range of motion at the wrist.

Monitoring Efficacy

Efficacy should be evaluated in three ways: (1) whether BTX helps in reducing involuntary muscle contractions; (2) whether BTX helps to relieve symptoms of pain and abnormal posturing; and (3) whether the patient obtains overall functional improvements. Measurement of efficacy should include measurement of all these aspects.

1. The effects of BTX on spastic muscle contractions may be monitored by recording spasticity before and after treatment. The most popular scale for measurement of spasticity is the Ashworth scale (Ashworth, 1964), and modifications of this scale can be made to suit different parts of the body. The scale consists of clinical assessment

of muscle tone and frequency of spasms per day. Positive results are reflected by improvement in tone and reduction of frequency of spasm.

2. Improvement in posture may be measured by evaluating the actual deviation in terms of angles from the normal posture at various joints. The absolute range of movement of joints in the extremities may be measured with a goniometer. In the upper limbs, the interphalangeal joints, metacarpophalangeal joints, and wrist and elbow joints may all be evaluated in this way. Similarly in the lower limbs, the joints in the toes, ankles, and knees may be measured. For the hip, abduction, adduction, flexion, and extension may also be assessed. However, for regions of the body with more complex movements, such as the neck, shoulders, and axial skeleton, it may be necessary to develop other systems for measuring range of movement and degree of deformity. Video analysis systems may be employed for such purposes.

3. Evaluating whether the treatment benefits the patient overall is important, since this is a symptomatic therapy. The cost of the treatment should be weighed against the benefits obtained. Functional use of the part of the body treated should be assessed before and after therapy. Patient diaries are useful in assessing the functional improvement achieved after therapy. The diaries should be simple and easy to fill in for better compliance and cooperation from the patients. The functions assessed should be designated specifically for each study, depending on the objectives. In treating spasticity of the feet, improvement in pain, standing, and walking should be recorded. The ease of wearing shoes or fitting braces is also an index of improvement. Treatment of spastic hands should be directed toward improving functional capacities such as holding objects, writing, and feeding.

Objective measurements of functions may sometimes be made with clinical rating scales. Patients are instructed to perform standard sets of tasks, and scores are given clinically according to the rating scales. Sometimes elaborate equipment may be used to assess functional capacities, but such systems may be expensive and not generally available. An example is gait analysis systems.

Double-blind studies are preferable. Within-patient comparison will provide improved statistical power with smaller number of patients. Typically, each patient is given at least two treatments, one of them with a placebo. Treatments should be spaced at least 3 months apart. Double-blindness may be ensured if the patients are videotaped during each visit and the tapes are scored by physicians who are blind to the order of treatment.

Follow-up clinical rating should be performed at 2 weeks and 6 weeks after each treatment. The amount of muscle weakness and atrophy induced in the muscles injected should be recorded.

Monitoring Safety

Published reports on the use of BTX in various conditions indicate that this drug is safe in doses up to 400 mouse units (MU) per treatment (Snow et al., 1990). In spastic condition, however, especially in the lower limbs, the enormous muscle masses involved might require much larger doses of BTX to achieve useful reduction in spasticity. It is unclear at present what the maximum tolerated dose per treatment is. Primate experiments suggest that the LD_{50} for humans is approximately 39 MU/kg (Scott and Suzuki, 1988), or 2500–3000 MU for an adult of average weight. Doses higher than 400 MU per treatment should be used extremely cautiously and are best avoided. Optimum treatment consists of delivering the minimum required dose to the appropriate muscles causing problems for the patient. The starting dose for different muscles varies. Guidelines are available for most neck muscles and distal limb muscles from studies in dystonia.

Patients should be instructed on the average time course of clinical response, which usually occurs within the first 2 weeks of treatment, as well as the potential side effects of BTX. They should be encouraged to keep a diary of any adverse reactions noted. Local pain and ecchymoses are infrequent and transient. Weakness in the muscles injected is an expected effect, although excessive weakness should be recorded as a side effect. Weakness in untreated muscles should be noted. Dysphagia is a complication in treating neck muscles. Diplopia, bulbar weakness, and generalized weakness are potentially signs of botulism and patients should be instructed to report them immediately through a 24-hour emergency phone number, and should be attended to as soon as possible.

Botulinum Toxin Injections

Injections may be done with or without electromyographic (EMG) guidance, depending on the surface anatomy of the muscles.

Safety in Children

Data about safety in children are scanty. One of the conditions on which interest is focused is cerebral palsy.

STUDY IN MULTIPLE SCLEROSIS

Chronic multiple sclerosis has been employed as a clinical model for spasticity. Patients who are bedridden may suffer from severe adductor spasms in their legs causing discomfort and pain. Hygienic care of the perineum and changing of catheters become difficult.

Patients

In a double-blind study, 10 patients with chronic multiple sclerosis (MS) were studied. The patients, one man and nine women, had a mean age of 40.2 years (range 23–61). They were inpatients in two long-stay institutions. All had chronic MS with a mean duration of 18.2 years (range 9–35). All patients were either confined to wheelchair or bed-bound. These patients had lower limb adductor spasms that interfered with sitting, positioning in bed, and perineal care. They had been treated before with oral medications and all were resistant to therapy. One patient had adductor tenotomy 10 years earlier, but the adductor spasm recurred.

Injections

Only the lower limb adductor muscles on the right side were injected, to minimize variation. On the basis of previous experience with dystonic muscles, a total dose of 400 MU of BTX-A (Smith-Kettlewell Eye Research Institute preparation) was selected. The toxin was given in divided doses of 50 MU (1 MU = 0.4 ng) into the adductor brevis (100 MU), adductor longus (100 MU), and adductor magnus (200 MU). The dilution was 100 MU/ml of normal saline with no preservatives. An equal volume of normal saline alone was used as the placebo treatment. The injection sites are illustrated in Fig. 1. Injections were given to patients in two separate treatments spaced 3 months apart. Only one treatment was with BTX, and the other was with placebo, in random order. The patients and the physician carrying out injections, as well as two other physicians performing the rating scales, were all blind to the order of treatment.

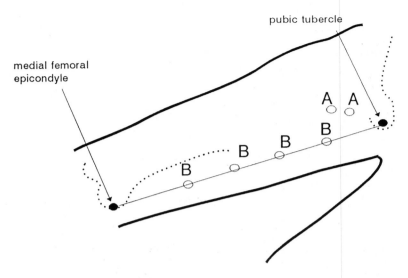

Figure 1   Injection sites (right thigh).

Rating Scales

A rating scale on spasticity (RSP) was designed as a modification of the Ashworth rating scale (Ashworth, 1964) and is shown in Table 1. In addition, a functional rating scale (FRS) (Table 2) was designed to assess the ease of hygienic care by nursing staff. The spasticity score in the RSP was the product of the degree of spasm and spasm frequency. The RSP was performed by two physicians who were blind to the order of treatment. These were done before and 2 and 6 weeks after each treatment. The FRS was performed by two nurses taking care of the patients.

Results

The injections were performed easily without EMG guidance and were well tolerated by all patients. No side effects were observed for either BTX or placebo injections. One patient developed left-sided numbness and weakness about 5 weeks after the first treatment. She was withdrawn from the study, and the code revealed that she had received a placebo treatment. Clinically she had a relapse of her MS. The results were analyzed for the remaining nine patients.

The scores on the RSP and FRS recorded by two separate physicians and two separate nurses, respectively, had good correlations. The correlation coefficients were 0.93 and 0.81, respectively, applying Spearman's rank correlation. The mean scores of the two observers for each scale were used for computing the results.

On the RSP, spasticity scores were reduced from 7.9 ± 4.9 to 4.7 ± 4.3 six weeks after treatment in the BTX group. This change was significant ($p = 0.009$, Wilcoxon signed rank test). For the placebo group, the change was from 6.8 ± 5.3 to 7.1 ± 4.8 after 6 weeks, and this was not significant. Comparison of BTX and placebo groups at 6 weeks also showed a significant difference between the two groups ($p = 0.009$) (Fig. 2). The reduction in spasticity scores in the BTX group was contributed by reduction in the degree of muscle tone (from 2.6 ± 0.9 to $1.4 \pm 0.9, p = 0.008$) rather than decrease in

Table 1   Rating Scale for Spasticity in Hip Adductors

Degree of muscle tone
    0   No increase
    1   Increased tone, hips easily abducted to 45° by one person
    2   Hips abducted to 45° by one person with mild effort
    3   Hips abducted to 45° by one person with major effort
    4   Two people required to abduct the hips to 45°
Spasm frequency score
    0   No spasms
    1   One or fewer spasms per day
    2   Between 1 and 5 spasms per day
    3   Five to <10 spasms per day
    4   Ten or more spasms per day, or continuous contractions

spasm frequency (from 2.9 ± 1.0 to 2.7 ± 1.3, not significant). Carry-over effect was not present ($p = 0.6$).

Hygienic care also improved 6 weeks after treatment in the BTX group ($p = 0.009$), with no significant changes in the placebo group. Comparison of BTX and placebo treatments also yielded significant differences between the two groups ($p = 0.02$) (Fig. 3).

Pain was present in two patients and was reduced in both after BTX treatment, requiring less use of analgesics. This improvement was not observed in the placebo group.

Discussion of Results

This study demonstrated that BTX is effective in reducing muscle spasms. It acts by reducing the force of the spasms rather than by reducing the spasm frequency. This may suggest that BTX does not have a significant action on the intrafusal fibers of muscle spindles, blockade of which should reduce stretch reflexes and reduce spasm frequency.

No local or systemic side effects were observed with BTX injections of up to 400 MU. By the end of 3 months, improvements in scores were no longer observed. This appears to correspond to the duration of effectiveness of treatment in dystonia. It should be noted that this study was performed under a rigid protocol. Better results may be expected with more experience and some variation in the muscles injected. On the other hand, a total dose of 400 MU was sufficient to reduce adductor spasms on one side only. This means that much larger doses are required to treat both sides, and this becomes a limitation to the maximum effects that may be achieved with BTX. Further studies with repeated treatment are necessary to establish the role of BTX in treating adductor spasms in MS.

Table 2   Functional Rating Scale (Hygiene Score)

    0   Independent with self-care.
    1   One person is able to clean and catheterize with ease.
    2   One person is able to clean and catheterize with effort.
    3   One person is able to clean and catheterize with major difficulty.
    4   Two people required, but together they can clean and catheterize
        easily.
    5   Two people clean and catheterize with difficulty.

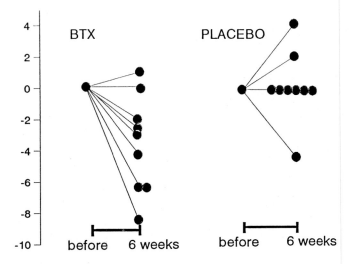

Figure 2 Changes in spasticity scores.

STUDY IN POST-STROKE SPASTICITY

At present, no double-blind, placebo-controlled trials have been published on the use of BTX in post-stroke spasticity. An open-label trial is under way at the Colorado Neurological Institute including patients with hemidystonia, dystonia plus spasticity, and spasticity with adequate muscle bulk. The preliminary results are encouraging. In the initial 10 patients, injections were given for a variety of patterns of abnormal posturing summarized in Table 3. Patients were selected because of the disabling nature of their symptoms. All had had symptoms for more than 5 months since the onset of stroke. The mean time of symptoms since stroke was 13 months (range 6–24). All had demonstrable motor function

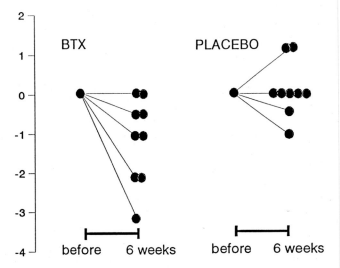

Figure 3 Changes in hygiene scores.

Table 3 Postural Abnormalities in 10 Patients with Post-Stroke Spasticity

Patient #	Postural abnormality
Lower limbs	
1	Inversion of foot with limited dorsiflexion
2	Inversion of foot with limited dorsiflexion
3	Inversion of foot with limited dorsiflexion
4	Fixed plantar flexion
5	Isolated inversion
6	Inversion and excessive dorsiflexion
Upper limbs	
7	Elbow flexion
8	Shoulder anteriorly displaced + elbow flexion
9	Wrist and elbow flexion
10	Wrist and elbow flexion

in the antagonistic muscle groups, but function was limited because of spasticity with or without dystonia. In patient 4, there was fixed dorsiflexion with marked contracture of the Achilles tendon. None had previous surgical treatment, and medical therapy had failed in all.

Injections of BTX were carried out with EMG guidance. Table 4 summarizes the doses employed for these patients in different muscles. The procedure was well tolerated by all patients, with no complications at the time of injection.

The results (summarized in Table 5) demonstrated significant improvement in spasticity as measured by the Ashworth scale. Two-thirds of the patients were very pleased about the results and were eager to receive repeat injections when the effects wore off. Patients who failed to benefit from the treatment appeared to have trouble because of either fixed contractures or disappointment in the lack of functional improvement despite adequate reduction of spasticify.

A carefully designed placebo-controlled, double-blind study must be carried out. Objective measurements of upper and lower limb functions should be performed to monitor response. As post-stroke spasticity typically emerges from 6–20 weeks following insult, the timing of BTX injections may be critical. It has been our anecdotal experience that BTX injections in the 3- to 9-month period after stroke may have the greatest potential for benefit. This may allow for the most effective intervention by rehabilitation therapists.

STUDY IN CEREBRAL PALSY

In a study (Koman et al, 1990), 48 children with cerebral palsy were treated with BTX injections over a 28-month period. The dose employed was 1–2 MU/kg body weight. Evaluation was done by a physician with a physician rating scale and by a physiotherapist with a physical therapist rating scale. Gait stride and video analysis were also employed.

The results showed that reduction in spasticity lasted for 3 to 6 months, without any weakness in any noninjected muscles. There was no evidence of clinical resistance to BTX injections after repeated treatment for 28 months. Other than some local soreness at injection sites, fatigue, and expected weakness in the muscles injected, no significant side effects were observed. The improvement achieved included reduced pain and greater ease of positioning in patients with paraspinal spasms, improved positioning and hygienic care

Table 4 Botulinum Toxin Doses
in Patients with Post-Stroke Spasticity

Muscle	Dose (MU)
Gastrocnemius	50–100
Soleus	50–100
Tibialis posterior	50–150
Tibialis anterior	25–75
Flexor carpi radialis	10–50
Flexor carpi ulnaris	10–50
Flexor digitorum	5–50
Brachioradialis	25–75
Biceps	25–100
Pectoralis	75

for nonambulatory patients, and improved gait dynamics in patients with ankle deformities without contractures.

DISCUSSION

Effectiveness

Injections of BTX are effective in relieving involuntary muscle contractions due to
spasticity. Short-term efficacy has been demonstrated in clinical trials, and muscles
injected are invariably weakened. Similar to applications in dystonia, the duration of
effects is about 3 months, and treatment has to be repeated.

Safety

Serious systemic side effects have not been described in clinical trials so far published for
spasticity. In the treatment of dystonia involving injections into facial or neck muscles,
side effects are usually due to local diffusion of the toxin into neighboring muscles. In the
treatment of spasticity, however, BTX is usually injected into larger muscles in the
extremities.

Table 5 Results of Treatment for Post-Stroke Spasticity

	Before treatment	After treatment
Lower limb group		
Ashworth scale (0–5)	4.2	2.8
Patient satisfaction		80% moderately to very satisfied
Upper limb group		
Ashworth scale (0–5)	4.0	2.5
Patient satisfaction		80% moderately to very satisfied

Limitations

Spasticity is usually secondary to disturbance of the pyramidal tract, and frequently there is accompanying muscle weakness. Reducing spasticity may be helpful in alleviating pain, discomfort, and abnormal posturing but may reduce muscle strength. This may make standing or walking more difficult, since some patients may be relying on spasticity to perform these functions. In conditions such as MS, patients are affected by spasticity and muscle weakness, as well as ataxia. Taking away one component does not necessarily help the patient to improve functional capacity. Treatment has to be individualized. The overall expected functional improvement and actual benefits achieved should be the most important consideration in deciding whether this treatment is to be given or not.

The timing of treatment may be important in conditions such as post-stroke spasticity, which usually emerges about 6 to 20 weeks after central injury. Injections of BTX in the 3- to 9-month period after stroke may have the greatest potential for benefit.

CONCLUSION

Botulinum toxin can reduce spasticity in selected groups of muscles and is superior to spasmolytic agents in that no significant adverse reactions occur at doses below 400 MU per treatment. It does not produce permanent disfiguring deformities, and treatment may be repeated when effects re wearing off. It is potentially a good alternative for treatment of troublesome muscle spasms. Further studies are desirable to establish the role of BTX in spasticity.

Future Considerations

The long-term effects of repeated BTX injections remain unknown. Experience may be gained from the published data obtained in treating dystonia, in which it has been employed for about 8 years. The treatment appears safe and remains effective for this period of time. There is scanty information on its safety in infants and children. Its safety in pregnancy is unknown.

A dose-response curve for BTX has never been satisfactorily established in the treatment of dystonia. There is considerable variability in sensitivity to BTX in different patients. Different muscles in the same patient may also vary in sensitivity of response. It is hoped that more carefully controlled studies may outline the dose-response relationship to arrive at optimal doses for individual muscles.

Antibody formation is a potential problem that may limit the effectiveness of BTX treatments in the long run. Very large doses and frequent injections should be avoided. Other serotypes of BTX, such as types F and B, should be explored for their applications in spasticity.

REFERENCES

Ashworth B. Preliminary trial of carisoprodol in multiple sclerosis. Practitioner 1964;192:540–542.

Dykstra DD, Sidi AA. Treatment of detrusor-sphincter dyssynergia with botulinum A toxin: a double-blind study. Arch Phys Med Rehabil 1990;71:24–26.

Koman LA, Mooney J, Smith B, Goodman A. Cerebral palsy management by neuromuscular blockade with botulinum-A toxin. NIH Consensus Development Conference on Clinical Use of Botulinum Toxin. Program and abstracts 142–145, November 1990.

Penn RD, Savoy SM, Corcos D, et al. Intrathecal backofen for severe spinal spasticity. N Engl J Med 1989;320:1517–1521.

Rice GP. Pharmacotherapy of spasticity: some theoretical and practical considerations. Can J Neurol Sci 1987;14(suppl):510–512.

Scott AB, Suzuki D. Systemic toxicity of botulinum toxin by intramuscular injection in the monkey. Mov Disord 1988;3:333–335.

Snow BJ, Tsui JKC, Bhatt MH, et al. Treatment of spasticity with botulinum toxin: a double-blind study. Ann Neurol 1990;28:512–515.

Young RR, Delwade PJ. Drug therapy: spasticity (first of two parts). N Engl J Med 1981;304: 28–33.

Young RR, Delwade PJ. Drug therapy: spasticity (second of two parts). N Engl J Med 1981;304:96–99.

42

Effects of Botulinum Toxin Type A on Detrusor-Sphincter Dyssynergia in Spinal Cord Injury Patients

Dennis D. Dykstra
University of Minnesota, Minneapolis, Minneapolis, Minnesota

INTRODUCTION

Detrusor-sphincter dyssynergia is a significant problem for patients after spinal cord injury. The resulting high intravesical pressures and poor emptying of the bladder may lead to autonomic dysreflexia, serious infection of the urinary tract, renal damage, and premature death. Detrusor-sphincter dyssynergia is currently managed by medication, condom or indwelling catheters, intermittent catheterization, electrical stimulation, or surgery to destroy sphincter function. All of these methods of treatment have associated complications (1). A safe, effective, and reversible treatment that allows low-pressure drainage of the bladder has not been developed.

ANATOMY AND PHYSIOLOGY OF MICTURITION

The two functions of the urinary bladder are storage and active expulsion of urine (2). During bladder filling, intravesical pressure rises slowly despite an increase in volume, a phenomenon that is due, initially at least, to the viscoelastic properties of the smooth muscle and connective tissue of the bladder wall. There is little neural efferent activity to the bladder until a critical intravesical pressure is reached, after which any further pressure increase stimulates a reflex arc. The afferent impulses of this reflex arc travel via the pelvic nerve, and the efferent impulses travel via the hypogastric nerve (Fig. 1). This sympathetic spinal reflex results in active stimulation of the functional internal sphincter; in addition, it inhibits bladder activity by a direct effect on smooth muscle and an indirect effect on parasympathetic ganglia, which allow more complete bladder filling.

Although many factors are involved in the micturition reflex, it is intravesical pressure, producing the sensation of distention, that primarily initiates bladder contraction. The pelvic nerve, which is the parasympathetic neural outflow to the bladder, has its origin in

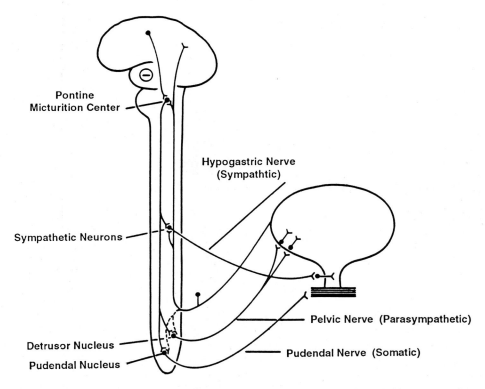

Figure 1   Neuronal interactions between lower urinary tract and the nervous system. Before micturition, vesical afferents ascend to the pontine micturitional center, which normally inhibited by higher centers. Efferents from the pons descend to the thoracolumbar sympathetic center and the detrusor and pudendal nuclei to coordinate vesical contraction with relaxation of the smooth muscle and striated muscle sphincter. (From Ref. 29.)

the sacral spinal cord. However, it appears that the actual organizational center for the micturition reflex is in the brain stem, and that the complete neural circuit for normal micturition includes ascending and descending spinal cord pathways to and from this area. The final step in micturition involves a highly coordinated, parasympathetically induced contraction of the bladder body, the shaping or funneling of a relaxed bladder outlet, the depression of the sympathetic inhibitory outflow, and the inhibition of the tonic somatic discharge to the striated pelvic floor musculature surrounding the bladder neck and urethra. Other reflexes that are elicited by bladder contraction and the passage of urine through the urethra may reinforce these primary reflexes and facilitate complete bladder emptying. Superimposed on the autonomic and somatic reflexes are complex modifying supraspinal inputs from other central neuronal networks. These facilitory and inhibitory impulses, which originate at several levels of the nervous system—including the brain stem, the cerebellum, and the cerebral cortex—allow for full conscious control of micturition.

Detrusor hyperreflexia is characterized by involuntary detrusor contractions during bladder filling that cannot be consciously suppressed and that produce an increase in intravesical pressure greater than 15 cm H_2O (3). Other terms that have been used to describe this disorder include motor unstable bladder, automatic bladder, and uninhibited neurogenic bladder (4). Detrusor hyperreflexia may be associated with a variety of clinical entities (5). Neurogenically induced detrusor hyperreflexia is almost always associated with a lesion that effects the sacral cord outflow.

Several theories have been offered to explain the neurophysiological basis of detrusor hyperreflexia following suprasacral neurological lesions. The normal micturitional reflex is not a simple segmental phenomenon; rather, it involves synapsing of long spinal tracts, presumably in the region of the pontine reticular formation (6–8). After suprasacral spinal cord transection, the micturitional reflex changes in nature from a long-tract reflex to a segmental reflex. Whether this segmental pathway is normally present in humans and is unmasked by a suprasacral lesion, or whether it represents a new reflex pathway formed by collateral sprouting, is not known (9,10). Whatever the cause, the end result is a new micturitional reflex center located in the sacral cord. The threshold for firing of this reflex center is reduced, which accounts for involuntary detrusor contractions at low intravesical volumes.

Reflex interactions between the detrusor and the external striated urethral sphincter must also be taken into account. Bladder filling will lead to increased external urethral sphincter activity. Conversely, a bladder contraction will normally be associated with reflex inhibition of all activity in the external urethral sphincter (11–13). In an intact nervous system, reflex coordination between the bladder and the external sphincter is thought to occur at a surpasacral level. Experimentally, it is known that centers for coordination of such long-tract reflexes exist in the region of the pons (6–8). Thus, suprasacral lesions between the sacral cord and pons (i.e., spinal cord injury) may result not only in detrusor hyperreflexia as described above, but also in lack of appropriate coordination between the detrusor and external sphincter (vesicosphincter dyssynergia) (14) (Fig. 2). As may be the case for detrusor hyperreflexia, vesicosphincter dyssyngergia may represent unmasking of a facilitative reflex between the detrusor and external sphincter or the formation of a new reflex by neural reorganization (collateral sprouting).

On rare occasions, detrusor hyperreflexia may be associated with a neurogenically mediated obstruction at the level of the smooth muscle sphincter (15,16). A detrusor contraction is normally accompanied by synchronous neurogenic relaxation of the smooth muscle sphincter. A lesion situated above the sympathetic spinal cord outflow (T6) may result in the loss of this appropriate inhibition of sympathetic discharge to the smooth muscle sphincter.

USE OF BOTULINUM TOXIN

Botulinum toxin type A (BTX-A) inhibits transmitter release at the neuromuscular junction. Low doses have been injected into the extrinsic ocular muscles in an attempt to control strabismus (17). Results of this treatment have been excellent, and toxin injections are now used at numerous medical centers instead of surgery to treat strabismus, blepharospasm (18), dystonia (19), and torticollis (20).

We evaluated the ability of low doses of BTX-A, an inhibitor of acetylcholine release at the neuromuscular junction, to denervate and relax the spastic external striated urethral sphincter in 11 men with spinal cord injury and detrusor-sphincter dyssynergia (21). Toxin concentration, injection volume, percutaneous versus cystoscopic injection of the sphincter, and number of injections were evaluated in three treatment protocols.

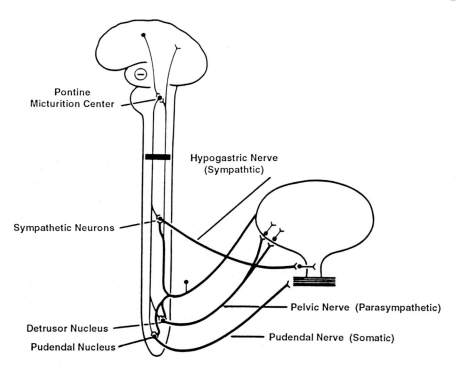

Figure 2 A lesion above the thoracolumbar sympathetic outflow, resulting in detrusor hyper-reflexia and loss of coordination between the detrusor and striated muscle sphincter (the smooth muscle sphincter may also be involved in this lesion). Facilitative segmental reflexes between the bladder and the external sphincter will result in detrusor-sphincter dyssynergia. The degree of dyssynergia between the detrusor and either sphincter will depend on the degree of neuronal damage to descending pathways that normally are present to coordinate detrusor and sphincter function. (From Ref. 29.)

All 10 patients evaluated by electromyography after injection showed signs of sphincter denervation. Bulbosphincteric reflexes in the 10 patients evaluated after injection were more difficult to obtain, and they showed a decreased amplitude and normal latency. The urethral pressure profile in the seven patients in whom it was measured before and after treatment decreed an average of 27 cm H_2O after toxin injections. Postvoiding residual urine volume decreased by an average of 146 ml after the toxin injections in eight patients. In the eight patients for whom it could be determined, toxin effects lasted an average of 50 days. The toxin also decreased autonomic dysreflexia in five patients.

The ability of BTX-A to denervate and relax a spastic external urethral sphincter was further evaluated in a double-blind study involving five men with high spinal cord injuries and detrusor-sphincter dyssynergia (22). The sphincter was injected with either BTX-A or normal saline once a week for 3 weeks. Electromyography of the external urethral sphincter indicated denervation in the three patients who received toxin injections. The urethral pressure profile decreased an average of 25 cm H_2O, postvoiding residual volume of urine decreased an average of 125 ml, and bladder pressure during voiding decreased to an average of 30 cm H_2O. Bulbosphincteric reflexes were more difficult to obtain, and they showed a decreased amplitude with normal latency. In the two patients who received normal saline injections, parameters were unchanged from baseline values until subsequent injection with BTX-A once a week for 3 weeks, when their responses were similar to those of the other three patients. Mild generalized weakness lasting 2–3 weeks was noted by three patients after initial toxin injections. The duration of the toxin's effect averaged 2 months.

METHOD OF INJECTION

An initial dose of 140 U of toxin (5 U of toxin per 0.1 ml normal saline) is injected into the rhabdosphincter through a cystoscope with a 23-gauge, 35-cm polytetrafluorethylene (Teflon)-coated monopolar needle electrode (Fig. 3). The electrode is connected to the TECA Model M two-channel electromyography machine. A urine sample is obtained for culture before cystoscopy. After cystoscopy a Foley catheter is left in place for 24 h, and the patients are treated prophylactically for 4 days with trimethoprim and sulfamethoxazole or nitrofurantoin. All subsequent weekly doses of toxin are 240 U (5 U toxin per 0.1 ml normal saline). An average of three injections are needed to produce a maximum decrease in postvoiding residual urine volume.

Because indirect sympathetic stimulation caused by bladder dilatation during cystoscopy puts patients at risk for autonomic hyperreflexia during the injection procedure (23), blood pressure and mean arterial pressure are measured before and during cystoscopy. Patients who develop symptoms of autonomic hyperreflexia are given 10 mg of nifedipine, a calcium channel blocker (24,25), by mouth 30 min before the next cystoscopy injection or are treated during cystoscopy by sublingual administration of 10 mg of

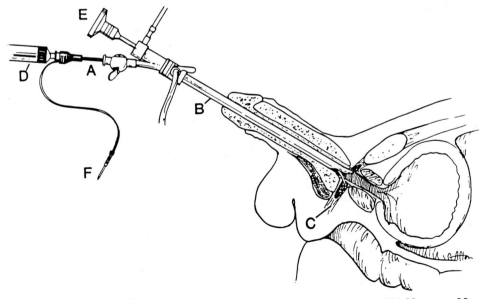

Figure 3 Technique used to inject toxin into the external urethral sphincter. (A) 23-gauge, 35-cm Teflon-coated monopolar needle electrode (TN needle). (B) Cystoscope. (C) External urethral sphincter. (D) Syringe containing toxin for injection. (E) Eyepiece of cystoscope. (F) Electrode to electromyography machine.

nifedipine to relax vascular smooth muscle and thereby control autonomic hyperreflexia (26,27).

CONCLUSION

Drawbacks to our present protocol are the requirement for two to three initial injections by cystoscopy and that at the current dose and volume the toxin's effects last only about 60 days before another single injection is needed.

It must be emphasized that options for bladder management in spinal cord injury patients are limited. Medications are unreliable and the side effects are troublesome. Long-term indwelling catheters are convenient, but they encourage chronic urinary tract infections. Intermittent catheterization is difficult for many patients, especially those with poor hand function. Surgical sphincterotomy is rejected by many spinal cord injury patients who do not want to undergo an irreversible surgical procedure. Electrical stimulation of the bladder does not reliably produce simultaneous sphincter relaxation. Condom catheters keep patients dry but they are not a treatment for detrusor-sphincter dyssynergia or dysreflexia if it exists.

Injections of BTX-A offer a new option in bladder management for the spinal cord injury patient with detrusor-sphincter dyssynergia who can wear a condom catheter but cannot perform intermittent catheterization and does not want a surgical sphincterotomy. It is in a sense a nonsurgical, reversible sphincterotomy. The effects of the toxin last longer than those of an anesthetic pudendal nerve block, and the toxin does not cause the tissue injury that a phenol block does (28). We believe that the results of our studies are most encouraging. Controlled studies of improved injection techniques, dosage schedules, use of other toxin types or combinations of toxin types, possible long-term toxin effects, and possible toxin interactions with other medications that decrease urethral pressure are warranted.

REFERENCES

1. Yalla SV. Neurology and urodynamics: principles and practice. New York: Macmillan, 1988.
2. Wein AJ, Raezer DM. Physiology of micturition. In: Krane RJ, Siroky MD, eds. Clinical neuro-urology. Boston: Little, Brown, 1979:26–29.
3. Bates P, Bradley WE, Glen E, Griffith D. Standardization of terminology of lower urinary tract function.Urology 1977;9:237–241.
4. Lapides J. Neuromuscular vesical and ureteral dysfunction. In: Campbell MF, Harrison JH, eds. Urology. Philadelphia: W.B. Saunders, 1976.
5. Krane RJ, Siroky MD. Classification of neuro-urologic disorders. In: Krane RJ, Siroky MD, eds. Clinical neuro-urology. Boston: Little, Brown, 1979:144–147.
6. Barrington FJF. The nervous mechanism of micturition. Q J Exp Physiol 1914;8:3–71.
7. Barrington FJF. The component reflexes of micturition in the cat: part III. Brain 1941;64:239–243.
8. DeGroat NC. Nervous control of the urinary bladder of the cat. Brain Res 1975;87:201–211.
9. Anderson JT. Detrusor hyperreflexia in benign infravesical obstruction: a cystometric study. J Urol 1976;115:532–534.
10. Liu CN, Chambers WW. Intraspinal sprouting of dorsal root axons. Arch Neurol Psychiatry 1958;79:46–61.
11. Diokno AC, Koff SA, Bender LF. Periurethral striated muscle activity in neurogenic bladder dysfunction. J Urol 1974;112:743–749.

12. Gary RC, Roberts TDM, Todd JK. Reflexes involving the external urethral sphincter in the cat. J Physiol (Lond) 1959;149:653–665.
13. Kuru M. Nervous control of micturition. Physiol Rev 1965;45:426–484.
14. Yalla SV, Rossier AB, Fam B. Dyssynergic vesicourethral responses during bladder rehabilitation in spinal cord injury patients: Effects of suprapubic percussion, Credé method and bethanechol chloride. J Urol 1976;115:575–579.
15. Scott MD, Morrow JW. Phenoxy-benzamine in neurogenic bladder dysfunction after spinal cord injury: I. Voiding dysfunction. J Urol 1978;119:480–482.
16. Scott MB, Morrow JW. Phenoxy-benzamine neurogenic bladder dysfunction after spinal cord injury: II. Automatic dysreflexia. J Urol 1978;119:483–484.
17. Scott AB. Botulinum toxin injection of eye muscles to correct strabismus. Trans Am Ophthalmol Soc 1981;79:734–770.
18. Scott AB, Kennedy RA, Stubbs HA. Botulinum A toxin injection as a treatment for blepharospasm. Arch Ophthalmol 1985;103:347–350.
19. Ludlow CL, Naunton RF, Sedory SE, Schultz GM, Hallett M. Effects of botulinum toxin injections on speech in adductor spasmodic dysphonia. Neurology 1988;38:1220–1225.
20. Taui JK, Eisen A, Mak E, Carruthers T, Scott A, Calne DB. A pilot study on the use of botulinum toxin in spasmodic torticollis. Canad J Neurol Sci 1985;12:314–316.
21. Dykstra DD, Sidi AA, Scott AB, Pagel JM, Goldish GD. Effects of botulinum A toxin on detrusor-sphincter dyssynergia in spinal cord injury patients. J Urol 1988;139:919–922.
22. Dykstra DD, Sidi AA. Treatment of detrusor-sphincter dyssynergia with botulinum A toxin: a double blind study. Arch Phys Med Rehabil 1990;71:24–26.
23. Erickson RP. Autonomic hyperreflexia: pathophysiology and medical management. Arch Phys Med Rehabil 1980;61:431–440.
24. Bartorelli C, Magrini F, Moruzzi P, Olevari MT, Polese K, Fiorentini C, et al. Haemodynamic effects of a calcium antagonistic agent (nifedipine) in hypertension: therapeutic implications. Clin Sci Mol Med 1978;55(suppl):291S–292S.
25. Beer N, Gallegos I, Cohen A, Klein N, Sonnenblick F, Fishman W. Efficacy of sublingual nifedipine in the acute treatment of systemic hypertension. Chest 1981;79:571–574.
26. Dykstra DD, Sidi AA, Anderson LC. The effect of nifedipine on cystoscopy-induced autonomic hyperreflexia in patients with high spinal cord injuries. J Urol 1987;138:1155–1157.
27. Linden R, Leffler EJ, Kedia KR. A comparison of the efficacy of an alpha 1-adrenergic blocker in the slow calcium channel in the control of autonomic dysreflexia. Paraplegia 1985;23:34–38.
28. Mooney V, Frykman G, McLamb J. Current status of intraneural phenol injections. Clin Orthop 1969;63:122–131.
29. Krane RJ, Siroky MB. Classification of neuro-urologic disorders. In: Krane RJ, Siroky MB, eds. Clinical neuro-urology. Boston: Little Brown, 1979;144–147.

43

Botulinum Toxin in the Treatment of Gastrointestinal Disorders

Pankaj Jay Pasricha and Anthony N. Kalloo
Johns Hopkins University and Hospital, Baltimore, Maryland

INTRODUCTION

Several decades have passed since the therapeutic potential of botulinum toxin (BTX) was first realized. The last few years have seen a virtual explosion of applications of this treatment in a variety of skeletal muscle disorders, as discussed in the other chapters of this book. However, until very recently there had been no attempt to explore the use of this unique biological agent in the treatment of disorders of gastrointestinal *smooth* muscle. This discrepancy becomes even more conspicuous when one realizes that the effects of BTX on cholinergic traffic within the enteric nervous system have been known for a long time. In this chapter we will attempt to summarize our knowledge of these effects and provide a glimpse of the exciting therapeutic opportunities that are only just beginning to emerge.

BACKGROUND

Regulation of Gastrointestinal Motility*

The enteric nervous system is an extremely complex network of nerves and muscles that resides within the gastrointestinal wall and orchestrates the entire digestive process, including motility, secretion, and absorption. The gut is a tubular organ whose wall is organized in a pattern of layers that is essentially consistent from the esophagus to the anus (Fig. 1). Within this wall, smooth muscle is organized into two main layers, a thick, inner circular layer and a thinner outer longitudinal layer. At certain sites along the length of the gut, the circular muscle becomes organized into physiologically distinct regions

---

*The reader is encouraged to refer to Furness and Costa (1) for an excellent and detailed review of the subject.

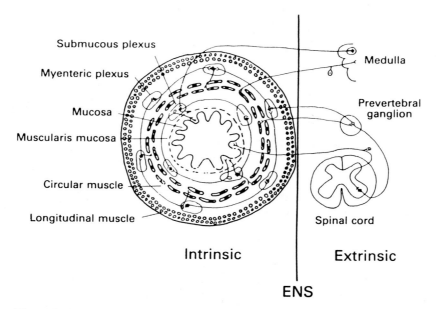

Intrinsic   Extrinsic

ENS

Figure 1 Transverse section of the gut showing the muscle layers and plexuses, along with some extrinsic and intrinsic interconnections. (From Kumar D, Gustavsson S. An illustrated guide to gastrointestinal motility. Chichester, England: John Wiley & Sons, 1988.)

called sphincters. Sphincters function to regulate forward movement of luminal contents and limit or prevent retrograde movement (or reflux). Sphincteric dysfunction is an important cause of gastrointestinal motility disorders, as will be discussed below.

The neuromuscular unit in the gut wall differs fundamentally from that of skeletal muscle in several ways. First, it lacks a discrete end plate, with nerve fibers from each axon running parallel to the muscle bundle and ending somewhat arbitrarily at various points along its length. Second, muscle cells are coupled electrically within large bundles by means of connecting bridges. An electrical event at any region in the bundle is therefore conducted in a decremental fashion to other regions. Third, each muscle bundle receives input from multiple axons in the form of either excitatory or inhibitory signals (see below).

The enteric nerves are also organized into interconnected networks called plexuses. Of these, the myenteric plexus, situated between the circular and longitudinal muscle layers, is the main modulator of gastrointestinal smooth muscle motility. It receives input from both the central nervous system (via vagal and sympathetic pathways) and local reflex pathways. Its output consists of both inhibitory and excitatory signals to the adjacent muscle.

The final neural pathway regulating smooth muscle activity in the gut is therefore represented by the neurons of the myenteric plexus. On the basis of their neurotransmitter content, these neurons can be broadly divided into two categories (2,3):

1. SP/SK/ACh, containing substance P, substance K, and acetylcholine (ACh), and constituting about 40–45% of the total number. Of these, acetylcholine is probably the most important. *These are the excitatory neurons*, stimulating the smooth muscle to contract.

2. The nonadrenergic, noncholinergic (NANC) system, which comprises the inhibitory neurons, constituting another 40–45%. Their main neurotransmitter appears to be VIP/PHM (vasoactive intestinal peptide and peptide with histidine and methionine) or NO (nitric oxide).

A useful, if somewhat simplistic, concept is to visualize *net* smooth muscle tone as that resulting from a balance between the opposing effects of these two neuronal systems (2). Support for this theory can be inferred from the results of various studies (4,5). Although the two main types of effector neurons within the myenteric plexus (ACh and NANC) have opposing effects on smooth muscle (excitation and relaxation, respectively), both types are activated by cholinergic excitation, albeit via different receptors (muscarinic and nicotinic, respectively) (Fig. 2). The role of the cholinergic system in the regulation of smooth muscle tone is therefore complex. Acetylcholine directly released by effector nerves near the muscle causes contraction; within the myenteric plexus, however, it may result in inhibition or excitation.

Apart from the ACh and NANC systems, at least 20 other potential neurotransmitters of lesser importance have been identified within the enteric nervous system, including adenosine triphosphate (ATP), serotonin (5-HT), somatostatin, dynorphin, and enkephalin, to name a few (1). The effect of any putative neurotransmitter in this system is determined by the sum of its effects at both the myenteric plexus and the neuromuscular

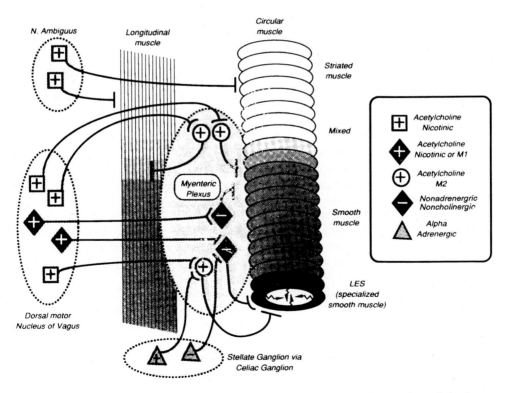

Figure 2 Diagrammatic representation of the intrinsic and extrinsic innervation of the lower esophageal sphincter. (From Castell DO, ed. The esophagus. Boston: Little, Brown, 1992.)

junction as well as by the nature of the receptor on the muscle cell. The role these substances play in the normal physiology is far from settled, but their sheer number and variety attests to the bewildering nature of the enteric nervous system.

Finally, it is important to remember that the myenteric plexus is probably the most important but is not the only determinant of muscle (particularly sphincter) tone in the gastrointestinal tract. In fact, basal sphincter tone may be visualized as resulting from the sum of many different factors, including intrinsic (myogenic) tone and circulating hormones, in addition to nerve activity (6).

It should be clear from even this brief overview that the regulation of smooth muscle motility is far more complex than that of skeletal muscle. The effects of cholinergic blockade by BTX therefore may not be straightforward and can have unexpected physiological consequences.

Botulinum Toxin and the Enteric Nervous System

There is both direct and indirect evidence to suggest that BTX may affect the cholinergic stimulation of visceral musculature as well as that of skeletal muscle. To begin with, symptoms and signs suggestive of inhibition of cholinergic transmission in smooth muscle are common in clinical botulism, as manifested by constipation, abdominal cramps, and heartburn, along with blurred vision, dry mouth, disturbances of micturition, and sexual dysfunction (7,8). Second, there is considerable experimental evidence to show that within the autonomic nervous system, BTX blocks ganglionic nerve endings, postganglionic parasympathetic nerve endings, and those parasympathetic nerve endings at which ACh is the transmitter (9). As far back as 1923, Dickson and Shevky showed that the toxin blocks intestinal motility induced by the splanchnic nerve (10).

More recently, Habermann and colleagues studied the effects of BTX on isolated myenteric plexus–muscle strips from guinea pig ileum and showed that the effects were very similar to those on a mouse phrenic nerve–hemidiaphragm preparation (11,12). The almost complete paralysis that resulted was associated with a decreased release of ACh and was partially reversed by 4-aminopyridine (a promoter of Ach release from cholinergic nerve endings). Strips retained their sensitivity to ACh, indicating that the toxin acted at a presynaptic level. The detection limit for toxin in their assay was around 0.01–0.1 μg/ml. Although interspecies comparisons may be fallacious, the detection limit in a mouse phrenic nerve–hemidiaphragm preparation is 0.001 μg/ml (11), suggesting that the myenteric plexus may be less sensitive by a factor of 10.

When considering the effects of BTX on the entric nervous system, a logical question that arises is whether the toxin affects the release of mediators other than ACh, particularly that of the putative NANC agent. In fact, this question has been addressed by at least two studies. First, Paul and Cook (13) examined the NANC inhibitory response of guinea pig fundic muscle to electric field stimulation and found that BTX had no effect. Later, McKenzie et al., using a guinea pig ileum preparation, also showed that NANC transmission was probably not inhibited by BTX (14). The effects of BTX on noradrenergic transmission are somewhat more controversial. Early studies done by Ambache (15,16) showed that peripheral noradrenergic synapses are resistant to BTX. These findings have since been challenged by other workers (17,18). However, this issue has not been examined specifically in the enteric nervous system. Further, the net effect of adrenergic stimulation in control of sphincter tone may be of only minor physiological importance (2). There is no information on the effects of BTX on other neurotransmitters in this system.

Summary

The effects of BTX on the enteric nervous system have not been extensively studied. However, it is clear that the toxin blocks release of ACh and can cause partial paralysis of gastrointestinal smooth muscle. This effect also appears to be relatively specific in that NANC transmitter release is not affected. The effects on other neurotransmitters within the gut are not known.

IN VIVO EFFECTS OF BOTULINUM TOXIN ON THE LOWER ESOPHAGEAL SPHINCTER

On the basis of these historic reports, we proceeded to investigate the effects of local (intrasphincteric) injection of BTX on lower esophageal sphincter (LES) pressure in piglets (19). This was the first time that the effects of BTX on gastrointestinal smooth muscle had been demonstrated in a live animal model. As can be seen from Fig. 3, intrasphincteric BTX caused a 70% reduction in resting baseline LES pressure, while intrasphincteric normal saline had no significant effect.

In other experiments, we have found that intrasphincteric BTX did not alter the LES response to intravenous injection of pentagastrin or bethanechol (a modest increase in LES pressure was seen in all cases). The fact that the LES retains its ability to contract in response to bethanechol and pentagastrin (both agents act directly on the LES) proves that the site of action of BTX is not the muscle itself.

Intrasphincteric BTX not only decreases basal LES pressure but also appears to alter the response of the sphincter to various pharmacological maneuvers. In untreated piglets, intravenously administered cholecystokinin (CCK) did not cause any significant change in LES pressure. However, after intrasphincteric BTX injection, a significant increase in

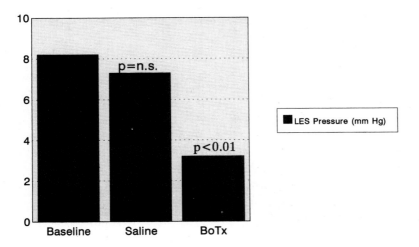

Saline = 1 week after normal ; BTX = 1 week after botulinum toxin

Figure 3 The effects of intrasphincteric injection of botulinum toxin (BTX) and normal saline (as control) on resting lower esophageal sphincter (LES) pressure in piglets. Intrasphincteric BTX caused a 70% reduction in resting baseline LES pressure, while intrasphincteric normal saline had no significant effect.

LES pressure was seen to occur in response to CCK, Cholecystokinin is known to have a dual effect on the LES: a direct stimulatory effect on smooth muscle and an indirect inhibitory one mediated via the myenteric plexus (3). In normal piglets, these effects may balance each other. However, by blocking the indirect pathway of inhibition (which is mediated cholinergically), BTX unmasks the direct excitatory effect of CCK on the LES muscle. This is similar to the reported effect of CCK in patients with achalasia, in which denervation of the inhibitory limb to the LES is thought to occur (20).

No evidence of adverse effects of BTX injection was apparent. The pigs appeared healthy, had a hearty appetite, and continued to gain weight. Follow-up endoscopy 1 week after injection did not reveal any evidence of esophagitis or other mucosal damage. At necropsy, performed 1 week after the injection, the gastroesophageal junction appeared normal, without any serosal inflammation. Histologically, the distal esophagus appeared normal under light microscopy.

These experiments were important for several reasons. First, they showed that gastrointestinal sphincteric smooth muscle can be partially paralyzed by BTX. Second, *net* cholinergic impulses (i.e., both in the myenteric plexus and at the neuromuscular junction) appear to play a dominant role in the maintenance of basal LES tone. This had been an area of controversy in previous reports (4,21). Finally, local injection of BTX appeared to be safe and well tolerated in these animals.

APPLICATION OF BOTULINUM TOXIN THERAPY IN MOTILITY DISORDERS OF THE GUT

Encouraged by the results of these animal studies, we decided to embark on a pilot trial to test the effect of intrasphincteric BTX in patients with achalasia. Although there are several important human diseases that result from derangements in motility, achalasia appeared particularly likely to respond to this form of treatment. This will become apparent in a brief review of the nature of this disease.

Achalasia

Achalasia is a disorder of esophageal motility characterized by an absence of peristalsis of the esophageal body accompanied by failure of the LES to relax with swallowing. The abnormalities of the LES are considered to be the most important feature of this disease because they are potentially amenable to treatment. Thus, despite the existence of disordered or absent propulsion, the success of any treatment for achalasia depends on its effects on the lower esophageal sphincter (22).

Traditionally, such treatment has taken one of three forms:

1. *Pharmacological therapy*, aimed at relaxation of the smooth muscle of the LES, and consisting mainly of nitroglycerin derivatives and calcium channel blockers. Despite initial enthusiasm for the latter, drug therapy has in general proved disappointing. Trials have shown mixed results, and benefit, when demonstrated, has been modest at best. Apart from the intrinsic efficacy of the drugs, other factors that have limited the role of pharmacotherapy include short-peaked duration of effect, tachyphylaxis, and the problem of delivery of adequate amounts of drug to the target site without the risk of systemic side effects.
2. *Surgery* (myotomy of the LES). While this may relieve symptoms in more than 90% of patients, it has been associated with an incidence of reflux greater than 25% (23).

In addition to the risks of anesthesia and thoracotomy, surgery has the added problems of cost, long recovery time, and prolonged hospitalization (24).

3. *Pneumatic (balloon) dilatation*, to produce a disruption of the muscle fibers of the LES. This is currently considered by most authorities to be the treatment of choice in the majority of cases. Its disadvantages include a lower efficacy rate (65–80%) in comparison with surgery and the significant risk of esophageal perforation, ranging from 1% to 13% (25), with attendant morbidity and mortality.

It is clear, therefore, that none of the current methods of treatment of achalasia is completely satisfactory. We hypothesized that blockade of cholinergic signals to the LES may be a more physiological (and perhaps more effective) approach. This was based on several observations previously reported in the literature. In patients with achalasia, one of the most striking pathological features in the region of the LES is the paucity of ganglion cells in the myenteric plexus (26). There is growing evidence to suggest that this ganglion loss is selective and predominantly involves the VIP/PHM neurons (i.e., the inhibitory system). Thus, ganglionic stimulation or cholecystokinin-octapeptide (CCK-OP) infusion, which usually reduces LES pressure in healthy subjects, either fails to do so or causes a paradoxical increase in patients with achalasia (20,27). Further, immunocytochemistry has revealed that there is a marked decrease in VIP-staining neurons in patients with achalasia (28). On the other hand, the LES contracts strongly when treated with the ACh analogue mecholyl (29) as well as with the cholinesterase inhibitor edrophonium (30), suggesting that the cholinergic (stimulatory) limb is preserved. Thus an imbalance of neural input to the smooth muscle, in favor of the excitatory stimulus, may be responsible for the LES abnormalities (31).

If this hypothesis is correct, one would expect anticholinergic therapy to be of benefit in this condition. In fact, this has been shown by at least one study using the anticholinergic drug dicyclomine HCl. In a double-blind, randomized trial the investigators showed that this drug caused significant clinical and manometric improvement (32). However, as with other anticholinergics, use of dicyclomine may be limited by its side-effects. In addition, it shares the general problems of pharmacological treatment that have been discussed above.

Ideally therefore, a desirable drug for achalasia should have the following properties:

1. It should be directed against the underlying physiological derangement. If one cannot restore the intrinsic inhibitory neurons that have been lost, this means counteracting the unopposed cholinergic system at the LES by some other means.
2. It should be site-specific, thus limiting systemic side effects.
3. It should maintain a constant effect, thus not limiting ingestion of food or drink to particular times of the day.
4. It should be relatively long-lasting.
5. Tachyphylaxis should not occur or be insignificant.

Initial results of our pilot trial (33) indicate that intrasphincteric BTX appears to meet most or all of these expectations. The treatment is carried out during the course of routine upper endoscopy. After a satisfactory examination of the esophagus, stomach, and duodenum, BTX is injected via a 5-mm sclerotherapy needle into the LES as estimated endoscopically. Four injections of 1.0 ml (20 U BTX/ml) into each quadrant are made, for a total of 80 U. The total duration of the procedure should not be more than about 15 minutes. Recovery is unremarkable, and the patients are usually able to go home within 2 hours of the procedure.

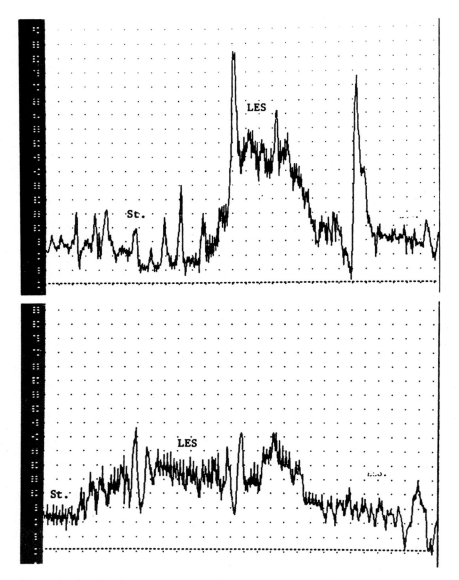

Figure 4 Baseline lower esophageal sphincter (LES) pressures in a patient with achalasia before (top panel) and one week after (bottom panel) treatment with intrasphincteric botulinum toxin. Pressures were recorded as the manometric catheter was slowly withdrawn from the stomach (st) to the esophagus. Note the approximately 50% reduction in LES pressures after treatment.

   The first patient to be treated in this fashion was a 71-year-old woman with achalasia who had failed to respond to drug treatment and balloon dilatation (34). One week after treatment, the patient's symptoms had completely resolved. Clinical improvement was accompanied by improvement in the esophagogram, as well as by a 50% reduction in resting LES pressure (Fig. 4), a change that compares favorably to the figures (41–50%) reported after balloon dilatation (35,36). With the exception of one patient who had only a partial response, all the other patients treated so far have had complete resolution of dysphagia. Most of these patients had undergone previous balloon dilatation, with only partial or temporary response. Symptomatic recovery has been accompanied by improvement in at least one of three objective criteria used to assess response, i.e., esophageal manometry, cine-esophagography, or esophageal transit time measured by radionuclide transit time (Fig. 5). The longest follow-up has been more than 8 months, with the patient having gained over 35 pounds of weight and remaining symptomatic. No adverse effects were seen except for one case of possible reflux esophagitis in a patient who had undergone a previous surgical myotomy.

On the basis of these encouraging results, we feel that local injection of BTX has the potential of being a safe and relatively simple form of therapy for achalasia. The clinical response is expected to wane with time, and thus further injections may be necessary. Nevertheless, it may provide a useful alternative for patients who either are not suitable for or refuse conventional treatment. This novel therapy for achalasia is being further evaluated at our institution in a randomized, placebo-controlled trial.

The Future: Other Gastrointestinal Applications

Table 1 shows a partial list of muscular disorders of the gut that may be potentially amenable to local injection with BTX. While such a list is certainly speculative, it provides a glimpse of the exciting possibilities that have been raised by the availability of an effective site-specific agent against smooth muscle spasm. Work is currently being done by our group on several of the disease entities mentioned in the table. We have recently reported the first patient with sphincter of Oddi dysfunction and chronic abdominal pain treated with BTX, with encouraging results (50). Sphincter pressure was reduced by nearly 50% following the injection, accompanied by complete relief of pain.

As can be seen, not all the disorders in Table 1 are of smooth muscle origin. Anismus (or rectosphincteric dyssynergia) results from an inability of the puborectalis and other skeletal muscles forming the external anal sphincter to relax during defecation (45). This condition is associated with characteristic findings on anorectal manometry or defecography. Surgical division of the puborectalis muscle has been disappointing, with a high incidence of incontinence (46). This disorder has been reported to respond to local injection of BTX. Using an electromyography-guided technique, Hallan et al. injected small amounts of BTX in seven patients with anismus and chronic severe constipation (47). Transient (about 8 weeks) symptomatic improvement, accompanied by objective evidence of muscle weakening, occurred in the majority of patients, but at the cost of incontinence in two of them. While the target in this study was skeletal and not smooth muscle, this was the first report of the clinical use of BTX in anorectal disorders.

Although this discussion has largely been restricted to gastrointestinal sphincters, it is conceivable that one day other targets will be found. Thus, in disorders of gastric dysrhythmias, one could envision a role for interfering with cholinergic mechanisms within the gastric electrical pacemaker.

CONCLUSIONS

While still in its experimental stages, the use of BTX injection to alleviate smooth muscle spasm is an exciting new development in the treatment of gastrointestinal disorders. If initial impressions about safety are upheld, its simplicity, effectiveness, and site-specificity may make it an attractive candidate for first-line therapy in several disorders of

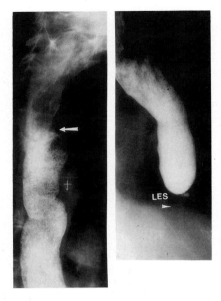

(a)

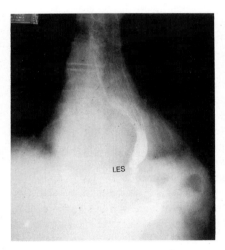

(b)

Figure 5   Esophagograms of a patient with achalasia before (a) and one week after (b) treatment with intrasphincteric botulinum toxin. Note the prominent air-fluid column high in the esophagus (arrow) and hold-up of contrast at the level of the lower esophageal sphincter (LES) before treatment. After treatment the esophagus is seen to be emptying almost completely and the LES appears more open.

Table 1 Motility Disorders of the Gut That May Be Potentially Amenable to Treatment with Local Injection of Botulinum Toxin

Disorder[a]	Symptoms	Proposed target muscle
Esophagus		
Upper esophageal sphincter (31)	Dysphagia, aspiration	Cricopharyngeus
Achalasia (see text)	Dysphagia, regurgitation	LES
Isolated disorders of the LES (37,38)	Dysphagia, chest pain	LES
Stomach		
Gastroparesis (39–42)	Pain, nausea, vomiting	Pylorus
Hypertrophic pyloric stenosis (43)	Vomiting	Pylorus
Biliary		
Sphincter of Oddi dysfunction (44)	Abdominal pain, pancreatitis	Sphincter of Oddi
Anorectal		
Anismus[b] (45–47)	Constipation	Levator ani, puborectalis
Levator syndrome[b] (48)	Pain	Levator ani, puborectalis
Short-segment Hirschsprung's disease (49)	Constipation	Internal anal sphincter
Anal fissure (48)	Pain, discharge	Internal anal sphincter
? Hemorrhoids (48)	Pain, bleeding discharge	Internal anal sphincter
Proctalgia fugax (48)	Pain	? Internal anal sphincter

[a]references listed are general discussions of the subject.
[b]Skeletal muscle.
LES = lower esophageal sphincter.

gastrointestinal sphincters. Further, if its effects on neurotransmitter release are truly specific for acetylcholine, it may provide a valuable investigative tool to understand the intricate workings of the enteric nervous system, in both normal and pathological states.

REFERENCES

1. Furness JB, Costa M. The enteric nervous system. Edinburgh: Churchill Livingstone, 1987.
2. Makhlouf GM. Smooth muscle of the gut. In: Yamada T, ed. Textbook of gastroenterology. 1st ed. Philadelphia: J.B. Lippincott, Philadelphia 1991:60.
3. Kahrilas P. Functional anatomy and physiology of the esophagus. In: Castell DO, ed. The esophagus. Boston: Little, Brown, 1992:1.
4. Dodds WJ, Dent J, Hogan WJ, Arndorfer RC. Effect of atropine on esophageal motor function in humans. Am J Physiol 1981;240:G290–296.

5. Biancani P, Walsh JH, Behar J. Vasoactive intestinal polypeptide—a neurotransmitter for lower esophageal sphincter relaxation. J Clin Invest 1984;73:963–967.
6. Goyal RK, Paterson WG. Esophageal motility. In: Handbook of physiology. Vol. 1. Bethesda, Maryland: American Physiological Society, 1989:865.
7. Jenzer G, Mumenthaler M, Ludin HP. Autonomic dysfunction in botulism B: a clinical report. Neurology 1975;25:150–153.
8. Koenig MG, Spickard A, Cardella MA, Rogers DE. Clinical and laboratory observations in type E botulism in man. Medicine 1964;43:517–545.
9. Simpson LL. The origin, structure, and pharmacological activity of botulinum toxin. Pharmacol Rev 1981;33:155–188.
10. Dickson EC, Shevky R. Botulism, studies on the manner in which the toxin of Clostridium botulinum acts upon the body. I. the effect upon the autonomic nervous system. J Exp Med 1923;37:711–731.
11. Habermann E. Botulinum A and tetanus toxin—similar actions on neurotransmitter systems in vitro. In: Lewis GE Jr, ed. Biomedical aspects of botulism. New York: Academic Press, 1981:129.
12. Bigalke H, Habermann E. Blockade of tetanus and botulinum A toxin of postganglionic cholinergic nerve endings in the myenteric plexus. Naunyn-Schmeidebergs Arch Pharmacol 1980;31:255–263.
13. Paul ML, Cook MA. Lack of effect of botulinum toxin on nonadrenergic, noncholinegic inhibitory responses of the guinea-pig fundus in vitro. Can J Physiol Pharmacol 1980;58:88–92.
14. MacKenzie I, Burnstock G, Dolly JO. The effects of purified botulinum neurotoxin type A on cholinergic, adrenergic and non-adrenergic, atropine-resistant autonomic neuromuscular transmission. Neuroscience 1982;7:997–1006.
15. Ambache N. The peripheral action of Cl. botulinum toxin. J Physiol (London) 1949;108:127–141.
16. Ambache N. A further survey of the action of Clostridium botulinum toxin upon different types of autonomic nerve fibre. J Physiol (London) 1951;113:1–17.
17. Holman ME, Spitzer NC. Action of botulinum toxin on transmission from sympathetic nerves to the vas deferens. Br J Pharmacol 1973;47:431–433.
18. Westwood DA, Whaler BC. Postganglionic paralysis of the guinea-pig hypogastric nerve–vas deferens preparation by Clostridium botulinum type D toxin. Br J Pharmacol 1968;33:21–31.
19. Pasricha PJ, Ravich WJ, Kalloo AN. Injection of botulinum toxin into the distal esophageal sphincter in piglets—a unique investigative tool with potential therapeutic uses (abstr). Am J Gastroenterol 1992;87:1255.
20. Dodds WJ, Dent J, Hogan WJ, Patel GK, Toouli J, Arndorfer RC. Paradoxical lower esophageal sphincter contraction induced by cholecystokinin-octapeptide in patients with achalasia. Gatroenterology 1981;80:327–333.
21. Goyal RK, Rattan S. Neurohormonal, hormonal, and drug receptors for the lower esophageal sphincter. Gastroenterology 1978;74:598–619.
22. Traube M. On drugs and dilators for achalasia. Dig Dis Sci 1991;36:257–259.
23. Csendes A, Braghetto I, Henriquez A, et al. Late results of a prospective randomized study comparing forceful dilatation and oesophagomyotomy in patients with achalasia. Gut 1989;30:299–304.
24. Richter JE. Achalasia: whether the knife or the balloon? Not such a difficult question. Am J Gastroenterol 1991;81:810–811.
25. Richter JE, Castell DO. Balloon dilatation for the treatment of achalasia. In: Bennet JR, Hunt JH, eds. Therapeutic endoscopy and radiology of the gut. 2d ed. Baltimore: Williams & Wilkins, 1990:82.
26. Csendes A, Smok G, Braghetto I, Ramirez C, Velasco N, Henriquez A. Gastroesophageal sphincter pressure and histological changes in distal esophagus in patients with achalasia of the esophagus. Dig Dis Sci 1985;30:941–45.

27. Misiewicz JJ, Waller SL, Anthony PP, Gummer JWP. Achalasia of the cardia: pharmacology and histopathology of isolated cardiac sphincteric muscle from patients with and without achalasia. Q J Med 1969;38:17–30.

28. Aggestrup S, Uddman R, Sundler F, et al. Lack of vasoactive intestinal peptide nerves in esophageal achalasia. Gastroenterology 1983;84:924.

29. Heitman P, Espinoza J, Czendes A. Physiology of the distal esophagus in achalasia. Scand J Gastroenterol 1969;4:1–11.

30. Holloway RH, Dodds WJ, Helms JF, Hogan WJ, Dent J, Arndorfer RC. Integrity of cholinegic innervation to the lower esophageal sphincter in achalasia. Gastroenterology 1986;90:924–992.

31. Richter JE. Motility disorders of the esophagus. In: Yamada T, ed. Textbook of gastroenterology. 1st ed. Philadelphia: J.B. Lippincott, 1991:1083.

32. Lobis IF, Fisher RS. Anticholinergic therapy for achalasia: a controlled trial. Gastroenterology 1976;90:76.

33. Pasricha PJ, Ravich WJ, Hendrix TR, Kalloo AN. Treatment of achalasia with intrasphincteric injection of botulinum toxin—results of a pilot trial (abstr). Gastroenterology 1993;104:A168.

34. Pasricha PJ, Ravich WJ, Kalloo AN. Botulinum toxin for achalasia. Lancet 1993;341: 244–245.

35. Coccia G, Bortolotti M, Michetti P, Dodero M. Prospective clinical and manometric study comparing pneumatic dilatation and sublingual nifedipine in the treatment of oesophageal achalasia. Gut 1991;32:604–606.

36. Robertson CS, Hardy JG, Atkinson M. Quantitative assessment of the response to therapy in achalasia of the cardia. Gut 1989;30:768–773.

37. Samelson SL, Nyhus LM. Hypertensive lower esophageal sphincter. In: Jamieson GG, ed. Surgery of the esophagus. Churchill Livingstone, 1988:511.

38. Aliperti G, Clouse RE. Incomplete lower esophageal sphincter relaxation in subjects with peristalsis: prevalence and clinical outcome. Am J Gastroenterol 1991;86:609–614.

39. Horowitz M, Harding PE, Maddox A, et al. Gastric and esophageal emptying in insulin-dependent diabetes mellitus. J Hepatol Gastroenterol 1986;1:97.

40. Mearin F, Camilleri M, Malagelada J-R. Pyloric dysfunction in diabetics with recurrent nausea and vomiting. Gastroenterology 1986;90:1919.

41. Camilleri M, Malagelada J-R. Abnormal intestinal motility in diabetics with the gastroparesis syndrome. Eur J Clin Invest 1984;14:420.

42. Jian R, Ducrot F, Ruskoff A, et al. Symptomatic radionuclide and therapeutic assessment of chronic idiopathic dyspepsia. Dig Dis Sci 1989;34:657.

43. Milla PJ. Gastric outlet obstruction in children. N Engl J Med 1992;327:558–560.

44. Venu RP, Geenen JE. Postcholecystecomy syndrome. In: Yamada T, ed. Textbook of gastroenterology. 1st ed. Philadelphia: J.B. Lippincott, 1991:2033.

45. Preston DM, Lennard-Jones JE. Anismus in chronic constipation. Dig Dis Sci 1985;30:413.

46. Barnes PRH, Hawley PR, Preston DM, Lennard-Jones JE. Experience of posterior division of the puborectalis in the management of chronic constipation. Br J Surg 1985;72:475.

47. Hallan RI, Melling J, Womack NR, Williams NS, Waldron DJ, Morrison JFB. Treatment of anismus in intractable constipation with botulinum A toxin. Lancet 1988;2:714–717.

48. Barnett JL, Raper SE. Anorectal diseases. In: Yamada T, ed. Textbook of gastroenterology. 1st ed. Philadelphia: J.B. Lippincott, 1991:1813.

49. Reynolds JC, Ouyang A, Lee CA, et al. Chronic severe constipation: prospective motility studies in twenty-five consecutive patients. Gastroenterology 1987;92:414.

50. Pasricha PJ, Miskovsky EP, Kalloo AN. Treatment of sphincter of Oddi dysfunction with botulinum toxin injection—case report (abstr). Gastrointest Endosc 1993;39:319.

44

Botulinum Toxin for Spasms and Spasticity in the Lower Extremities

Reiner Benecke
Heinrich Heine University, Düsseldorf, Germany

INTRODUCTION

The therapeutic scope of botulinum toxin (BTX) has continued to expand, and it now includes a variety of diseases associated with inappropriate muscle tone, muscular contractions, or spasms (1–14). The wide spectrum of therapeutic use of BTX results from its relatively unspecific effect, i.e., muscle paralysis by inhibition of the exocytosis of acetylcholine at the neuromuscular junction. Recent results indicate that BTXs block neurotransmitter release by cleaving synaptobrevin-2, a protein that seems to play a key part in neurotransmitter release (15).

Surprisingly, focal dystonia is the symptom most frequently treated with BTX, although other hyperactivity states of the muscles, such as spasticity, are much more common and induced by a long list of diseases. The reason for the dominant use in focal dystonia may be historical, because BTX was first used for treatment of strabismus by ophthalmologists, who also often saw patients with blepharospasm (3,13,16), the first focal dystonia treated with this toxin. Other reasons may be the relative insufficiency of drug treatment, and the focality of BTX treatment, which makes therapeutic weakness of all muscles involved possible in focal dystonias.

Spasticity is a motor disorder characterized by a velocity-dependent increase of muscle tone combined with exaggerated monosynaptic tendon reflexes and polysynaptic tonic reflexes (17). Clinically, the increase of monosynaptic stretch reflexes is often combined with reflex irradiation, i.e., the application of a phasic stretch by a reflex hammer, and the mechanical effects of the primarily contracting muscle lead to excitations of muscle spindles in distant muscles. Most clinicians also regard Babinski's reflex as a representative symptom of spasticity.

In clinical practice spasticity occurs as a constituent part of the upper motor neuron syndrome. In addition to spasticity, flexor withdrawal reflexes and flexor and extensor spasms appear as positive phenomena. Negative phenomena include weakness, impaired control of distal muscle groups, particularly in the upper extremity, and hypotonia and hyporeflexia during the acute stages following injury to the brain or spinal cord. The weakness often assumes a pyramidal distribution, with greater involvement of flexor muscle groups than of extensors in the lower extremity and the opposite pattern in the upper extremity.

Whether spasticity and exaggerated stretch reflexes interfere with voluntary movement is an important practical question, because it forms at least part of the rationale for the treatment that has been directed at spasticity. At first glance it would seem obvious that if there were a velocity-dependent increase in the response to stretching of a muscle and a spastic subject attempted to execute a rapid movement, then a stretch reflex would be activated in the antagonist muscle and would oppose the movement. Such a mechanism has been shown in passive lengthening of muscles and also when muscles are actively stretched during the performance of natural movements (18).

Landau (19) addressed this issue when he did not observe any improvement in motor performance after abolishing spasticity in spastic limbs by infiltration of local anesthetic. He questioned the rationale of therapeutic approaches aimed solely at reducing muscle tone and hyperreflexia.

In the light of these considerations the question arises whether BTX, which similarly to local anesthetics may reduce spasticity by a decrease of muscle power, can improve motor performance. Oral medications that are used to treat spasticity include dantrolene, baclofen, and tizanidine (20). In addition to a decrease of spasticity these drugs also produce weakness, especially at higher doses and in those muscles that are affected already by negative phenomena of the upper motor neuron syndrome. Clinical experience suggests that these compounds are relatively inappropriate in as many as 50% of patients because worsening of weakness is of more pronounced functional relevance than concomitant decrease of spasticity. It has, however, to be emphasized that the principles of treatment for upper motor neuron syndrome also include prevention of complications such as contractures and secondary damage to joints. Furthermore, spasticity and flexor spasms may give rise to pain in the muscles, tendons, and connective tissues. On the basis of these considerations local injections of BTX may be of therapeutic value in those situations where spasticity and flexor spasms lead to these secondary complications and where improvement of motor performance is not of major importance. This is especially the case for patients who are severely affected by both negative and positive phenomena of the upper motor neuron syndrome. An advantage of BTX injections over conventional oral treatment and intrathecal baclofen therapy (21) is the focality of muscle relaxation and the lack of side effects such as drowsiness, confusion, seizures, and gastrointestinal problems. It is also possible that the neuromuscular junctions of the intrafusal muscle fibers of muscle spindles are blocked by local BTX injections, which would enhance the relaxing effect in spasticity.

In a recent investigation, Snow and coworkers (8) studied the effect of botulinum toxin type A on spasticity of the leg adductors in nine patients who were either chair-bound or bed-bound with chronic stable multiple sclerosis. They injected toxin (400 mouse units; Smith-Kettlewell Eye Research Institute, San Francisco, California) or placebo into the adductor muscles in a randomized, crossover, double-blind design. They found that BTX produced a significant reduction in spasticity and a significant improvement in the ease of nursing care. There were no adverse effects during this short-term trial.

EFFECTS OF BOTULINUM TOXIN IN ADDUCTOR SPASTICITY

Patients and Rating Scales

In 1991 and 1992, 14 patients with a prominent disabling spasticity of adductor muscles were treated with botulinum toxin type A (Dysport; Porton Products, Maidenhead, England) in Düsseldorf. All patients were chair-bound or bed-bound because of stable cervical and/or thoracic myelopathy. Myelopathies were caused by bacterial or viral myelitis, spinal cord trauma, or encephalomyelitis disseminata. In all patients with myelopathy the lesion was incomplete, with residual sensorimotor functions.

The rating protocol is shown in Table 1. The degree of muscle tone in the adductors was assessed by means of a modified Ashworth scale (22). The intensity of spasms was rated on the basis of the patient's report. The frequency of spasms per day and the severity of pain were averaged over a 1-week observation period before the BTX injections or at regular reexaminations that were performed at 4-week intervals. A global clinical score was assessed by summation of separate scores for spasticity, spasms, and pain. Clinical data for all patients are summarized in Table 2.

Injections

Dysport was used for intramuscular BTX injections. Dysport is supplied as a white freeze-dried pellet containing 500 mouse units (12.5 ng) of *Clostridium botulinum* type A toxin-hemagglutinin complex in a clear glass vial. For injection, the compound was diluted with saline to a concentration of 10 ng/ml. Botulinum toxin was injected through a 0.9-inch 40-gauge needle that was Teflon-coated except for the tip and that was simultaneously used as an electromyographic recording electrode. The adductor longus, gracilis, adductor brevis, and adductor magnus muscles were localized according to electromyographic

Table 1 Rating Scales

Degree of spastic muscle tone
- 0 = Normal
- 1 = Increased tendon reflexes, slightly increased muscle tone, hips actively abducted > 45°
- 2 = Increased tendon reflexes, moderately increased muscle tone, hips passively but not actively abducted > 45°
- 3 = Increased tendon reflexes, severe spastic muscle tone, hips passively abducted < 45°
- 4 = Severe spastic muscle tone, hips cannot be passively abducted, tendon reflexes cannot be tested

Spasms
- 0 = No spasms
- 1 = One or fewer spasms at night only
- 2 = Up to 5 spasms by night or day
- 3 = Up to 10 spasms by night or day
- 4 = More than 10 spasms, or continuous hip adduction

Pain
- 0 = No pain
- 1 = Occasionally, often in conjunction with spasms
- 2 = Longer than 3 hr a day
- 3 = Severe and continuous

Table 2 Clinical Data for 14 Patients Suffering from Adductor Spasticity

Patient	Sex	Age (yr)	Disease	Duration (yr)	Pain (0–3)	Spasticity (0–4)	Spasms (0–4)
1	M	44	Ed	14	2	4	3
2	M	52	Ed	30	2	3	3
3	F	32	Ed	10	3	2	4
4	F	52	My	5	2	3	2
5	F	30	Ed	4	3	4	4
6	M	32	Tr	6	2	3	3
7	M	42	Tr	15	2	3	3
8	F	35	Ed	10	3	2	4
9	M	42	My	4	3	4	4
10	F	44	Tr	10	2	3	3
11	M	28	Tr	6	1	3	2
12	M	32	Ed	8	2	4	4
13	M	48	Ed	20	3	4	4
14	F	38	My	8	1	2	2

F = female; M = male; Ed = encephalomyelitis disseminata; My = viral/bacterial myelitis; Tr = spinal cord trauma; for definition of scores see Table 1.

procedures (23) (Fig. 1). When the correct positioning of the needle was ascertained by recording of exaggerated tonic activity at slow passive lengthening and/or of phasic bursts at reflex release, intramuscular injections were performed at two injection sites per muscle about 2 cm apart. Injections were performed on both body sides with standard doses: adductor longus, gracilis, and adductor brevis 5 ng each, adductor magnus 10 ng. The total dose therefore amounted to 50 ng.

Evaluations

Patients were examined before and 4, 8, and 12 weeks after BTX injections. During the examination 12 weeks after injection the next injection was performed. Four injections at 12-week intervals have been performed in all 14 patients who are included in this study. During each examination a conventional neurological examination and the ratings of spasticity, spasms, and pain were performed by the same examiner. Furthermore, the patients were asked about any side effects. The effects of BTX were assessed by calculation of sum scores for spasticity, spasms, and pain for all patients.

Results

In Fig. 2 the global scores including all patients and rated symptoms before the first injection and 4 weeks after each of four injections are illustrated. It can be seen that BTX led to a significant ($p < 0.001$; paired t-test) improvement in the overall state after the first injection. Subsequent injections did not induce a further significant improvement.

In Figs. 3, 4, and 5 the changes in scores for individual symptoms are demonstrated. Similar to the global score, the scores for spasticity, spasms, and pain were all significantly ($p < 0.001$; paired t-test) decreased 4 weeks after the first injection, and thereafter they remained constant. The percentage improvement was most pronounced for the pain scores. On average the improvement of spasticity, spasms, and pain started 4.4 days

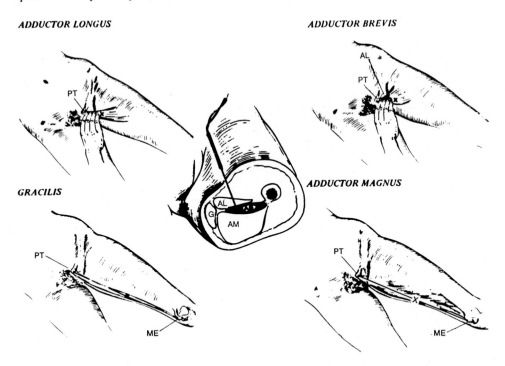

ADDUCTOR LONGUS

ADDUCTOR BREVIS

GRACILIS

ADDUCTOR MAGNUS

Figure 1 Injection sites for botulinum toxin in adductor spasticity. PT: pubic tubercle. ME: femoral epicondyle. AL: adductor longus; G: gracilis; AM: adductor magnus; AB: adductor brevis. X: injection site; injections were performed about 1 cm proximal and 1 cm distal to this point. For gracilis and adductor magnus X was defined as the point midway between the pubic tubercle and the medial femoral epicondyle.

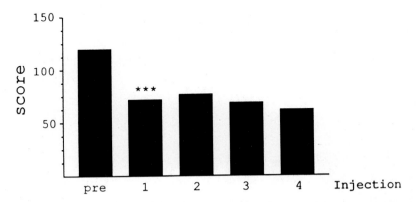

Figure 2 Improvement in global score after botulinum toxin injections. Columns indicate the sum of the scores for spasticity, spasms, and pain of all 14 patients. Ratings were performed before and 4 weeks after each of four consecutive injections. The decrease in the global score after the first injection was highly significant ($p < 0.001$; paired t-test for global scores in individual patients).

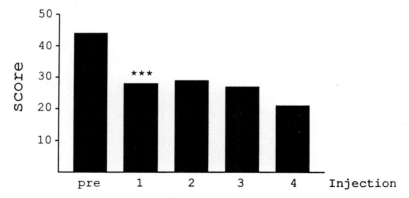

Figure 3   Ratings of spasticity before and 4 weeks after each of four injections. Scores are the sum for all 14 patients.

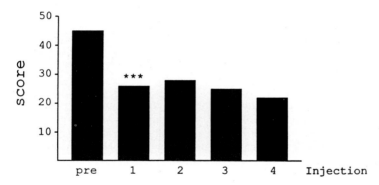

Figure 4   Ratings of spasms before and 4 weeks after each of four injections. Scores are the sum for all 14 patients.

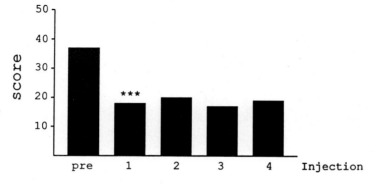

Figure 5   Ratings of pain before and 4 weeks after each of four injections. Scores are the sum for all 14 patients.

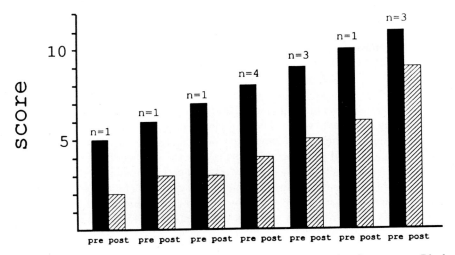

Figure 6 Improvement in global scores (see Fig. 2) in separated patient groups. Black columns show the mean global scores of patients with identical scores before treatment. Hatched columns indicate the mean score 4 weeks after the first injection. Note that the percentage decrease is more pronounced in less severely affected patients.

(range 2–12 days) after the injections. There was no significant difference in onset of improvements after the various injections ($p > 0.1$; paired t-test). In the examinations 8 weeks after the injections, scores for all rated symptoms increased again but were significantly different neither from the values before injection nor from the values 4 weeks after the injections ($p > 0.1$; paired t-test). Figure 6 shows the mean improvements in global scores in patients with differing scores at the beginning of BTX treatment. It can be seen that the percentage improvement is most pronounced in patients with less disturbed motor functions and minor pain.

Table 3 summarizes the frequency, duration, and onset of side effects that occurred during this investigation. Some patients suffered from muscle pain that they could differentiate from the preexisting pain resulting from spasticity and spasms. A minority of the patients experienced mild weakness of arm muscles that could not be objectified by conventional grading of muscle power within the conventional neurological examinations. The patients reported early fatigue or decreased muscle power, especially when maximal muscle strength was required during the performance of natural movements. The occur-

Table 3 Side Effects (56 Injections)

Side effect	Duration (range; days)	Onset (range; days)	Percentage frequency
Intermittent injection pain	2–22	1–3	14%
Weakness of the arms	1–14	3–12	8%
Dysphagia	3–18	3–5	5%

rence of dysphagia, which is a common side effect in BTX treatment of cervical dystonia (14), was surprising, and it was interpreted as a result of toxin diffusion after injection into the sternocleidomastoid muscle.

DISCUSSION

The present investigation shows that intramuscular injections of BTX reduce the disability of adductor spasticity in patients who are bed- or chair-bound and suffering from severe residuals of myelopathy in multiple sclerosis and other diseases. The severity of spasticity, spasms, and pain could be reduced by this treatment. The beneficial effects were more pronounced in more mildly than in severely affected patients, and pain was the more improved sign of adductor spasticity than spasticity and spasms. The doses used in the present study were much higher that those administered in the treatment of blepharospasm and cervical dystonia (1–6,12–14). In previous pilot trials it could be observed that at lower doses (30-ng and 40-ng total doses tested in three patients each) effects were marginal. The reason for the higher doses required in adductor spasticity might be the enormous amount of exaggerated activity in this condition and the higher absolute muscle power of the adductor muscles. Nevertheless, side effects were relatively rare in the spastic patients. The reason for this might be the insignificance of toxin-induced paresis, because the patients were chair- or bed-bound and did not expect a restoration or an unaffected performance of natural voluntary movements, as is the case in patients with blepharospasm or cervical dystonia.

The occurrence of dysphagia after three injections in two different patients was surprising. From this observation it can be concluded that dysphagia is not the result of toxin diffusion, as was suspected in the treatment of cervical dystonia (14), but results from a systemic effect of BTX. It may well be that the pharyngeal muscles react as sensitively to BTX as they do in the pharyngeal manifestation of myasthenia gravis with systemic action of autoantibodies. The onset and duration of BTX action in the treatment of adductor spasticity are similar to those seen in the treatment of blepharospasm and cervical dystonia. The clinical action of the toxin disappears after about 3 months even after four injections, and repeated injections are therefore required. It is most doubtful that a permanent effect will be achieved after more than four injections.

The present study confirms the investigations by Snow and co-workers (8) and Dengler and co-workers (9), who also described beneficial effects of BTX in spasticity states. Snow and co-workers (8) emphasized the beneficial effects of BTX treatment on hygiene and patient care. In the present study also, cleaning and catheterizing the patient was clearly made easier, but this effect is difficult to quantify.

In summary, BTX seems to be helpful for patients with pronounced adductor spasticity who do not sufficiently improve with orally administered antispastic drugs. Whether local injections of BTX are superior to intrathecal applications of baclofen (21) for these patients is still an open question and has to be clarified in future comparative studies.

REFERENCES

1. Tsui JKC, Eisen A, Stoessl AJ, Calne S, Calne DB. Double-blind study of botulinum toxin in spasmodic torticollis. Lancet 1986;2:245–247.
2. Tsui JKC, Calne DB. Botulinum toxin treatment in cervical dystonia. Adv Neurol 1988;49: 473–478.

3. Stell R, Thompson PD, Marsden CD. Botulinum toxin in spasmodic torticollis. J Neurol Neurosurg Psychiatry 1988;51:920–923.

4. Gelb DJ, Lowenstein DH, Aminoff MJ. Controlled trial of botulinum toxin injections in the treatment of spasmodic torticollis. Neurology 1989;39:80–84.

5. Blackie JD, Lees AJ. Botulinum toxin treatment in spasmodic torticollis. J Neurol Neurosurg Psychiatry 1990;53:640–643.

6. Greene P, Kang U, Fahn S, Brin MF, Moskowitz C, Flaster E. Double-blind, placebo-controlled trial of botulinum toxin injections for the treatment of spasmodic torticollis. Neurology 1990;40:1213–1218.

7. Dykstra DD, Sidi A, Scott AB, Pagel JM, Goldish GD. Effects of botulinum A toxin on detrusor-sphincter dyssynergia in spinal cord injury patients. J Urol 1988;139:912–922.

8. Snow BJ, Tsui JKC, Bhatt MH, Varelas M, Hashimoto SA, Calne DB. Treatment of spasticity with botulinum toxin: a double-blind study. Ann Neurol 1990;28:512–515.

9. Dengler R, Neyer U, Wohlfarth K, Bettig U, Janzik K. Local botulinum toxin in the treatment of spastic drop foot. J Neurol 1992;239:375–378.

10. Marsden CD, Sheehy MP. Writer's cramp. Trends Neurosci 1990;13:148–153.

11. Ludlow CL, Naunton RF, Fujita M, Sedory SE. Spasmodic dysphonia: botulinum toxin injection after recurrent nerve surgery. Otolaryngol Head Neck Surg 1990;102:122–131.

12. Brin MF, Fahn S, Moskowitz C, et al. Localized injections of botulinum toxin for the treatment of focal dystonia and hemifacial spasm. Mov Discord 1987;2:237–254.

13. Elston JS. Botulinum toxin treatment of blepharospasm. Adv Neurol 1988;50:579–581.

14. Jankovic J, Schwartz K, Donovan DT. Botulinum toxin treatment of cranial-cervical dystonia, spasmodic dysphonia, other focal dystonias and hemifacial spasms. J Neurol Neurosurg Psychiatry 1990;53:633–639.

15. Schiavo G, Benfenati F, Poulain B, Rossetto O, et al. Tetanus and botulinum-B neurotoxins block neurotransmitter release by proteolytic cleavage of synaptobrevin. Nature 1992;359:832–835.

16. Scott AB. Botulinum toxin injection into extraocular muscles as an alternative to strabismus surgery. Ophthalmology 1980;87:1044–1049.

17. Lance JW. Symposium synopsis. In: Feldman RG, Young RR, Koeller WP, eds. Spasticity: disordered motor control. Chicago: Year Book Medical Publishers, 1980:485.

18. Benecke R, Conrad B, Meinck HM, Höhne J. Electromyographic analysis of bicycling on an ergometer for evaluation of spasticity of lower limbs in man. In: Desmedt JE, ed. Motor control in health and disease. New York: Raven Press, 1983:1035–1046.

19. Landau WM. Spasticity: the fable of a neurological demon and the emperors's new therapy. Arch Neurol 1977;31:217–219.

20. Davidoff RA. Antispasticity drugs: mechanisms of action. Ann Neurol 1985;17:107–116.

21. Penn RD, Kroin JS. Long-term intrathecal baclofen infusion for treatment of spasticity. J Neurosurg 1987;66:1981–1985.

22. Ashworth B. Preliminary trial of carisoprodol in multiple sclerosis. Practitioner 1964;192:540–542.

23. Delagi EF, Perotto A, Iazzetti J, Morrison D. Anatomic guide for the electromyographer. Springfield, Illinois: CC Thomas, 1980.

45

Botulinum Toxin Treatment of Palatal Tremor (Myoclonus)

Günther Deuschl and E. Löhle
University of Freiburg, Freiburg, Germany

Camilo Toro and Mark Hallett
National Institute of Neurological Disorders and Stroke,
National Institutes of Health, Bethesda, Maryland

Robert S. Lebovics
National Institute on Deafness and Other Communication Disorders,
National Institutes of Health, Bethesda, Maryland

INTRODUCTION

Palatal tremor is a rare disorder characterized by involuntary rhythmic movements of the soft palate and sometimes of brain stem or extremity muscles. As the available data indicate that this movement disorder is a type of tremor, former names such as palatal myoclonus and palatal nystagmus are less appropriate. Subjective complaints directly related to this hyperkinetic movement include oscillopsia when the extraocular muscles or the oculomotor control systems are involved. Sometimes an extremity tremor or objective clicking noises may occur. Generally, these hyperkinetic movements are time-locked with the palatal movements. Therefore, a common central oscillator has been assumed to underlie these rhythmic movements.

The clinical symptom amenable to treatment with BTX in this condition is the earclick, which is clearly the most distressing symptom. Some general remarks about the disease are necessary to understand the clinical rationale for this treatment.

CLINICAL AND PATHOPHYSIOLOGIC BACKGROUND OF THE DISEASE

Recent work has suggested that palatal tremor has to be separated into two different conditions called symptomatic palatal tremor (SPT) and essential palatal tremor (EPT) (Table 1). This distinction is based on several observations in a large group of patients reported in the literature (1). One major difference was that patients with SPT all had neurological signs or symptoms indicating a brain stem or cerebellar affection at the time

Table 1 The Separation of Symptomatic Palatal Tremor (SPT) and Essential Palatal Tremor (EPT)

	SPT	EPT
Underlying brain stem or cerebellar lesion	Yes	No
Symptoms (other than palatal tremor)	Pendular nystagmus, extremity tremors (no earclick)	Only earclick
Age at onset (yr)	45.1 ± 17.3	24.8 ± 12.9
Influence of narcosis	No	Yes
Influence of sleep	No	Yes
Remissions	Never	Seldom described
MRI-evidence of hypertrophic degeneration of the inferior olive	Yes	No
Pathology	Hypertrophic degeneration of the inferior olive	Unknown

MRI = magnetic resonance imaging.

of presentation or in the past. In contrast, the patients with EPT had an uneventful medical history, with a sudden onset of earclicks unrelated to any other clearly defined disease. Patients may discover the palatal movements by accident while looking in their mouths. Otherwise, the physician may find it for the first time on clinical examination.

The major clinical difference between the two conditions, however, was the occurrence of an earclick in patients with EPT but not in patients with SPT. This symptom is the typical presenting complaint of patients with EPT. Patients with SPT usually present with symptoms of the underlying brain stem or cerebellar disease that causes palatal tremor. Occasionally the patients suffer from two other symptoms that can be directly related to the involuntary rhythmic activity and its extension to other brain stem or extremity muscles. These are oscillopsia due to a pendular nystagmus (2) and extremity tremors (3). Neither ever occurs in EPT. Further differences between the two conditions have been delineated on the basis of this literature survey. The mean age at onset of EPT is about 25 years, whereas it is 45 years in SPT. The mean frequency of palatal tremor is usually lower in patients with EPT (107 ± 41 jerks/min) than in patients with SPT (139 ± 51 jerks/min). The rhythm of EPT seems to be less stable than that of SPT and can be more easily disturbed: during sleep there is usually cessation of the palatal rhythm in EPT but not in SPT. Remissions of palatal tremor have never been described in SPT but have been reported in several cases of EPT, especially in children. These observations prompted us (1) to suggest that the two conditions are different diseases based on different mechanisms, which are briefly summarized as follows.

The pathophysiological basis of SPT is believed to be spontaneous oscillations of the nerve cells of the inferior olive. This hypothesis is based on several observations.

The first is the finding that the inferior olive undergoes a so-called hypertrophic pseudodegeneration. This is a macroscopic abnormality of the inferior olive with swelling of the nerve cells and astrocytic proliferation (4–6). It develops secondary to a lesion of the dentato-olivary pathway mediated through the superior cerebellar peduncle and the central tegmental tract (7–9). This degeneration has been studied in patients with brain stem hemorrhages, showing a typical time course for the different stages of these changes, with full-blown development after about 1 year (10). Clinical observations about the onset of palatal tremor after a brain stem stroke or hemorrhage suggest that the hyperkinesia develops with a time delay varying between a few weeks and several months after the primary lesion (11). Thus, the development of oscillatory activity shows a time course similar to the pathoanatomical development of hypertrophic degeneration. Moreover, it was recently reported that in a patient in whom magnetic resonance imaging (MRI) revealed signs of hypertrophic degeneration, these morphologic abnormalities preceded the onset of palatal hyperkinesia (12). Hence, the development of palatal tremor and hypertrophic degeneration are most likely related, and the rhythmic activity may be generated in the inferior olive.

A second line of evidence comes from single unit recordings of inferior olive neurons in different species, which have shown that these neurons are able to generate rhythmic spontaneous oscillations under certain conditions (13–15). This oscillatory mode of activation is due to distinct changes of the membrane conductance to calcium at somatic and dendritic levels (16). The oscillatory action of different cells could be linked together by electronic coupling through the gap junctions (17,18) and could thereby produce synchronized rhythmic activity.

A third line of evidence suggesting involvement of the inferior olive on palatal tremor comes from positron emission tomography data in patients with palatal tremor showing abnormal metabolic activity of the medulla (19), which could reflect abnormal rhythmic activity of the inferior olive. These hypotheses are likely to explain the background of SPT, and further evidence has been gained in recent years.

Essential palatal tremor appears to be due to other mechanisms. There are several arguments against a contribution of the inferior olive to EPT. The first is that we have no evidence for a hypertrophic degeneration of the inferior olive in EPT. Since the available autopsies are from patients with SPT (1), we do not know the microscopic anatomy of the brain stem in EPT. Recently, MRI has provided some relevant information. Abnormal, hyperintense signals in the upper medulla have been found in all our patients with SPT exactly at the location where the inferior olives are located (20). Therefore, hypertrophic degeneration is most likely visible with high-resolution MRI. In contrast, none of our patients with EPT exhibited a similar abnormality, suggesting that they do not have this type of olivary degeneration. These observations suggest that, if EPT has a morphological basis, it must be different from that of SPT. Future pathoanatomical studies are mandatory to draw final conclusions.

A further argument against a common pathophysiology of SPT and EPT is the different distributions of the rhythmic activity in these two conditions. In SPT, various supra-nuclear motor centers such as the eye movement control centers or intraspinally descending motor tracts can be involved, because pendular nystagmus or extremity tremors occur in this condition. In EPT, only the involvement of muscles innervated by cranial nerves has been described, and as far as can be deduced from the involved regions, the territory could be limited to muscles innervated by the trigeminal nerve (1,21).

In conclusion, all the available clinical and laboratory evidence suggests that two different pathophysiological mechanisms and two different clinical entities underlie SPT and EPT.

THE DIFFERENTIAL DIAGNOSIS OF PALATAL TREMOR

Palatal tremor is a rare condition, and a few comments are necessary about other diseases that could be confused with it (Table 2). The major clinical symptoms besides rhythmic palatal contractions are the rhythmic earclick, pendular nystagmus, and slow extremity tremors.

There are different sources of a pulse-synchronous tinnitus that can be confused with earclicks. These include congenital or acquired arteriovenous malformations (fistulae or tumors), and venous hums or other arterial bruits (22). They can be identified by the relation of the sounds to the heartbeat and the absence of palatal movement. A movement similar to palatal tremor has been described as a manifestation of focal epilepsy (23–25), but earclick was not part of this syndrome. An occasional episode of convulsion or electroencephalographic abnormalities should be expected in such a condition.

We have observed two patients who developed a syndrome of psychogenic palatal tremor presenting with "voluntary" activation of palatal muscles with smacking noises for periods of up to several minutes. Both are known to have had contact with patients suffering from palatal tremor or to have heard of the syndrome before the onset of their complaints. They both had a gross morphological movement of the palate and the pharynx, and the noises had a smacking instead of a clicking quality. Neither could maintain this symptom for longer than a few minutes, and one of them stopped it while complaining about the exhausting quality of the movement disorder. The psychiatric background was most likely a personality disorder in both conditions.

Acquired pendular nystagmus most often occurs in multiple sclerosis and is usually not accompanied by palatal tremor (26). Hereditary pendular fixation nystagmus is a mono-symptomatic familial disease without palatal movements. Rhythmic vergence movements together with facial and masseter contractions are observed in oculomasticatory myorhythmia. This syndrome has been described hitherto only in Whipple's disease and consist of the triad of rhythmic hyperkinesia of various brain stem muscles, gaze paralysis (sometimes intermittent), and episodic somnolence (27). The latter two symptoms are not seen in SPT. Rhythmic myoclonias of isolated brain stem muscles or muscle groups have been described in single cases often termed branchial myoclonus (28–30). Their separation from or relation to SPT may be difficult. Another rare differential diagnosis is masticatory spasms (31). Furthermore, tremors of various origins of other muscles than the palate may cause confusion, such as isolated tongue tremors, hereditary chin tremor (32), or the rabbit syndrome (a rare type of tardive dyskinesia). Whenever palatal

Table 2 Differential Diagnosis of Palatal Tremor

Essential palatal tremor
  Arteriovenous malformation with rhythmic sounds
  Focal epilepsia partialis continua
  Psychogenic palatal tremor
Symptomatic palatal tremor
  Oculomasticatory myorhythmia
  Isolated branchial myoclonus
  Masticatory spasms
  Isolated tremors of cranial nerve muscles
  Generalized myoclonias with cranial manifestations

movements occur in the setting of a myoclonic syndrome, they are mostly not rhythmic and can be separated by the generalized nature of the myoclonic disease (33).

THE ORIGIN OF THE EARCLICK

The major symptom to treat in palatal tremor is the earclick. This can be heard usually as an objective short rhythmic sound with a frequency of 40–200/min (mean ± standard deviation: 107 ± 41). The loudness of the click varies interindividually and intraindividually over time, and we have measured a sound pressure of up to 75 dB in the external auditory meatus. Clicking noises can be heard from both ears at either the same or different frequencies. In all our patients the clicks occurred continuously when the mouth was closed. Our sleep recordings demonstrated that the click stopped completely in sleep stage II. Different maneuvers have been reported by the patients to decrease the loudness of the click or stop the noise. One patient had cessation of the click during singing, while another patient could stop the click during forceful breathing with open mouth. Another patient with a left-sided click could stop the click when lying horizontally with the right side down. None of these maneuvers except sleep showed a consistent effect on the click in all the patients.

The origin of the earclick has long been discussed. A contraction of the stapedius muscle (34,35) or of the levator veli palatini muscle (36) has been proposed. Several lines of evidence suggest the tensor veli palatini muscle is responsible for the click.

The first is the observation that the palatal movements systematically differ in EPT and SPT. In the latter, only the dorsal free edge of the soft palate moves, whereas in EPT the roof of the soft palate moves (21). This is because different muscles are active. The levator veli palatini muscle originates at the petrous portion of the temporal bone in front of the carotid canal and inserts at the palatal midline aponeurosis. The tensor veli palatini muscle originates with a broad insertion at the sphenoid spine to the scaphoid fossa, but three-quarters of the fibers originate at the lateral wall of the cartilaginous portion of the auditory tube. The fibers or tendons, respectively, then turn around the hamulus to the rostral part of the palatal aponeurosis. Therefore, the contraction of the tensor lifts (or extends) the rostral part of the palate and opens the Eustachian tube (37,38). Thus, the click must be due to the activity of the tensor veli palatini muscle.

In order to understand the exact mechanism, we have recorded (39) the electromyogram (EMG) of the tensor muscle and the earclick in parallel (Fig. 1).

The earclick occurred about 150 msec after the onset of the tensor EMG. Therefore, the click is produced during opening of the Eustachian tube and is most likely due to the sudden breakdown of the surface tension between the walls of the Eustachian tube. This is in line with sonotubometric recordings showing an opening of the Eustachian tube after the occurrence of the click (40).

PROPOSED THERAPIES FOR THE CLICK

As the click is an extremely distressing symptom for the patients, it has been subjected to many different therapeutic attempts. There are only single case reports except for one study (41), because of the rare occurrence of the syndrome. The oral medications that have been proposed are summarized in Table 3 (for references see Ref. 1). Some medications have been used successfully, but from our own experience we cannot recommend any of these drugs as very likely to work. Among the surgical approaches it can be

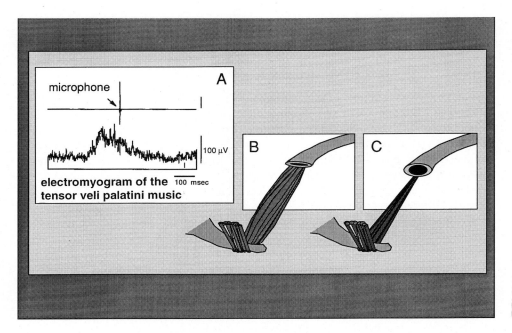

Figure 1 Mechanisms producing the earclick. (A) Relation of the rectified electromyographic (EMG) activity of the tensor veli palatini and its relation to the earclick (modified after Ref. 39). The latter occurs 150 msec after the onset of the EMG burst, indicating that the click is produced during the contraction phase of the muscle. (B,C) Schematic illustration of the position of the Eustachian tube during relaxation (B) and contraction (C).

expected that cutting of the tensor veli palatini or aeration of the Eustachian tube should help, in accordance with the mechanisms underlying the disease. In conclusion, we have not had encouraging experience with these therapies, although others may have found them helpful.

BOTULINUM TOXIN TREATMENT OF THE CLICK

In the absence of a curative treatment, efforts are necessary to develop new approaches to alleviate this distressing symptom. In accordance with the physiology and mechanisms producing the earclick, the most straightforward way could be to prevent the contraction of the tensor veli palatini muscle. This has been accomplished by using botulinum toxin (BTX).

Compared with other indications for BTX, the application of the toxin is more critical, as other muscles in the vicinity, especially the levator veli palatini, should not be injected with the substance. Therefore, delivery of the toxin has to be performed through a special needle that allows recording of the EMG activity. The needles have to be electrically shielded except for their tip. We use this needle as a monopolar recording device with a surface electrode positioned at the tip of the nose as a reference. In our experience, there are two ways to find the tensor muscle (Fig. 2). One approach is a transpalatal technique (39). After surface anesthesia of the pharynx, the needle has to be inserted at the lateral aspect of the rostral soft palate aiming toward the hamulus. Under continuous EMG

Table 3 Therapeutic Attempts to Treat the Earclick

Treatment	Number of patients[a]
Medications	
Phenytoin	2/3
Carbamazepine	2/4
Barbiturates	1/2
Diazepam	2/2
5-HTP	1/1
Trihexyphenidyl	2/2
Surgical approaches	
Perforation of the tympanic membrane	0/1
Aeration of the Eustachian tube	2/2
Cutting of the levator veli palatini muscle	1/1
Cutting of the tensor veli palatini muscle	1/1
Microsurgical decompression of the posterior fossa	1/1

[a]Number of successfully treated patients/number of tested patients. For references, see Refs. 1,30.

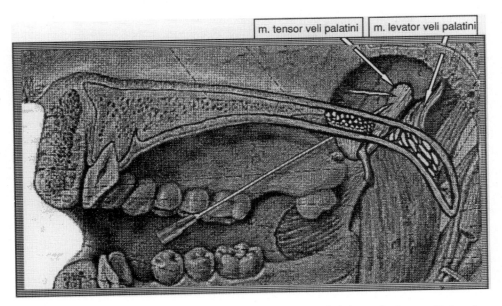

Figure 2 Anatomical location of the tensor and levator veli palatini muscles in a sagittal section. The two needles indicate the possible approaches to the tensor muscle.

control, the electrode has to be slowly pushed forward until a sharp rhythmic signal is obtained typical for the tremor bursts of palatal muscles. If possible, the patient should attempt to swallow, because this helps to identify the levator veli palatini muscle, which is mainly active in this condition. Whenever there are sharp EMG signals during choking, the position of the needle has to be corrected. A second approach is through the nose. Under endoscopic control, the contracting muscle can be seen and injected. We prefer to guide the injection electromyographically with this approach as well. Any uncontrolled injection with result in either an insufficient blockade of the tensor muscle or an unspecific paresis of all the muscles on the injected side of the palate. The patient should not be exposed to general anesthesia or strong sedatives, as the clicking stops in these circumstances. Control of the injection with endoscopic devices may be helpful but is not mandatory. As a number of critical anatomical structures are near the injection site, the cooperation of an otolaryngolist and an experienced electromyographer is desirable.

To our knowledge, three patients (39,42) have been treated with this approach (Table 4). In all of them a good or excellent response was obtained. The clicking noise usually stops after 1–3 days, provided sufficient amounts of toxin have been injected. The duration of the effect was reported to be between 4 and 12 weeks. Reinjections can be performed. Two patients have been followed now for more than 1 year. They have been repeatedly injected whenever they experienced recurrence of the clicks.

The dosages applied for one tensor muscle is indicated in Table 4. The first two patients were treated with the British BTX (Dysport), and the third was treated with the American BTX (Botox). All the patients were treated first on one side and, after intervals between 2 and 6 weeks, on the other side. After treatment of one side, an increase of the loudness of the click on the other side was sometimes observed. Complete relief from clicking could be achieved in all the patients.

Side effects of the treatment were limited. During the first injections in patient 2 a slight weakness of the lifting movement of the palate was observed by clinical inspection. The patient complained at that time of occasional transnasal regurgitation of fluids when drinking rapidly. A similar complaint was observed in patient 3 for short periods after the second and third injection. A possible complication of this treatment is the development of otitis media with effusion. It has been shown experimentally in rhesus monkeys that otitis developed after injection (43) of BTX because of impairment of the physiological function of the tensor veli palatini, which is aeration of the middle ear. It is not clear why we did not see this complication. Perhaps the paresis that we have induced was incomplete, preventing involuntary openings of the tube but still allowing opening of the tube with voluntary effort. A possible treatment of such a complication would be to position a Teflon tube in the eardrum.

In conclusion, the present experience with this new treatment is still limited. It seems possible to maintain a continuous satisfying treatment with this approach. Possible

Table 4 Clinical Data for Three Patients Treated with Botulinum Toxin for Earclick

Patient no.[a]	Age at onset (yr)	Duration of the click (yr)	Laterality	Dosage for effective unilateral injections	Bilateral injections	Authors
1	20	21	Bilateral	0.33 mg (=13 U)	Yes	Le Pajolev et al. (42)
2	52	1	Bilateral	0.42 mg (=17 U)	Yes	Deuschl et al. (39)
3	23	25	Bilateral	25 U	Yes	Toro et al. (in preparation)

[a]Patients 1 and 2 were treated with the British toxin preparation Dysport and patient 3 with the American preparation Botox.

complications are minor regurgitation and otitis media. Further experience is necessary to draw conclusions about its long-term application.

ACKNOWLEDGMENTS

We thank Mrs. W. Vasold for her editorial assistance and Dr. E. Feifel for preparing the figures.

REFERENCES

1. Deuschl G, Mischke G, Schenck E, Schulte-Mönting J, Lücking CH. Symptomatic and essential rhythmic palatal myoclonus. Brain 1990;113:1645–1672.
2. Nakada T, Kwee IL. Oculopalatal myoclonus. Brain 1986;109:431–441.
3. Massucci E, Kurtzke J. Palatal myoclonus associated with extremity tremor. J Neurol 1989; 236:474–477.
4. Gautier JC, Blackwood W. Enlargement of the inferior olivary nucleus in association with lesions of the central tegmental tract or dentate nucleus. Brain 1961;84:341–361.
5. Koeppen AH, Barron KD, Dentinger MP. Olivary hypertrophy in man. In: Courville J, de Montigny C, Lamarre Y, eds. The inferior olivary nucleus. Anatomy and physiology. New York: Raven Press, 1980:309–314.
6. Koeppen AH, Barron KD, Dentinger MP. Olivary hypertrophy: histochemical demonstration of hydrolytic enzymes. Neurology 1980;30:471–480.
7. Lapresle J, Ben Hamida M. Correspondance somatotopique, secteur par secteur, des dégénérescences de l'olive bulbaire consécutives à des lésions limitées du noyau dentelé controlatéral. Rev Neurol 1965;113:439–448.
8. Lapresle J, Ben Hamida M. Contribution à la connaisance de la voie dento-olivaire. Etude anatomique de deux cas de dégénérescence hypertrophique des olives bulbaires secondaire à un ramollissement limité de la calotte mésencéphalique. Presse Médicale 1968;76:1226–1230.
9. Lapresle J. Palatal myoclonus. Adv Neurol 1986;43:265–273.
10. Goto N, Kaneko M. Olivary enlargement; chronological and morphometric analyses. Acta Neuropathol (Berlin) 1981;54:275–282.
11. Matsuo F, Ajax ET. Palatal myoclonus and denervation supersensitivity in the central nervous system. Ann Neurol 1979;5:72–78.
12. Yokota T, Tsukagoshi H. Olivary hypertrophy precedes the appearance of palatal myoclonus. J Neurol 1991;238:408.
13. Llínas RR. Rebound excitation as the physiological basis for tremor: a biophysical study of the oscillatory properties of mammalian central neurones in vitro. In: Findley LJ, Capildeo R, eds. Tremor. London: Macmillan Press, 1984:165–182.
14. Llínas RR, Yarom Y. Oscillatory properties of guinea-pig inferior olivary neurones and their pharmacological modulation: an in vitro study. J Physiol 1986;376:163–182.
15. Llínas RR, Mühlethaler M. Electrophysiology of guinea-pig cerebellar nuclear cells in the in-vitro brainstem cerebellar preparation. J Physiol 1988;404:241–258.
16. Steriade M, Jones EG, Llínas RR. Thalamic oscillations and signaling. New York: John Wiley & Sons, 1990.
17. Sotelo C, Llínas RR, Baker R. Structural study of the inferior olivary nucleus of the cat. Morphological correlates of electronic coupling. J Neurophysiol 1974;37:522–532.
18. Llínas RR, Baker R, Sotelo C. Electronic coupling between neurons in the cat inferior olive. J Neurophysiol 1974;37:560–571.
19. Dubinsky RM, Hallett M, Di Chiro G, Fulham M, Schwankhaus J. Increased glucose metabolism in the medulla of patients with palatal myoclonus. Neurology 1991;41:557–562.
20. Deuschl G, Toro C, Valls-Sole J, Zeffiro T, Zee D, Hallett M. Symptomatic and essential palatal tremor: 1. Clinical, physiological and MRI-analysis. (In preparation.)

21. Deuschl G, Toro C, Hallett M. Symptomatic and essential palatal tremor. 2. Differences of palatal movements. (In preparation.)
22. Hazell JWP. Tinnitus II: surgical management of conditions associated with tinnitus and somatosounds. J Otolaryngol 1990;1:6–10.
23. Thomas JE, Reagan TJ, Klass DW. Epilepsia partialis continua. Arch Neurol 1977;34:266–275.
24. Tatum WO, Sperling MR, Jacobstein JG. Epileptic palatal myoclonus. Neurology 1991; 41:1305–1306.
25. Emre M. Palatal myoclonus occurring during complex partial status epilepticus. J Neurol 1992;239:228–230.
26. Gresty MA, Ell JJ, Findley LJ. Acquired pendular nystagmus: its characteristics, localising value and pathophysiology. J Neurol Neurosurg Psychiatry 1982;45:431–439.
27. Schwartz MA, Selhorst JB, Ochs AL, et al. Oculomasticatory myorhythmia: a unique movement disorder occurring in Whipple's disease. Ann Neurol 1986;20:677–683.
28. Silfverskiöld BR. Rhythmic myoclonias including spinal myoclonus. In: Fahn S, Marsden CD, Van Woert M, eds. Myoclonus. Advances in neurology, vol. 43. New York: Raven Press, 1986:275–285.
29. Dubinsky RM, Hallett M. Palatal myoclonus and facial involvement in other types of myoclonus. In: J Jankovic, E Tolosa, eds. Facial dyskinesias. New York: Raven Press, 1988: 263–278.
30. Deuschl G, Mischke G, Schenck E, Lücking CH. Rhythmic palatal myoclonus: aetiology and differential diagnosis. In: Berardelli A, Benecke R, Manfredi M, Marsden CD, eds. Motor Disturbances II. London: Academic Press 1990:261–272.
31. Kaufman MD. Masticatory spasm in facial hemiatrophy. Ann Neurol 1980;7:585–587.
32. Rosenberg ML, Clark JB. Familial trembling of the chin. Neurology 1987;37(suppl 1):190.
33. Marsden CD, Hallett M, Fahn S. The nosology and pathophysiology of myoclonus. In: Marsden CD, Fahn S, eds. Movement Disorders. London: Butterworth Scientific, 1982: 196–248.
34. Müller J. Eine willkürliche Contraction des M. tensor tympani. Archiv für Ohrenheilkunde 1866;1:5.
35. Tateishi J. Über einen Fall von Hirnnervenmyorhythmie. Clin Neurol 1968;8:128.
36. Cancura W. Myoklonus der Gaumenmuskulatur als Ursache eines objektivierbaren Ohrgeräusches. Laryngol Rhinol Otol (Wien) 1969;103:19–25.
37. Brodal A. Neurological anatomy in relation to clinical medicine. New York, Oxford: Oxford University Press, 1981.
38. Hollinshead W. Anatomy for surgeons, 3d ed. New York: Harper and Row, 1982.
39. Deuschl G, Löhle E, Heinen F, Lücking CH. Earclick in palatal tremor: its origin and treatment with botulinum toxin. Neurology 41;1991:1677–1679.
40. Slack RWT, Soucek SO, Wong K. Sonotubometry in the investigation of objective tinnitus and palatal myoclonus: a demonstration of Eustachian tube opening. J Laryngol Otol 1986; 100:529–531.
41. Jabbari B, Scherokman B, Gunderson CH, Rosenberg ML, Miller J. Treatment of movement disorders with trihexyphenidyl. Mov Dis, Vol 4, 1989;3:202–212.
42. Le Pajolec C, Marion MM, Bobin S. Acouphène objective et myoclonies vélaires. Nouvelle approche thérapeutique. Ann Oto-Laryngol 1990;107:363–365.
43. Casselbrant ML, Cantekin EI, Dirkmaat DC, Doyle WJ, Bluestone CD. Experimental paralysis of tensor veli palatini muscle. Acta Otolaryngol 1988;106:178–185.

46

Botulinum Toxin in the Treatment of Glabellar Frown Lines and Other Facial Wrinkles

Alastair Carruthers and Jean D. A. Carruthers
University of British Columbia, Vancouver, British Columbia, Canada

INTRODUCTION

Aging is associated with the development of lines and wrinkles on the face. This association may be of great concern, and considerable efforts may be made to reverse these changes. Analysis of the face will show that the lines and wrinkles are due to a number of different causes (1):

1. Aging (intrinsic and photoaging)
2. Gravity (vertical and sleep lines)
3. Muscular action (lines of facial expression)

Botulinum toxin (BTX) reversibly paralyzes striated muscle. It is therefore rational to use this toxin for the treatment of facial lines and wrinkles that are due, in whole or in part, to muscular action. However, it is important to avoid paralyzing functional muscles completely. For example, upper lip wrinkles are caused by photoaging and the action of the orbicularis oris muscle. Botulinum toxin therapy sufficient to reduce the muscle-induced wrinkling would probably also produce an incompetent mouth, which is even more distressing than the upper lip wrinkles, On the other hand, "crow's-feet" wrinkles are due to "squinting" or overcontraction of the orbicularis oculi. Selective weakening of parts of this muscle will ameliorate the crow's-feet but still allow full functional closure of the eyelids.

Wrinkles and lines on the face give two separate messages to the observer. First, they can produce an appearance of aging, and second, they can express emotions. Fine wrinkling on the upper lip, cheeks, and crow's-feet area as well as deeper lines in the nasolabial area are a signal of aging, whereas wrinkling in the glabellar area is associated with anger, anxiety, and sadness, all "negative" emotions. Much of the glabellar wrinkling is due to the corrugator superciliaris, a muscle that has no essential function other than to express emotion.

In this chapter we first describe our experience with the treatment of glabellar wrinkling by reversible chemodenervation of corrugator muscle. We began with this "safe" muscle because of its lack of significant function. We shall then describe the early experience of ourselves and others with the treatment of other lines and wrinkles of the face.

GLABELLAR FROWN LINES

Anatomy

Corrugator Superciliaris

The belly of the corrugator superciliaris lies buried at the medial end of the eyebrow beneath the frontal belly of the frontalis and the orbicularis. Its origin is from the medial end of the superciliary arch and fibers pass upward and laterally to insert into the deep surface of the skin above the middle of the orbital arch.

There are variations in the arrangement of these structures as well as in the individual's expressive use of the muscle. This probably accounts for the variation in the degree of glabellar furrowing and particularly for the familial nature of some of these furrows. We estimate that in one-third of our subjects the glabellar frown lines are familial.

Other Muscles

Pierard and Lapierre (2) have described striated muscle inserted into the dermis at the base of deep facial lines. Two of our patients get an improved result when BTX is injected

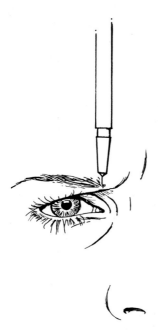

Figure 1   Injection technique for glabellar frown lines showing approximately half of a 30-gauge, half-inch needle inserted in the muscle at the level of the inner canthus.

beneath the furrow rather than into corrugator, and in these patients the muscle described by Pierard and Lapierre may be of greater significance than corrugator contraction.

Study of Botulinum Toxin Therapy for Glabellar Frown Lines

Subjects, Materials, and Methods

Thirty-one subjects on whom we have adequate follow-up data are included. There is one North American Indian in the trial, the remainder being Caucasian, and there is one man. Their ages at first injection range from 28 to 69 years, with an average of 42.4 years. All subjects underwent a full ophthalmological examination, and informed consent was obtained.

Until September 1990 the purified *Clostridium botulinum* A exotoxin was obtained from Dr. Alan Scott (Smith-Kettlewell Institute of Visual Sciences, San Francisco) as part of the multicenter trial of BTX therapy for strabismus, benign essential blepharospasm, hemifacial spasm, and spastic age-related lower eyelid entropion. After this date it has been obtained through Allergan Pharmaceuticals (Markham, Ontario, Canada).

The toxin is kept freeze-dried at $-4°C$. Immediately before use, the vial, containing 100 U of toxin, is diluted with 1 ml of sterile normal saline without preservative, to produce a solution with a concentration of 100 U. This is used within several hours of preparation, and the remainder, including the needles and syringes, is disposed of in a manner appropriate for biohazardous waste.

Subjects are treated in the sitting position. The cutaneous region over the muscles to be injected is cleansed with an alcohol swab. Glabellar furrows were initially treated with injections along the length of the furrow. A 30-gauge needle on a tuberculin syringe containing the toxin is inserted at the superior portion of the furrow, and the needle is passed down the length of the furrow in the deep subdermal plane. The plunger is depressed as the needle is withdrawn so the toxin is evenly distributed along the length of the furrow.

Starting early in 1990 the glabellar furrows were treated with injection into the belly of the corrugator superciliaris. The technique was slightly different, insofar as the subject was asked to frown and to maintain this expression throughout the procedure. The contracted corrugator can easily be felt between the examiner's finger and thumb as well as seen as a bulge beneath the medial aspect of the brow. At the same time the glabellar furrows are at their deepest. The injection is made into the contracted corrugator muscle by again passing the needle inferiorly from just above the brow. The needle tip lines up vertically with the inner canthus when the subject frowns.

If a ½-inch 30-gauge needle is used, approximately half of its length will be in the skin and subcutaneous tissue if it is correctly positioned. (See Fig. 1)

Results

Figures 2 and 3 demonstrate the effect of successful injection of *Clostridium botulinum* A exotoxin into the corrugator muscles.

Figure 2a shows the subject at rest with a glabellar frown line. When the subject is asked to frown (Fig. 2b), the line becomes a deep furrow. In addition, the eyebrow moves inferomedially, there is bunching up of the soft tissue overlying the contracting corrugator muscle, and there is increased "hooding" of the lateral part of the palpebral aperture as a result of contraction of part of the orbicularis oculi.

Figure 3a shows the same subject one month after injection of 10 U of *Clostridium botulinum* toxin into each corrugator muscle. The line is improved at rest (Fig. 3a), but the

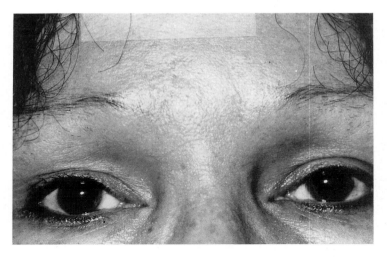

(a)

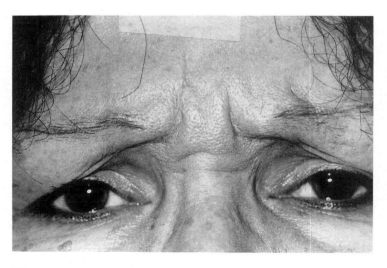

(b)

Figure 2   (a) Previously treated subject at rest prior to treatment. (b) After voluntarily frowning, full corrugator function is demonstrated with formation of glabellar lines, ''procerus line,'' inferomedial displacement of the brow, and lateral hooding.

change is most obvious when the subject is asked to frown (Fig. 3b). Increased hooding laterally shows that the subject is indeed attempting to frown, but there are none of the medial features of the frown, indicating paralysis of the corrugator muscles.

Table 1 shows the number of injection sessions that were performed on each subject. We began by injecting the toxin beneath the furrow but, as previously mentioned, in early 1990 switched to injecting the corrugator muscle directly. Table 2 shows the duration of the response to the first injection, comparing these two sites.

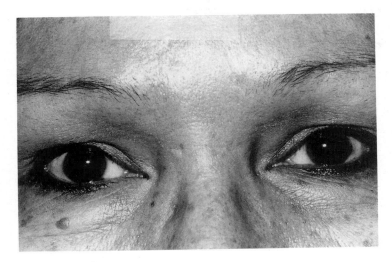

(a)

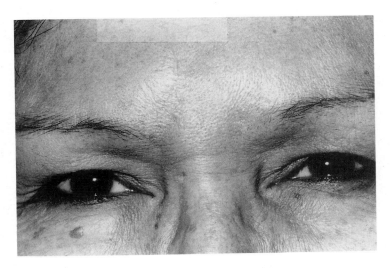

(b)

Figure 3 (a) Subject at rest 1 month after a further injection of 10 U of botulinum toxin into each corrugator muscle. (b) On attempting to frown, subject shows only orbicularis oculi function; corrugator supercilii muscles are paralyzed.

Of the 16 subjects who were initially injected under the line/furrow, six have discontinued BTX therapy and 10 continue. Of these 10, eight now have the injection into the corrugator muscle, but two think their response is better with the injection under the furrow. Of the 15 subjects initially injected into the corrugator, two have discontinued therapy, and all the others still have their injections into the corrugator. In addition, one of these has had an injection under the furrow in an attempt to further attenuate a particularly deep furrow.

Table 1 Number of Injection Sessions
Performed on Each Subject[a]

Number of injection sessions	Number of subjects
1	10
2	6
3	4
4	1
6	3
7	2
8	1
9	2
10	1
11	1

[a]Number of subjects = 31; total number of injection
sessions = 117.

Table 3 compares the cumulative data on all injection sessions with injection responses
after the fifth and subsequent injections. The duration of response in Table 3 was
measured as either the response reported by the subject or the interval between injections,
whichever was shorter. The effectiveness of the injection was crudely measured both
subjectively and objectively. Subjective assessment was made by asking the subjects to
assess their response by comparison with their expectations after they had discussed BTX
therapy with the physician. A scale of 0–7 (0 = no correlation, 7 = excellent correlation
with expectations) was used (see Table 4).

The two subjects who gave a score of 0 had no response subjectively, although one had
a response objectively (Table 5 and Fig. 4a and b) and the subject who gave it a score of 1
had developed brow ptosis.

Table 5 presents the objective assessment, in which the physician, in a nonmasked
manner, documented the response of the furrow at rest to the injection.

Four subjects developed complications, as shown in Table 6.

Eleven of our subjects have also been treated with injectable collagen for glabellar
frown lines. Eight of these prefer BTX to injectable-collagen therapy, one because she is

Table 2 Correlation of Length of Initial Response
with Injection Site

Length of Response	Initial injection site (no. of patients)	
	Furrow	Corrugator
No response	1	1
8 weeks or less	7	2
9–12 weeks	4	2
13–16 weeks	0	5
17 weeks or more	4	6
Total	16	15

Table 3 Duration of Corrugator Paralysis or Time Between Injections; All Injections Compared with Later Injections

Duration of interval	All injections		Injection #5 and over	
	Number	%	Number	%
8 weeks or less	24	24.7	2	6.9
9–12 weeks	15	15.5	4	13.8
13–16 weeks	20	20.6	6	20.7
17–20 weeks	16	16.5	6	20.7
21–30 weeks	13	13.4	6	20.7
31–52 weeks	9	9.3	5	17.2
Total	97	100	29	100

allergic to injectable collagen. One subject prefers the combination of BTX therapy with collagen; one felt that neither was very effective; and one had a better response to collagen. Eight subjects have discontinued BTX therapy for the reasons shown in Table 7.

OTHER LINES

Anatomy, Materials, Methods, and Results

The Treatment of Acquired Facial Lines

It is important to understand the subcutaneous muscular anatomy of the face to give the appropriate treatment for the presenting facial lines. In Table 8 and Figs. 5 and 6 we present the relevant anatomy of the facial muscles. Table 8 also indicates which muscles are to be avoided when BTX injections are given.

1. Crow's-feet. Crow's-feet are well established, deep, radiating, horizontal and oblique furrows at the temporal aspect of each eye due to the squeezing action of the orbicularis oculi. Denervation of the temporal orbital and palpebral fibers of the orbicularis oculi collapses these lines. We have injected only two subjects with 5 U of purified BTX into this area on each side, with reasonable improvement in each.

Table 4 Correlation of Subject's Expectations with Actual Experience (0 = no correlation; 7 = excellent response)

Correlation	No. of subjects[a]
0	2
1	1
4	2
5	3
6	6
6.5	5
7	12

[a]Total = 31.

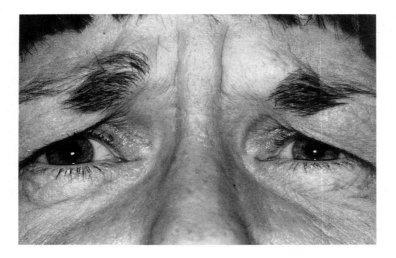

(a)

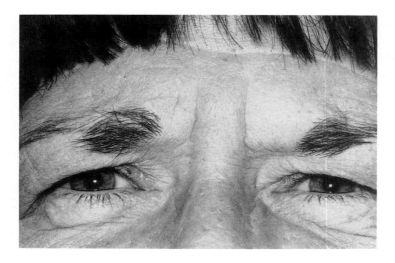

(b)

Figure 4   An individual attempting to frown who subjectively had no response to botulinum toxin injection into corrugator superciliaris before (a) and one month after (b) injection.

2.   Nasal muscles.
  a.   Procerus. The procerus groove can be a marked horizontal line at the base of the nose. Denervation of the procerus muscle collapses this line, and usually 5 U of purified BTX are needed.
  b.   Dilator naris. We have one subject who had a persistent over–action of his dilator naris, so that he was continually embarrassed socially by his flaring nostrils (Fig. 7a and b). Five U of BTX was injected into each dilator naris, and he has had a good, prolonged response from this for 10 weeks to date.

Table 5 Objective Response of Glabellar Frown Lines
to Botulinum Toxin Injection

Response	No. of subjects
Nil	1
Improved line	11
Slight line	11
Smooth	8
Total	31

Table 6 Complications of Botulinum Toxin Therapy
for Glabellar Frown Lines[a]

Complication	No. of subjects
Brow ptosis	1
Lid ptosis	2
Numbness	1

[a]Number of injection sessions = 117.

Table 7 Reasons for Discontinuing Botulinum Toxin
Therapy for Glabellar Frown Lines

Reason	No. of subjects
Did not work	2
Moved away	2
Brow ptosis	1
Cost	1
BT risk	1
"Wooden brow"	1

    c. Compressor naris. We have had no experience injecting this muscle in order to make the nostrils become more dilated. However, we feel that there may be some call for this, particularly within the acting profession.

    d. Levator labii superioris alaeque nasi. This muscle enhances the upper aspect of the nasolabial furrow. It is possible to inject directly into this muscle with 2½ U of toxin to give a beneficial response. It is important not to overdo the injection, because it could lead to a flattening of the upper lip. The use of electromyographic control during injection is very helpful so that the toxin goes accurately into the muscle.

3. Mental crease. We have treated two subjects with "mental creases." In the first subject, 10 U of BTX was injected along the length of the crease. The subject found that she had some drooling and incompetence of her orbicularis oris as well as some difficulty with her speech. Presumably the dose was too great and affected the orbicularis oris as well as the mentalis and depressor labii inferioris muscles. In the

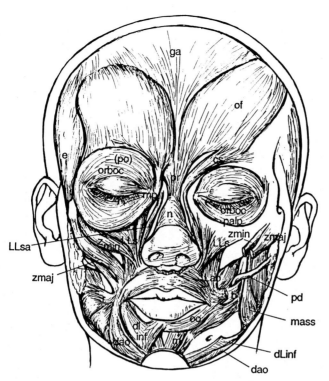

Figure 5 Anterior view of the muscles of facial expression. ga = galea aponeurotica; of = frontal belly, occipitafrontalis muscle; cs = corrugator supercilii; pr = procerus; dsup = depressor supercilii; orboc = orbicularis oculi; orboc palp = orbicularis oculi, palpebral part; e = epicranius (temporoparietalis muscle); mp = medial palpebral ligament; n = nasalis muscle; LLs = levator labii superioris; LLsa = levator labii superioris alaequs nasi; zmin = zygomaticus minor; zmaj = zygomaticus major; pd = parotid duct; dsept = depressor septi; Lao = levator anguli oris; b = buccinator; r = risorius muscle; mass = masseter; oor = orbicularis oris; dLinf = depressor labii inferioris; dao = depressor anguli oris; m = mentalis muscle.

second subject, 5 U of BTX was used. The effect lasted about 3 months, and the subject was very pleased. This reiterates the important point that one must be careful not to compromise the physiological function of muscles in the treated areas.

DISCUSSION

The effectiveness of *Clostridium botulinum* A exotoxin in blocking neuromuscular transmission is well established. In addition, the disappearance of facial lines after damage to the facial nerve, for example on the forehead, is also well known. That we have shown (3) that *Clostridium botulinum* A exotoxin can smooth facial lines is not therefore surprising. The questions to be answered are

1. How effective is it?
2. How long is it effective?
3. What delivery technique is most appropriate?

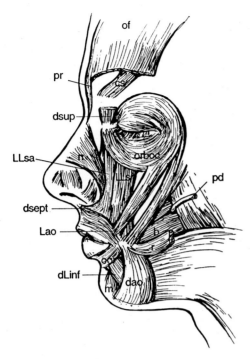

Figure 6 Lateral view of the muscles of facial expression. See legend for Fig. 5.

4. What complications occur?
5. What facial lines can be treated?
6. How does it compare with other treatments?

How Effective Is It?

Assessment of facial lines and wrinkles is notoriously difficult. Photography can vary so much from day to day, camera to camera, film batch to film batch, etc., that strict control of all variables and professional techniques is necessary to get a meaningful result. We have used photography only to illustrate the inability of the subject to frown, although using still photographs to demonstrate a lack of movement is not ideal.

Subjective and objective assessment by the subject and a trained observer are more likely to give an adequate measure of improvement without complicated photographic equipment. In our study of treatment of glabellar furrows we have asked patients to assess the response of their frown lines by comparison with their expectations after discussing the procedure with the physician and being injected. Table 4 shows their response. Apart from three subjects, all the remaining 28 gave it a score of 4 or higher on a scale of 0–7. Of the three who gave it a low score, two felt they had no response and one developed a complication (transient brow ptosis). Of the two subjects who gave it a score of 4, one has had 7 injections and the other 11. This may represent a declining satisfaction with the result, perhaps due to the impermanent nature of the therapy.

The other seven patients who have had six or more injections all gave it a score of 6 or higher (average 6.8).

Table 8 Relevant Anatomy of the Facial Muscles[a]

Muscle	Origin	Trajectory	Insertion	Action	What happens if totally paralysed
Orbicularis oculi					
Palpebral head	Medial palpebral tendon	Hemispheric on ciliary side of tarsal sulcus	Lateral palpebral raphe	Blinking, ocular lubrication	Keratoconjunctivitis sicca
Orbital head	Medial palpebral tendon	Hemispheric on orbital side of tarsal sulcus	Lateral palpebral raphe and spread to corrugator, frontalis and depressor supercilii	Forceful closure of the lids	Keratoconjunctivitis sicca, severe ocular exposure, possible loss of globe
Levator palpebrae superioris[b]	Above annulus of Zinn at the superior/posterior orbit	Forward above superior rectus and behind the orbital septum	By broad levator aponeurosis to upper tarsal plate superior palpebral furrow	Elevation of upper lid	Eyelid ptosis
Medial rectus[b]	Annulus of Zinn	Forward well behind orbital septum	Medial wall of globe, 5.5 mm behind limbus	Adduction of globe	Exotropia
Frontalis[b]	Occipitofrontalis	From the nuchal area projecting in a sagittal direction from the occiput forward to the frontal area via an intermediary aponeurosis	Insertion into the brow and fascial tissue of the frontal bone	To elevate brow	Brow ptosis
Corrugator supercilii	Medial end of superciliary arch	Upward and lateral	Deep surface of skin of brow (above middle of orbital arch)	Draws medial brow down and medially, furrowing the overlying skin	Inability to frown, smoothing of glabellar lines
Procerus	Upper nasal cartilage and lower nasal bone	Vertical over bridge of nose	Skin between brows and frontal belly of occipitofrontalis	Draws down medial brows and makes a transverse groove across bridge of nose	No horizontal procerus line

Muscle	Origin	Direction	Insertion	Action	Effect
Dilator naris	Maxilla latral to incisor tooth	Horizontal	Lower part of cartilaginous ala	Dilates nostrils	Nostril dilates poorly
Compressor naris	Maxilla above and lateral to incisive fossa	Up and medial	Mutual aponeurosis across bridge of nose and aponeurosis of procerus	Constricts nostrils	Nostril constricts poorly
Levator labii superioris (LLS)	Broad origin lower margin orbit above infraorbital foramen	Convergent	Muscles of upper lip between LAO and LLSAN	Lifts upper lip, enhances nasolabial furrow	Flattening of the nasolabial furrow
Levator labii superioris alaeque nasi (LLSAN)	Narrow origin frontal process of maxilla	Vertical	Alar cartilage upper lip with LLS	Lifts upper lip and nose, enhances nasolabial furrow	Flattening of nasolabial furrow
Levator anguli oris (LAO)	Canine fossa below infraorbital foramen	Vertical	Angle of mouth intermingling with zygomaticus major, depressor anguli oris, and orbicularis oris	Lifts angle of mouth	Inability to smile
Zygomaticus minor	Malar surface of zygomatic bone immediately behind zygomaticomaxillary suture	Down	Upper lip between LLS and zygomaticus major	Deepens nasolabial furrow	Flattening of the nasolabial furrow
Zygomaticus major	Anterior to zygomatico-temporal suture	Oblique to angle of mouth	Blends with fibers of levator and depressor anguli oris and orbicularis oris	Corner of mouth drawn up and back (laughing)	
Mentalis	Incisive fossa of mandible	Descends	Skin of chin	Raises and protrudes the lower lip (e.g. pouting)	Obliterates mental furrow

Table 8 Relevant Anatomy of the Facial Muscles[a] (Cont'd)

Muscle	Origin	Trajectory	Insertion	Action	What happens if totally paralysed
Orbicularis oris Deep stratum	Buccinator and fibers crossing at the angle of the mouth and transverse nondecussating fibers	Complex horizontal, vertical, oblique, confluence of muscle fibers around the mouth		Direct lip closure. Deep fibers yield closely apply to lips to teeth and alveolar arches. Speech, feeding, drinking	Incompetent sphincter action, difficulty with speech, feeding, drinking, etc.
Superficial stratum	Levator and depressor anguli oris, oblique intermingling fibers from LLS, ZM, and DLI				
Proper fibers	Pass full thickness from skin to mucous membrane				

[a]The facial muscles usually originate from fascia or facial bone and insert into facial skin confluent with the merging insertions of other facial muscles.
[b]Muscle to be avoided when botulinum toxin injections are given.

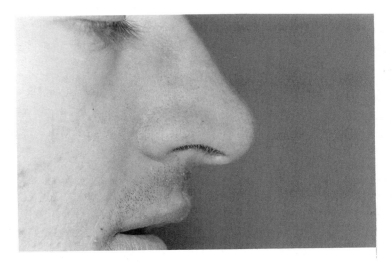

(a)

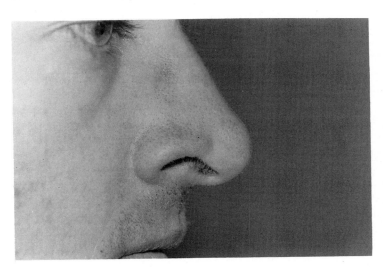

(b)

Figure 7 Individual with cosmetically dissatisfying "flaring" of the ala nasi, at rest and on flaring.

Objectively, one subject had no response, even after a second injection. The other patient who subjectively had no response was noted by the physician to have decreased ability to frown and a shorter (improved) line (Fig.4a and b). We estimated the response as shown in Table 5. It can be seen that approximately equal numbers of subjects had an improved line, a slight or faint line, and a smooth glabellar area.

More accurate objective assessment of the line can best be managed by taking casts of the line and serially analyzing them (4). This painstaking work will be necessary for the further study of the effectiveness of BTX therapy in facial lines.

How Long Is It Effective?

The longevity data are found in Tables 2 and 3. We had difficulty assessing the longevity of this therapy. Essentially we are measuring the length of time the subject is unable to frown. Unfortunately, this ability comes back slowly, almost imperceptibly. It was our impression that many of our subjects did not have full corrugator function when they returned for a further injection. We therefore used the length of time between injections or the subject's assessment of the period of effectiveness as an imperfect but nonetheless valid measure of the length of effectiveness. We have previously used the retreatment rate as a measure of the success of therapy (5).

From Table 3 it can be seen that approximately one-quarter of injections produced either no response or a response lasting 8 weeks or less. Many of these injections were under the furrow, which in our study is a less effective placement site. However, even if we look only at the response of patients after their fifth or later injections, when route, dose, etc., should have been well worked out, 6.9% of injections produced a response lasting 8 weeks or less. Looking at all injection sessions, 21% of responses lasted 13 to 16 weeks, and 39% more than 17 weeks. For the fifth subsequent injections, 21% lasted 13 to 16 weeks, but 59% lasted 17 weeks or longer. Interestingly, there is a small number of injection sessions that are effective for greater than 30 weeks. These super-long responses tend to occur in subjects whose normal response is longer than usual.

What Delivery Technique Is Most Appropriate?

From the longevity data, it can be seen that we have found that injection into the corrugator is more effective than injection under the furrow. Table 2 shows that of initial injections, eight of 16 into the furrow remained effective for 8 weeks or less, by comparison with only three of 15 into corrugator. Of the 10 subjects who have been injected into both areas, eight prefer the injection into corrugator, one prefers it under the line, and one likes injection into both areas. We have another subject who has only had injection under the line, for a total of three of 31 subjects who currently have the injection under the furrow. We have done some informal dose studies, and some of our subjects require a dose greater than 10 U per side, but this is adequate for 80–90% of subjects.

We inject from above the brow down toward the furrow or corrugator (Fig.1). This risks minor trauma to the branches of the frontal nerve (one subject complained of transient numbness above the brow lasting less than 2 weeks). However, a superior, rather than direct, approach allows pressure to be applied over the puncture site without applying pressure to the site of toxin placement. The toxin is rapidly bound to its receptors (6), but we advise subjects not to apply pressure to the area and to remain vertical for 3 to 4 hours during this binding.

Is a delivery system other than injection possible for this indication? As with other indications, placement of the toxin is important, especially in the glabellar area, where spread of the toxin can produce ptosis or ophthalmoplegia. In areas where the toxin is injected subcutaneously over the muscle, as in the lateral crow's-feet area, it is possible that a topical delivery system could be effective with minimal systemic effects.

What Complications Occur?

In our 31 subjects treated for glabellar frown lines in 117 injection sessions, we had four complications, an overall rate of 3.5%. Brow ptosis occurred in one subject in whom the toxin was presumably placed too deep under the furrow and produced partial paralysis of the brow levators. This cleared after approximately 2 weeks. Two subjects had minimal lid ptosis, lasting less than 2 weeks, and one subject had a small area of numbness of the brow. Considering the rich blood supply and innervation in this area, it is possible that more damage to these structures might be anticipated.

Inaccurate placement of the toxin or overdosage can produce temporary paralysis of any striated muscle in the area. One of us (JDAC) has been contacted about a subject injected with toxin by another physician for glabellar frown lines. The subject developed complete ptosis and medial rectus paralysis. This indicates placement of the toxin behind the orbital septum and behind the levator aponeurosis. Physicians are encouraged to attend a course to receive practical instruction in injection technique before treating their subjects.

The use of *Clostridium botulinum* A exotoxin for benign essential blepharospasm is analogous to its use for glabellar frown lines. The difference between them is that, in treating benign essential blepharospasm, a larger dose of toxin is injected via multiple injections into the brow and also into the orbicularis oculi, including the lower eyelid. In a large series of injections for benign essential blepharospasm (7), there was an 11% incidence of ptosis. This is higher than the two out of 31 subjects (6.5%) reported in this series, but similar in that the effect is transient. The ptosis is due to migration of toxin through the orbital septum, with consequent weakening of the levator palpebrae superioris muscle. Of great concern in the treatment of blepharospasm and hemifacial spasm are the reports of ectropion, entropion, and keratoconjunctivitis sicca (8). These complications are seen only with injection of the orbicularis, particularly in the lower eyelid, which is not intentionally treated when the corrugator muscles are injected.

The systemic toxicity of BTX and the development of antibodies or other allergic responses to the toxin therapy are dealt with in other chapters. Suffice it to say that in our experience using BTX toxin therapy for this indication as well as for benign essential blepharospasm, strabismus, hemifacial spasm, and age-related spastic entropion, we have seen no systemic complications.

What Facial Lines Can Be Treated?

We have established that *Clostridium botulinum* A exotoxin is effective in the treatment of glabellar frown lines (3). In addition, we have treated the mental crease, crow's-feet area, procerus line, and dilator naris levator. Blitzer et al. (9), have reported treating frontalis/ corrugator muscles, lateral canthus, nasolabial fold and upper lip muscles, and platysma muscles in 26 subjects. These subjects had 3–6 months of partial or total resolution of their ''hyperfunctional facial lines.'' Others have reported treating the unaffected side in subjects with Bell's palsy in order to produce a symmetrical appearance (10).

We have documented above many of the facial muscles that we think may be satisfactorily treated as well as describing some of the muscles to be avoided. As we have stated previously, accurate placement of the toxin is essential for both effectiveness and a low level of complications. We do not use electromyography routinely except for injecting extraocular muscles. Brin has indicated to us that he does use electromyography on occasion for accurate toxin placement in facial muscles. Undoubtedly greater experience will elucidate other areas suitable for treatment and the appropriate technique to be used.

How Does It Compare with Other Treatments?

There is no treatment for glabellar frown lines that is entirely satisfactory. The simplest and most widely used form of therapy is with ''fillers'' injected into or beneath the dermis to elevate the furrow. Injectable collagen and ''Fibrel'' (Mentor Corporation, Goleta, California) are both used extensively in this area, smoothing out the line temporarily. Collagen can produce allergic reactions as well as idiosyncratic reactions (11). Many practitioners have stopped injecting Zyplast (Collagen Corporation, Palo Alto, California) into the glabellar area because of the incidence of vascular occlusion in this area. In addition, collagen injected into the glabella has been reported to cause blindness (12), as may any particulate matter that is injected under pressure into this area. However, long-term use of injectable collagen (principally Zyderm; Collagen Corporation, Palo Alto, California) continues to be the most widely used therapy for glabellar frown lines in North America.

Subcutaneous injectable fat will ''puff up'' the whole glabellar area but is not precise enough to fill in the line specifically. In addition, two cases of blindness have been reported (13,14), so that this is no longer considered satisfactory treatment for any but exceptional subjects. Injectable silicon has been used in the past but is currently banned by both the Food and Drug Administration in the United States and the Health Protection Branch in Canada.

Surgical removal of the corrugator muscle during a brow lift is the ultimate treatment for glabellar frown lines, but because this is a significant operation with risks and complications, it is generally used for therapy of brow ptosis rather than just for glabellar frown lines. Chemical destruction of the corrugator and other muscles is possible. Doxorubicin has been described as a more permanent form of treatment for blepharospasm than BTX (15).

REFERENCES

1. Stegman SJ, Tromovitch TA, Glogau RG. Cosmetic dermatologic surgery. 2d ed. St. Louis: Mosby Year Book, 1990:5–15.
2. Pierard GE, Lapierre CM. The microanatomical basis of facial frown lines. Arch Dermatol 1989;125:1090–1092.
3. Carruthers JDA, Carruthers JA. Treatment of glabellar frown lines with C. botulinum-A exotoxin. J Dermatol Surg Oncol 1992;18:17–21.
4. Grove BL, Grove MJ, Leyden JJ, Lufrano MS, Schuab B, Perry BH, Thorne EG. Skin replica analysis of photodamaged skin after therapy with tretinoin emollient cream. J Am Acad Dermatol 1991;25:231–237.
5. Carruthers JDA, Kennedy RA, Bagaric D. Botulinum vs. adjustable suture surgery in the treatment of horizontal misalignment in adult subjects lacking fusion. Arch Ophthalmol 1990; 108:1432–1435.
6. Burgen ASV, Dickens F, Zatman LJ. The action of botulinum toxin on the neuromuscular function. J Physiol (London) 1949;109:10–24.
7. Carruthers JDA, Stubbs HA. Botulinum toxin for benign essential blepharospasm, hemifacial spasm and age-related lower eyelid entropion. Can J Neurol Sci 1987;14:42–45.
8. Therapeutics and Technology Assessment Committee of the American Academy of Neurology. The clinical usefulness of botulinum toxin A in treating neurologic disorders. Report of the Therapeutics and Technology Assessment Committee of the American Academy of Neurology. Neurology 1990;40:1332–1333.
9. Blitzer A, Brin MF, Keen MS. Botulinum toxin for the treatment of hyperfunctional lines of the face. Arch Otolaryngol Head Neck Surg. In press.

10. Clark RP, Berris CE. Botulinum toxin; a treatment for facial asymmetry caused by facial nerve paralysis. J Plast Reconst Surg 1989;84:353–535.

11. Stegman SJ, Chu S, Armstrong R. Adverse reactions to bovine collagen implant: clinical and histologic features. J Dermatol Surg Oncol 1988;13(suppl 1):39.

12. Cucin RL, Barek O. Complications of injectable collagen implant. Plast Reconstr Surg 1983;71:731.

13. Driezen NG, Framm L. Sudden unilateral visual loss after autogenous fat injection into the glabellar area. Am J Ophthalmol 1989;107:92:361.

14. Teimourian B. Blindness following fat injection. Plast Reconstr Surg 1988;92:361.

15. Wirtschafter JD. Chemical doxorubicin chemomyectomy. An experimental treatment for benign essential blepharospasm and hemifacial spasm. Ophthalmology 1991;98:357–366.

Index

About the Editors

JOSEPH JANKOVIC is a Professor of Neurology and Director of the Parkinson's Disease Center and Movement Disorders Clinic at Baylor College of Medicine, Houston, Texas. Dr. Jankovic received his neurologic training at the Neurologic Institute, Columbia University, New York, New York. The author or coauthor of over 350 original articles, chapters, and professional papers, and the editor or coeditor of eight books, Dr. Jankovic has served on the editorial board of *Clinical Neuropharmacology* and *Movement Disorders*. A President-Elect of the Movement Disorders Society, he is a Fellow of the American Academy of Neurology and a member of the American Neurological Association and the Society for Neuroscience, among others. He is also a current or past member of scientific and medical advisory boards of several national foundations, including the Dystonia Medical Research Foundation, Benign Essential Blepharospasm Research Foundation, the United Parkinson Foundation, the International Tremor Foundation, and the Tourette Syndrome Association. Under his direction, the Parkinson's Disease Center has been selected as a center of excellence by the National Parkinson Foundation.

MARK HALLETT is Chief of the Human Motor Control Section, Chief of the Medical Neurology Branch, and Director of the Clinical Neuroscience Program in the Division of Intramural Research at, and Clinical Director of, the National Institute of Neurological Disorders and Stroke, National Institutes of Health, Bethesda, Maryland. A Consultant in Neurology at the Naval Hospital and Clinical Professor of Neurology at the Uniformed Services University for the Health Sciences, both in Bethesda, Maryland, Dr. Hallett serves on the editorial boards of numerous journals and is the author or coauthor of over 200 research papers and chapters. He is a Fellow of the American Academy of Neurology and a member of the American Neurological Association, the Society for Neuroscience, and the Movement Disorders Society, among others. Focusing his research interests on clinical neurophysiology and movement disorders, Dr. Hallett is a former President of the American Association of Electrodiagnostic Medicine. He is also a current or past member of the medical advisory boards of several national foundations, including the Dystonia Medical Research Foundation, the National Parkinson Foundation, and the Benign Essential Blepharospasm Research Foundation, Inc. He received the A.B. degree (1965) in biology from Harvard University, Cambridge, Massachusetts, and the M.D. degree (1969) from Harvard Medical School, Boston, Massachusetts.